GENERAL PHARMACOLOGY

Hana Smalley

ALLIED
HEALTH
PRESS

General Pharmacology

Author: **Hana Smalley**

Allied Health Press
4164 Lakeshore Road
Burlington ON L7L 1A4
Canada
www.alliedhealthpress.com
Email: orders@arclereducation.com

ISBN: 978-1-77956-233-3

ABOUT THE AUTHOR

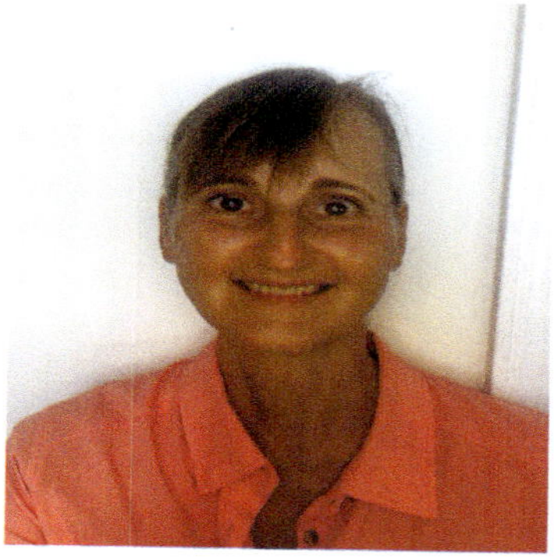

Hana Smalley is a pharmacist with a passion for optimizing medications for her patients and educating her audiences in the field of pharmacology. Hana has a diverse background in hospital care, long term care, geriatric and palliative care, pain management, and education. With her expertise in pharmacology, she has been working with multi-disciplinary care teams along with patients and care-givers to adjust medications, including collaborating with prescribers to select medications, identify and prevent adverse reactions, and educate medical staff and patients about the risks and benefits of medications. She also creates and teaches pharmacology courses for beginner and advanced levels. Hana's academic journey includes earning her pharmacy degree from the "Université de Montréal". She further obtained a doctorate of pharmacy (Pharm.D) at the Medical University of South Carolina in Charleston, USA. Hana has vast experience as a clinician, a manager and pharmacology instructor. Her knowledge of pharmacology and passion for health makes her an asset to a care team and a key educator for health care students.

Word Roots, Prefixes, and Suffixes by Chapter

Chapter 1 General Principles of Pharmacology

pharmac-, pharmakon, drug, medication

rhod(o)-, denoting a rose-red color

-floxacin, quinolone antibiotic

-mab, monoclonal antibody

Chapter 2 Drugs Acting on the Autonomic Nervous System

encephal/o-, (brain)

psych/o-, mind

-itis, inflammation

-lysis, loosening, dissolution, separating

-oma, tumor

Chapter 3 Cardiovascular-Renal Drugs

Hydr/o-, water

Adren/o-, gland

Angi/o-, blood vessel

-osis, condition, usually abnormal

Chapter 4 Drugs Acting on the Respiratory System

-cycline, broad spectrum antibiotics that treat bacterial infections

-azine, treat and prevent nausea and vomiting

-tidine, Block the action of histamine in the stomach

-ium, structure, tissue

lymph(o)-, lympha, lymph

Chapter 5 Drugs Used in Gastrointestinal Diseases

urin-, of or pertaining to urine, the urinary system

ventr(o)- , of or pertaining to the belly

pne-, pneum-, air, breath, lung

pulmon(i)-, (pulmo-), lungs

Chapter 6 Drugs Acting on the Central Nervous System

cephal/o-, head

encephal/o-, brain

esthesi/o-, sensation, sensitivity, feeling

-algia, pain

-cele, hernia, protrusion

-malacia, softening

Chapter 7 Chemotherapeutic Drugs

carcin/o-, cancer

Hepat/o-, hepatico-, liver

-ium, structure or tissue

fluoro-, indicates the presence of fluorine

doxo-, refers to doxorubicin

Chapter 8 Endocrine Pharmacology

thyr/o-, thyroid gland

para-, alongside; abnormal

arthr-, of or pertaining to the joints, limbs

lymph/o-, lymph

Meta-, beyond; change

Chapter 9 Pharmacological Management of Urinary Incontinence: Current and Emerging Treatments

ur-, of or pertaining to urine, the urinary system

cyst(o)-, cyst(i)-, of or pertaining to the urinary bladder

lip(o)-, fat

Prostat-, prostate

Chapter 10 Lower Urinary Tract Disorders Due to Adverse Drug Reactions

uro-, pertaining to the urinary system

-cillin, indicates penicillin antibiotics

-floxacin: refers to fluoroquinolone antibiotics

-dine, used in medications that treat overactive bladder or urinary frequency

Table of Contents

5 Drugs Used in Gastrointestinal Diseases 157

6 Drugs Acting on the Central Nervous System 201

LIST OF FIGURES

LIST OF TABLES

PREFACE

Pharmacology is a vital branch of medicine that delves into the myriad uses, effects, and mechanisms of action of drugs. This discipline is fundamentally concerned with understanding how various chemical substances interact with biological systems, shaping physiological and behavioral outcomes. It synthesizes a broad array of knowledge from essential scientific disciplines, including physiology, biochemistry, and cellular and molecular biology. As the array of available medicines expands, the role of pharmacology has grown significantly, particularly in assessing the potential interactions among multiple drugs—whether they are prescribed, over-the-counter, or even homeopathic—that patients might take simultaneously.

The relevance of pharmacology is underscored by findings such as those from a 2008 survey by the Centers for Disease Control and Prevention (CDC), which reported that nearly half of Americans had used at least one prescription drug in the preceding month. Moreover, a higher percentage of Americans had utilized over-the-counter medications along with dietary and herbal supplements during the same period. Pharmacology is pivotal in evaluating the safety and efficacy of these various medications, ensuring that they deliver intended benefits without undue risk. In its scope, pharmacology examines the influence of chemical agents on everything from subcellular mechanisms to systemic processes, encompassing both physiological and behavioral effects. The field also plays a crucial role in disease prevention and treatment, evaluating the safety of chemical substances like pesticides and herbicides that are widely used in various industries.

Pharmacologists contribute significantly to science and medical advancements across diverse settings, including universities, government agencies, healthcare, and industries related to pharmaceuticals and biosciences. Their work is crucial not only in understanding drug mechanisms but also in developing new therapies that can significantly improve health outcomes.

Within the field of research, pharmacologists are found in academia, industry, and healthcare. In academic and industrial settings, these professionals primarily engage in basic research to elucidate how drugs work, often employing animal disease models. Meanwhile, clinical research pharmacologists bridge the gap between laboratory discoveries and clinical applications, aiding in the development of new drugs that are safe and effective for patient use. Additionally, the specialty of clinical pharmacology and therapeutics trains medical doctors to focus on the precise and beneficial use of pharmaceuticals. This specialty emphasizes the importance of understanding drug interactions, side effects, and the optimal use of pharmaceuticals in clinical settings to ensure patient safety and treatment efficacy.

Beyond laboratory and clinical settings, pharmacologists also pursue careers in areas such as scientific publishing, education, science communication, policy-making, and regulatory affairs. These roles allow them to extend their impact by shaping scientific discourse, educating the next generation of scientists, and influencing policies and regulations in drug development and safety. This diversity of career paths highlights the broad influence and importance of pharmacology in advancing medical science and improving healthcare outcomes globally.

This textbook "*General Pharmacology*" is designed to serve as a comprehensive introductory resource for students and professionals in the fields of medicine, pharmacy, and health sciences. Its primary aim is to provide a thorough grounding in the fundamental principles of pharmacology, including the origins, chemical properties, biological effects, and mechanisms of action of various drugs. By covering a wide spectrum of topics, from the molecular basis of drug action to the systemic effects on the human body, the book equips readers with the necessary knowledge to understand the complex interactions between drugs and biological systems.

This text will be beneficial for both newcomers to the field and those seeking to refresh or expand their knowledge. The book caters to a diverse readership, including undergraduate and graduate students in pharmacology and related disciplines, as well as healthcare professionals like physicians, nurses, and pharmacists. Through clear explanations, detailed diagrams, and real-world examples, the textbook aims to make the science of pharmacology accessible and applicable, enhancing the ability of readers to apply this knowledge in clinical settings, research, and further studies in pharmacology and related fields.

Chapter 1

GENERAL PRINCIPLES OF PHARMACOLOGY

Contents

Introduction

The science of pharmaceuticals and medicines, encompassing the pharmacokinetics, toxicology, origin, and composition of a substance, is known as pharmacology. More precisely, it is the study of how substances interact with living things to influence normal or aberrant biochemical function. Substances are classified as pharmaceuticals if they have therapeutic qualities.

The area includes drug composition and properties, sources, functions, synthesis, and drug design. It also includes information on organ/system mechanisms, molecular and cellular mechanisms, signal transduction and cellular communication, chemical biology, therapy, molecular diagnostics, and medical applications. Pharmacodynamics and pharmacokinetics are the two primary subfields of pharmacology. Pharmacokinetics examines how a drug affects biological systems, while pharmacodynamics studies how a drug affects biological systems. Broadly speaking, pharmacokinetics studies the absorption, distribution, metabolism, and excretion (ADME) of chemicals from biological systems, while pharmacodynamics studies chemicals having biological receptors.

Although the terms are commonly used interchangeably, pharmacy and pharmacology are not the same. As a biomedical science, pharmacology studies the identification, investigation, and characterization of substances that exhibit biological effects as well as the clarification of how cells and organisms function in connection to these substances. Pharmacy, a health services profession, on the other hand, focuses on applying the concepts of pharmacology in clinical settings, whether in a role related to dispensing or clinical care. The main differences between the two fields in either case are how they classify direct patient care, pharmacy practice, and the science-based, pharmacology-driven research field. (Rang, 2006; Krska & Cox, 2019)

Orientation and Directional Terms

Term	Definition	Illustration
ADME	ADME is the abbreviation for Absorption, Distribution, Metabolism and Excretion. ADME studies are designed to investigate how a chemical (e.g., a drug compound) is processed by a living organism. Toxicology tests are often a part of this process, yielding the acronym ADMET.	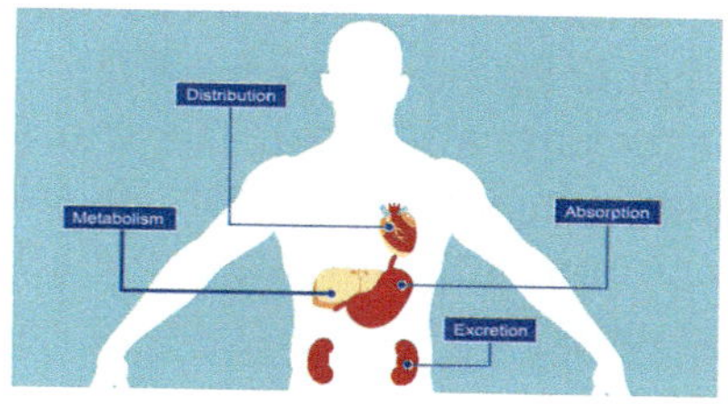
Acetylcholine	Acetylcholine (ACh) is a neurotransmitter that plays a role in many parts of the body, including the brain, spinal cord, and nerves. It's most commonly associated with the neuromuscular junction, where motor neurons in the spinal cord connect with muscles to activate them. ACh also functions in the autonomic nervous system, regulating heart rate, blood pressure, and gut motility.	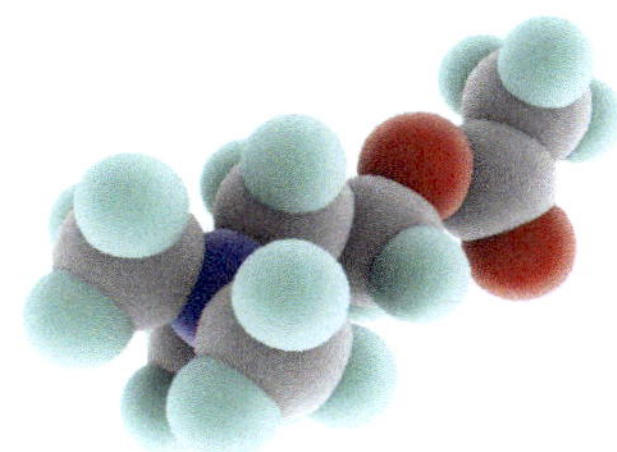
GABA	GABA (gamma Aminobutyric acid, γ-Aminobutyric acid) is the chief inhibitory neurotransmitter in the developmentally mature mammalian central nervous system. Its principal role is reducing neuronal excitability throughout the nervous system.	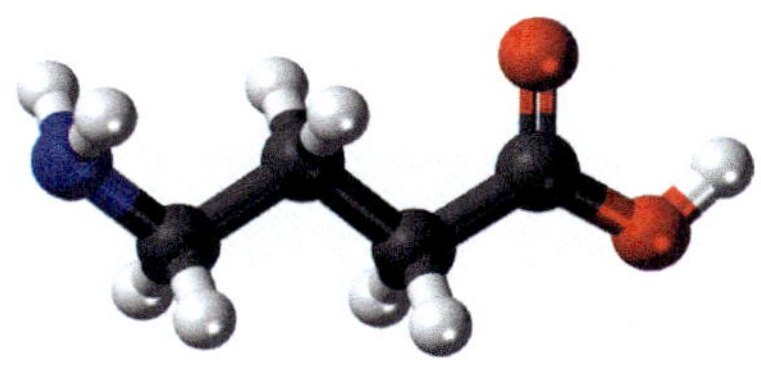
Epinephrine	Epinephrine is a hormone and medication which is involved in regulating visceral functions. It appears as a white microcrystalline granule. Adrenaline is normally produced by the adrenal glands and by a small number of neurons in the medulla oblongata.	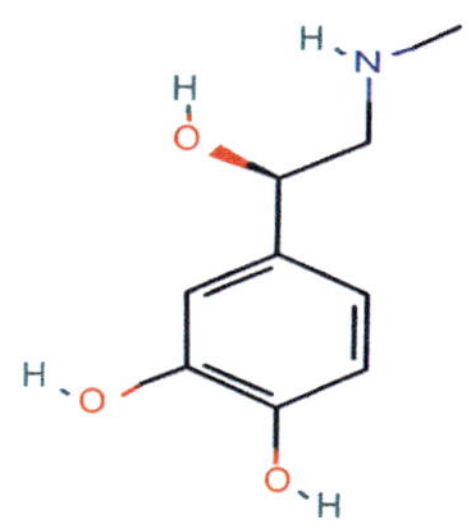
Redox enzymes	Redox enzymes are enzymes that catalyze biological electron transfer reactions, or redox reactions, between two molecules. These reactions involve the transfer of electrons, the addition of an oxygen atom, and the movement of a pair of hydrogen atoms.	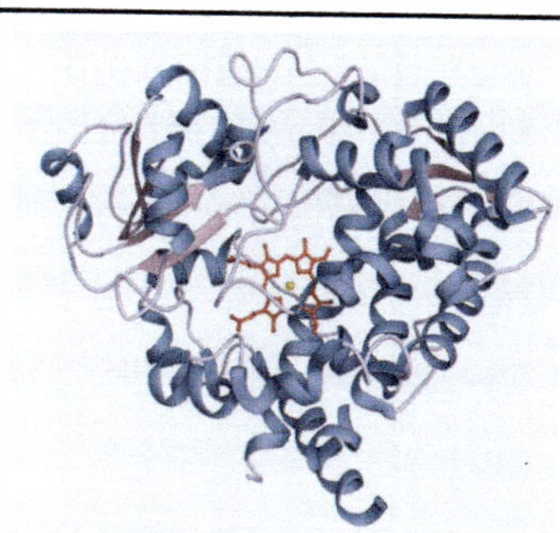

1.1. Pharmacodynamics

The study of a drug's physiological and biochemical effects is known as pharmacodynamics (PD) (especially pharmaceutical drugs). The consequences may appear in microbes, animals (including humans), or combinations of organisms (for instance, infection).

The two main subfields of pharmacology are pharmacodynamics and pharmacokinetics. Pharmacology is a branch of biology that studies how chemicals interact with living things, both endogenous and exogenous.

Specifically, pharmacodynamics studies how a drug acts on an organism, while pharmacokinetics studies how the drug acts on the organism. Together, they affect dosage, advantages, and side effects. Sometimes, particularly in combined references, pharmacodynamics is shortened to PD and pharmacokinetics to PK.

The relationships between drug concentration and effect, or dose-response relationships, are of special importance in pharmacodynamics. One dominant example is drug-receptor interactions as modeled by (Figure 1.1):

where; L, R, and LR represent ligand (drug), receptor, and ligand-receptor complex concentrations, respectively. This equation is a mathematically study able simplified model of reaction dynamics that can be investigated using resources like free energy maps.

The way that medications affect target cells to change cellular function is known as pharmacodynamics

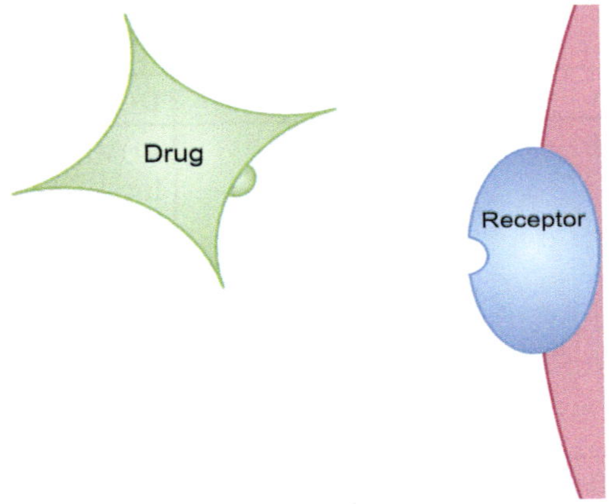

Figure 1.1. *Pharmacodynamics: Drug and receptor binding.*

Source: *Open Resources for Nursing (Open RN); Ernstmeyer K, Christman E, editors. Nursing Pharmacology [Internet]. 2nd edition. Eau Claire (WI): Chippewa Valley Technical College; 2023. Chapter 1 Pharmacokinetics & Pharmacodynamics. Available from: https://www.ncbi.nlm.nih.gov/books/NBK595006/.*

1. **Receptor and non-receptor mechanisms**

The majority of medications work by interacting with receptors, which are parts of cells. Certain drugs don't interact with receptors; instead, they work through straightforward chemical or physical processes.

- Receptors are protein molecules present either on the cell surface or within the cell e.g. adrenergic receptors, cholinoceptors, insulin receptors, etc.
- The endogenous neurotransmitters, hormones, autacoids and most of the drugs produce their effects by binding with their specific receptors.
- Aluminum hydroxide and magnesium trisilicate, which are used in the treatment of peptic ulcer disease act by non-receptor mechanism by neutralizing the gastric acid.

Numerous drugs share similar chemical structures with naturally occurring chemicals and can bind to receptors, leading to either a response from the receptor or blocking its activity.

A drug is said to have an affinity for a receptor if it can attach itself to it. A drug's efficacy is determined by its capacity to elicit a response at a receptor. Whereas an antagonist possesses affinity but neither efficacy nor intrinsic activity, an agonist possesses both. A medication is referred to as an agonist when it has the ability to stimulate a receptor, imitating the endogenous transmitter in the process. An antagonist drug is one that inhibits the action of an endogenous transmitter by blocking a receptor (for example, it will stop a natural chemical from acting on the receptor). There will be competition between the drug and the natural stimulus to the receptor, because the majority of drug binding is reversible. Chemical bonds are the forces that draw a drug to its receptor; they are: (a) hydrogen bond; (b) ionic bond; (c) covalent bond; and (d) Vander Waals force. The strongest type of bond is covalent, and the drug-receptor complex is typically irreversible.

Second messengers, also known as intracellular regulatory molecules, are synthesized and released when first messengers, such as neurotransmitters, hormones, autacoids, and most drugs, bind to their respective receptors to form drug-receptor complexes e g, cyclic AMP, calcium, cyclic GMP, diacylglycerol, inositol triphosphate (IP3), and calmodulin, which subsequently result in a subcellular or molecular mechanism of action for the drug.

2. Site of drug action

A drug may act:

- Extracellularly e.g.: osmotic diuretics, plasma expanders.
- On the cell surface e.g.: digitalis, penicillin, catecholamines
- Inside the cell e.g.: anti-cancer drugs, steroid hormones.

3. **Dose-Response Relationship**

- The biological object being observed and the medication used determine the precise relationship between the dose and the response. The "S" shaped or sigmoid-type curve is produced when the logarithm of the dose as the abscissa and the responses as the ordinate are graphically constructed. A drug's minimal dose is its lowest concentration at which a response is elicited, and its maximal dose is its highest concentration at which an additional increase in concentration does not alter the response.

i. Graded dose effect

The pharmacological response rises in a graded manner up to the ceiling effect as the dose given to a single subject or tissue increases.

- It is used for the characterization of the action of drugs. The concentration that is required to produce 50% of the maximum effect is termed as EC_{50} or ED_{50}.

ii. Quantal dose effect

It is all or none response, the sensitive objects give a response to small doses of a drug while some will be resistant and need very large doses. The median effective dose and the median lethal dose are frequently used to describe the quantal dose-effect curve.

- Median lethal dose or LD_{50}: This is the dose (mg/kg), which would be expected to kill one-half of a population of the same species and strain.
- Median effective dose or ED_{50}: This is the dose (mg/kg), which produces a

desired response in 50% of the test population.

- Therapeutic index: It is an approximate assessment of the safety of the drug. It is the ratio of the median lethal dose and the median effective dose. Also called therapeutic window or safety.

$$T_I = \frac{TD_{50}}{ED_{50}}$$

A drug is considered safer the higher its therapeutic index. Penicillin has a very high therapeutic index, but the digitalis preparation has a much lower one.

4. Structural activity relationship

The activity of a drug is intimately related to its chemical structure. Knowledge about the chemical structure of a drug is useful for:

- Synthesis of new compounds with more specific actions and fewer adverse reactions
- Synthesis of competitive antagonist and
- Understanding the mechanism of drug action.

A slight modification of the structure of the compound can change the effect completely.

1.1.1. Physiological Influences on Pharmacodynamics

Big proteins called receptors are crucial to the study of pharmacodynamics. Because receptors can amplify physiological signals, they could be targets for pharmaceuticals. The two main jobs of receptors are to bind to their particular molecules, or ligands, and to transmit signals, or signal transduction, to trigger a chain of events. This dual function suggests that a receptor needs to have both an effector domain and a ligand-binding domain. Receptors are special because they function as proteins that can detect and accept both endogenous and exogenous ligands. However, the structures of exogenous ligands (xenobiotics or drug products) ought to resemble those of endogenous ligands. Physiological receptors are those that are able to identify and accept exogenous ligands.

A drug's effect can be stopped when it separates from a receptor, just as it can be produced after binding to a receptor. A drug will continue to have an effect as long as the receptor–drug complex is intact even if it is bound so tightly (such as by a covalent bond). The latter process, though, is not very long-lasting because eventually a new free receptor is synthesized and the receptor–drug complex is broken down and removed.

The size of a drug molecule is significantly less than that of a receptor. It is possible to locate and investigate a receptor's particular binding site. Important characteristics of receptors, their binding sites, and their roles in pharmacodynamics have been revealed by extensive crystallography studies and genetic alterations (mutations) in wild-type receptors. The effects of drugs depend on a combination of physiological and physicochemical factors because the chemical structure and affinity of a drug for a receptor both play significant roles in producing a physiological effect. Additionally, a drug's effect may be influenced by the pathophysiology. In other words, in a person without any abnormalities in cellular or physiological function, a drug may have a different effect on them or have no effect at all. On the other hand, a disease state may alter how a drug acts. For example, oral administration of drugs that are extensively metabolized by the liver will increase the systemic bioavailability (plasma level) of those drugs in patients with cirrhosis who also have reduced hepatic metabolism. In addition to having decreased renal plasma flow and glomerular filtration rate, patients with liver cirrhosis also have decreased renal elimination of medications like ofloxacin (Apo-Oflox, from Canada), lithium (Lithobid), and fluconazole (Diflucan).

Pharmacology, pharmacodynamics, pharmacokinetics, biochemistry, and pharmaceutics are all influenced by a range of physiological and physicochemical factors. When a drug action is investigated, these fields are frequently integrated, so it is not surprising to find overlapping factors that can have an impact on all of the fields.

1.1.2. Receptors

Chemical messengers, such as hormones, ions, and neurotransmitters released by nerve cells, are responsible for a multitude of vital physiological and biological processes. Receptors pick up these messengers. Numerous hydrophilic hormones (e.g. peptide hormones like glucagon and insulin) interact with plasma membrane receptors to send signals to the cytoplasm. We refer to the entire mechanism as transmembrane signaling. Thyroid, steroid, and retinoid hormones, on the other hand, are hydrophobic hormones that can pass through cell membranes and interact with intracellular receptors found inside cells. Because of this, the hydrophobic ligands have intracellular receptors instead of transmembrane receptors.

Similar to an enzyme-substrate interaction, the messenger-receptor interaction is typically accomplished noncovalently. The "second messengers"—Ca^{2+}, cAMP, IP3, diacylglycerol, and cGMP—are produced or released when a hormone binds to its receptor. Hormones are ligands that act as the "first messengers." Second messengers function in the cytoplasm or nucleus to either stimulate or inhibit a variety of biochemical processes.

Many medications can bind to physiological receptors by imitating the endogenous ligands. Like endogenous ligands, these medications cause biochemical alterations in a cell that lead to pharmacological reactions by binding to receptors and starting a chain of events. A change in a receptor's affinity for its ligand can have an instantaneous effect on biochemistry and physiology because receptors are crucial for both receiving extracellular signals and converting them into intracellular signals.

Not every protein found in plasma membranes functions as a receptor. Proteins can function as transporters, ion channels, enzymes, or receptors. These proteins also serve vital purposes. For example, anions and cations cannot easily cross plasma membranes because of the hydrophobic nature of the lipid bilayer of the membrane. Critical regulatory events in both excitable and non-excitable cells are the ingress and egress of ions. All cells express ion transporters for Na^+, K^+, Ca^{2+}, and Cl^- to maintain the electrochemical gradients necessary to produce or maintain a membrane potential. The human body, for example, expresses over 200 distinct ion channels that precisely control the flow of Na+, K^+, Ca^{2+}, and Cl^- across cell membranes.

The names of the ligands (or a class of ligands) that receptors bind are frequently used to designate the names of the receptors. For example, norepinephrine (ligand) binds to adrenergic receptors whereas insulin (ligand) binds to an insulin receptor. Different ligands may bind to different receptors in a single cell; for instance, hepatocytes have receptors for glucagon and insulin ligands. Additionally, distinct cells may express the same ligand-binding receptor. For instance, hepatocytes, myocytes, and adipocytes are the main cell types that express insulin receptors.

Signal transduction refers to the movement of chemical signals (e.g., neurotransmitters, hormones, and second messengers) from the outside of a cell into its interior. Signals can travel in two ways: either along a straightforward path, as in the case of the plasma membrane's ion channels, which open and close in response to a chemical ligand, or along a more intricate one, such as the coupling of ligand–receptor interactions that results in a series of steps that alter protein conformations and enzyme activities in the cytoplasm of a cell. (Rang, 2006; Krska & Cox, 2019)

1.1.3. Transmembrane Signaling and Signal Transduction

Despite a small distinction between the two, transmembrane signaling and signal transduction are frequently used synonymously. Transmembrane signaling is the process of transmitting an extracellular signal via a receptor located on the cell membrane. Sending a signal through a cell membrane, where the receptor may be an intracellular rather than an embedded cell membrane receptor, is referred to as signal transduction, a much more general term.

Six signal transduction systems are employed by receptors:

- Gated ion channels;
- Receptor enzymes;
- Serpentine receptors;
- Receptors for hydrophobic ligands;
- Receptors without intrinsic enzyme activity and
- Adhesion receptors

1.1.3.1. Gated Ion Channels

Numerous medications stimulate or block the influx of ions through cell membrane channels by acting on their receptors. For example, certain medications that induce calcium influx can impact gene expression and neurotransmitter release.

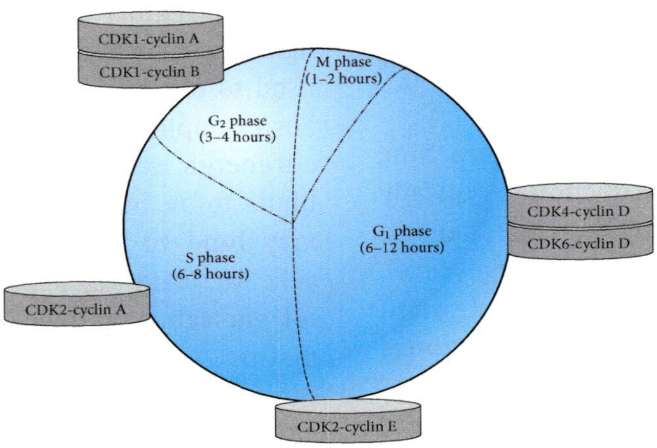

Figure 1.2. *The eukaryotic cell cycle and the points where cyclin-dependent protein kinases (CDKs) are activated by different cyclins.*

Source: https://samples.jbpub.com/9781449621087/9781449621087_ch06.pdf.

Ion channels can also be opened by endogenous ligands binding to their receptors. For example, acetylcholine, an endogenous ligand, binds to the acetylcholine receptor to increase the amount of Na^+ that enters the cells from the extracellular fluid.

The gated ion channels are divided into voltage-gated and ligand-gated categories according to their gating mechanisms. When ions flow through these two gates, cations enter the cell, causing depolarization, or anions enter the cell, causing hyperpolarization (Figure 1.2).

1.1.3.1.1. Voltage-Gated Ion Channels

As their name suggests, voltage-gated ion channels respond to changes in the membrane potential rather than directly binding to their ligands. Put differently, the membrane voltage determines the likelihood of these channels opening. In many different types of cells, voltage-gated ion channels are a major pathway for K^+, Cl^-, Na^+, and Ca^{2+} ions. For example, the voltage-gated Na^+ channels close at a membrane voltage of -60 mV (i.e. when the membrane is in its resting state), but they become open when the membrane becomes depolarized (i.e. when the cell's interior is positive). The binding of acetylcholine to its receptor causes the depolarization effect to occur. These ion channels have a high rate of influx and are highly selective. One such channel is the Na+ channel, whichhas an ion influx rate of more than 10 million Na^+ ions per second and is 100 times more selective for Na^+ ions than for Ca^{2+} or K^+ ions.

The use of verapamil (Calan), a calcium channel blocker, illustrates how blocking these channels results in a physiological alteration. Verapamil lowers blood pressure and has antiarrhythmic effects by blocking voltage-gated calcium channels in the heart and vascular smooth muscle. Various anticonvulsants function by means of voltage-gated sodium channels. For example, carbamazepine (TEGretol) and phenytoin (Dilantin) reduce seizure activity by reducing the flow of Na^+ ions across cell membranes.

1.1.3.1.2. Ligand-Gated Ion Channels

One can use the neurotransmitter acetylcholine as an example to better understand this class of gated ion channels. Many studies have been conducted on the acetylcholine receptor, its ligand acetylcholine, and their functions in signal transduction. The postsynaptic membrane of neurons at specific synapses and the myocytes at neuromuscular junctions contain the nicotinic acetylcholine receptor. A synaptic knob's synaptic vesicles hold roughly 10,000 acetylcholine molecules each. Na^+ enters the cell as a result of the released acetylcholine binding to its receptor on the postsynaptic neuron.

Comparing it to the voltage-gated ion channel, which opens in response to a change in the membrane potential, the acetylcholine receptor functions as an ion channel and opens in response to the neurotransmitter acetylcholine (a ligand). Five subunits make up the receptor (ion channel): two α subunits, one subunit each of β, γ, and δ, and the neurotransmitter acetylcholine is bound by the N termini of the two α subunits. Protein conformational changes are the primary cause of acetylcholine's effects on the postsynaptic ion channel. Acetylcholine causes its receptor to change from a closed to an open conformation when it binds to it. Consequently, only Na^+, Ca^{2+}, or K^+ can enter; other ions are unable to do so. Because of the positive cooperative nature of ligand binding, acetylcholine binding affinity is increased when other α subunits are bound to the first α subunit (Figure 1.3).

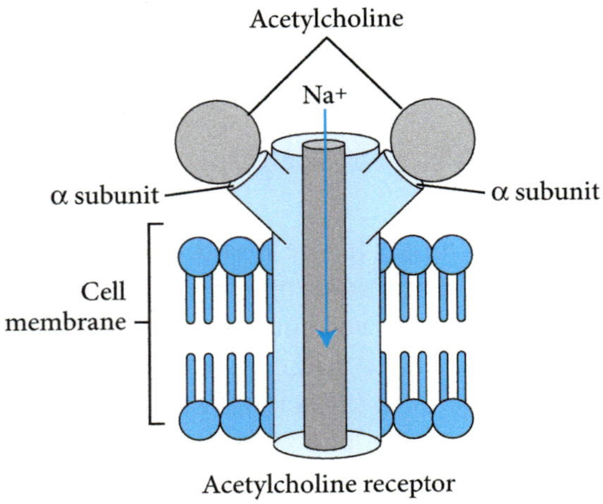

Figure 1.3. *A ligand-gated ion channel reacting to its ligand, acetylcholine.*

Source: https://samples.jbpub.com/9781449621087/9781449621087_ch06.pdf.

While ligand-gated ion channels, such as the acetylcholine receptor channel, are primarily responsible for facilitating ion influx, serotonin neurotransmitter and amino acid ligands, including glutamate and glycine, have also been studied as potential ligand-gated ion channels. For example, ion entry of K^+, Na^+, and Ca^{2+} is facilitated by the binding of the serotonin or glutamate ligands to their receptor channels; ion entry of Cl^- is facilitated by the binding of the glycine ligand to its receptor channel. Another illustration is the major inhibitory neurotransmitter gamma-aminobutyric acid (GABA) binding to its receptor channel, which opens the channel for Cl^-ion entry and causes the neuron to become hyperpolarized. It has also been proposed that benzodiazepines increase the entry of Cl^- ions through the GABA receptor because GABA inhibits the action potential (through Cl^- ion entry and neuronal hyperpolarization). Benzodiazepines, on the other hand, bind to their own binding site on the GABA receptor rather than competing with GABA for the GABA binding site.

1.1.3.2. Receptor Enzymes

Receptor enzymes consist of two domains: a catalytic domain that faces the cell cytosol and a single membrane-spanning domain that faces the extracellular environment to receive signals. A protein tyrosine kinase, a serine kinase, or a guanylyl cyclase could make up the catalytic domain, also known as the intracellular domain. The enzymatic domain is activated by ligand binding, and this phosphorylation of various target proteins has an impact on cellular metabolism.

Important receptors in the receptor enzyme signal transduction system are insulin receptor, epidermal growth factor (EGF), and numerous other trophic hormone receptors. The glycoprotein insulin receptor is composed of two α and two β subunits, which are held together by disulfide bonds. Tyrosine kinase activity occurs in the β chains' intracellular domain. Tyr residues in the β subunit's C-terminal domain auto phosphorylate to initiate the β subunit's tyrosine kinase activity. The phosphoryl group from ATP molecules is subsequently transferred by this tyrosine kinase to the hydroxyl group of Tyr residues in other target proteins, including insulin receptor substrate (IRS).

Since numerous tyrosine kinases play a role in signaling pathways in neoplastic diseases, therapeutic agents targeting these signaling pathways could effectively target some of the receptor enzymes. For instance, the monoclonal antibody trastuzumab (Herceptin) binds to the extracellular domain of the human epidermal growth factor receptor 2 (HER-2) and suppresses the expression of HER-2 receptors on cancerous cells by inhibiting the S phase of the cell cycle. This results in cellular cytotoxicity.

Approximately thirty percent of patients with breast cancer have overexpressed HER-2 receptors. Furthermore, this receptor is present in other cancers such as lung, prostate, and ovarian cancers, albeit to varying degrees (Figure 1.4).

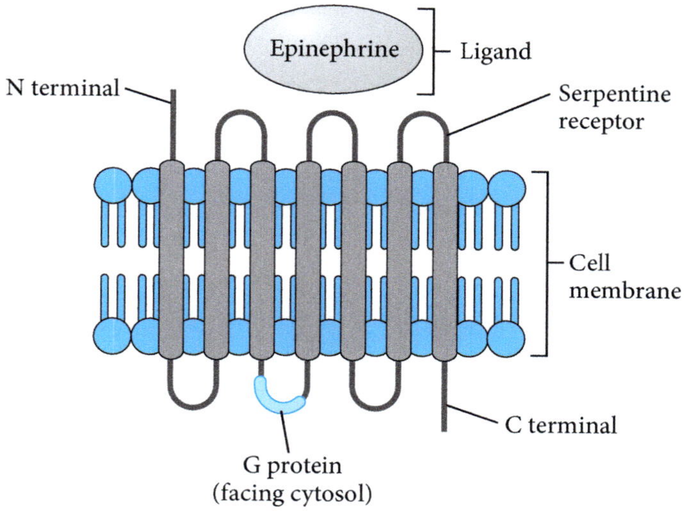

Figure 1.4. *A serpentine receptor that has been folded back and forth seven times inside of the cell membrane.*

Source: https://samples.jbpub.com/9781449621087/9781449621087_ch06.pdf.

1.1.3.3. Serpentine Receptors

Serpentine receptors increase the amounts of second messengers like cAMP, Ca^{2+}, and phosphoinositides inside cells by binding to extracellular ligands. Small molecules or ions known as second messengers attach to a range of proteins, altering their structures and functionalities in the process. A G protein on the cytoplasmic face of the plasma membrane is activated when a ligand binds to a serpentine receptor. Thus, the term "G-protein receptor" refers to these receptors. The name "serpentine receptor" refers to a special property of these receptors: they are embedded and folded seven times across the cell membrane.

Numerous medications, such as antihistamines, neuroleptics, antidepressants, and antihypertensive agents, target serpentine receptors. The β-adrenergic receptor is an illustration of a serpentine receptor. Two scientists, Brian Kobilka and Robert Lefkowitz, were awarded the 2012 Nobel Prize in Chemistry for their contributions to the understanding of serpentine receptor signaling.

Epinephrine is an adrenergic ligand that attaches itself to the β-adrenergic receptor, a particular type of cell surface receptor. The receptor's cytosolic domain changes conformation as a result of this binding, and the Gs protein is then bound by the receptor. The binding site for either GDP or GTP is located on the α subunit of the Gs protein. GTP replaces GDP when a ligand-bound receptor is present, activating the Gs protein. The synthesis of cAMP is then catalyzed by adenylate cyclase, which is activated by the Gs protein. cAMP causes the protein kinase PKA, which is dependent on cAMP, to become active. Glycogen phosphorylase b kinase is activated by PKA, and this process ultimately results in glycogenolysis by converting glycogen phosphorylase b to glycogen phosphorylase a. Numerous physiological targets, such as metabolic enzymes, transport proteins, regulatory proteins, other protein kinases, ion channels, and transcription factors, can be phosphorylated by PKA.

The way that different serpentine receptors use the G proteins may vary. In fact, it is known that G proteins help over 500 receptors send signals to each other.

"Here are some examples of serpentine receptors:

- Gq activates phospholipase C to produce diacylglycerol and IP3 when oxytocin or vasopressin hormones bind to their serpentine receptors.
- Gs activates adenylate cyclase (AC) when epinephrine binds to its β-adrenergic receptors. On the other hand, the inhibition of AC's enzymatic activity occurs when epinephrine binds to an α_2-adrenergic receptor because this receptor is coupled to Gi, an inhibitory G protein, rather than Gs.
- In vertebrates, serpentine receptors are also used for the detection of light (vision), smells (olfaction), and tastes (gustation). These receptors modify the electrical potential of sensory neurons by acting through G proteins. Three layers of cells make up the retina: (1) rods and cones; (2) bipolar cells, which connect neurons; and (3) ganglion cells. Cone cells allow us to see color and are active in bright light. About 6 million cone cells make up a human retina. Cones only work during the daytime because they need a sufficient amount of light to be stimulated. Because of this, we can only see color during the daytime, or when the light is strong enough to activate the cone receptors.
- Before the light can reach and affect the photoreceptors (rod and cone cells), it must first pass through the bipolar cells and the ganglion cells. In the retina, rhodopsin and photopsin are found in rod and cone cells, respectively. Both photopsin and rhodopsin, which share a similar structure, have a pigment that absorbs light. The structure of rhodopsin is a typical serpentine one. It is composed of a prosthetic group called 11-cis retinal, a derivative of vitamin A, and a protein called opsin. Rhodopsin's retinal component absorbs photons of energy, which modifies the prosthetic group's conformation. This modifies rhodopsin's conformation, which is the first step in the visual transduction process. Cyclic GMP concentration falls as a result of conformational changes in rhodopsin caused by photons of energy. Na^+- and Ca^{2+}-gated ion channels in the rod cell's outer segment close in response to a drop in cGMP. This causes the cell membrane to become hyperpolarized, which sends an electrical signal to the brain.

Gq activates phospholipase C to produce diacylglycerol and IP3 when oxytocin or vasopressin hormones bind to their serpentine receptors, whereas Gs activates adenylate cyclase (AC) when epinephrine binds to its β-adrenergic receptors. Furthermore, the inhibition of AC's enzymatic activity occurs when epinephrine binds to an α_2-adrenergic receptor because this receptor is coupled to Gi, an inhibitory G protein, rather than Gs.

In vertebrates, serpentine receptors are also used for the detection of light (vision), smells (olfaction), and tastes (gustation). These receptors modify the electrical potential of sensory neurons by acting through G proteins. Three layers of cells make up the retina: (1) rods and cones; (2) bipolar cells, which connect neurons; and (3) ganglion cells.

Cone cells ~~are what~~ allow us to see color and are active in bright light. About 6 million cone cells make up a human retina. Cones only work during the daytime because they need a sufficient amount of light to be stimulated. Because of this, we can only see color during the daytime, or when the light is strong enough to activate the cone receptors.

Before the light can reach and affect the photoreceptors (rod and cone cells), it must first pass through the bipolar cells and the ganglion cells. In the retina, rhodopsin and photopsin are found in rod and cone cells, respectively. Both photopsin and rhodopsin, which share a similar structure, have a pigment that absorbs light. The structure of rhodopsin is a typical serpentine one. It is composed of a prosthetic group called 11-cis retinal, a derivative of vitamin A, and a protein called opsin. Rhodopsin's retinal component absorbs photons of energy, which modifies the prosthetic group's conformation. This modifies rhodopsin's conformation, which is the first step in the visual transduction process. Cyclic GMP concentration falls as a result of conformational changes in rhodopsin caused by photons of energy. Na^+- and Ca^{2+}-gated ion channels in the rod cell's outer segment close in response to a drop in cGMP. This causes the cell membrane to become hyperpolarized, which sends an electrical signal to the brain.

Sildenafil and tadalafil, two drugs used for erectile dysfunction, inhibit cGMP phosphodiesterase (PDE). This raises cGMP levels and impairs color discrimination in a dose-related manner.

1.1.3.4. Receptors for Hydrophobic Ligands

Certain ligands target proteins that have intracellular receptors; they lack plasma membrane receptors because they are hydrophobic. Thyroid hormones and steroids, including corticosteroids, mineralocorticoids, sex steroids, and vitamin D, are included in this class. Gene expression is influenced by these receptors. These ligands are hydrophobic, meaning that for them to move from the location of their synthesis to the site of their action via blood circulation, other proteins must help. For example, transthyretin helps thyroid hormones travel and reach their target cells, while transcortin, androgen-binding proteins, and sex-hormone-binding proteins help steroid hormones in the blood do the same.

The steroid hormones separate from their transport proteins as soon as they get to their target cells, enter the cytoplasm by breaking free of the cell membrane, attach to their receptor, and move toward the nucleus. Their job in the nucleus is to stimulate (or, to a lesser degree, repress) the transcription of particular genes. The steroid hormone-binding receptors have a high affinity for ligands. These receptors belong to a large family of structurally similar DNA-binding proteins. Depending on the nature of the steroid hormones, the receptor-binding complex may occur in the cytoplasm (e.g., for glucocorticoids) or in the nucleus (e.g., for estrogen and androgen). (Rang, 2006; Krska & Cox, 2019)

The conformation of these receptors is altered when steroids bind to them, allowing the hormone-receptor complex to bind to particular DNA sequences known as hormone response elements (HRE). The transcription of nearby genes can be either activated or repressed by binding to HRE.

There are some structural similarities amongst steroid receptors. Zinc is a necessary component for DNA binding and is present in a small DNA-binding domain found in all known steroid receptors. Without zinc, the domain's structure would unravel; zinc stabilizes the domain's structure.

A hormone can alter the expression of multiple genes by binding to multiple HREs through a hormone-receptor complex. Every kind of HRE has the ability to affect between 50 and 100 genes' transcription. Because of this, the impact on cellular function of a steroid hormone-receptor complex binding to its HRE is greatly amplified.

Steroid hormones act relatively slowly compared to peptide hormones, which act on membrane receptors quickly (think of the functions of insulin and glucagon). Their slow action is caused by the fact that activating a gene's expression for the synthesis of an enzyme or protein takes longer than directly acting on preexisting enzymes, ranging from 30 minutes to several hours. The gradual action helps to explain why steroids (e.g. budesonide, fluticasone) are not suitable for treating acute bronchial asthma symptoms quickly. But compared to peptide hormones, the effects of steroid hormones last longer—from hours to days. The majority of the enzymes and proteins that these ligands express have a slow turnover rate, which accounts for the longer effect.

1.1.3.5. Receptors without Intrinsic Activity

Certain receptor proteins lack intrinsic enzymatic activity. For example, cells have cytokine receptors that react to γ-interferon, growth hormone, and erythropoietin. These receptors' intracellular domains bind Janus kinase (JAK), a soluble tyrosine kinase. To control the transcription of a gene, JAK phosphorylates additional proteins known as signal transducers and activators of transcription, or STAT, upon ligand binding. The JAK-STAT pathway is the name given to the entire pathway. Four JAKs and six STATs, which activate gene transcription differently in various cell types, are found in mammals.

The kidney synthesizes erythropoietin, a hormone consisting of 165 amino acid residues. Erythrocyte production is stimulated by EPO binding to its receptor. There is no enzymatic activity in the EPO receptor. But the EPO-bound receptor complex's intercellular domain binds a soluble JAK, which phosphorylates a number of the EPO receptor's tyrosine residues. A STAT domain is bound by these phosphorylated tyrosine residues. Through this process, the STAT domain becomes sufficiently close to JAK for JAK to phosphorylate it as well. After entering the cell nucleus, the phosphorylated STAT domain increases the expression of genes necessary for erythrocyte maturation. Ninety percent of patients receiving dialysis and having end-stage renal failure have an erythropoietin deficiency as their underlying cause of anemia.

1.1.3.6. Adhesion Receptors

Numerous signaling pathways involve adhesion molecules like immunoglobulin-like cell adhesion molecules (Ig-CAM) and selectins, cadherins, and integrins. The extracellular and intracellular domains of these receptors are present. The intracellular domain of a protein is linked to the cytoskeleton of the cytoplasm, primarily actin and filaments, whereas the extracellular domain is linked to macromolecule proteins like collagen and fibronectin. These adhesion receptors mediate tissue repair, promote cell migration, cell-cell adhesion, and platelet aggregation at the site of tissue injury, and carry out other vital tasks to return the body to homeostasis when they receive the proper signals. An integrin receptor, for example, consists of two subunits, α and β (the β subunit is also referred to as CD18). Leukocyte adhesion deficiency is an immune disease caused by a genetic mutation that encodes a nonfunctional β subunit (LAD). The disease is caused by the nonfunctional β subunit, which prevents leukocytes from adhering to the blood vessel and preventing them from migrating through it to reach the infection site. LAD is an inherited illness. Affected newborns frequently experience recurrent infections, and many pass away from infections before turning two.

1.1.4. Regulation of Receptors

The body regulates the quantity, sensitivity, location, and intensity of receptors because they are essential to signaling pathways. For certain receptors, the regulation happens instantly, but for others, it might take several days.

Receptor responses may be diminished if a ligand (agonist) is continuously applied to the receptor; this is known as tachyphylaxis. For example, while β-adrenergic receptors are continuously binding to their agonistic ligands, an intracellular component of the receptors binds to a molecule known as β-arrestin. β-arrestin functions to obstruct the Gs protein's entry, which could potentially cause the receptor to become desensitized in a matter of minutes. β-arrestin also separates from the intracellular part of β-adrenergic receptors when the agonist is removed, enabling the receptors to regain their full sensitivity.

An additional instance of regulation occurs when an endocytosis process internalizes an agonist-bound receptor. The ligand cannot bind to the receptor due to endocytosis. Because the internalized receptor may be delocalized into the membrane (as is the case for morphine receptors) or may be permanently degraded (as is the case for epidermal growth factor receptors), the removal of the receptor from the membrane may only be temporary. In the latter scenario, it could take a few hours or a day for a new receptor to express its gene.

Furthermore, receptors may be both up- and down-regulated in addition to these processes. If a receptor is exposed to an agonistic ligand on a regular basis, its expression may be down-regulated. Conversely, if an antagonist blocks the receptor for a few days, there may be an up-regulation of receptor expression. However, pathophysiological factors may also be the cause of these changes in receptor expressions. (Rang, 2006; Krska & Cox, 2019)

1.2. Pharmacokinetics

A subfield of pharmacology called pharmacokinetics studies how a drug interacts with the body after it is administered. Any chemical xenobiotic, such as prescription medications, insecticides, food additives, cosmetics, etc., is one of the substances of interest. It makes an effort to examine chemical metabolism and ascertain a substance's fate from the time of administration until it is entirely removed from the body. The foundation of pharmacokinetics is mathematical modeling, which emphasizes the correlation between drug plasma concentration and time since administration. Pharmacodynamics (PD) is the study of how the drug affects the organism, whereas pharmacokinetics is the study of how an organism affects a drug. As demonstrated in PK/PD models, the combination of the two affects dosage, advantages, and side effects.

1.2.1. ADME

The abbreviation ADME, which stands for absorption, distribution, metabolism, and excretion, is an acronym that is commonly used in the fields of pharmacology and pharmacokinetics. The four letters represent descriptors, which measure the way a drug interacts with the body over time. Since its initial use in the 1960s, the term "ADME" has gained widespread usage in scientific literature, education, drug regulations, and clinical practice.

The term "ADME" refers to a pharmaceutical compound's internal distribution within an organism. The four factors all affect the drug's concentration and the rate at which it enters the tissues, which in turn affects the compound's therapeutic efficacy and activity. Occasionally, toxicity and/or liberation are also taken into account, producing LADMET, ADMET, or LADME.

1.2.1.1. Components

1. Absorption/administration

A substance typically needs to enter the bloodstream through mucous surfaces, such as the digestive tract (intestinal absorption), to reach a tissue, where it is then absorbed by the target cells. The degree to which a medication is absorbed following oral administration can be decreased by a number of factors, including inadequate compound solubility, gastric emptying time, intestinal transit time, chemical instability in the stomach, and inability to penetrate the intestinal wall. The compound's absorption has a major impact on its bioavailability. Medications that do not absorb well when taken orally have to be administered in less ideal ways, such as intravenously or through inhalation (e.g. zanamivir). Administration routes are a crucial factor to take into account.

2. Distribution

The compound must be transported, usually by the bloodstream, to its effector site. From there, the substance may spread, usually to varying degrees, into the muscles and organs. Upon entering the bloodstream through intravascular injection or absorption from different extracellular locations, the medication undergoes multiple distribution processes that typically result in a decrease in its plasma concentration.

The reversible transfer of a drug from one compartment to another is known as distribution. Drug distribution is influenced by various factors such as molecular size, polarity, binding to serum proteins, and complex formation. At certain natural barriers, such as the blood–brain barrier, distribution can pose a significant challenge.

3. Metabolism

As soon as compounds enter the body, they start to degrade. Cytochrome P450 enzymes are redox enzymes that do most of the liver's work in the metabolism of small molecules. The original (parent) compound is changed into new ones known as metabolites during metabolism. Metabolism deactivates the parent drug dose when metabolites are pharmacologically inert, which typically lessens the effects on the body. Additionally, metabolites have the potential to have greater pharmacological activity than the parent drug.

4. Excretion

Substances and their metabolites must be eliminated from the body by excretion, which typically occurs in the form of feces or urine from the kidneys. Accumulation of foreign substances can negatively impact normal metabolism unless excretion is completed. Drug excretion takes place in three primary locations. The most significant location is the kidney, which is where products are eliminated through urine. The process known as biliary excretion, also known as fecal excretion, starts in the liver and moves through the gut before the products are eventually expelled along with waste materials or feces. The lungs are the final major route of excretion (e.g. gases used in anesthesia).

Excretion of drugs by the kidney involves 3 main mechanisms:

- Glomerular filtration of unbound drug.
- Active secretion of (free & protein-bound) drug by transporters (e.g. anions such as urate, penicillin, glucuronide, sulfate conjugates) or cations such as choline, histamine.
- Filtrate 100-fold concentrated in tubules for a favorable concentration gradient so that it may be secreted by passive diffusion and passed out through the urine.

5. Toxicity

Occasionally, the compound's actual or potential toxicity is considered (ADME-Tox or ADMET). The therapeutic index and median lethal dose (LD50) are two metrics used to describe toxicity. Using techniques like QSPR or QSAR, computational chemists attempt to predict the ADME-Tox properties of compounds. The administration route has a major impact on ADME.

1.2.2. Factors Affecting Drug Absorption and Bioavailability

Drug absorption and bioavailability are the mechanisms through which a drug is absorbed into the bloodstream and made ready to exert its intended effects.

1. Physico-Chemical Properties of the Drug:

i. **Physical State:** Liquids are absorbed better than solids and crystalloids are absorbed better than colloids.

ii. **Lipid or Water Solubility:** Compared to an oily solution, drugs in an aqueous solution mix more easily. On the other hand, lipid-soluble medications enter cells at the cell surface more quickly than water-soluble medications.

iii. **Ionization:** Drugs are mostly made of organic compounds. The organic medications are partially ionized in the fluid, in contrast to inorganic substances. A unionized component is primarily lipid soluble and absorbs quickly, whereas an ionized component is frequently water-soluble and absorbs slowly. The majority of medications are weak bases or acids. It may be assumed for all practical purposes, that the mucosal lining of the G.I.T is impermeable to the ionized form of a weak organic acid or a weak organic base. These drugs exist in two forms.

- **Acidic drugs:** rapidly absorbed from the stomach e.g. salicylates and barbiturates.
- **Basic drugs:** Not absorbed until they reach the alkaline environment i.e. small intestine when administered orally e.g. pethidine and ephedrine.

2. Dosage Forms:

i. **Particle Size:** Small particle size is important for drug absorption. Drugs given in a dispersed or emulsified state are absorbed better e.g. vitamin D and vitamin A.

ii. Disintegration Time and Dissolution Rate:

- **Disintegration time:** The rate of breakup of the tablet or capsule into the drug granules.
- **Dissolution rate:** The rate at which the drug goes into solution.

iii. **Formulation:** When creating powders or tablets, inert diluents such as lactose, sucrose, starch, and calcium phosphate are typically utilized. Although fillers might not be completely inert, they could still have an impact on the medication's stability and absorption. Therefore, a poorly formulated medication may completely lose its therapeutic value.

3. Physiological Factors:

i. **Gastrointestinal Transit Time:** When the medication is administered on an empty stomach, rapid absorption takes place. To reduce gastrointestinal irritation, some medications that cause irritation, such as salicylates and iron preparations, are purposefully administered after meals. However, sometimes the presence of food in the GI tract aids the absorption of certain drugs e.g. griseofulvin, propranolol and riboflavin.

ii. **Presence of Other Agents:** Vitamin C enhances the absorption of iron from the G.I.T. Calcium present in milk and in antacids forms insoluble complexes with the tetracycline antibiotics and reduces their absorption.

iii. **Area of the Absorbing Surface and Local Circulation:** Drugs can be absorbed better from the small intestine than from the stomach because of the larger surface area of the former. Increased vascular supply can increase the absorption.

iv. **Enterohepatic Cycling:** Some drugs move in between the intestines and the liver before they reach the site of action. This increases the bioavailability e.g. phenolphthalein.

v. **Drug Metabolism/First Pass Effect:** The bioavailability of a medication is also impacted by the drug's quick breakdown by the liver during the first pass (propranolol) or the intestinal wall (isoprenaline). As a result, a medication that is well absorbed when taken orally may not work due to extensive first pass metabolism.

4. **Pharmacogenetic Factors:** Individual variations occur due to the genetically mediated reason in drug absorption and response.

5. **Disease States:** Absorption and first pass metabolism may be affected in conditions like malabsorption, thyrotoxicosis, achlorhydria and liver cirrhosis.

1.2.3. Modeling

To make the many processes involved in the interaction between an organism and a chemical substance easier to conceptualize, models have been developed. It is possible to carry out pharmacokinetic modeling using either noncompartmental or compartmental techniques. Although multi-compartmental models offer the most accurate representations of reality, they are less commonly used than monocompartmental and, more importantly, two-compartmental models due to the difficulty of adding parameters to such models. The results of a drug's model can be applied in the clinical setting to pharmacokinetic concepts or in industry (e.g., to calculate bioequivalency when designing generic drugs). For both human health professionals and veterinary medicine, clinical pharmacokinetics offers a wealth of performance guidelines regarding the safe and efficient use of medications.

Typically, models are expressed mathematical formulas with a corresponding graphical representation. By using these models, one can comprehend the properties of molecules and the behavior of specific drugs based on information about their basic properties, such as their distribution within the organism, acid dissociation constant (pKa), bioavailability, and solubility. To create models, a range of analysis methods, including curve stripping and nonlinear regression, may be applied.

1.2.3.1. Non-compartmental Analysis

PK parameters are directly estimated by noncompartmental methods using a table of concentration-time measurements. Noncompartmental methods are flexible because they don't rely on any particular model and typically yield reliable results that meet the requirements of bioequivalency studies. The most popular technique for estimating total drug exposure is the trapezoidal rule (numerical integration), which is based on area under the curve (AUC) methods. The area estimation depends heavily on the blood/plasma sampling schedule because of the trapezoidal rule's dependence on the length of x. In other words, the trapezoids more closely resemble the real concentration-time curve shape the closer the time points are. To successfully complete an NCA analysis, there should be sufficient time points available to cover the drug's absorption, distribution, and elimination phases. In addition to AUC exposure measurements, NCA techniques can also be used to report values for Cmax (maximum concentration), Tmax (time to maximum concentration), CL, and Vd.

1.2.3.2. Compartmental Analysis

Compartment model approaches use a system of differential equations to model the concentration-time graph and estimate it. These models are predicated on the idea that an organism consists of several related compartments. There are models with one and multiple compartments in use. Comparable to kinetic models found in other scientific fields like chemical kinetics and thermodynamics are PK compartmental models. Compartmental analysis has an advantage over noncompartmental analysis in that it allows for parameter modification and extrapolation to new scenarios. The challenge of creating and verifying the appropriate model is the drawback. While compartment models can accurately simulate the state of affairs within an organism, they will always include simplifying assumptions and be limited in their applicability. Regardless of how intricate and accurate a model is, despite the work required to determine different drug distribution values, it still does not accurately reflect reality. The reason for this is that distribution volume is a relative concept that does not accurately represent reality. Choosing a model thus boils down to determining which one gives the drug in question the smallest margin of error.

1. Single-compartment model

The one-compartmental PK model is the most basic PK compartmental model. This represents an organism as a single, uniform compartment. According to this monocompartmental model, the drug's concentration in blood plasma serves as the sole indicator of the drug's concentration in other bodily fluids and tissues. For instance, there may be known, constant factors that roughly relate the blood plasma concentration to the concentration in other areas.

In this one-compartment model, the most common model of elimination is first-order kinetics, where the elimination of the drug is directly proportional to the drug's concentration in the organism.

This is often called linear pharmacokinetics, as the change in concentration over time can be expressed as a linear differential equation $\frac{dC}{dt}=-k_{el}C$. Assuming a single IV bolus dose resulting in a concentration $C_{initial}$ time t=0, the equation can be solved to give:

2. Two-compartment model

The drug's distribution will be slower in some body tissues than in others with better blood supplies because different body tissues have different blood supplies. Furthermore, depending on the properties of the drug, certain tissues—like the brain tissue—present a true barrier to drug distribution, which can be overcome more easily or less easily. When the rate of elimination is taken into account along with these relative conditions for the various tissue types, the organism can be thought of as functioning like two compartments: a peripheral compartment consisting of organs with a lower blood flow and a central compartment, which we can refer to as having a more rapid distribution and containing systems and organs with a well-developed blood supply. Depending on a drug's capacity to penetrate the blood-brain barrier, other tissues, like the brain, may occupy a variable position. Depending on which compartment elimination takes place in, two-compartment models differ. The liver and kidneys are organs with an excellent blood supply, so the most frequent scenario is that elimination takes place in the central compartment. Elimination, however, might sometimes take place in the peripheral compartment or even in both. This could imply that the two-compartment model has three possible versions, which may not account for all scenarios.

3. Multi-compartment models

Every tissue will have unique distribution characteristics in the real world, and none of them will be strictly linear. When an active elimination mechanism exists that is independent of the drug's plasma concentration or when some of the enzymes responsible for metabolizing the drug become saturated, the two-compartment model might not work as intended. Labeling the drug's volume of distribution within the organism as Vd_F and its volume of distribution in a tissue as Vd_T will allow us to describe the former using an equation that accounts for all the tissues with varying actions, which is:.

$$Vd_F = Vd_{T1} + Vd_{T2} + Vd_{T3} + \cdots + Vd_{Tn}$$

This is a representation of the multi-compartment model, where an overall curve is obtained by expressing complex equations through multiple curves. For the purpose of plotting these equations, several computer programs have been created. Physiological data is used in the most sophisticated PK models (referred to as PBPK models) to facilitate development and validation.

The relationships between the factors can then be determined by computing the dimensions of various areas under the curve, which represents the graph for the non-linear relationship between the various factors as a curve. Michaelis-Menten kinetics serves as the foundation for many of the models used in non-linear pharmacokinetics. A reaction's factors of non-linearity include the following:

- **Multiphasic absorption:** There are two main ways that drugs injected intravenously are eliminated from the plasma: (1) distribution to bodily tissues, and (2) drug metabolism and excretion. The drug's plasma concentration subsequently drops in a biphasic manner.
  - o **Beta phase:** After the alpha phase, there is a progressive drop in plasma concentration known as the beta phase. Drug clearance, or metabolism

and excretion, is the main cause of the decline.

- o Additional phases (gamma, delta, etc.) are sometimes seen.
- A drug's characteristics make a clear distinction between tissues with high and low blood flow.
- **Enzymatic saturation:** The enzymes in charge of a drug's metabolism become saturated when the dosage of a drug whose removal depends on biotransformation is raised above a particular threshold. The drug will then no longer be eliminated continuously and its plasma concentration will rise disproportionately.
- **Induction or enzymatic inhibition:** Certain medications can either positively or negatively feedback-react by inhibiting or stimulating their own metabolism. As is the case with phenytoin, fluoxetine, and fluvoxamine. The elimination half-life and plasma concentrations of the unmetabolized drug both rise with higher dosages of these medications. Therefore, when a high dosage is required, the dose or other treatment parameters must be changed.

Certain medications can also be actively eliminated by the kidneys, regardless of plasma concentrations. Thus, it is clear that non-linearity can arise for a variety of causes affecting the absorption, distribution, metabolism, and elimination phases of the pharmacokinetic sequence.

1.2.4. Bioavailability

Practically speaking, the percentage of a medication that reaches its site of action is known as its bioavailability. According to this viewpoint, administering a medication intravenously offers the highest bioavailability and is thought to produce a bioavailability of 1 (or 100%). In a specific study, the bioavailability of alternative delivery methods is compared to either an intravenous injection standard value (absolute bioavailability) or to that of the other delivery methods (relative bioavailability) (Figure 1.6).

$$B_A = \frac{[ABC]_P \cdot D_{IV}}{[ABC]_{IV} \cdot D_P}$$

$$B_R = \frac{[ABC]_A \cdot dose_B}{[ABC]_B \cdot dose_A}$$

Once a drug's bioavailability has been determined, the dosage adjustments necessary to achieve the necessary blood plasma levels can be computed. Therefore, for each drug, bioavailability is a mathematical factor that affects the dose that is administered.

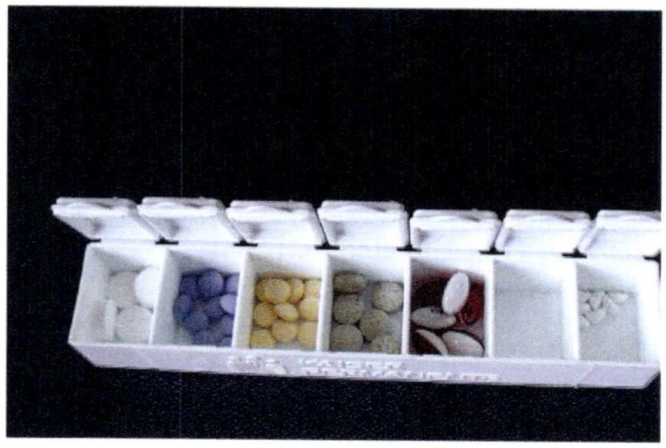

Figure 1.5. *Different forms of tablets, which will have different pharmacokinetic behaviors after their administration.*

Source: https://en.wikipedia.org/wiki/Pharmacokinetics.

It is possible to calculate the amount of a drug in the blood plasma that has a real potential to bring about its effect using the formula:

$$De = B \cdot Da$$

where; *De* is the effective dose, *B* bioavailability and *Da* is the administered dose.

Therefore, if a drug has a bioavailability of 0.8 (or 80%) and it is administered in a dose of 100 mg, the equation will demonstrate the following:

$De = 0.8 \times 100 \text{ mg} = 80 \text{ mg}$

That is the 100 mg administered represents a blood plasma concentration of 80 mg that has the capacity to have a pharmaceutical effect.

This concept depends on a series of factors inherent to each drug, such as:

- Pharmaceutical form
- Chemical form
- Route of administration
- Stability
- Metabolism

These concepts, which are discussed in detail in their respective titled articles, can be mathematically quantified and integrated to obtain an overall mathematical equation:

$$De = Q \cdot Da \cdot B$$

where; Q is the drug's purity.

$$Va = \frac{Da \cdot B \cdot Q}{\tau}$$

where; Va is the drug's rate of administration and τ is the rate at which the absorbed drug reaches the circulatory system.

Finally, using the Henderson-Hasselbalch equation, and knowing the drug's pKa (pH at which there is an equilibrium between its ionized and non-ionized molecules), it is possible to calculate the non-ionized concentration of the drug and therefore the concentration that will be subject to absorption:

$$pH = pKa + \log \frac{B}{A}$$

Biological equivalents, sometimes known as bioequivalents, are pharmaceuticals that have the same bioavailability. Because it is currently used as a yardstick in many countries for the authorization of generic drugs, the concept of bioequivalency is significant. (Rang, 2006; Krska & Cox, 2019)

1.2.5. Analysis

1.2.5.1. Bioanalytical Methods

A concentration-time profile cannot be created without the use of bioanalytical techniques. To determine the drug concentration in the biological matrix, most commonly plasma, chemical techniques are used. Appropriate bioanalytical techniques ought to be sensitive and selective. One technique that can be used to measure the impact of the biological matrix or liquid on a drug's affinity for its target is microscale thermophoresis.

1.2.5.2. Mass Spectrometry

Because of the complex nature of the matrix (typically plasma or urine) and the requirement for high sensitivity to monitor concentrations after a low dose and a long time period, pharmacokinetics is frequently studied using mass spectrometry. The most often utilized equipment in this application is a triple quadrupole mass spectrometer coupled with LC-MS. Typically, tandem mass spectrometry is used to increase specificity. Internal standards and standard curves are typically used to quantify a single pharmaceutical in the samples. The samples show various stages of the administration, metabolism, and excretion of a medication from the body. With such intricate sample matrices, blank samples obtained before administration are crucial for establishing background and guaranteeing data integrity. Although the linearity of the standard curve receives a lot of attention, most mass spectrometers do not respond linearly over wide concentration ranges, so curve fitting with more complicated functions like quadratics is frequently used. Currently, there is a lot of interest in the application of very high-sensitivity mass spectrometry as a potential substitute for animal testing

in microdosing studies. The utilization of Secondary electrospray ionization (SESI-MS) in drug monitoring has been demonstrated in recent research, offering the benefit of not requiring animal sacrifice.

1.3. Theoretical Pharmacokinetics

Pharmacokinetics—the mathematical expression of the time course of drug absorption, distribution, and elimination—has helped us better understand and plan medication regimens. Drug dosage schedule selection and modification are made easier by pharmacokinetic principles.

1.3.1. Half-Life

A drug's half-life ($t_{1/2}$) is the amount of time it takes for the drug's concentration in blood or plasma to drop to half of its initial value or for the drug's total body amount to decrease by 50%. The half-lives of distribution and elimination are its two phases.

For the majority of drugs, a half-life value can be easily ascertained by giving a subject a dose of the drug, drawing blood at different intervals, and then assaying the samples. For instance, if drug A's blood level is 8 points 6 mg/ml at 10 minutes and 4 points 3 mg/ml at 60 minutes, then its half-life is 50 minutes.

Most of the time, a drug's rate of elimination from the body is represented by how quickly its plasma concentration falls after a single intravenous dose; in most cases, this drug's plasma concentration falls exponentially. The biological half-life of medications whose elimination is exponential is unaffected by the dosage, mode of administration, or plasma concentration. It is dependent on VD in addition to the drug's metabolism and renal excretion.

1.3.2. Order of Kinetics

Although there are various ways to administer drugs, they are used to treat diseases. For instance, whereas paracetamol, For North American customers, also known as acetaminophen, requires administration three to four times daily, atenolol only needs to be given once. Subcutaneous insulin administration is more effective than intramuscular morphine administration. The absorption, distribution, metabolism, and excretion (ADME) of pharmaceuticals is the foundation upon which the mode of administration is designed. When it comes to their pharmacokinetic behavior in the body, drugs typically go through two processes. First-order and zero-order processes are these.

1. First-order

This is the most common process for many drugs. The rate at which absorption, distribution, metabolism and excretion occur are proportional to the concentration of drugs i.e. constant fraction of this drug in the body disappears in each equal interval of time.

2. Zero order kinetic

It is independent of the amount of drug present at the particular sites of drug absorption or elimination. Few drugs follow this process e.g. ethanol, phenytoin. Here constant amount of the drug is eliminated in each equal interval of time. Repeated administration of the drug after a certain stage, it accumulates in the body and leads to toxic reactions.

3. Steady state plasma concentration

A steady state is eventually reached when a drug dose is administered repeatedly over a predetermined amount of time. At this point, the amounts of drug absorbed and eliminated from the body are in balance.

For most drugs that follow first-order kinetics, steady state is reached after four to five half-lives. For instance, a medication with a six-hour half-life should reach a steady state after being administered for more than twenty-four hours. The accumulation pattern of a drug after it is repeatedly administered at intervals equal to its half-life of elimination.

Certain drugs have hard-to-measure effects, a narrow therapeutic window, and/or potential hazards from toxicity and ineffectiveness. Under these conditions, loading and maintenance doses must be administered to carefully adjust the doses to a desired steady-state concentration.

- **Loading dose:** To quickly reach the target concentration, the loading dose is one or more doses that may be administered at the beginning of therapy.
- **Maintenance dose:** To maintain the chosen steady-state or target concentration, the rate of drug administration is adjusted such that the rate of input equals to rate of loss (Rang, 2006; Krska & Cox, 2019).

1.4. Drug Safety (Pharmacovigilance) and Effectiveness

Pharmacovigilance, also known as drug safety, is the branch of pharmacy science that deals with the gathering, identification, evaluation, tracking, and avoidance of side effects from pharmaceuticals. Pharmacovigilance places a great deal of emphasis on adverse drug reactions (ADRs), which are defined as any unpleasant and unexpected reaction to a medication, including ineffectiveness (the most recent amendment to the relevant legislation excluded the condition that this definition applies only to doses typically used for prophylaxis, diagnosis, or therapy of disease, or for the modification of physiological disorder function). Even in the absence of an adverse event, medication errors such as overdosing, drug abuse and misuse, and drug exposure during pregnancy and lactation are of interest because they may result in an adverse drug reaction.

The data required for pharmacovigilance is largely provided by information obtained from patients and healthcare providers through pharmacovigilance agreements, as well as from other sources like the medical literature. Most countries require adverse event data received by the license holder, typically a pharmaceutical company, to be submitted to the local drug regulatory authority before allowing the marketing or testing of a pharmaceutical product.

Pharmacovigilance is ultimately focused on reducing the possibility of patient injury and identifying the risks connected to pharmaceutical products. To evaluate their compliance with international laws, regulations, and guidelines, companies need to perform a thorough audit focused on drug safety and pharmacovigilance.

1.4.1. Factors Modifying the Dosage and Action of Drugs

The degree and nature of the response that a drug may elicit vary from person to person, and as a result, there is variation in the ideal dosage of a drug that yields the intended therapeutic effect.

The important factors which influence the effect of a drug are:

1. **Drug Intolerance**: It is a quantitative deviation from the anticipated response to a given dose of a drug. Thus drug intolerance is the inability of the individual to tolerate a drug. It is also called hyper susceptibility.
2. **Sex Difference**: Special care should be exercised when drugs are administrated during menstruation, pregnancy and lactation.

a. ***Menstruation***: Drugs producing pelvic congestion should be avoided during menstruation e.g. drastic purgatives.

b. ***Pregnancy***: All medications during pregnancy should be used cautiously, except for those required to sustain pregnancy. Pregnancy should not be combined with the use of medications that may stimulate the uterine smooth muscle. Furthermore, a lot of medications given to the mother have the potential to affect the fetus by crossing the placenta. When taken during pregnancy, most medications have the potential to cause teratogenicity. Teratogenicity refers to birth defects.

i. Drugs known to produce teratogenicity e.g. thalidomide, cyclophosphamide, methotrexate, tetracyclines, phenytoin, carbamazepine and progestogens.

ii. drugs may be teratogenic e.g. Warfarin, lithium, quinine, primaquine, trimethoprim, rifampicin, and anesthetic agents.

c. ***Breastfeeding***: Almost every agent that a mother receives is likely to be present in her milk and may potentially be harmful to the child. The majority of lipid-soluble medications end up in breast milk. Therefore, nursing moms should refrain from giving their infants drugs that are excreted in milk and negatively impact their health e.g. sulphonamides, tetracyclines, nalidixic acid, isoniazid, diazepam, lithium, Indomethacin, aspirin, etc.

3. **Body Weight:** The average dose is expressed as the total single dose for an adult weighing between 50 and 100 kg, or as mg per kg of body weight. The dose stated in this way, however, might not apply to people who are extremely obese, edematous, or dehydrated. Nutritional factors can also change a drug's ability to be metabolized, so patients who are malnourished should be aware of this.

4. **Age:** The pharmacokinetics alter as people age. As a result, in newborns and neonates, the amount of body water is higher, the gastric pH fluctuates, and the gastric emptying process is prolonged. Additionally, the liver's ability to metabolize drugs is reduced. Children therefore might not respond to all drugs in the same way that young adults do. With a few notable exceptions, newborns are more sensitive to the effects of drugs than adults are.

The dosages for children are stated as mg/kg per dose or day for body weight, or mg/m2 per day for body surface area. The child's weight and height can be used to compute the body surface area.

Similar to children, elderly individuals may experience difficulties with dosage adjustments, and these differences can be substantial. As people age, their kidney function deteriorates and their ability to metabolize drugs may also decrease. Drugs like hypnotics, tranquilizers, phenylbutazone, diazepam, pethidine, etc. can cause sensitivity in the elderly.

5. **Disease state:** Some antimicrobial agents penetrate the cerebrospinal fluid well across the normal meninges while other antimicrobials penetrate well only when the meninges are inflamed (meningitis) e.g. sulphonamides, metronidazole, chloramphenicol, isoniazid and rifampicin penetrate well through the normal meninges and other antimicrobial agents like benzyl penicillin, ampicillin, tetracycline, streptomycin, gentamicin and cephalosporin penetrate only when the meninges are inflamed.

Drug biotransformation is significantly altered by acute or chronic liver diseases, both in terms of rate and volume. Patients with liver cirrhosis have significantly higher $t^{1/2}$ values for diazepam and chlordiazepoxide, which results in a corresponding prolongation of their effects.

Cardiac disease by limiting blood flow to the liver may impair the disposition of those drugs whose biotransformation is flow-limited e.g. imipramine, isoniazid, lignocaine, morphine and propranolol.

Analogously, illnesses of the kidneys and lungs can alter how medications like insulin or isoprenaline are bio transformed. Drug excretion is compromised by chronic renal disease.

6. **Pharmacogenetics**: The science of pharmacogenetics is concerned with the genetically-mediated variations in drug responses.
7. **Drug interactions**: It is usual for patients to receive many drugs at the same time. It is a phenomenon that occurs when the effects of one drug are modified by the prior or concurrent administration of another drug(s).

1.4.2. Risk Management

The risk management discipline is in charge of tracking the risk-benefit profile of medications and identifying signals. The creation of risk management plans (RMPs) and aggregate reports, such as the Development Safety Update Report (DSUR), Periodic Benefit-Risk Evaluation Report (PBRER), and Periodic Safety Update Report (PSUR), are additional crucial tasks in the field of risk management.

1.4.2.1. Causality Assessment

The determination of causality is a crucial and intricate issue in the field of pharmacovigilance. The relationship between a particular adverse event and a particular drug is known as causality. Causality determination (or assessment) is often difficult because of the lack of clear-cut or reliable data. While one may assume that a positive temporal relationship might "prove" a positive causal relationship, this is not always the case. Indeed, a "bee sting" Adverse Event — where the AE can clearly be attributed to a specific cause — is by far the exception rather than the rule. This is due to the complexity of human physiology as well as that of disease and illnesses. By this reckoning, to determine causality between an adverse event and a drug, one must first exclude the possibility that there were other possible causes or contributing factors.

If the patient is taking multiple medications, it's possible that the AE is caused by the combination of these medications rather than any one of them alone. There have been several high-profile recent cases where an individual's death was caused by an adverse event. The patients' numerous prescriptions were not overdosed on by any one of them; rather, the combination of them seemed to be what caused the adverse event. Therefore, it is crucial to include in your/one's adverse event report not just the medication that is being reported, but also all other medications the patient was taking.

For example, one might be tempted to blame Drug X if a patient started taking it and three days later experienced an adverse event. To search for potential risk factors for the adverse event, the patient's medical history must be examined first. Is the adverse event (AE) related to the medication or did it happen as a result of the medication? This is because patients taking any kind of medication may get sick or be diagnosed with a condition that has nothing to do with the medication. This is particularly true for illnesses like cancer, which take time to manifest and are diagnosed in patients who have taken medication for a comparatively short time. On the other hand, some medications can cause short-term exposure to certain adverse events, like blood clots (thrombosis). However, identifying risk factors is a crucial first step in establishing or disproving a causal connection between a medication and an occurrence.

Often, an observational study comparing the incidence of an event in a patient population taking the drug to a control group is the only way to verify the existence of a causal relationship between an event and a drug. This may be necessary to determine if the background incidence of an event is less than that found in a group taking a drug. If the incidence of an event is statistically significantly higher in the "active" group versus the placebo group (or other control group), it is possible that a causal relationship may exist to a drug, unless other confounding factors may exist.

1.4.2.2. Signal Detection

Signal detection involves a range of techniques (CIOMS). The WHO defines a safety signal as: "Reported information on a possible causal relationship between an adverse event and a drug, the relationship being unknown or incompletely documented previously." Usually more than a single report is required to generate a signal, depending upon the event and quality of the information available.

With the proliferation of large data sources and low-cost computing resources, one method that has gained popularity is data mining pharmacovigilance databases. A pharmaceutical company, a drug regulatory body, or a sizable healthcare provider may own the data sources (databases). These databases contain individual case safety reports that are retrieved, formatted, and statistically analyzed (often using a mathematical algorithm) to determine statistical measures of association. An arbitrary threshold is crossed by the statistical measure to declare a signal for a particular drug linked to a specific adverse event. Any signal that is judged worthy of examination needs to be further examined using all of the information at hand in an effort to validate or disprove the signal. Further information, such as a post-marketing observational trial, might be required if the analysis is unsatisfactory.

A crucial component of drug use and safety surveillance is signal detection. Identifying adverse drug reactions that were previously thought to be unexpected and being able to advise in product labeling regarding how to reduce the risk of using the drug in a particular patient population are the ideal goals of signal detection.

1.4.2.3. Risk Management Plans

A risk management plan is a written plan that outlines the risks (possible and actual adverse drug reactions) related to using a medication and how they are being managed. For example, warnings about possible side effects on drug labels or packet inserts should prompt patients to consult their doctor, pharmacist, the manufacturer of the medication, the FDA, or the European Medicines Agency if they are noticed. The overall goal of a risk management plan is to assure a positive risk-benefit profile once the drug is (has been) marketed. The document is required to be submitted, in a specified format, with all new market authorization requests within the European Union (EU). Although not necessarily required, risk management plans may also be submitted in countries outside the EU. One of three categories applies to the risks mentioned in a risk management plan: identified risks, potential risks, and unknown risks. The steps that the Market Authorization Holder, typically a pharmaceutical company, will take to reduce the risks connected with the use of the drug are also covered in a risk management plan. These measures are usually focused on the product's labeling and healthcare professionals. Indeed, the risks that are documented in a pre-authorization risk management plan will inevitably become part of the product's post-marketing labeling. Since a drug, once authorized, may be used in ways not originally studied in clinical trials, this potential "off-label use," and its associated risks, is also described within the risk management plan. Risk management plans can be very lengthy documents, running in some cases hundreds of pages and, in rare instances, up to a thousand pages long.

When a drug has a particular risk that the FDA feels has to be mitigated, it may, in certain cases, require a company to submit a document known as a Risk Evaluation and Mitigation Strategy (REMS). A Risk Evaluation and Mitigation Strategy, while not as comprehensive as a risk management plan, may still require a sponsor to carry out specific tasks or adhere to a set of guidelines known as Elements to Assure Safe Use to ensure that a favorable risk-benefit profile for the medication is maintained for the specific conditions under which the product is marketed.

1.4.2.4. Risk/benefit Profile of Drugs

Most nations have laws requiring pharmaceutical companies to conduct clinical trials, which test new medications on humans before they are released to the general public. This happens following a medication's initial toxicity screening, which occasionally involves testing on animals. Typically, a control group and a representative sample of patients (up to a few thousand) are chosen by the drug's manufacturers or their representatives. The control group may receive a placebo and/or another drug, often a so-called "gold standard" that is the "best" drug marketed for the disease.

The purpose of clinical trials is to determine:

- if a drug works and how well it works
- if it has any harmful effects, and
- if it does more good than harm, and how much more? If it has a potential for harm, how probable and how serious is the harm?

Overall, clinical trials provide valuable insights into a medication's effectiveness. Although target clinical populations are usually very different from trial populations in terms of such characteristics, they provide information that should be reliable for larger populations with the same characteristics as the trial group – age, gender, state of health, ethnic origin, and so on.

The variables in a clinical trial are carefully defined and monitored, however, a clinical trial can never provide a complete understanding of the effects of a drug in every possible scenario. In fact, nothing could tell you the whole story, but a clinical trial must tell you enough; "enough" being determined by legislation and by contemporary judgements about the acceptable balance of benefit and harm. In the end, a medication that is marketed may be used to patients who were not included in clinical trials, such as young children, the elderly, expectant mothers, patients with co-morbidities not present in the trial population, etc. Maintaining a positive risk/benefit profile in all known populations using the drug may require a different set of warnings, precautions, or contraindications (where the drug should not be used at all) for the product's labeling.

1.5. Development and Evaluation of New Drugs

Finding a therapeutic agent appropriate for clinical evaluation in humans is the ultimate goal of pharmacological research conducted on animals. Without a doubt, research on animals offers comparisons and valuable models. Even the most meticulous and thorough animal testing cannot completely eliminate the element of risk involved in administering biologically active agents to humans.

Researchers worldwide are constantly working to create novel medications, despite the fact that this process is highly complex and costly. Pharmacologists are among those who contribute to the creation of new drugs, and they are particularly interested in assessing "new chemical entities" (NCE). Before new medications can be released onto the market, thousands of NCEs must typically be synthesized and evaluated. Over the past few decades, there has been a significant increase in government regulations governing the research and development of new drugs.

Drug development comprises two steps.

- Preclinical development and
- Clinical development

1.5.1. Preclinical Development

Synthesis of new chemical entities is done as per the research policy decision which is based on:

- Random synthesis
- Structure activity relationship (SAR)
- Biochemical and pharmacological insight and
- Chance finding.

Examining a drug's safety and efficacy before patient administration is the goal of the preclinical development stage of a possible new medication. Different drug dosages are tested on animals and/or *in vitro* systems during this preclinical stage.

If active compounds are identified, animal studies must be conducted to assess pharmacodynamics, pharmacokinetics, toxicology, and specific toxicological studies such as mutagenicity and carcinogenicity. Single doses are used for acute toxicity assessments, while repeated doses are used for sub chronic and chronic toxicity studies. Preclinical testing must be conducted in compliance with established standards.

1.5.2. Clinical Development

About one in 1000 NCEs reach this stage. The steps to be studied in this stage include:

a. **Pharmaceutical study** covers the stability of formulation and compatibility of the NCEs with other tablet or infusion ingredients.

b. **Pharmacological study** includes further chronic toxicological study in animals, initially animal metabolic and pharmacokinetic study. When studies in animals predict that an NCE may be useful medicine i.e. effective and safe in relation to its benefits, then the time has come to put it to the test in man i.e. clinical trial.

c. **Studies on humans or clinical trial:** A clinical trial is a means by which the efficacy of a drug is tested on human beings. It may also give some idea about the risk involved. It is divided into 4 phases. With each phase, the safety and efficacy of the compound are tested progressively.

Phase – I: This is the first exposure of the new drug on man which is usually conducted in healthy volunteers and which is designed to test the tolerable dose, and duration of action. This phase is usually carried out in only one center on 20 to 50 subjects.

Phase – II: This phase comprises small-scale trials on patients used to determine dose levels and establish that the treatment offers some benefit. It usually involves 100–500 patients and is usually conducted in several centers.

Phase – III: Full-scale evaluation of treatment comparing it with standard treatment is done in this phase. It involves randomized control trials on 250 to 2000 patients and is done in multiple centers. Information from all studies is received by the "Committee of Safety of Medicines" (CSM). If the drug is satisfied by the CSM, the product license is issued then the drug is marketed.

Phase – IV: It is also called phase of post-marketing surveillance. Reports about efficacy and toxicity are received from the medical practitioners and reviewed by the committee of review of medicines. Renewal or cancellation of the product license depends on the comment of the review committee (Shankar et al, 2006; World Health Organization).

A Closer Look

Tackling Pharmacovigilance Issues in the Clinical Trial Stage of Product Development

To satisfy their needs for safety, medical information, and compliance with regulations, manufacturers of pharmaceuticals and devices frequently contract out their pharmacovigilance (PV) operations to suppliers and consultants. These businesses are required by law to monitor the conduct and caliber of their vendors while doing so. However, due to variations in auditors, scope, and comprehension of PV principles and operations, vendor audits carried out by these companies can produce a wide range of results. The same holds true for regulatory agencies inspecting different companies. PV professionals and company leadership are deeply engaged in a heated debate about important goals such as finding ways to achieve quality compliance and consistency in PV, as well as streamlining the process of signal detection and risk management by shifting the focus to premarket product development and the clinical trial stage.

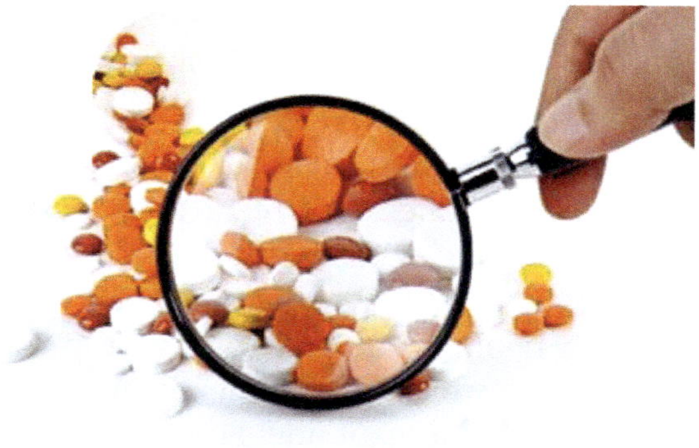

Ø ***Tackling Inconsistencies***

- **The Issue:** A large portion of PV's efforts are directed toward finding, gathering, assessing, and turning pertinent safety data into information that businesses and regulators can use. Pharmaceutical companies often outsource a large portion of their PV activities to consultants, contractors, and vendors who specialize in these activities to maintain growth and keep up with the growing volumes of data and overall workload. However, after a business activity is contracted out, the vendor needs to undergo regular audits for quality control and oversight. Many companies use the PV services provided by vendors, particularly the large pharmaceutical support services that can host large safety databases. Contrary to popular belief, however, company audits of the same vendor don't always produce the same results. Similarly, a company may receive different results for the same PV system from each regulatory body that conducts audits and inspections (e.g., the FDA, Health Canada, MHRA, Swiss Medic, and ANSM).

These discrepancies can be caused by a variety of factors, but they are frequently attributable to the auditors and inspectors themselves, who may have differing professional backgrounds and levels of experience with PV and the related requirements. An auditor with primary experience in manufacturing or quality assurance (QA) might, for instance, undertake a PV audit. Because of this, the resulting audit did not specifically look into the safety system or the metrics and procedure for case processing, even though it could have focused heavily on the CAPA (corrective and preventive action) and deviation process.

- **Possible resolution:** Although reconciling these disparities is difficult, it presents as yet unexplored chances for increased cooperation and coordination between the regulatory agencies and business sectors. For example, creating quality standards or checklists that businesses can follow may be the most crucial requirement in terms of PV operations and quality compliance. Moreover, a PV quality group, or entity, made up of people nominated or elected by a group of businesses, could guarantee a more efficient and uniform auditing procedure. Other businesses or regulatory bodies may choose not to audit the same vendor or company in the same year if the results of the group's vendor and company audits are made publicly available. Establishing a PV quality group or consortium would not only result in more consistent results but also in lower overhead both internally and externally. For instance, if such a procedure or program were in place, businesses might be able to lessen the financial strain of routinely auditing popular vendors, which would ultimately lower the overall costs of a PV audit program. Additionally, it might lessen the expense and strain on our vendors to conduct, maintain, and correct numerous audits, CAPAs, and deviations for various clients.
- **Challenges:** For example, representatives of pharmaceutical companies frequently collaborate to establish best practices. As a result, they currently have a platform in place that might, in theory, also handle quality standards. However, these kinds of consortia might not be interested in establishing data standards. Furthermore, all work done by a working group toward a common objective is usually voluntary and unpaid, and any member may choose to end the working relationship at any time. Experience is yet another barrier, and perhaps the most significant one. Finding experts with a broad background in photovoltaics (PV) is crucial but challenging, as very few possess both genuine operational experience and the necessary knowledge and experience throughout the PV development life cycle. The ideal candidates for these positions would have a wide range of experience in the clinical, data management, statistical, medical, and regulatory domains throughout the product life cycle. Finding this breadth is very difficult since many organizations lock their staff members into a specific path without exposing them to experience in other functional areas.

Furthermore, the primary obstacle would be persuading businesses to adopt this model and be more open with the community regarding their inefficiencies and deviations. While some might worry about trade secrets or proprietary information, others might think that increased transparency could hurt the market. On the other hand, there is hope that this stigma and perception of hoarding audit and inspection results and quality events will disappear because the components of a PV system should be relatively harmonized.

Ø ***Tackling Inefficiencies***

- **The issue:** PV activity inefficiencies are slowing down pre- and post-market product development and creating operational and financial burdens, which will eventually be passed on to patients. Some significant "missing links" in the corporate structures of some pharmaceutical companies and a top-level lack of knowledge about the various PV requirements are among the main causes of these inefficiencies. For instance, senior management frequently lacks awareness of the financial commitment required to keep PV staff competent and capable of handling increasing workloads, as well as the legal requirements for managing a product. The PV department frequently becomes involved too late in the drug development process—for example, after the submission of an NDA—due to a lack of planning and communication between departments. But once they're in the market, businesses are usually inundated with cases, and to keep up with the workload, they eventually find themselves in dire need of consultants and contractors. However, addressing PV at this point is very expensive and inefficient.
- **Potential solution:** Companies should prioritize premarket development and involve the PV department in clinical trials to plan ahead for potential signals, audits, and inspections. This is a crucial first step in addressing these inefficiencies. Companies that prepare their PV systems in advance will be better positioned to enter the market safely and compliantly with regulations, as well as gather better and more consistent data before market release. It's also crucial to include PV leadership in talks about business development. For instance, businesses should ensure that they have enough personnel in place, such as QPPVs (qualified persons responsible for pharmacovigilance) and local PV support, before extending access into the European Economic Area (EEA). This will help them get ready for any system modifications that may occur. Global PV needs are different and can occasionally necessitate a large staffing level to maintain, even for a single product.
- **Challenges:**

  Planning ahead and making upfront investments in personnel and high-quality PV systems may present serious financial and budgetary challenges. Bringing in the right team at the right time is a balanced approach that is necessary for early planning. Finding the possible cost savings and return on investment (ROI) of doing so, however, is frequently challenging. Not only do businesses usually not realize the overhead and administrative load that comes with managing the results of audits and inspections when multiple findings are made, but it's also challenging to assign a specific "cost" to those activities. Determining the most effective strategy for bringing in the right team at the right time may also result in a brief period of extremely low work. In this case, team building and training are crucial initiatives that could close those gaps.

Not having a proper understanding of the roles and responsibilities of each department and an organizational structure that is clearly defined presents another challenge. For example, quality and regulatory departments frequently push back and don't participate in important discussions because they might not understand why PV needs to be involved.

Summary

- Pharmacology is the science of medical drugs and medications, including a substance's origin, composition, pharmacokinetics, therapeutic use, and toxicology.
- Pharmacodynamics studies the effects of a drug on biological systems, and pharmacokinetics studies the effects of biological systems on a drug.
- Pharmacodynamics (PD) is the study of the biochemical and physiologic effects of drugs (especially pharmaceutical drugs). The effects can include those manifested within animals (including humans), microorganisms, or combinations of organisms (for example, infection)
- Receptors are large proteins that play an important role in the field of pharmacodynamics. Receptors can amplify physiological signals and, as a result, they are potential targets for drugs.
- Signal transduction is a much broader concept, referring to sending a signal through a cell membrane where the receptor may not be an embedded cell membrane receptor, but rather an intracellular receptor.
- Adhesion molecules such as integrins, cadherins, and selectins and immunoglobulin-like cell adhesion molecules (Ig-CAM) are involved in a variety of signaling pathways.
- Pharmacokinetics is a branch of pharmacology dedicated to describing how the body affects a specific substance after administration. The substances of interest include any chemical xenobiotics such as pharmaceutical drugs, pesticides, food additives, cosmetics, etc.
- ADME is the four-letter abbreviation (acronym) for absorption, distribution, metabolism, and excretion, and is mainly used in fields such as pharmacokinetics and pharmacology.
- Drug safety or pharmacovigilance is the pharmaceutical science relating to the "collection, detection, assessment, monitoring, and prevention" of adverse effects with pharmaceutical products.
- Risk management is the discipline within pharmacovigilance that is responsible for signal detection and the monitoring of the risk-benefit profile of drugs.

References

1. Alcorn, J., & McNamara, P. J. (2003). Pharmacokinetics in the newborn. *Advanced Drug Delivery Reviews, 55*(5), 667–686. https://doi.org/10.1016/S0169-409X(03)00059-3.
2. Bari, N. (1995). Salicylate poisoning. *Journal of the Pakistan Medical Association, 45*(6), 160–161.
3. Cahill, C. M., Walwyn, W., Taylor, A. M. W., Pradhan, A. A., & Evans, C. J. (2016). Allostatic mechanisms of opioid tolerance beyond desensitization and downregulation. *Trends in Pharmacological Sciences, 37*(11), 963–976. https://doi.org/10.1016/j.tips.2016.08.007.
4. Cirillo, P., Taglialatela, V., Pellegrino, G., Morello, A., Conte, S., Di Serafino, L., & Cimmino, G. (2020). Effects of colchicine on platelet aggregation in patients on dual antiplatelet therapy with aspirin and clopidogrel. *Journal of Thrombosis and Thrombolysis, 50*(2), 468–472. https://doi.org/10.1007/s11239-020-02205-2.

5. Dumas, E. O., & Pollack, G. M. (2008). Opioid tolerance development: A pharmacokinetic/pharmacodynamic perspective. *AAPS Journal, 10*(4), 537–551. https://doi.org/10.1208/s12248-008-9054-1.

6. Goutelle, S., Maurin, M., Rougier, F., Barbaut, X., Bourguignon, L., Ducher, M., & Maire, P. (2008). The Hill equation: A review of its capabilities in pharmacological modelling. *Fundamental & Clinical Pharmacology, 22*(6), 633–648. https://doi.org/10.1111/j.1472-8206.2008.00605.x.

7. Gray, K., Adhikary, S. D., & Janicki, P. (2018). Pharmacogenomics of analgesics in anesthesia practice: A current update of literature. *Journal of Anesthesiology Clinical Pharmacology, 34*(2), 155–160. https://doi.org/10.4103/joacp.JOACP_124_17.

8. Jonsson, M., Dabrowski, M., Gurley, D. A., Larsson, O., Johnson, E. C., Fredholm, B. B., & Eriksson, L. I. (2006). Activation and inhibition of human muscular and neuronal nicotinic acetylcholine receptors by succinylcholine. *Anesthesiology, 104*(4), 724–733. https://doi.org/10.1097/00000542-200604000-00019.

9. Keller, F., & Hann, A. (2018). Clinical pharmacodynamics: Principles of drug response and alterations in kidney disease. *Clinical Journal of the American Society of Nephrology, 13*(9), 1413–1420. https://doi.org/10.2215/CJN.01850218.

10. Krska, J., & Cox, A. R. (2019). Adverse drug reactions. In C. Whittlesea & K. Hodson (Eds.), *Clinical Pharmacy and Therapeutics* (6th ed., pp. 66–80). Elsevier.

11. Lees, P., Cunningham, F. M., & Elliott, J. (2004). Principles of pharmacodynamics and their applications in veterinary pharmacology. *Journal of Veterinary Pharmacology and Therapeutics, 27*(6), 397–414. https://doi.org/10.1111/j.1365-2885.2004.00622.x.

12. Mangoni, A. A., & Jackson, S. H. (2004). Age-related changes in pharmacokinetics and pharmacodynamics: Basic principles and practical applications. *British Journal of Clinical Pharmacology, 57*(1), 6–14. https://doi.org/10.1046/j.1365-2125.2003.01977.x.

13. Mei, H., Wang, J., Che, H., Wang, R., & Cai, Y. (2019). The clinical efficacy and safety of vancomycin loading dose: A systematic review and meta-analysis. *Medicine, 98*(43), e17639. https://doi.org/10.1097/MD.0000000000017639.

14. Meng, J., Xiao, G., Zhang, J., He, X., Ou, M., Bi, J., Yang, R., Di, W., Wang, Z., Li, Z., Gao, H., Liu, L., & Zhang, G. (2020). Renin-angiotensin system inhibitors improve the clinical outcomes of COVID-19 patients with hypertension. *Emerging Microbes & Infections, 9*(1), 757–760. https://doi.org/10.1080/22221751.2020.1831304.

15. Nancarrow, C., & Mather, L. E. (1983). Pharmacokinetics in renal failure. *Anesthesia and Intensive Care, 11*(4), 350–360. https://doi.org/10.1177/0310057X8301100406.

16. Pillans, P. I. (2008). Clinical perspectives in drug safety and adverse drug reactions. *Expert Review of Clinical Pharmacology, 1*, 695–705. https://doi.org/10.1586/17512433.1.5.695.

17. Preuss, C. V., & Quick, J. (2023). Ixekizumab. In *StatPearls* [Internet]. StatPearls Publishing. Retrieved from: https://www.statpearls.com (accessed on 30 July 2024).

18. Ramamoorthy, S., & Cidlowski, J. A. (2016). Corticosteroids: Mechanisms of action in health and disease. *Rheumatic Diseases Clinics of North America, 42*(1), 15–31, vii. https://doi.org/10.1016/j.rdc.2015.09.007.

19. Rang, H. P. (2006). The receptor concept: Pharmacology's big idea. *British Journal of Pharmacology, 147*(Suppl 1), S9–S16. https://doi.org/10.1038/sj.bjp.0706400.

20. Shankar, P. R., Subish, P., Mishra, P., & Dubey, A. K. (2006). Teaching pharmacovigilance to medical students and doctors. *Indian Journal of Pharmacology, 38*, 316–319. https://doi.org/10.4103/0253-7613.29080.

21. Sharma, A., & Jusko, W. J. (1998). Characteristics of indirect pharmacodynamic models and applications to clinical drug responses. *British Journal of Clinical Pharmacology, 45*(3), 229–239. https://doi.org/10.1046/j.1365-2125.1998.00713.x.

22. Slørdal, L., & Spigset, O. (2005). Basic pharmacokinetics–absorption. *Tidsskrift for den Norske Laegeforening, 125*(7), 886–887. https://doi.org/10.4045/tidsskr.05.0165.

23. Slørdal, L., & Spigset, O. (2005). Basic pharmacokinetics–distribution. *Tidsskrift for den Norske Laegeforening, 125*(8), 1007–1008. https://doi.org/10.4045/tidsskr.05.0183.

24. Starkey, E. S., & Sammons, H. M. (2015). Practical pharmacokinetics: What do you really need to know? *Archives of Disease in Childhood Education and Practice Edition, 100*(1), 37–43. https://doi.org/10.1136/archdischild-2014-307973.

25. Trescot, A. M., Datta, S., Lee, M., & Hansen, H. (2008). Opioid pharmacology. *Pain Physician, 11*(2 Suppl), S133–S153.

26. Trontell, A. (2004). Expecting the unexpected—Drug safety, pharmacovigilance, and the prepared mind. *New England Journal of Medicine, 351*, 1385–1387. https://doi.org/10.1056/NEJMp048187.

27. Westervelt, P., Cho, K., Bright, D. R., & Kisor, D. F. (2014). Drug-gene interactions: Inherent variability in drug maintenance dose requirements. *P&T, 39*(9), 630–637.

28. Zhivkova, Z. D., Mandova, T., & Doytchinova, I. (2015). Quantitative structure-pharmacokinetics relationships analysis of basic drugs: Volume of distribution. *Journal of Pharmaceutical Sciences, 18*(3), 515–527. https://doi.org/10.18433/J3P34T

Chapter

2

DRUGS ACTING ON THE AUTONOMIC NERVOUS SYSTEM

Contents

Introduction

Every major bodily function is under the control of the nervous system. The nerve systems are separated into the central and peripheral regions. The somatic and autonomic nervous systems, which regulate voluntary and involuntary functions, respectively, are components of the peripheral nervous system. The body's vegetative processes are managed by the ANS. These include processes like breathing, digestion, circulation, and body temperature regulation.

Based on both anatomical and physiological principles, the ANS is classified into two major sub-divisions: parasympathetic (craniosacral) and sympathetic (thoracolumbar). The preganglionic and postganglionic neuron systems, which are named after their anatomical positions in relation to the ganglia, are what make up the autonomic nerves. The brain or spinal cord contains the cell body of a preganglionic neuron. The preganglionic fibers of the parasympathetic nervous system originate from the cranial and sacral nerves, while the sympathetic nervous system is derived from the thoracic and lumbar regions of the spinal cord. The effector organs, also known as the peripheral involuntary visceral organs, receive direct axon transmission from postganglionic neurons. Regardless of whether it is a part of the sympathetic or parasympathetic nervous systems, autonomic innervation is made up of a myelinated preganglionic fiber that synapses with the cell body of a second, non-myelinated neuron known as the post-ganglionic fiber. A synapse is characterized as a structure created when two neurons align closely, either with effector cells or with other neurons. The preservation and restoration of function are the parasympathetic nervous system's main goals in terms of function.

The sympathetic nervous system, on the other hand, is focused on energy expenditure, it functions nearly in opposition to parasympathetic nerve stimulation and is typically connected to arousal or emergency scenarios, for instance. gets the body ready for fight-or-flight reactions. It is crucial to comprehend the autonomic nervous system's operation and to pinpoint the underlying mechanisms to comprehend the pharmacology of the system.

The autonomic nervous system contains two key neurotransmitters. Acetylcholine and noradrenaline, also known as norepinephrine, are these.

Acetylcholine is a neurotransmitter that is released after stimulation of the parasympathetic nervous system to act on effector organs (cells) to elicit their response, but it also acts as a neurotransmitter:

- At the ganglia of both sympathetic and parasympathetic nervous system;
- At postganlionic sympathetic nerve endings to blood vessels of skeletal muscles and sweat glands(eccrine);
- At the neuromuscular junction of skeletal muscles (somatic motor fibers to skeletal muscle);
- Between some neurons in the CNS; and
- At preganglionic nerve endings to the adrenal medulla

An impulse must cross a synapse for neurotransmission to take place.

The enzyme choline acetyltransferase catalyzes the conversion of choline and acetyl coenzyme A into acetylcholine inside the cytoplasm of nerve fibers. Acetylcholine is released into the synaptic cleft upon the transit of synthesized acetylcholine from the cytoplasm into vesicles for storage upon the arrival of an action potential at the terminal and subsequent stimulation of the latter. Following its release from the presynaptic terminal, the molecule attaches to an effector cell's acetylcholine receptor (also known as a cholinergic receptor) and activates it. Ultimately, the transmitter's action is stopped when the acetyl cholinesterase enzyme hydrolyzes it into choline and acetate.

Muscarinic and nicotinic cholinergic receptors are the two types of cholinergic receptors.

Most autonomic effector cells in peripheral visceral organs normally have muscarinic responses, while skeletal muscle and the parasympathetic and sympathetic ganglia respond with nicotinic responses.

Acetylcholine or other parasympathomimetic can be applied to the effector cells to produce the effect of parasympathetic nervous system activity in an organ, or the parasympathetic nerve fibers supplying the organ can be stimulated. We refer to this as cholinergic activity.

The neurotransmitter that postganglionic sympathetic nerves release to affect effector cells is noradrenaline. Adrenergic or noradrenergic sympathetic fibers are found in the post-ganglionic region. The application of noradrenaline, adrenaline, or other sympathomimetics, i.e., sympathetic nerve stimulation, can be used to demonstrate sympathetic nerve activity. e. the release of acetylcholine as a neurotransmitter from sweat glands and blood vessels to skeletal muscles, which is not considered "adrenergic activity."

Table 2.1. *Distribution of Adrenoceptor Subtypes and Their Actions*

Type	Tissue	Actions
$Alpha_1$	Most vascular smooth muscles	Contraction
	Pupillary dilator muscle	Mydriasis
	Heart	Increase force of contraction
$Alpha_2$	Adrenergic nerve terminals	Inhibition of transmitter release
	Platelets	Aggregation
$Beta_1$	Heart	Increased rate and force of contraction
$Beta_2$	Respiratory, uterine, and vascular smooth muscle	Relaxation
	Human liver	Glycogenolysis
$Beta_3$	Fat cells	Lipolysis

Source: https://www.cartercenter.org/resources/pdfs/health/ephti/library/lecture_notes/health_science_students/pharmacology.pdf.

Noradrenaline is produced by adrenalinergic neuron terminals, which then encapsulate and release it into effector cells in response to nerve stimulation. There are multiple processes involved in the synthesis of the transmitter from the precursor amino acid, tyrosine, which may serve as sites of drug action. Noradrenaline exerts its effects upon binding to receptor sites. Many processes, including reuptake into the nerve terminal (reuptake1), diffusion out of the synaptic cleft and subsequent reuptake into the perisynaptic glia or smooth muscle (reuptake2), or enzyme degradation, cause the termination of noradrenergic transmission. The primary mechanism by which noradrenaline's effects are terminated is reuptake into the nerve terminal.

Adrenergic receptors are receptors that react to the adrenergic nerve transmitter. Based on both agonist and antagonist selectivity, these receptors are separated into alpha and beta-adrenoreceptor types. Subclasses of the receptors exist based on drug selectivity. These are beta 1, 2, and 3, as well as alpha 1 and 2. (Gerretsen & Pollock, 2011; Ehret & Chamberlin, 2015; Wiercinski & Jackson, 2022) (Table 2.1).

Five essential aspects of neurotransmitter function serve as possible targets for pharmaceutical treatment. These include the processes of synthesis, storage, release, receptor activation, and transmitter action termination (Figure 2.1).

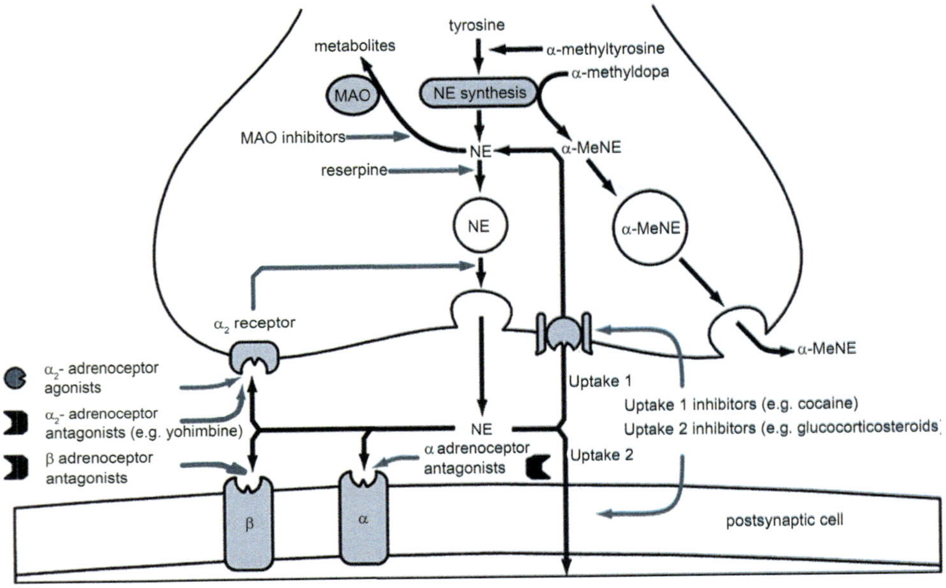

Figure 2.1. *Drug actions on the sympathetic nervous system.*

Source: https://www.researchgate.net/profile/Boris-Zanolari/publication/33681407/figure/fig9/AS:669507110567960@1536634342901/4-Drug-actions-on-the-sympathetic-nervous-system-Drugs-may-affect-synthesis-storage.png.

Orientation and Directional Terms

Term	Definition	Illustration
Choline acetyltransferase	Choline acetyltransferase is a transferase enzyme responsible for the synthesis of the neurotransmitter acetylcholine. ChAT catalyzes the transfer of an acetyl group from the coenzyme acetyl-CoA to choline, yielding acetylcholine.	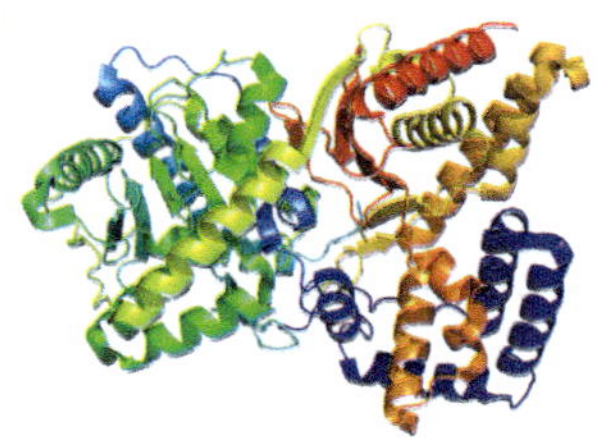
Muscarinic agonists	Muscarinic agonists are drugs that activate the body's muscarinic acetylcholine receptors, which are part of the parasympathetic nervous system. These receptors have different subtypes, labeled M1–M5, and the mechanism of action of a muscarinic agonist depends on which receptor is activated. The M1, M2, and M3 receptors are the most clinically significant.	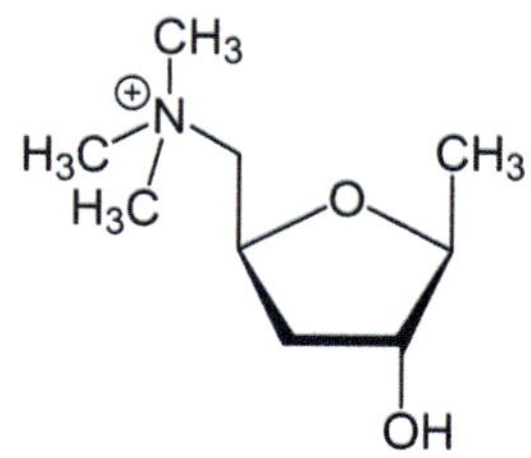
Parasympathetic nervous system (PNS)	The parasympathetic nervous system (PNS) is a part of the autonomic nervous system (ANS) that helps the body relax and conserve energy during quiet periods. It's also known as the "rest and digest" system, and its opposite is the sympathetic nervous system (SNS), which controls the "fight or flight" response	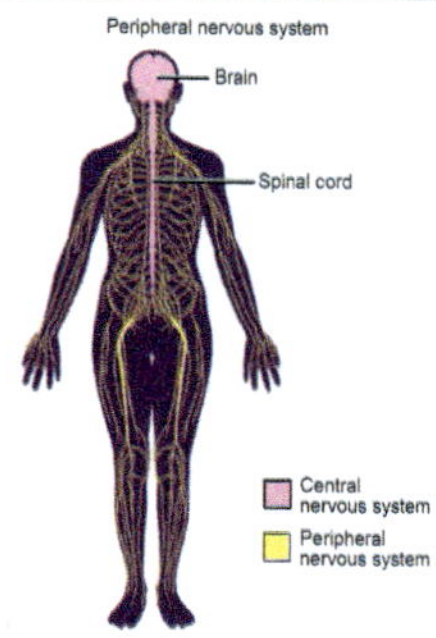
Dementia	Dementia is a general term for a group of diseases that affect a person's ability to think, remember, and make decisions, which can interfere with their daily activities. It's not a normal part of aging, but the risk of developing dementia increases with age, especially after 65.	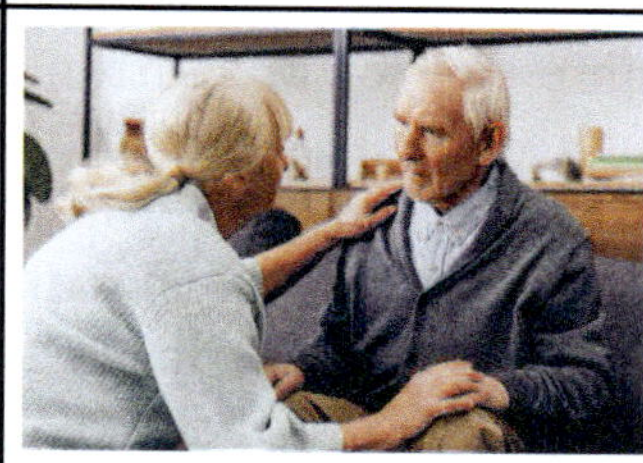
Sarin	Sarin is a human-made chemical warfare nerve agent and is one of the most toxic and rapidly acting of known nerve agents. Sarin is also known by the military designation GB. Sarin, like all nerve agents, interferes with the operation of an enzyme that stops muscles from contracting.	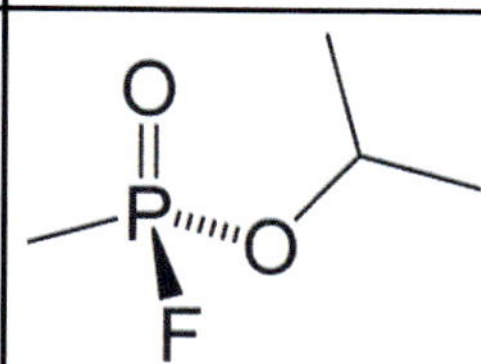

2.1. Autonomic Drug

The effects of autonomic drugs on the parasympathetic and sympathetic nervous systems can vary. This kind of medication is useful in treating a variety of illnesses, including asthma, glaucoma, kidney, gastrointestinal, and heart conditions.

2.1.1. Drugs Acting on the Parasympathetic Nervous System

One of the targets of autonomic medications is the parasympathetic nervous system. The nervous system can be inhibited or stimulated to produce therapeutic effects.

2.1.1.1. Mechanism of Action

Major physiological effects that can result from activating the parasympathetic nervous system include an increase in glandular secretion, an increase in smooth muscle contraction, and a decrease in heart rate and contractility. Nicotinic and muscarinic receptors are the two types of receptors involved in neurotransmission that work together to produce the physiological effects mentioned above. To relay the neurotransmission in the synapse, these two groups of receptors can bind to the same neurotransmitter, acetylcholine. Acetylcholine is released from the presynaptic neuron at the synapse. Acetylcholine can bind to receptors on postsynaptic neurons to carry on nerve signal transmission, or it can bind to receptors on organ tissues to trigger an organ-specific physiological response. The action of acetylcholine is terminated when acetylcholinesterase breaks down the molecule after it binds to the receptors, converting it to choline and acetate.

To produce therapeutic effects, autonomic drugs can be used to either stimulate or inhibit the parasympathetic nervous system by acting on the receptors and acetylcholinesterase involved in nerve signal transmission.

It is possible to stimulate the parasympathetic nervous system by taking anticholinesterase medications or muscarinic agonists. Muscarinic agonists have the ability to bind to muscarinic receptors, which enhances the nerve impulses' ability to reach organs and facilitates the physiological effects of the parasympathetic nervous system. Acetylcholinesterase and anticholinesterase medications interact to stop acetylcholine from binding to the enzyme. This prevents acetylcholine from breaking down, preserving neurotransmission and the physiological effects that follow.

Acetylcholine release inhibitors or muscarinic antagonists can be used to inhibit the parasympathetic nervous system. Muscarinic receptors can be bound by muscarinic antagonists, which then block the receptors. Since acetylcholine does not bind to muscarinic receptors, nerve impulses cannot be transmitted from neurons to organs in a way that would cause the initial physiological reaction. The release of acetylcholine from the presynaptic nerve fiber can be hampered by acetylcholine release inhibitors. This results in a decrease in neurotransmission and a corresponding reduction in the physiological effect.

2.1.1.2. Medical Uses

Clinically, autonomic drugs are used to treat disorders involving the parasympathetic nervous system.

1. Bethanechol

One such muscarinic agonist is bethanechol. It is a part of the treatment for underactive bladder and weak detrusor muscle contraction. Because the parasympathetic nervous system regulates the contraction of the bladder's detrusor muscle, bethanechol can bind to muscarinic receptors to trigger the parasympathetic nervous system's activation and restore the contraction of the detrusor muscle. Since increasing the dosage of bethanechol can result in adverse effects like nausea, diarrhea, and headaches, a low dose is frequently used in treatment.

2. Physostigmine

An anticholinesterase medication called physostigmine is used to treat glaucoma. An increase in intraocular pressure is typically observed in glaucoma patients. Physostigmine has the ability to inhibit acetylcholinesterase, which lessens acetylcholine's disintegration. Acetylcholine is more readily available to support parasympathetic nervous system neurotransmission, which encourages smooth muscle contraction in the ciliary body. Patients with glaucoma experience a decrease in intraocular pressure as a result of the widening of Schlemm's canal and the trabecular meshwork, which increases the outflow of aqueous humor. Physostigmine use can result in many negative side effects, including increased spasms of accommodation and intestinal cramps.

3. Atropine

Atropine is used to treat patients with bradycardia. As a muscarinic antagonist, atropine can block the muscarinic receptor, making it impossible for acetylcholine to bind to the receptor and continue sending nerve signals to the heart via the parasympathetic nervous system. This permits an elevation in heart rate. The adverse effects of atropine include dry mouth, dilated pupils, and hyperthermia.

4. Botulinum toxin A

One example of an acetylcholine release inhibitor is botulinum toxin A, a medication used to treat overactive bladder. It prevents acetylcholine from being released from the presynaptic neuron, which prevents it from interacting with postsynaptic neuron receptors to continue neurotransmission in the parasympathetic nervous system. This causes the bladder's detrusor muscle contraction to decrease and restores normal bladder function. Using this medication to treat an overactive bladder may increase the risk of hematuria, lower urinary tract infections, and urine retention.

2.1.2. Drugs Acting on the Sympathetic Nervous System

Another area that autonomic medications target is the sympathetic nervous system. Therapy effects can be attained by activating or inhibiting the sympathetic nervous system.

2.1.2.1. Mechanisms of Action

1. Sympathetic nervous system

The body's fight-or-flight response is triggered in part by the sympathetic nervous system. The sympathetic nervous system is responsible for many physiological responses, such as an accelerated heartbeat, an increase in heart contraction force, noradrenaline and adrenaline secretion by the adrenal gland, relaxation of the bronchi, and inhibition of gastrointestinal and peristalsis. To produce these physiological effects, neurotransmission is relayed by neurotransmitters. A class of neurotransmitter called acetylcholine is discharged from the preganglionic nerve and binds to the nicotinic receptors in the autonomic ganglion. Another class of neurotransmitter secreted by the postganglionic nerve is noradrenaline, which elicits physiological reactions by binding to adrenergic receptors in target organ tissues.

2. Adrenergic receptor

Many autonomic drugs that affect the sympathetic nervous system target the adrenaline receptors. Adrenergic receptors are primarily categorized into five types: β_1, β_2, β_3, and α_1, α_2. These adrenergic receptors stimulate various physiological reactions and are distributed throughout various tissues.

Since smooth muscles contain the majority of $\square_1$ receptors, activating them causes smooth muscle constriction as well as vasoconstriction. Presynaptic nerve endings contain α_2 receptors, which when activated reduce the release of noradrenaline at the presynaptic level. This functioned as a negative feedback mechanism. The heart contains the majority of β_1 receptors, which when activated, cause the heart to contract more forcefully and beat faster. Smooth muscles contain β_2 receptors, which when activated cause the smooth muscles to vasodilate and relax. This action is in contrast to that of the β_1 receptor. The majority of β_3 receptors are found in adipocytes and the bladder's detrusor muscles. When these receptors are activated, the detrusor muscles relax and lipolysis—the process that breaks down fat molecules into fatty acids—is stimulated.

Sympathomimetic drugs, which mimic the action of sympathetic nervous system activation, and sympatholytic drugs, which lessen or stop the action of sympathetic nervous system activation, are the two main categories of drugs that affect the sympathetic nervous system.

2.1.2.2. Sympathomimetic Drug

Drugs known as sympathomimetics are stimulants that replicate the actions of endogenous sympathetic nervous system agonists. There are two categories for the actions of sympathomimetic medications: direct and indirect. The indirect mode of action involves mechanisms that increase or decrease noradrenaline release, breakdown, and removal. The direct mode of activation of adrenergic receptors involves mimicking endogenous molecules through agonist molecules.

2.1.2.3. Sympatholytic Drug

Drugs that are sympathomimetic have the opposite effect as those that are sympatholytic. They lessen or stop the action of the sympathetic nervous system. The two main ways that sympatholytic medications work are through direct blocking of adrenoreceptor activation by receptor antagonists (blockers) and indirect inhibition of noradrenaline synthesis, storage, and release.

2.1.2.3. Medical Uses

Autonomic drugs that act on the sympathetic nervous system are widely used in medicine to treat heart failure, angina, asthma, hypertension, and hypotension.

1. Terbutaline

Terbutaline is a sympathomimetic drug that acts as a selective β_2 receptor agonist in the treatment of asthma. By activating β_2 receptors in smooth muscles, it stimulates sympathetic responses that lead to the relaxation of muscles. This relaxation in the bronchi and trachea helps widen the airways, making it an effective bronchodilator for asthma. Unlike other medications, terbutaline's selectivity for β_2 receptors means it has minimal impact on the heart, reducing the risk of heart-related side effects. Common side effects of terbutaline include peripheral vasodilation, tremors, and increased heart rate. To minimize these side effects, terbutaline is most often administered through inhalation, targeting the lungs directly. Additionally, terbutaline can be used to prevent premature labor by relaxing uterine smooth muscles.

2. Atenolol

One class of sympatholytic medication is atenolol. A selective β_1 antagonist, atenolol is used clinically to treat cardiac dysrhythmias, angina, and hypertension. Atenolol exclusively acts on β1 receptors found in the heart because it is selective to these receptors. It opposes the effect of activation of the sympathetic nervous system as an antagonist. Myocardial contractility and heart rate are reduced as a result of atenolol's actions, which also lower blood pressure and cardiac output. Patients with heart failure should not use atenolol because of its side effects, which include cold extremities and an aggravation of cardiac failure. Patients with asthma can use atenolol because it does not cause bronchoconstriction because it does not act on β_2 receptors.

2.2. Cholinergic Medications

2.2.1. Indications

Pharmacological agents classified as cholinergic medications work on acetylcholine, the main neurotransmitter in the parasympathetic nervous system (PNS). Cholinergic medications fall into two main categories: direct-acting and indirect-acting. The muscarinic receptors are directly bound to and activated by the direct-acting cholinergic agonists. Choline esters (acetylcholine, methacholine, carbachol, and bethanechol) and alkaloids (muscarine, pilocarpine, cevimeline) are a few examples of direct-acting cholinergic agents. Acetylcholine is more readily available at cholinergic receptors when an indirect cholinergic agent is used. These comprise irreversible agents such as echothiophate, parathion, malathion, diazinon, tabun, sarin, soman, carbaryl, and propoxur, and reversible agents such as physostigmine, neostigmine, pyridostigmine, edrophonium, rivastigmine, donepezil, and galantamine. Because cholinergic agonists have the potential to have negative effects on any organ that is under the parasympathetic nervous system's control, their use is limited.

Some indications for use are listed below:

- **Myasthenia gravis:** The initial first-line therapy for most patients is anticholinesterase medication, usually pyridostigmine. Neostigmine is also available but not commonly used.
- **Dementia:** Cholinesterase inhibitors like rivastigmine, donepezil, galantamine are the available medications for cognition and global functioning in patients with dementia of all causes. Their primary use is in mild to moderate Alzheimer's disease. These medications have off label use for dementia from-Parkinson's disease and Lewy body dementia.
- **Ophthalmology:** Pilocarpine and carbachol work by increasing the aqueous outflow and hence decrease the intra-ocular tension in open-angle glaucoma. Miotics are used as an add-on therapy and are now third-choice drugs. Carbachol has utility with intraocular use as a miotic in surgery. Sequential use of atropine (mydriatic) and pilocarpine (miotic) is used to break iris-lens adhesions. Pilocarpine is used off label to counter the effects of cycloplegics.
- **Reversal of nondepolarizing neuromuscular blockade after surgery:** Neostigmine preceded by atropine to block muscarinic effects, rapidly reverses muscle paralysis induced by neuromuscular blockers and is approved by the FDA.
- **Postoperative urinary retention:** For both prevention and treatment of urinary distention and retention, neostigmine is a common option. Bethanechol is the indicated pharmaceutical treatment of acute postoperative and postpartum non-obstructive urinary retention.
- **Neurogenic bladder:** Bethanechol may help complete bladder emptying in those with a hypotonic bladder.
- **Acute colonic pseudo-obstruction:** Off-label use of neostigmine is acute colonic pseudo-obstruction.

- **Xerostomia:** Use of muscarinic agonists in patients with an inadequate response to artificial saliva and mechanical stimulation in Sjogren syndrome or patients post-radiation treatment associated with head and neck cancer. Cevimeline is FDA-approved for the treatment of symptoms of dry mouth in Sjogren syndrome.
- **Anticholinergic overdose:** Physostigmine is the specific antidote for poisoning with belladonna or other anticholinergics. It should only be used to reverse toxic, life-threatening delirium caused by an anticholinergic agent (atropine, scopolamine, diphenhydramine).
- **Tensilon test:** Edrophonium was previously a bedside test in patients with suspected myasthenia gravis, has been discontinued and is no longer available in the United States of America.
- **Snakebite:** Neostigmine also has found use in patients with neurotoxic snakebite for whom antivenom is not available or is ineffective.

2.2.2. Mechanism of Action

One of the body's primary neurotransmitters is acetylcholine. The peripheral effects of acetylcholine are classified as acting on either muscarinic (M_1, M_2, M_3, M_4, M_5) or nicotinic (N_m, N_n) receptors, depending on the type of receptors through which it undergoes mediation. Both the central nervous system and the stomach parietal cells have M_1 receptors. The muscle of the heart contains M2 receptors. Smooth muscle, exocrine glands, and bladder receptors all have M_3 receptors. The adrenal medulla, autonomic ganglia, central nervous system, and neuromuscular junction all contain nicotinic receptors. The autonomic and somatic nervous systems make up the peripheral nervous system. The sympathetic and parasympathetic nervous systems are subsets of the autonomic nervous system. Like all cholinomimetics, the parasympathetic nervous system primarily uses acetylcholine as its primary neurotransmitter to regulate the functions of various organs and glands.

Drugs classified as anticholinesterase agents block choline esterase, prevent acetylcholine from hydrolyzing and have cholinergic effects. Anticholinesterases are further divided into agents that are irreversible (organophosphates) and reversible (carbamates).

2.2.3. Administration

There are several different formulations of cholinergic medications. For instance, ophthalmic eye drops are used to administer physostigmine and pilocarpine when used as miotic agents. Pyridostigmine is taken orally to treat myasthenia gravis. Patients who are unable to take it orally may receive it parenterally. Galantamine, rivastigmine, and donepezil are taken orally to treat Alzheimer's disease. All sites of absorption, including the lungs and intact skin, are used by organophosphates. Inducing bowel evacuation in individuals with spinal cord injury appears to be a successful use of transdermal administration of neostigmine via iontophoresis. Parenteral administration is the usual method for administering the other anticholinesterase agents that are used to treat different conditions.

2.2.4. Adverse Effects

Medication containing cholinergic agents may have nicotinic or muscarinic side effects. Through the heart's M_2 receptors, acetylcholine causes the SA nodal cells to become hyperpolarized. Bradycardia or even cardiac arrest could consequently happen. Conduction slows at the A-V node and Purkinje fibers, and an entire A-V block could happen. People may be more susceptible to atrial fibrillation or flutter because of non-uniform vagal innervation of the atrial fibers.

The blood vessels' M_3 receptors mediate dilatation, which lowers blood pressure and causes flushing. An erection is brought on by stimulating the cholinergic nerves in the penis. However, when using injected cholinomimetic medications, this reaction is negligible. M_3 receptors mediate the contraction of smooth muscle in different organs of the body. Abdominal cramps and bowel evacuation result from the gastrointestinal tract's increased tone and peristalsis as well as the relaxation of sphincters. Urinating the bladder is caused by the contraction of the detrusor muscle and the relaxation of the bladder's sphincter and trigone. An attack of bronchial asthma is brought on by constriction of the bronchial muscles.

Through the M_3 and M_2 receptors, gland secretions are increased, leading to increased sweating, salivation, lacrimation, gastric secretions, and tracheobronchial secretions. The iris contracts as a result of pilocarpine eye drops, resulting in miosis and accommodation spasm.

When administered intravenously, acetylcholine does not pass through the blood-brain barrier and has no effect. On the other hand, cholinergic medications that penetrate the brain cause a complicated pattern of stimulation that is followed by depression.

Anticholinesterases block the breakdown of acetylcholine, thus increasing the activation of muscarinic receptors that are located there. Acetylcholine released by nerve impulses in skeletal muscles may result in twitching and fasciculations by repetitive firing following treatment with an anticholinesterase. Increased dosages of anticholinesterase drugs inhibit impulse transmission in the neuromuscular junction, resulting in muscle weakness or paralysis.

Physostigmine, a reversible anticholinesterase and organophosphates, which are irreversible anticholinesterases, enhance acetylcholine levels to stimulate ganglia and have more pronounced muscarinic and central nervous system effects; their effects on skeletal muscles are less pronounced. The skeletal muscles are more strongly affected by neostigmine and other agents, which also stimulate the ganglia; however, the muscarinic effects are not as evident.

The most frequent causes of cholinergic crises are overdoses or inappropriate drug dosages, as well as unintentional exposure to pesticides like parathion and malathion. Sarin, a nerve gas, is one of the additional sources.

2.2.5. Monitoring

Medical supervision is recommended for agricultural workers who handle organophosphates for extended periods of time. It is advised to conduct appropriate testing to determine overexposure before the development of a clinical illness. Cholinesterase in serum and red blood cells needs to be measured. One of the following schedules can be followed to obtain baseline blood samples and compare them with the samples:

- On a routine 30-day basis(or)
- Within three days at the end of each qualifying period where the employee meets the exposure threshold.

Examine the worker's work practices to find and address possible sources of pesticide poisoning if the worker's serum or RBC cholinesterase concentrations are more than 20% below baseline.

2.2.6. Toxicity

Anticholinesterase agents are widely accessible and commonly used as insecticides in agriculture and household settings (e.g. malathion, parathion). Accidental, suicidal, and homicidal poisoning incidents are frequent, manifesting as severe cholinergic toxicity from ingestion or skin contact with these substances. Some of these agents have been utilized in chemical warfare, like nerve gases (e.g. sarin, soman). Anticholinesterases also have medicinal applications in treating conditions such as myasthenia gravis, reversing neuromuscular blockade, and managing Alzheimer's disease.

Acute toxicity caused by organophosphate agents is characterized by excess cholinergic behavior. The neuromuscular junction, autonomic nervous system, and central nervous system are the primary targets of toxic effects. Miosis, salivation, lacrimation, emesis, bradycardia, bronchospasm, bronchorrhea, urination, and diarrhea are among the clinical signs of acute cholinergic toxicity. Diaphoresis is brought on by the regulation of sweat glands by sympathetic activation of postganglionic muscarinic receptors. However, because sympathetic ganglia have nicotinic receptors, mydriasis and tachycardia can occasionally be seen. Nicotine stimulates receptors at the neuromuscular junction, resulting in acetylcholine-induced muscle weakness, fasciculations, and paralysis. It has also been discovered that the brain contains nicotinic and muscarinic receptors, which may be involved in coma, central respiratory depression, seizures, and lethargy. In organophosphorus agent poisoning, cardiac arrhythmias such as QTc prolongation and heart block are occasionally seen. Acute poisoning usually results in respiratory failure, which is caused by a confluence of factors including neuromuscular weakness, bronchoconstriction, depression of the CNS respiratory center, and excessive respiratory secretions. Overstimulation of the cholinergic and glutamatergic nervous systems is brought on by oxidative stress, which can have long-term negative health effects.

Acetylcholinesterase is bound by organophosphorus agents, rendering the enzyme inactive. The process known as "aging" occurs when the acetylcholinesterase-organophosphorus compound becomes resistant to antidote reactivation over time. Therefore, it is important to start the treatment as soon as possible.

2.2.6.1. Intoxication Management

Medical professionals should completely undress the patient and rinse their skin and mucous membranes to stop their exposure. Individuals exhibiting altered mental status necessitate endotracheal intubation and 100% oxygen. If the patient is experiencing respiratory distress, keep them breathing under positive pressure. supportive actions include maintaining blood pressure, staying hydrated, and using diazepam to stop convulsions. It has also been demonstrated that prophylactic diazepam can avert cognitive function impairment following organophosphorus poisoning. Atropine and pralidoxime are used to treat cholinergic toxicity caused by organophosphate agents. Atropine inhibits cholinergic activation by competing with acetylcholine at muscarinic receptors. A cholinesterase-reactivating medication called pralidoxime is useful in the treatment of nicotinic and muscarinic symptoms. As a particular counteragent for organophosphate poisoning, pralidoxime is effective. There is a dosage form that can be injected intramuscularly and contains both pralidoxime and atropine.

2.2.7. Enhancing Healthcare Team Outcomes

A wide range of illnesses can benefit from the use of cholinergic medications. Healthcare workers, such as nurses and pharmacists, should be aware of the typical side effects of cholinergic drugs. Follow-up visits should be scheduled for patients taking cholinesterase inhibitors every three and six months to evaluate drug response, and tolerance, and to avoid any signs of cholinergic excess. Employers in agriculture should be subject to strict measures to prevent unintentional exposure to insecticides that have cholinergic properties. Blood tests should be performed on a regular basis to measure cholinesterase concentrations after establishing a baseline. Emergencies such as poisoning and overexposure can be avoided with prompt intervention. At all institutions receiving presentations of intoxication, all emergency department staff members as well as primary care physicians should be trained in and have easy access to drug intoxication procedures. All new medications should come with comprehensive information for patients about common potential side effects.

It is imperative to use an interprofessional team approach when prescribing cholinergic medications. The adverse effect profile of these agents is required as mentioned above. When prescribing cholinergic medications, clinicians must understand both their advantages and disadvantages. A pharmacist consult is helpful because they can check for drug interactions, confirm dosage, reconcile medications, and let the prescriber know if there are any problems. Since nurses frequently interact with patients for the first time during follow-up visits, it is imperative that they are knowledgeable about the adverse effect profile. They can assess treatment efficacy and medication compliance in addition to keeping an eye out for these side effects. To achieve the best possible patient outcomes with cholinergic therapy, an interprofessional team approach involving doctors, specialists, specialty-trained nurses, and pharmacists is imperative (Gerretsen & Pollock, 2011; Ehret & Chamberlin, 2015; Wiercinski & Jackson, 2022).

2.3. Anticholinergic Medications

Many different diseases are managed and treated with anticholinergic medications. This exercise demonstrates the use of anticholinergic medications as effective treatments for cholinergic toxicity, urogenital tract infections, Parkinson's disease, respiratory conditions, cardiovascular disease, and a host of other illnesses. The mechanism of action, adverse event profile, and other important elements (e.g. relevant interactions, monitoring, pharmacodynamics, pharmacokinetics, off-label uses, and dosing) are important for the interprofessional team members treating patients with the aforementioned disorders and related conditions.

2.3.1. Indications

Acetylcholine (ACh) is a neurotransmitter that is blocked and inhibited at synapses in the central and peripheral nervous systems by anticholinergic medications. In doing so, these drugs inhibit the actions of the parasympathetic nervous system (the "rest and digest" function of the autonomic nervous system) via selective blockade of ACh from binding to its receptors in neurons. The parasympathetic nervous system regulates the involuntary contractions of smooth muscle in the gastrointestinal tract, lungs, urinary tract, and other parts of the body.

Anticholinergic drugs affect circulation, breathing, alertness, and vision, among other physiological functions. Anticholinergic medications are helpful in the treatment of psychiatric conditions, depression, mydriasis, allergies, Parkinson's disease, urge incontinence, and respiratory disorders (asthma, COPD). With the exception of a few drugs, more than 600 medications have some degree of anticholinergic activity. Experts typically attribute side effects rather than therapeutic effects to the anticholinergic properties of these medications. Examples of specific anticholinergic medications where the anticholinergic activity is deemed to be therapeutic are listed below, along with the conditions they treat:

- **Ipratropium and tiotropium:** Function to dilate the bronchi and relieve shortness of breath and FDA approved for the use in patients with chronic obstructive pulmonary disease.
- **Benztropine and trihexyphenidyl:** Used to counter reduced dopamine levels and relieve symptoms of Parkinson's disease
- **Oxybutynin and tolterodine:** FDA-approved for the treatment of urge incontinence and detrusor hyperactivity
- Oxybutynin has an off-label use for the treatment of hyperhidrosis.
- **Diphenhydramine and other anti-histamines:** FDA-approved as a sleeping aid
- **Scopolamine:** Used as a prophylactic anti-emetic
- **Atropine:** Used to dilate the pupil during retina visualization and in the treatment of cholinergic toxicity
- **Vecuronium and Succinylcholine:** Antinicotinic medications used as a neuromuscular blockade in surgeries
- **Mecamylamine:** Used strictly in research settings as a ganglionic blocker
- **Glycopyrrolate:** A type of quaternary amine used in anesthesia to decrease salivary and tracheal secretions

Despite not being the cause of their therapeutic effects, medications such as antipsychotics, tricyclic antidepressants, and diphenhydramine (when used to treat allergies) have anticholinergic properties.

2.3.2. Mechanism of Action

Competitive antagonists of the neurotransmitter acetylcholine at cholinergic system receptor sites are known as anticholinergic drugs. The G protein-coupled muscarinic receptors that are bound to the plasma membrane and the ligand-gated nicotinic receptors that are ion channel-gated are the two types of receptors that the cholinergic system uses. The autonomic nervous system's postganglionic dendrites, nerve bodies, and motor endplate of the neuromuscular junction all contain nicotinic receptors.

Sweat glands in the sympathetic nervous system and target organ cells in the parasympathetic nervous system both have muscarinic receptors. The effects of cholinergic neurotransmission in peripheral and central nervous systems are lessened or, in certain situations, completely eliminated by antagonistic interactions with the cholinergic system. Medications that have an anticholinergic effect mostly target muscarinic receptors.

2.3.3. Administration

The vast majority of drugs with anticholinergic properties are available in oral and intravenous forms; the administration of these medications varies. For instance, ipratropium, which is used to treat COPD, can be injected or taken orally. It is possible to give diphenhydramine intravenously (IV), intramuscularly (IM), or orally. Atropine is available in IV and IM dose forms, while antipsychotics are available in oral and IM forms. Trihexyphenidyl and oxybutynin are administered orally, while vecuronium and succinylcholine are available intravenously.

2.3.4. Adverse Effects

Anticholinergic drugs have two categories of side effects: central and peripheral. Excessive cholinergic receptor blockade in the central nervous system causes central effects, while peripheral parasympathetic nervous system end-organ targets, muscle contraction, and exocrine glandular secretion blockade cause peripheral adverse effects. At low dosages, common side effects of central anticholinergic medications include headache, memory loss, reduced cognitive function, behavioral abnormalities, anxiety, and insomnia.

Symptoms of agitation, confusion, delirium, and seizures are central adverse effects that occur at high dosages and are on the verge of anticholinergic toxicity. Adverse effects on the central nervous system are more common in drugs with greater blood-brain barrier crossing ability than in those with less border crossing ability. Common peripheral adverse effects of medications with anticholinergic activity are described below, organized by organ system:

- General: Hyperthermia and anhidrosis
- Cardiovascular: Tachycardia, flushing, and arrhythmias
- Gastrointestinal: Reduced gut motility, constipation, vomiting, reduced saliva, and tear production
- Genitourinary: Urinary retention
- HEENT: Blurred vision, mydriasis, narrow-angle glaucoma, and potentially vision loss
- Skin: Inhibition of sweating
- Musculoskeletal: Diminished muscle contraction

Generally, a drug's affinity for cholinergic receptors determines its potential to cause anticholinergic side effects.

2.3.5. Contraindications

Anticholinergics should only be used with caution in the elderly, in people with high anticholinergic burdens, and in people with conditions like dementia that can lead to increased anticholinergic activity. Due to decreased acetylcholine-induced transmission within the central nervous system and increased permeability of the blood-brain barrier, elderly adults are more susceptible to the effects of anticholinergic medications. Furthermore, many ailments that call for anticholinergic medication therapy are common in the elderly (e.g. COPD, urine incontinence). They are therefore more likely to be using medications that have anticholinergic effects and are in danger.

When prescribing new medications, healthcare professionals should take the patient's overall anticholinergic burden into account because patients with high anticholinergic burdens are more susceptible to side effects and anticholinergic toxicity. Anticholinergic medication use is also somewhat contraindicated in patients with dementia. Since dementia is associated with decreased brain acetylcholine, anticholinergic medication use may exacerbate dementia symptoms. Anticholinergic medications can cause glaucoma, hyperthyroidism, tachyarrhythmia, and prostate hypertrophy, all of which are common in older people.

2.3.6. Monitoring

One method for calculating an individual's overall anticholinergic burden across all substances is the serum anticholinergic assay. This method has made it possible to scale the levels of anticholinergic activity in drugs from low to high. Drugs were previously classified as either anticholinergic or not; however, a more thorough drug scaling enables healthcare professionals to more effectively assess the benefits and drawbacks of prescribing anticholinergic medications, particularly for high-risk groups like the elderly and people with mental illnesses.

It is important to note that the assay lacks specificity for muscarinic receptor subtypes and is unable to directly detect CNS anticholinergic levels. The Anticholinergic Drug Scale is another instrument used to track the risk of anticholinergic drugs. On a scale from 0 to 3, the anticholinergic drug scale rates the anticholinergic activity of each medication; a score of 0 indicates no anticholinergic activity at all, while a score of 3 indicates high levels of anticholinergic activity. A final score is obtained by adding up all of the drug scores. It is hoped that ADS will help patients with a high anticholinergic burden by offering guidance on which medications to stop taking; however, more research is required to confirm a link between the score and clinical results.

2.3.7. Toxicity

Anticholinergic medication toxicity is essentially a severe form of the central and peripheral adverse effects that were previously discussed. Anhidrosis, anhidrotic hyperthermia, mydriasis, vasodilation-induced flushing, urine retention, and neurological symptoms such as delirium, agitation, and hallucinations are among the clinical features of anticholinergic toxicity. An effective memory aid for the common symptoms of anticholinergic toxicity is "red as a beet, dry as a bone, blind as a bat, mad as a hatter, hot as a hare, full as a flask." Tachycardia and absent bowel sounds are two of the earliest signs of acute anticholinergic toxicity. As of right now, there is no test to confirm the diagnosis of anticholinergic toxicity, which is thought to be a clinical diagnosis.

2.3.8. Enhancing Healthcare Team Outcomes

Throughout the healthcare system, anticholinergic drugs are widely used, and many more that are not specifically prescribed for their anticholinergic qualities nevertheless have anticholinergic side effects. All members of the interprofessional healthcare team, such as nurses, pharmacists, and clinicians (MDs, DOs, NPs, and PAs), must be knowledgeable about the benefits and drawbacks of anticholinergic medications. This is particularly significant in light of the role anticholinergics play in side effects. The group should keep an eye on the total amount of anticholinergic burden, make an effort to reduce the overuse of anticholinergic drugs and give extra consideration to high-risk populations like the elderly and people undergoing treatment for schizophrenia and depression.

When prescribing anticholinergic medications, doctors must be aware of any additional medications the patient may be taking. A pharmacist can help with this by doing a thorough medication reconciliation and providing the prescriber with updates. In addition to guiding appropriate administration, nurses can also offer patients advice on potential adverse events so that, should they arise, they will be able to identify them early and seek appropriate intervention from other members of the interprofessional team. This may involve contacting the pharmacist or other members of the nursing staff where they pick up their medication. Any team member who notices or becomes aware of a problem has a duty to notify the other members of the healthcare team and document the information in the patient's chart or electronic health record (EHR). Improved patient outcomes can result from the use of these medications, which have a lower potential for side effects when used in conjunction with interprofessional communication and collaborative efforts. (Gerretsen & Pollock, 2011; Ehret & Chamberlin, 2015; Wiercinski & Jackson, 2022)

2.4. Anticholinergics and Central Nervous System Effects

Behavioral and pharmacologic therapy is currently the standard of care for older patients with overactive bladder (OAB). Pharmacological therapy relies primarily on anticholinergic agents. These substances are known as antimuscarinics (AMs) because they work by preventing acetylcholine's effects on bladder muscarinic receptors. One acknowledged group of side effects associated with the AM medication class is the possibility of central nervous system (CNS) effects. Many adverse CNS events are regarded by most doctors as "safety events."

A significant portion of the elderly—at least 25% of those over 65—are afflicted with OAB. Cognitively impaired individuals may be more vulnerable to further cognitive decline and CNS events. A portion of the elderly population may also be more vulnerable due to additional medical conditions, drug-drug interactions, metabolism changes, and the use of other pharmacologic agents with AM activity (referred to as anticholinergic load). Cognitive abnormalities, vertigo, sleeplessness, and sedation are among the CNS events that can occur in even a younger population.

Notable publications on the CNS effects of some of these drugs include positive case reports, anomalies in surrogate measures of CNS function, and changes in performance on computerized cognitive tests. Unsolicited CNS adverse-event reporting, phase III placebo-controlled and community-use studies, enrollment of a heterogeneous patient population with varying susceptibility and risk, and the use of a methodology underpowered to detect a difference from placebo for a given adverse event are some of the reasons why these studies have not reported a population effect for CNS events.

2.4.1. AM Pharmacology

According to recent reviews, AMs may function by inhibiting both the efferent pathways that cause the bladder to contract and void as well as the afferent pathways that change the bladder's sensory feedback. It is known that there are five different muscarinic receptor subtypes (M_1–M_5). M_2 and M_3 receptors predominate in the bladder's detrusor muscle, with the M_2 subtype accounting for about 80% of receptors. It has been observed that M_2 receptors are involved in the process of accommodating urine during urinary storage, while the smaller subset of M_3 receptors is thought to be principally in charge of bladder muscle contraction. It has been observed, nevertheless, that these capacities can change depending on the illness. Because AMs have the ability to bind to muscarinic receptors in a variety of organ systems throughout the body and are the cause of the drug class's frequently reported adverse events, blockade will not only impair detrusor muscle activity but also interfere with other organ systems. For example, salivary glands, the smooth muscle of the colon, and the eyes all contain M_3 muscarinic receptors. Constipation, dry mouth, and blurred vision may become more detrimental effects if these receptors are blocked. On the other hand, a relative increase in heart rate could result from heart M_2 receptor blockade.

The brain contains every subtype of muscarinic receptor (M_1–M_5). The M1 receptor subtype is the most prevalent in the central nervous system, hippocampal region, and neostratum. It is primarily found in the neocortex. The brain is also filled with M_2 receptors. The CNS is also home to the M_3 receptor, albeit at a comparatively lower density. M_5 receptors have been found in the hippocampus and projection neurons of the substantia nigra, pars compacta, and ventral tegmental nuclei. M_4 receptors are widely distributed in the neostriatum. It should be mentioned that potency or pharmacologic effects are not determined by the mere presence of receptors or by binding to them. According to clinical research, antagonistic interactions with M_1 and, to a lesser extent, M_2 or M_4 receptors in the central nervous system may lead to cognitive impairment, specifically memory loss. Clinically, patients who are already elderly and have cognitive impairment, as well as those who have dementia in the early stages, age-related memory impairment, or mild cognitive impairment, may be particularly susceptible to these cognitive side effects.

2.4.2. Central Nervous System Side Effects: The Blood-Brain Barrier

Depending on the drug's pharmacologic activity on CNS receptors and its capacity to cross the blood–brain barrier (BBB), AMs can have a variety of CNS side effects. The BBB requires both passive and active transport for penetration. The endothelial cells that line the capillaries in the brain are encircled by astroglial processes, a collagen matrix, pericytes, and zonulae occludentes and tight junctions. As a result, there is a high electrical resistance across the endothelium and a significant restriction on solute passage via the paracellular pathway. Only lipid-soluble, unpolarized, small molecules (400–600 Da) can easily diffuse from capillary blood to brain tissue.

BBB penetration by AMs may cause CNS side effects. The following variables affect how well any pharmacologically active parent compound or metabolite penetrates the body:

- Serum concentration (passive diffusion);
- Active transport ("in" or "out");
- Lipophilicity (predisposition to dissolve in fat vs water);
- The electrical charge (polarity); and
- Molecular size and configuration (bulk, not purely molecular weight) may influence the extent to which substances penetrate the CNS under normal conditions.

Once more, it is crucial to take into account the parent compounds' metabolites because these substances can be converted into more or less polar substances that change in lipophilicity and are more susceptible to transport, as well as larger or smaller molecules that vary in size (configuration) and weight (Da).

Without a doubt, tertiary ammonium groups—small, lipophilic, noncharged molecules—cross the blood-brain barrier (BBB) more easily than do quaternary ammonium groups. The current OAB medications rank in order of lipophilicity and likelihood of crossing the blood-brain barrier (BBB): Darifenacin is the most likely tertiary amine to cross the BBB, surpassing both oxybutynin and solifenacin, which are more likely to pass than tolterodine. The only quaternary amine in the group that causes both increased polarity and decreased permeability is trospium chloride. Transdermal delivery of oxybutynin is an intriguing illustration of how drug delivery affects a drug's potential to cause an adverse event. The parent compound oxybutynin is favorably altered to the metabolite N-desethyloxybutynin (DEO) levels by transdermal delivery, which also results in a more stable serum level. Transdermal delivery theoretically results in decreased systemic adverse events (and potentially CNS events) by:

- Decreasing the total anticholinergic load (less oxybutynin and DEO);

- Providing more stable serum levels (decreasing passive CNS diffusion); and
- Reducing the amount of DEO that may possibly penetrate the CNS more readily.

It has been demonstrated that several circumstances raise BBB permeability. These include growing older (over 45 years), using specific medications, having multiple illnesses, and stress. Compounds that are thought to be less likely to cross under normal conditions would be able to penetrate the CNS more readily through a permeable BBB because of modifications to passive barriers, active transport, or efflux mechanisms. It is crucial to realize that aging can cause changes in cell junctions, passive lipid barriers, and active transport mechanisms (enzyme systems). Therefore, regardless of their physiochemical characteristics, all AM agents that are currently prescribed for the treatment of OAB should be regarded as having the capacity to cross the blood-brain barrier and engage with the central nervous system's muscarinic receptors (Figure 2.2).

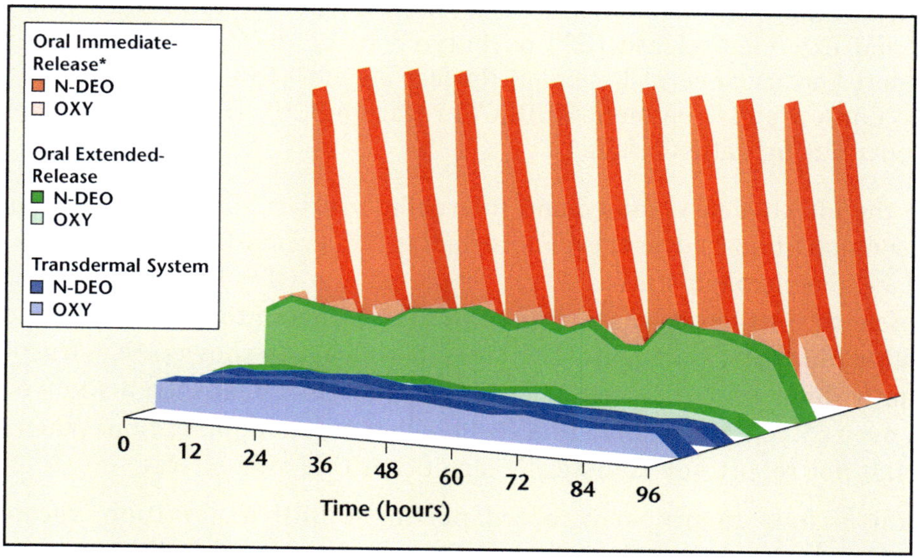

Figure 2.2. *OXY and N-DEO steady-state plasma concentrations.*

Source: https://www.researchgate.net/publication/5619581_Anticholinergics_and_Central_Nervous_System_Effects_Are_We_Confused.

2.4.3. Cognitive Effects of AMs: Measuring the Clinical Risk

An increased risk of cognitive impairment and other CNS side effects associated with AM agents is present in the older OAB patient population. There is evidence of a typical age-related decline in memory function, which may make people more vulnerable to AM medication's possible cognitive side effects. It is commonly known that M1 receptor density decreases with age. There is a chance that further hostility toward AM could hasten the deterioration of memory.

Other medications with AM activity, such as muscle relaxants, antiemetics, antihistamines, tricyclic antidepressants, and antispasmodics, are also likely to be taken by the elderly. The use of these drugs increases the burden of AM in older adults and may raise the risk of falls in the elderly. Finally, elderly patients may be more vulnerable to cognitive impairment and experience an exaggerated effect from AM drugs due to comorbid conditions such as Alzheimer's dementia, Parkinson's disease, cerebrovascular disease, and type 2 diabetes mellitus.

2.4.4. Phase III Clinical Data

None of the AM agents have shown statistically significant evidence of increased CNS events over placebo during phase III placebo-controlled clinical trials or head-to-head clinical trials. It should be mentioned that protocol visits are the means by which these CNS adverse events are collected, albeit uninvitedly. The small studies lack the power to discern a difference in the incidence of these reports between active agents and placebo, and the studies are conducted on a heterogeneous patient population, many of whom are not at high risk. Oxybutynin has been linked to cognitive impairment in the elderly, according to case studies and reports of what appears to be oxybutynin-induced delirium. Furthermore, there have been reports of tolterodine-related CNS case reports. Furthermore, no distinctions were found between immediate-release tolterodine, ER tolterodine, and extended-release (ER) oxybutynin twice daily in the head-to-head studies Overactive Bladder: Performance of Extended Release Agents (OPERA) and Overactive Bladder: Judging Effective Control and Treatment (OBJECT) regarding CNS effects recorded or nonelicited CNS adverse events during patient visits.

To evaluate the effectiveness, safety, and tolerability of darifenacin, Chapple and colleagues combined data on unintentional adverse events, including CNS events, from three sizable, multicenter, double-blind, placebo-controlled studies. Every single patient (N = 1049), who was over the age of 18, had experienced OAB for at least six months. CNS events in this group were comparable to placebo. Using uninvited adverse events, Staskin and colleagues showed that trospium chloride did not significantly differ from a placebo. Wagg and colleagues published a study on a cohort of elderly subjects over 65 years of age who received solifenacin administration. When compared to a placebo, they did not report any statistically significant CNS side effects.

The question of how to properly record pertinent BBB penetration, receptor binding, pharmacologic effect, and subclinical or clinical CNS changes arises if clinical phase III studies using an unsolicited CNS adverse events collection are not specific enough to elicit and analyze these events compared with placebo in a study population.

2.4.5. Sleep Studies for Potential CNS Effects

In a clinical context, the potential of AM agents used for OAB to influence the central nervous system has been assessed. Tests like electroencephalograms (EEG), sleep studies, reaction time tests, and more advanced imaging studies can be used to assess how a particular drug treatment affects receptor binding, brain activity, or cognitive function.

There is proof that AM compounds affect both the structure and quality of sleep based on sleep studies. Case reports of pavor nocturnus (night terror) following oxybutynin administration exist. The effects of trospium chloride, tolterodine, and oxybutynin on sleep parameters in healthy subjects were compared in two studies. The first study included young, healthy volunteers (ages 22 to 36). The second study included healthy participants over 50 years of age and had a similar design.

Following single doses of oxybutynin (15 mg), tolterodine (4 mg), trospium (45 mg), or placebo, polysomnographic recordings, sleep questionnaires, and psychometric tests (the number combination test and the d2 test of attention) were conducted. The main polysomnography parameter was the amount of rapid eye movement (REM) sleep relative to total sleep time. Compared to trospium chloride and placebo, oxybutynin significantly reduced the amount of REM sleep in young, healthy patients. It is noteworthy that no differences were found between the medications in the psychometric tests conducted during this study. In healthy young volunteers tested in some of these studies, the clinical significance was minimal, and it's possible that the findings couldn't be safely applied to the at-risk population.

In the second study, which included healthy participants over 50 years of age, the administration of oxybutynin and tolterodine resulted in a reduction in the median duration of REM sleep; however, the administration of trospium, when compared to placebo, did not significantly alter the duration of REM sleep. Subjective sleep metrics did not change significantly. The various medications had no effect on the quantity or quality of sleep. Once more, none of the study drugs had any effect on the volunteers' cognitive abilities. Compared to the younger patients, this group of patients experienced a more noticeable impairment of REM sleep following the administration of oxybutynin and tolterodine. However, the decrease in REM sleep in both trials did not become pathologically severe. Therefore, cognitive impairment was not anticipated. The next logical step would be to measure the effects of the various AM medications by administering these tests to elderly patients who already have sleep or cognitive impairments. Using this technique, the elderly patient population has not yet been studied.

2.4.6. EEG Studies for Potential CNS Side Effects

EEG data are frequently used as a physiological indicator of how drugs affect central nervous system function. In 1994, Pietzko and colleagues investigated potential CNS side effects of oral oxybutynin and oral and intravenous trospium chloride using quantitative assessment of the multichannel EEG from young, healthy volunteers. It was discovered that oxybutynin caused a noticeable and substantial power decrease in many EEG frequency bands. Trospium had no discernible effect on the EEG.

Trospium chloride, tolterodine, and oxybutynin are three AM medications whose possible CNS side effects were examined by Todorova and colleagues in 2001. Again, the participants were young, healthy volunteers who underwent three different tests: one at rest with their eyes open, one at rest with them closed, and one under mental pressure. Oxybutynin was found to cause notable alterations in EEG. There was a noticeable cumulative effect of the multiple doses administered; the difference from placebo became more noticeable after the second and third doses. On the other hand, following tolterodine and placebo administration, the EEG essentially stayed within the placebo range.

When darifenacin's EEG effects were investigated in healthy volunteers, they were discovered to be present, brief, and unrelated to any changes in cognitive function. Notably, the researchers deduced from the EEG alterations that brain activity linked to treatment-induced effects on dry mouth, vision, or bladder sensations.

2.4.7. Cognitive Studies for Potential CNS Effects

Around 150 healthy adults 60 years of age and above were randomly assigned to receive darifenacin, ER oxybutynin, or a placebo by Kay and colleagues. They used a series of computerized tests to evaluate cognitive function. The groups treated with darifenacin and placebo did not significantly differ in the delayed recall assessment; however, the group treated with oxybutynin ER had lower delayed recall scores. Interestingly, the subjects did not report any differences in memory between the medications when tested for self-rated memory. The authors explained this discrepancy as an extra risk factor for clinical screening in the absence of advanced testing, implying that the patients were impaired but were unaware of it. However, statistical changes might be a finding with little clinical significance in other quality-of-life studies involving OAB patients. Additionally, as an unsolicited adverse event, the rate of constipation with darifenacin over a 3-week period (7.5 mg, 15 mg) was observed to be 5 times higher (10/49 patients vs 2/50 patients) in this study, which is consistent with the selective M_3 activity of the agent, than in patients receiving oxybutynin ER (10 mg, 15 mg, 20 mg).

Darifenacin had no negative effects on the cognitive function of volunteers 65 years of age and older, according to research by Lipton and colleagues. In a different study, 400 patients older than 65 who received darifenacin treatment for 12 weeks saw similar outcomes. Once more, during the screening process for unwanted adverse events, no notable CNS side effects were observed. In a study, Perry and colleagues examined the postmortem brain morphology of patients older than 70 years who had been diagnosed with Parkinson's disease and were on AM medication. They concluded that, in comparison to patients who were untreated or receiving short-term treatment, those receiving long-term AM medication had amyloid plaque densities that were more than 2.5 times higher. Although these results have not been confirmed in other research, they have significant ramifications for how older adults, particularly those with Parkinson's disease, use AMs. Chronic AMs may not be suitable for elderly patients.

2.5. Adrenergic Drugs

Medications known as "adrenergic drugs" stimulate specific body nerves. They accomplish this by either inducing the release of norepinephrine and adrenaline or by imitating the action of these chemical messengers. These medications are used to treat a variety of potentially fatal illnesses, such as allergic reactions, asthma attacks, shock, and cardiac arrest.

2.5.1. Receptors

Adrenergic receptors are the target of directly acting adrenergic agonists. G-protein coupled adrenergic receptors all initiate signal transduction pathways. Adenylate cyclase or phospholipase C function can be influenced by the G-protein receptor; an agonist of the receptor will increase the effects on the downstream pathway, but not necessarily the pathway itself.

The receptors can be classified into two categories: α and β receptors. α-receptors are classified into two subclasses: α_1 and α_2, which are further separated into α_{1A}, α_{1B}, α_{1D}, α_{2A}, α_{2B}, and α_{2C}. Because of its higher homology with the α_2 class, the α_{2C} receptor was reclassified from the α_{1C} class, leading to the somewhat ambiguous nomenclature. There are three types of β receptors: β_1, β_2, and β_3. Though pharmacological selectivity for receptor subtypes exists and is crucial for the clinical use of adrenergic agonists (and, in fact, antagonists), the receptors are categorized physiologically.

Overall, α_1 receptors increase the activity of protein kinase C (PKC) by activating phospholipase C (via Gq); α_2 receptors inhibit the activity of protein kinase A (PKA) by activating adenylate cyclase (via Gi); and β receptors activate PKA via Gs. These downstream reactions are elicited by antagonists of each receptor class.

2.5.2. How Do They Work?

Adrenergic medications activate the sympathetic nervous system (SNS) of your body. This system assists in controlling how your body responds to emergencies or stress. The adrenal gland sends chemical messengers to the central nervous system (SNS) when under stress. Your body responds to these chemical messengers by speeding up breathing, sweating, and heart rate while slowing down digestion. This reaction is sometimes referred to as "fight or flight."

Adrenergic medications resemble the chemical messengers, such as norepinephrine and adrenaline, that your body releases when under stress. The messages from adrenaline and norepinephrine tell your body how to react, and they are received by specific regions known as adrenergic receptors. Adrenergic medications also have an effect on these receptors. They can bind to receptors and imitate norepinephrine and adrenaline, inducing the fight-or-flight response. Additionally, these medications have the ability to bind to receptors and cause the release of norepinephrine and adrenaline.

Adrenergic drugs can help do the following:

- increase blood pressure
- constrict blood vessels
- open the airways leading to the lungs
- increase heart rate
- stop bleeding

2.5.3. Types of Adrenergic Drugs and Their Uses

Depending on which receptors are targeted, different conditions are treated by different types of adrenergic drugs. Whether a medication acts as a chemical messenger directly or indirectly by inducing the release of chemical messengers will also determine its precise mode of action.

2.5.3.1. Bronchodilators

The bronchial tubes, or air passages, are made wider by bronchodilators. These adrenergic medications directly affect beta receptors. They open the airways that lead to the lungs when they bind to beta-2 receptors. This helps improve breathing in patients with respiratory diseases such as:

- asthma
- chronic obstructive pulmonary disease (COPD)
- emphysema
- bronchitis

Examples of bronchodilators include:

- albuterol
- formoterol
- levalbuterol
- olodaterol
- salmeterol

2.5.3.2. Vasopressors

The alpha-1, beta-1, and beta-2 adrenergic receptors are the sites of action for vasopressors. Moreover, they may function on dopamine receptors. These medications cause the blood vessels' smooth muscle contraction. Your blood vessels narrow as a result of this. Additionally, this effect raises your blood pressure.

Treating shock can involve raising blood pressure. Blood vessel narrowing can aid in halting bleeding. It can also prevent the spread of anesthetics, or medications that cause numbness in the body, by obstructing surrounding blood vessels.

Allergies and colds can also be treated with some vasopressors. They have the ability to reduce the enlarged blood vessels in your nasal mucous membranes. Oftentimes, these medications are referred to as nasal decongestants.

Examples of different vasopressors include:

- ephedrine
- epinephrine
- dopamine
- phenylephrine
- pseudoephedrine
- oxymetazoline

2.5.3.3. Cardiac Stimulators

The heartbeat can be stimulated and restored with the use of cardiac stimulators. They are used in cases of sudden cardiac arrest caused by drowning, suffocation, or electrocution. In such cases, an intracardiac injection of epinephrine can help your heart begin beating again. (Gerretsen & Pollock, 2011; Ehret & Chamberlin, 2015; Wiercinski & Jackson, 2022)

2.6. Adrenergic Blockers

Adrenergic receptor blockers may be considered in two groups:

- Drugs blocking the α adrenergic receptor
- Drugs blocking the β adrenergic receptor

These medications stop effector organs from responding to injected or naturally occurring sympathomimetic amines such as noradrenaline, adrenaline, and others. Catecholamines in circulation can be antagonistic more easily than they can be when sympathetic nerve stimulation is applied. The medications work by vying for the α or β receptors on the effector organs with catecholamines. They don't change how the substances are made or released.

2.6.1. Alpha Blocker

Pharmacological agents classified as alpha-blockers, also referred to as α-blockers or α-adrenoreceptor antagonists, function as antagonists on α-adrenergic receptors (α-adrenoceptors).

In the past, pharmacologic research employed alpha-blockers as a tool to gain a deeper comprehension of the autonomic nervous system. Researchers started characterizing central vasomotor control in the autonomic nervous system and arterial blood pressure using alpha-blockers. They are currently effective as clinical treatments for just a few ailments.

A limited number of conditions, including benign prostatic hyperplasia (BPH), erectile dysfunction, Raynaud's disease, and hypertension, can be treated with alpha-blockers. These medications usually work by attaching an α-blocker to smooth muscle and arterial α receptors. In the end, this relaxes the smooth muscle or blood vessels, increasing fluid flow in these entities, depending on the type of alpha receptor.

2.6.1.1. Classification

Without more explanation, the term "alpha blocker" can relate to α_1 or α_2 blockers, nonselective blockers (both α_1 and α_2 activity), or α blockers with some β activity. Nonetheless, α_1 blockers are typically the most prevalent kind of alpha blocker.

Non-selective α-adrenergic receptor antagonists include:

- Phenoxybenzamine
- Phentolamine
- Tolazoline
- Trazodone

Selective α_1-adrenergic receptor antagonists include:

- **Alfuzosin**
- **Doxazosin**
- **Prazosin (inverse agonist)**
- **Tamsulosin**
- **Terazosin**
- **Silodosin**

Selective α_2-adrenergic receptor antagonists include:

- Atipamezole
- Idazoxan
- Mirtazapine
- Yohimbine

Finally, the agents carvedilol and labetalol are both α and β-blockers.

2.6.1.2. Medical Uses

Although there are few clinical applications for α-blockers, most of which involve treating benign prostatic hyperplasia or hypertension, α-blockers can also be used to treat a few other conditions, including erectile dysfunction, Raynaud's disease, congestive heart failure (CHF), and pheochromocytoma.

Moreover, α-blockers are occasionally used to treat panic disorders and anxiety, including nightmares brought on by posttraumatic stress disorder (PTSD). Research has demonstrated significant interest in using alpha-blockers, particularly α_2 blockers, to treat mental depression and type II diabetes.

1. **Hypertension:** Vasoconstriction and increased vascular resistance are the causes of hypertension. Mild to moderate hypertension has been effectively treated with α1 selective antagonists like prazosin. This is due to their ability to lower blood pressure and vascular resistance. Although these medications are usually well tolerated, side effects like orthostatic hypotension and vertigo are possible. Alpha-blockers, on the other hand, have not shown the same mortality and morbidity benefits as other treatments for hypertension, such as ACE inhibitors, ARBs, calcium channel blockers, thiazide diuretics, or beta blockers. As a result, they are not typically used as first or even second-line agents.

Another option for treating hypertension is the use of drugs like Labetalol or carvedilol, which have both α_1 blocking and nonselective β activities. When taken in low doses, labetalol and carvedilol can lower peripheral resistance and counteract the effects of isoprenaline, helping to alleviate symptoms of hypertension.

2. **Pheochromocytoma:** A tumor that secretes catecholamines can develop into a phenochroma. Specifically, these tumors secrete adrenaline and norepinephrine either continuously or sporadically. Excessive catecholamine release stimulates the central nervous system, which raises vascular resistance in blood vessels and eventually results in hypertension. Patients who have these uncommon tumors also frequently experience headaches, palpitations in their hearts, and increased perspiration.

A nonselective α_1 and α_2 blocker, phenoxybenzamine, has been used to treat pheochromocytoma. By opposing the alpha receptors, this medication inhibits the effects of norepinephrine and adrenaline, lowering blood pressure overall, increasing vasodilation, and decreasing vascular resistance.

3. **Congestive Heart Failure:** Carvedilol, bucindolol, and labetalol are examples of blockers that can block both α and β receptors, which can help to lessen the symptoms of congestive heart failure. These medications work by binding to both the α and β receptors, which reduces cardiac output and increases blood vessel dilatation to lower blood pressure.

4. **Erectile Dysfunction:** Yohimbine, an α_2 blocker, has been tested to treat erectile dysfunction and increase libido. It is derived from the bark of the Pausinystalia johimbe tree. Yohimbine's suggested mechanism of action involves blocking adrenergic receptors, which are linked to the inhibition of neurotransmitters like dopamine and nitric oxide, thereby promoting libido and penile erection. They can then modify the flow of blood in the penis to help achieve an erection. However, there's a chance of experiencing some adverse effects, like anxiety, tremor, elevated blood pressure, and palpitations.

"α1 and α2 adrenergic receptors are blocked by alkaloids found in yohimbine bark."

Non-selective alpha-blockers like phentolamine have also been tried to treat erectile dysfunction. Penile erection appears to be aided by increased blood flow in the penis due to a reduction in vasoconstriction. Phentolamine side effects include nasal congestion, flushing, and headache.

5. **Benign Prostatic Hyperplasia:** Men with benign prostatic hyperplasia (BPH) have urinary obstruction, which makes it difficult for them to urinate and results in urine retention. It has been possible to relax the smooth muscle in the bladder and enlarged prostate by using α1 specific blockers. Patients with BPH have found particular benefit from doxazosin, terazosin, and prazosin, especially those who also have hypertension. These medications can treat both conditions concurrently in such patients. Tamsulosin can be used in patients without hypertension because it relaxes the smooth muscle in the bladder and prostate without significantly altering blood pressure.

6. **Raynaud's Disease:** The potential of α_1 and α_2 blockers as treatments for Raynaud's disease has been investigated. While α1 blockers, like prazosin, have shown some promise in improving the sclerotic symptoms associated with Raynaud's disease, using this medication comes with many side effects. On the other hand, α_2 blockers, like yohimbine, seem to significantly improve Raynaud's disease patients' sclerotic symptoms without having too many negative effects.

7. **Post-Traumatic Stress Disorder:** Even after taking medications designed specifically to treat posttraumatic stress disorder (PTSD), patients frequently still experience symptoms. In addition, even after receiving treatment, PTSD sufferers frequently experience incapacitating nightmares. Due to its ability to block norepinephrine's effects, high doses of the α1 blocker prazosin have proven effective in treating patients experiencing nightmares brought on by PTSD. When prazosin is used to treat PTSD nightmares, side effects might include fatigue, dizziness, nausea, weakness, and the first dose effect, which is a sudden loss of consciousness.

2.6.1.3. Adverse Effects

While some disease pathology can be reduced by alpha-blockers, these medications also have certain side effects. Nevertheless, each alpha-blocker has a unique set of side effects due to its various structural compositions. The first dose effect, cardiovascular side effects, genitourinary side effects, and other side effects can occur when taking alpha-blockers.

1. First dose effect

The first dose effect is among the most typical alpha blocker side effects. This phenomenon occurs when hypertension patients take an alpha blocker for the first time and notice a sharp drop in blood pressure. In the end, this results in a sharp drop in blood pressure, orthostatic hypotension, dizziness, and an abrupt loss of consciousness. These side effects are associated with alpha-blockers such as doxazosin, terazosin, and prazosin.

2. Cardiovascular side effects

Certain alpha-blockers have the potential to cause cardiovascular side effects, including the induction of reflex tachycardia, orthostatic hypotension, or palpitations of the heart through modifications to the QT interval. These side effects are possible with alpha-blockers such as yohimbine, phenoxybenzamine, and phentolamine.

3. Genitourinary side effects

When alpha-blockers are used to treat BPH, the blood vessels in the bladder and prostate dilate, which increases the need to urinate more frequently overall. Nevertheless, the exact opposite side effect—edema, or abnormal fluid retention—can also be brought on by these alpha-blockers.

Impotence and the inability to ejaculate are additional side effects that occur in men receiving treatment for benign prostatic hyperplasia (BPH) as a result of the prostate smooth muscle relaxing. When ejaculation does happen, though, it frequently leads to a condition known as retrograde ejaculation, in which semen enters the bladder rather than leaving through the urethra.

Medication that can cause these kinds of side effects includes doxazosin, prazosin, terazosin, and tamsulosin.

4. Other side effects

Lastly, the majority of alpha-blockers can also have other general side effects (though these occur more frequently in alpha-1 blockers). These adverse effects include dry mouth, psychiatric depression, weakness, drowsiness, and dizziness.

The use of alpha-blockers has been linked to pruritus, an uncomfortable, prolonged erection that lasts for several hours and is not caused by sexual arousal. Even though it's very uncommon, especially when using tamsulosin, it can result in irreversible impotence if left untreated in a hospital. This should be explained to male patients because it can happen after a single dose or develop gradually.

2.6.2. Beta Blocker

A class of drugs known as beta-blockers is primarily used to treat arrhythmias, or irregular heartbeats, and to prevent subsequent heart attacks by shielding the heart from damage after an initial attack (secondary prevention). They are also frequently used to treat high blood pressure, though most patients no longer choose them as their first line of treatment.

The endogenous catecholamines norepinephrine (noradrenaline) and epinephrine (adrenaline) mediate the fight-or-flight response by binding to adrenergic beta receptors of the sympathetic nervous system. This response is blocked by beta-blockers, which are competitive antagonists. Certain substances inhibit the activation of all β-adrenergic receptor types, while others exhibit selectivity towards one of the three recognized beta receptor types, identified as β_1, β_2, and β_3 receptors. The primary sites of β_1-adrenergic receptors are found in the kidneys and heart. The lungs, gastrointestinal tract, liver, uterus, vascular smooth muscle, and skeletal muscle are the primary locations of β_2-adrenergic receptors. Within fat cells are β_3-adrenergic receptors.

The sympathetic nervous system includes beta receptors on cells of the smooth muscle, heart, arteries, kidneys, and other tissues. These receptors can be stimulated by epinephrine (adrenaline), which can cause stress responses. The effects of stress hormones are lessened by beta-blockers because they prevent adrenaline and other stress hormones from binding to their receptors.

James Black created propranolol and pronethalol in 1964, which were the first clinically meaningful beta blockers. This groundbreaking discovery, which is regarded by many as one of the most significant contributions to clinical medicine and pharmacology of the 20th century, completely changed the way angina pectoris was treated medically.

Meta-analyses of studies that primarily used atenolol for the treatment of primary hypertension have demonstrated that while beta-blockers are more effective than placebo in preventing stroke and cardiovascular events overall, they are not as effective as diuretics, drugs that inhibit the renin-angiotensin system, or calcium channel blockers in treating primary hypertension.

2.6.2.1. Medical Uses

In addition to treating many other medical disorders, beta-blockers are used to treat many heart and vascular system disorders. Beta-blockers are widely used to treat many common heart conditions, such as angina pectoris, acute coronary syndromes, hypertension, and arrhythmias like atrial fibrillation and heart failure. They are also used to treat other heart conditions like dissecting aneurysm, hypertrophic obstructive cardiomyopathy, and mitral valve stenosis or prolapse. Furthermore, beta-blockers are used in vascular surgery, anxiety treatment, glaucoma, esophageal varices, thyrotoxicosis, and migraines.

1. Congestive heart failure

Studies conducted in the late 1990s demonstrated the effectiveness of beta-blockers in lowering morbidity and mortality, despite the fact that they were previously contraindicated in congestive heart failure due to their potential to exacerbate the condition by decreasing cardiac contractility. In congestive heart failure, bisoprolol, carvedilol, and sustained-release metoprolol are specifically recommended as adjuncts to standard ACE inhibitors and diuretic therapy, albeit usually at much lower doses than those recommended for other conditions. Only compensated, stable congestive heart failure is a good candidate for beta-blocker use; in acute decompensated heart failure, beta-blockers will worsen the patient's existing symptoms by further lowering the ejection fraction.

Although there are other important mechanisms of action for beta-blockers in congestive heart failure, their reductive effect on heart rate is the primary mechanism of action that is well-known. Apart from their sympatholytic β_1 action in the heart, beta-blockers also affect the renal renin-angiotensin system.

Beta-blockers lower renin secretion. This decreases extracellular volume, thereby lowering the workload of the heart and its oxygen requirements. Heart failure is typified by elevated catecholamine activity in the heart. This leads to many harmful outcomes, such as elevated oxygen demand, the spread of inflammatory mediators, and aberrant remodelling of the cardiac tissue, all of which reduce the effectiveness of cardiac contraction and lower the ejection fraction. Even though the ejection fraction initially decreases, beta-blockers eventually improve the ejection fraction by reducing this excessively high sympathetic activity.

Based on clinical trials, beta-blockers can lower the overall risk of death by 4.5% over a 13-month duration. The trials not only decreased the risk of death but also decreased the number of hospital visits and hospitalizations. Although there is little evidence to support the use of beta-blockers in children with congestive heart failure, a 2020 Cochrane review did find that they may be helpful based on the data that was available.

When administering beta-blockers therapeutically for congestive heart failure, the dose should be gradually increased starting at extremely low levels (1/8 of the target). The patient's heart must adapt to the decreasing stimulation of catecholamines by achieving a new balance at a lower adrenergic drive.

2. Acute myocardial infarction

Acute myocardial infarctions can be treated with beta-blockers. Circulating catecholamines rise as a result of systemic stress following a myocardial infarction. This raises blood pressure and heart rate, which raises the oxygen demand in the heart. By competitively inhibiting catecholamines that act on the β1-adrenergic receptors, beta-blockers mitigate these negative effects and lower the oxygen demand and consumption of the heart.

According to a 2019 Cochrane review, beta-blockers likely decreased the long-term risk of all-cause mortality and cardiovascular mortality as well as the short-term risk of reinfarction when compared to placebo or no intervention. According to the review, beta-blockers probably had negligible to no effect on cardiovascular and short-term all-cause mortality.

3. Hypertension

Many people use beta-blockers to treat hypertension. Non-selective beta-blockers reduced systolic and diastolic blood pressure in people with mild-to-moderate hypertension by −10/−7 mmHg without increasing the risk of adverse events, according to a 2014 Cochrane review. It was discovered that at higher dosages, there was a greater incidence of side effects, such as a drop-in heart rate, without a corresponding drop in blood pressure.

According to a 2017 Cochrane review, beta-blockers have a minor impact on cardiovascular disease but have little to no effect on mortality. This suggests that beta blockers' benefits are not as great as those of other anti-hypertensive drugs.

4. Anxiety

The United States Food and Drug Organization has not officially approved any beta-blocker for anxiety relief. Though the exact mode of action is unknown, numerous controlled trials conducted over the previous 25 years have shown that beta-blockers are helpful in treating anxiety disorders. Anxious people can focus on the task at hand because the physiological signs of the fight-or-flight response are greatly diminished.

Beta-blockers have been known to help performers such as musicians, actors, public speakers, and professional dancers prevent tremor, stage fright, and performance anxiety during public performances and auditions. The International Conference of Symphony Orchestra Musicians, which represents the 51 largest orchestras in the US, conducted a survey in 1987 and found that 27% of its musicians had used beta-blockers, with 70% of them obtaining them from friends rather than doctors. This study marked the first recognition of the application of beta-blockers to stage fright in the medical literature.

5. Surgery

The use of beta-blockers around the time of cardiac surgery may reduce the risk of atrial fibrillation and heart dysrhythmias, according to low certainty evidence. However, scheduling them at the same time as other surgeries could make the results worse. While there is moderate certainty evidence that using beta-blockers to prevent side effects may increase the risk of hypotension, there is very low certainty evidence that using them to prevent atrial fibrillation and myocardial infarctions may lower those risks. Beta-blockers used perioperatively in non-cardiac surgeries may raise the risk of bradycardia, according to low-certainty evidence.

2.6.2.2. Adverse Effects

Possible side effects of beta-blockers include nausea, diarrhea, bronchospasm, cold extremities, exacerbation of Raynaud's syndrome, bradycardia, hypotension, heart failure, heart block, fatigue, dizziness, hair loss, vision changes, hallucinations, insomnia, nightmares, sexual dysfunction, erectile dysfunction, and alterations in glucose and lipid metabolism. Orthostatic hypotension is commonly associated with mixed $\alpha 1/\beta$-antagonist therapy, while edema is a common side effect of carvedilol therapy. Lipophilic beta-blockers, like propranolol and metoprolol, may cause sleep disturbances due to their ability to penetrate the blood-brain barrier. Additional research is needed to support these claims.

Adverse effects associated with β_2-adrenergic receptor antagonist activity (bronchospasm, peripheral vasoconstriction, alteration of glucose and lipid metabolism) are less common with β_1-selective (often termed "cardioselective") agents, but receptor selectivity diminishes at higher doses. Beta blockade, especially of the beta-1 receptor at the macula densa, inhibits renin release, thus decreasing the release of aldosterone. This causes hyponatremia and hyperkalemia.

Because β_2-adrenoceptors normally stimulate the breakdown of glycogen (glycogenolysis) in the liver and the pancreatic release of the hormone glucagon, which work together to increase plasma glucose, hypoglycemia can occur with beta blockade. Thus, β_2-adrenoceptor blocking reduces plasma glucose. In diabetic patients, β_1-blockers have fewer metabolic side effects; however, they may mask the fast heart rate that is a warning sign of insulin-induced low blood sugar, leading to hypoglycemia unawareness. We refer to this as hypoglycemia unawareness induced by beta blockers. Beta-blockers should therefore be used with caution in diabetics.

According to a 2007 study, patients taking beta-blockers and diuretics for hypertension have a higher chance of developing diabetes mellitus, whereas patients taking ACE inhibitors and angiotensin II receptor antagonists (angiotensin receptor blockers) have a lower risk of the disease. Because of the risk of diabetes, clinical guidelines in Great Britain—but not in the United States—recommend against using beta-blockers and diuretics as the first line of treatment for hypertension.

It is not appropriate to treat selective alpha-adrenergic agonist overdose with beta-blockers. By preventing the alpha-adrenergic system from being stimulated, the blockade of solely beta receptors raises blood pressure, decreases coronary blood flow, left ventricular function, cardiac output, and tissue perfusion. Metoprolol and labetalol, two beta-blockers with lipophilic characteristics and CNS penetration, may be helpful in treating the CNS and cardiovascular toxicity resulting from a methamphetamine overdose. Labetalol, a mixed alpha- and beta-blocker, is particularly helpful in treating methamphetamine-induced concomitant tachycardia and hypertension. The phenomenon of "unopposed alpha stimulation" has not been reported with the use of beta-blockers for the treatment of methamphetamine toxicity. Other appropriate antihypertensive drugs to administer during hypertensive crisis resulting from stimulant overdose are vasodilators such as nitroglycerin, diuretics such as furosemide, and alpha-blockers such as phentolamine.

2.6.2.3. Pharmacology

1. **Intrinsic sympathomimetic activity**

This term, also known as the intrinsic sympathomimetic effect, is especially applied to beta blockers, which, depending on the concentration of the antagonized agent (usually an endogenous compound like norepinephrine) and the agent (beta blocker), can exhibit both agonism and antagonism at a given beta receptor. For a broader definition, see partial agonist.

There are several beta-blockers that show intrinsic sympathomimetic activity (ISA), including acebutolol, labetalol, penbutolol, oxprenolol, and pindolol. These substances have the ability to function as both a receptor site antagonist and a low-level agonist at the β-adrenergic receptor. Therefore, these drugs might be helpful for people on long-term beta-blocker therapy who are experiencing excessive bradycardia. Patients with any form of angina should not use agents containing ISA because they may worsen their condition or cause myocardial infarctions. Additionally, they might not be as successful in treating angina and tachyarrhythmia as other beta-blockers are.

2. **β-Adrenergic receptor antagonism**

The heart experiences a positive chronotropic and inotropic effect when β_1 receptors are stimulated by adrenaline and norepinephrine, which also raises cardiac conduction velocity and automaticity. Renin is released when the kidney's β_1 receptors are stimulated. β_2 receptor stimulation results in increased glycogenolysis in the liver and skeletal muscle, tremor in skeletal muscle, and relaxation of smooth muscle. Lipolysis is induced by β_3 receptor stimulation.

While they have little effect on subjects who are at rest, beta-blockers inhibit these typical sympathetic actions mediated by adrenaline and norepinephrine. In other words, they lessen the impact of excitement or physical exertion on heart rate, contraction force, tremor, and glycogen breakdown. Beta-blockers may constrict the bronchi in the lungs, potentially exacerbating or triggering symptoms of asthma.

Beta-blockers have the potential to cause vasoconstriction because β_2 adrenergic receptors can cause vascular smooth muscle dilation. The activity of β_2 receptors is often overshadowed by the more prevalent α1 receptors, which constrict blood vessels, therefore this effect is usually minimal. The heart continues to experience beta blockers' greatest effects. Third-generation beta blockers, which are more recent, can block alpha-adrenergic receptors, resulting ivasodilation.

Thus, antihypertensive effects of nonselective beta-blockers are anticipated. Though their main antihypertensive mechanism is unknown, beta-blockers may work by decreasing cardiac output (because of their negative inotropic and chronotropic effects). It might also result from a decrease in the kidneys' production of renin and a decrease in sympathetic activity caused by the central nervous system (for beta-blockers like propranolol that do cross the blood-brain barrier).

Negative chronotropic and inotropic effects reduce cardiac workload and oxygen demand, resulting in antianginal effects. The life-saving ability of beta-blockers to regulate heart rate is made possible by their negative chronotropic properties. In many pathologic states, beta-blockers can be easily titrated to achieve optimal rate control.

The sympathetic nervous system blockade that results in prolonged atrial refractory periods, depression of sinus node function and atrioventricular node conduction is the source of beta blockers' antiarrhythmic effects. Specifically, sotalol blocks potassium channels to lengthen action potential duration and possesses additional antiarrhythmic effects.

Reduced aldosterone via the renin-angiotensin-aldosterone pathway results from blocking the sympathetic nervous system's release of renin, which lowers blood pressure by reducing the retention of water and salt.

3. α1-Adrenergic receptor antagonism

Certain beta-blockers (e.g. carvedilol and labetalol) show mixed antagonistic activity against both β- and α_1-adrenergic receptors, resulting in an extra dose of arteriolar vasodilation.

4. Blood–brain barrier permeability

Different beta-blockers have different levels of lipophilicity, or fat solubility, which affects their capacity to penetrate the blood–brain barrier and influence the central nervous system. Increased blood-brain barrier permeability in beta-blockers can have negative cognitive effects in addition to therapeutic benefits and side effects related to neuropsychiatry. Beta-blockers may cause side effects and risks related to the central nervous system, such as depression, delirium, psychosis, insomnia, nightmares, fatigue, and visual hallucinations. They may also increase the risk of falling. On the other hand, beta-blockers may benefit the central nervous system by preventing or treating migraine, essential tremor, akathisia, anxiety, PTSD, aggression, and obsessive-compulsive disorder.

A few exceptions exist, but most beta-blockers are lipophilic and can enter the brain. Penbutolol, pindolol, propranolol, and timolol are examples of highly lipophilic beta blockers. Acebutolol, betaxolol, bisoprolol, carvedilol, metoprolol, and nebivolol are examples of moderately lipophilic beta blockers. Atenolol, carteolol, esmolol, labetalol, nadolol, and sotalol are examples of low lipophilicity or hydrophilic beta blockers. It is believed that beta-blockers with a high lipophilicity can enter the brain easily, while those with a moderate lipophilicity can enter the brain less easily, and those with a low lipophilicity or hydrophilicity can enter the brain very little. It is known that lipophilic beta-blockers can reduce melatonin release by 50–80%. Additionally, the β1-adrenergic receptor selectivity (or cardioselectivity) and intrinsic sympathomimetic activity of the previous beta-blockers differ, leading to further variations in their pharmacological profiles and suitability in various contexts. (Gerretsen & Pollock, 2011; Ehret & Chamberlin, 2015; Wiercinski & Jackson, 2022)

A Closer Look

Bethanechol – Clinical Pharmacology

The main way that bethanechol chloride works is by stimulating the parasympathetic nervous system. It raises the detrusor urinae muscle tone, which typically results in a contraction strong enough to start micturition and empty the bladder. It raises stomach tone, promotes gastric motility, and frequently improves irregular peristalsis.

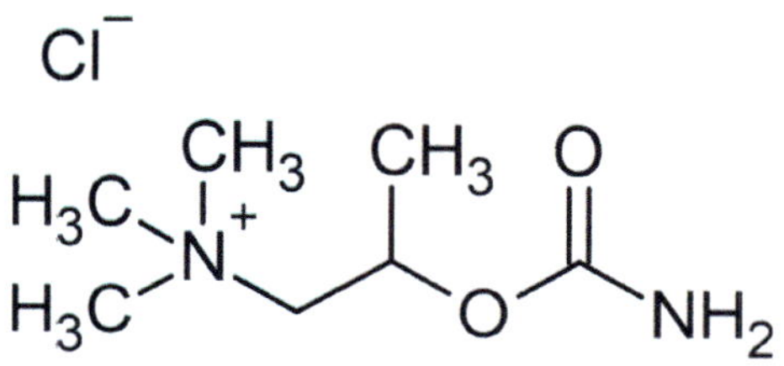

Acetylcholine is released at the nerve ends upon stimulation of the parasympathetic nervous system. Acetylcholine can be administered when spontaneous stimulation is reduced and therapeutic intervention is necessary, but its effects are temporary because cholinesterase quickly hydrolyzes it. Unlike acetylcholine, bethanechol chloride has longer-lasting effects and is not degraded by cholinesterase.

When bethanechol chloride is taken orally, effects on the gastrointestinal and urinary tracts can occasionally be felt within 30 minutes, but it usually takes 60 to 90 minutes to become fully effective. Betanechol chloride typically takes an hour to take effect when taken orally, but high doses (300–400 mg) have been known to have effects that last up to six hours. When the drug is administered subcutaneously, it acts on the bladder muscle more forcefully than when it is taken orally.

When administered orally or subcutaneously in therapeutic doses, bethanechol chloride's selective action usually results in muscarinic effects that are prominent, while nicotinic symptoms of cholinergic stimulation are either absent or very minimal. Following a subcutaneous injection, the effects of muscarinic agents typically manifest five to fifteen minutes later, peak fifteen to thirty minutes later, and then fade away in two hours. Usually, doses that promote micturition, defecation, and increased peristalsis do not activate voluntary muscles or ganglia. In healthy human subjects, therapeutic test doses have minimal impact on peripheral circulation, blood pressure, or heart rate.

Because bethanechol chloride contains a charged quaternary amine moiety, it is unable to pass through the blood-brain barrier. It is unknown how quickly the medication is metabolized or excreted.

A clinical trial compared the effectiveness of oral and subcutaneous doses of bethanechol chloride in stimulating the stretch response of bladder muscles in patients with urinary retention. The results indicated that a subcutaneous dose of 5 mg produced a faster and stronger response compared to oral doses of 50 mg, 100 mg, or 200 mg. However, the oral doses had a longer-lasting effect than the subcutaneous dose. While the 50 mg oral dose did not significantly impact intravesical pressure in this study, it has been shown to be effective in rehabilitating patients with decompensated bladders in other research.

Summary

- The nervous system controls all the major functions of the body. It is divided into central and peripheral nervous systems. The peripheral nervous system includes the somatic and autonomic nervous systems which control voluntary and involuntary functions respectively.
- Noradrenaline is the neurotransmitter released by post ganglionic sympathetic nerves to elicit its effect on effectors cells. The post-ganglionic sympathetic fibers are called noradrenergic or adrenergic.
- The parasympathetic nervous system is one of the targets of autonomic drugs. By inhibiting or stimulating this nervous system, therapeutic effects can be achieved.
- Cholinergic medications are a category of pharmaceutical agents that act upon the neurotransmitter acetylcholine, the primary neurotransmitter within the parasympathetic nervous system (PNS).
- Cholinergic medications are useful for a variety of medical conditions. Healthcare professionals, including pharmacists and nurses, need to be aware of the common adverse effects of cholinergic medications.
- Anticholinergic medications are used to manage and treat a wide range of diseases. This activity illustrates the indications, action, and contraindications for anticholinergic drugs as valuable agents in managing cholinergic toxicity, urinary incontinence, Parkinson's disease, respiratory disorders, cardiovascular disease, and numerous other diseases.
- The current standard of care for older patients with overactive bladder (OAB) is a combination of behavioral and pharmacologic therapy.

References

1. Abdel-Rahman, A., Abou-Donia, S. M., El-Masry, E. M., et al. (2004). Stress and combined exposure to low doses of pyridostigmine bromide, DEET, and permethrin produce neurochemical and neuropathological alterations in cerebral cortex, hippocampus, and cerebellum. *Journal of Toxicology and Environmental Health, Part A, 67*(2), 163–192. https://doi.org/10.1080/15287390490255195.
2. Abrams, P., Andersson, K. E., Buccafusco, J. J., Chapple, C., de Groat, W. C., Fryer, A. D., Kay, G., Laties, A., Nathanson, N. M., Pasricha, P. J., & Wein, A. J. (2006). Muscarinic receptors: Their distribution and function in body systems, and the implications for treating overactive bladder. *British Journal of Pharmacology, 148*(5), 565–578. https://doi.org/10.1038/sj.bjp.0706749.
3. Abrams, P., Cardozo, L., Fall, M., Griffiths, D., Rosier, P., Ulmsten, U., Van Kerrebroeck, P., Victor, A., Wein, A., & Standardization Sub-Committee of the International Continence Society. (2003). The standardization of terminology in lower urinary tract function: Report from the Standardization Sub-Committee of the International Continence Society. *Urology, 61*(1), 37–49. https://doi.org/10.1016/S0090-4295(02)02243-9.
4. Adeyinka, A., & Kondamudi, N. P. (2023). Cholinergic crisis. In *StatPearls* [Internet]. StatPearls Publishing. Retrieved from: https://www.statpearls.com (accessed on 30 July 2024).
5. Anagnostaras, S. G., Murphy, G. G., Hamilton, S. E., et al. (2003). Selective cognitive dysfunction in acetylcholine M1 muscarinic receptor mutant mice. *Nature Neuroscience, 6*(1), 51–58. https://doi.org/10.1038/nn985.

6. Andersson, K. E. (2002). Bladder activation: Afferent mechanisms. *Urology, 59*(Suppl 5A), 43–50. https://doi.org/10.1016/S0090-4295(02)02171-2.

7. Andersson, K. E., & Yoshida, M. (2003). Antimuscarinics and the overactive detrusor: Which is the main mechanism of action? *European Urology, 43*, 1–5. https://doi.org/10.1016/S0302-2838(02)00387-5.

8. Antonijevic, E., Kotur-Stevuljevic, J., Musilek, K., Kosvancova, A., Kuca, K., Djukic-Cosic, D., Spasojevic-Kalimanovska, V., & Antonijevic, B. (2018). Effect of six oximes on acutely anticholinesterase inhibitor-induced oxidative stress in rat plasma and brain. *Archives of Toxicology, 92*(2), 745–757. https://doi.org/10.1007/s00204-017-2061-4.

9. Appell, R. A., Chancellor, M. B., Zobrist, R. H., et al. (2003). Pharmacokinetics, metabolism, and saliva output during transdermal and extended-release oral oxybutynin administration in healthy subjects. *Mayo Clinic Proceedings, 78*(6), 696–702. https://doi.org/10.4065/78.6.696.

10. Arsura, E. L., Brunner, N. G., Namba, T., & Grob, D. (1987). Adverse cardiovascular effects of anticholinesterase medications. *American Journal of Medical Sciences, 293*(1), 18–23. https://doi.org/10.1097/00000441-198701000-00005.

11. Assis, C. R. D., Linhares, A. G., Cabrera, M. P., Oliveira, V. M., Silva, K. C. C., Marcuschi, M., Maciel Carvalho, E. V. M., Bezerra, R. S., & Carvalho, L. B. (2018). Erythrocyte acetylcholinesterase as a biomarker of pesticide exposure: New and forgotten insights. *Environmental Science and Pollution Research International, 25*(19), 18364–18376. https://doi.org/10.1007/s11356-018-1793-5.

12. Broderick, E. D., Metheny, H., & Crosby, B. (2023). Anticholinergic toxicity. In *StatPearls* [Internet]. StatPearls Publishing. Retrieved from: https://www.statpearls.com (accessed on 30 July 2024).

13. Campbell, N. L., Boustani, M. A., Lane, K. A., Gao, S., Hendrie, H., Khan, B. A., Murrell, J. R., Unverzagt, F. W., Hake, A., Smith-Gamble, V., & Hall, K. (2010). Use of anticholinergics and the risk of cognitive impairment in an African American population. *Neurology, 75*(2), 152–159. https://doi.org/10.1212/WNL.0b013e3181e52660.

14. Chew, M. L., Mulsant, B. H., Pollock, B. G., Lehman, M. E., Greenspan, A., Mahmoud, R. A., Kirshner, M. A., Sorisio, D. A., Bies, R. R., & Gharabawi, G. (2008). Anticholinergic activity of 107 medications commonly used by older adults. *Journal of the American Geriatrics Society, 56*(7), 1333–1341. https://doi.org/10.1111/j.1532-5415.2008.01782.x.

15. Clissold, S. P., & Heel, R. C. (1985). Transdermal hyoscine (scopolamine). A preliminary review of its pharmacodynamic properties and therapeutic efficacy. *Drugs, 29*(3), 189–207. https://doi.org/10.2165/00003495-198529030-00001.

16. De Wilde, S., Carey, I. M., Harris, T., Richards, N., Victor, C., Hilton, S. R., & Cook, D. G. (2007). Trends in potentially inappropriate prescribing amongst older UK primary care patients. *Pharmacoepidemiology and Drug Safety, 16*(6), 658–667. https://doi.org/10.1002/pds.1307.

17. D'hoedt, D., & Bertrand, D. (2009). Nicotinic acetylcholine receptors: An overview on drug discovery. *Expert Opinion on Therapeutic Targets, 13*(4), 395–411. https://doi.org/10.1517/14728220902853515.

18. Ehret, M. J., & Chamberlin, K. W. (2015). Current practices in the treatment of Alzheimer's disease: Where is the evidence after the phase III trials? *Clinical Therapeutics, 37*(8), 1604–1616. https://doi.org/10.1016/j.clinthera.2015.06.010.

19. Gerretsen, P., & Pollock, B. G. (2011). Drugs with anticholinergic properties: A current perspective on use and safety. *Expert Opinion on Drug Safety, 10*(5), 751–765. https://doi.org/10.1517/14740338.2011.596206.

20. Gorecki, L., Korabecny, J., Musilek, K., Nepovimova, E., Malinak, D., Kucera, T., Dolezal, R., Jun, D., Soukup, O., & Kuca, K. (2017). Progress in acetylcholinesterase reactivators and in the treatment of organophosphorus intoxication: A patent review (2006-2016). *Expert Opinion on Therapeutic Patents, 27*(9), 971–985. https://doi.org/10.1080/13543776.2017.1354841.

21. Gosens, R., & Gross, N. (2018). The mode of action of anticholinergics in asthma. *European Respiratory Journal, 52*(4). https://doi.org/10.1183/13993003.00797-2018.

22. Griebling, T. L. (2014). Re: Anticholinergic drug use, serum anticholinergic activity, and adverse drug events among older people: A population-based study. *Journal of Urology, 192*(2), 490. https://doi.org/10.1016/j.juro.2014.04.033.

23. Guay, D. R., & New, K. (2002). Poster presented at the 37th Annual Meeting of the American Society of Health-System Pharmacists. Atlanta, GA: December 8–12, 2002.

24. Haga, T. (2013). Molecular properties of muscarinic acetylcholine receptors. *Proceedings of the Japan Academy, Series B: Physical and Biological Sciences, 89*(6), 226–256. https://doi.org/10.2183/pjab.89.226.

25. Hegde, S. S., & Eglen, R. M. (1999). Muscarinic receptor subtypes modulating smooth muscle contractility in the urinary bladder. *Life Sciences, 64*(5), 419–428. https://doi.org/10.1016/S0024-3205(98)00716-0.

26. Houzé, P., Berthin, T., Raphalen, J. H., Hutin, A., & Baud, J. F. (2018). High dose of pralidoxime reverses paraoxon-induced respiratory toxicity in mice. *Turkish Journal of Anesthesiology and Reanimation, 46*(2), 131–138. https://doi.org/10.5152/TJAR.2018.52822.

27. Korsten, M. A., Lyons, B. L., Radulovic, M., Cummings, T. M., Sikka, G., Singh, K., Hobson, J. C., Sabiev, A., Spungen, A. M., & Bauman, W. A. (2018). Delivery of neostigmine and glycopyrrolate by iontophoresis: A nonrandomized study in individuals with spinal cord injury. *Spinal Cord, 56*(3), 212–217. https://doi.org/10.1038/s41393-017-0028-1.

28. Lott, E. L., & Jones, E. B. (2022). Cholinergic toxicity. In *StatPearls* [Internet]. StatPearls Publishing. Retrieved from: https://www.statpearls.com (accessed on 30 July 2024).

29. Malinak, D., Nepovimova, E., Jun, D., Musilek, K., & Kuca, K. (2018). Novel group of AChE reactivators—Synthesis, in vitro reactivation, and molecular docking study. *Molecules, 23*(9). https://doi.org/10.3390/molecules23092312.

30. Messer, W. S. Jr., Bohnett, M., & Stibbe, J. (1990). Evidence for a preferential involvement of M1 muscarinic receptors in representational memory. *Neuroscience Letters, 116*, 184–189. https://doi.org/10.1016/0304-3940(90)90223-6.

31. Miller, C. A. (2002). Anticholinergics: The good and the bad. *Geriatric Nursing, 23*(5), 286–287. https://doi.org/10.1067/mgn.2002.129387.

32. Milsom, I., Abrams, P., Cardozo, L., Roberts, R. G., Thüroff, J., & Wein, A. J. (2001). How widespread are the symptoms of an overactive bladder and how are they managed? A population-based prevalence study. *BJU International, 87*(9), 760–766. https://doi.org/10.1046/j.1464-410x.2001.02204.x.

33. Mirakhur, R. K., & Dundee, J. W. (1981). Glycopyrrolate. *General Pharmacology, 12*(6), 423–427. https://doi.org/10.1016/0306-3623(81)90052-5.

34. Ohbe, H., Jo, T., Matsui, H., Fushimi, K., & Yasunaga, H. (2018). Cholinergic crisis caused by cholinesterase inhibitors: A retrospective nationwide database study. *Journal of Medical Toxicology, 14*(3), 237–241. https://doi.org/10.1007/s13181-018-0677-3.

35. Pak, R. W., Petrou, S. P., & Staskin, D. (2003). Tropism chloride: A quaternary amine with unique pharmacological properties. *Current Urology Reports, 4*(5), 436–440. https://doi.org/10.1007/s11934-003-0015-1.

36. Pakulski, C., Drobnik, L., & Millo, B. (2000). Age and sex as factors modifying the function of the blood-cerebrospinal fluid barrier. *Medical Science Monitor, 6*(3), 314–318. https://doi.org/10.12659/MSM.923583.

37. Patel, P., Saab, H., & Aboeed, A. (2023). Ipratropium. In *StatPearls* [Internet]. StatPearls Publishing. Retrieved from: https://www.statpearls.com (accessed on 30 July 2024).

38. Pepeu, G., & Giovannini, M. G. (2009). Cholinesterase inhibitors and beyond. *Current Alzheimer Research, 6*(2), 86–96. https://doi.org/10.2174/156720509787846688.

39. Peters, N. L. (1989). Snipping the thread of life: Antimuscarinic side effects of medications in the elderly. *Archives of Internal Medicine, 149*(11), 2414–2420. https://doi.org/10.1001/archinte.1989.00390060064007.

40. Roe, C. M., Anderson, M. J., & Spivack, B. (2002). Use of anticholinergic medications by older adults with dementia. *Journal of the American Geriatrics Society, 50*(5), 836–842. https://doi.org/10.1046/j.1532-5415.2002.50206.x.

41. Ruggieri, M. R. Sr., & Braverman, A. S. (2006). Regulation of bladder muscarinic receptor subtypes by experimental pathologies. *Autonomic & Autacoid Pharmacology, 26*, 311–325. https://doi.org/10.1111/j.1474-8660.2006.00225.x.

42. Schweitzer, P., & Mark, H. (1980). The effect of atropine on cardiac arrhythmias and conduction. Part 1. *American Heart Journal, 100*(1), 119–127. https://doi.org/10.1016/0002-8703(80)90273-0.

43. Sicari, V., & Zabbo, C. P. (2023). Diphenhydramine. In *StatPearls* [Internet]. StatPearls Publishing. Retrieved from: https://www.statpearls.com (accessed on 30 July 2024).

44. Starr, J. M., Wardlaw, J., Ferguson, K., et al. (2003). Increased blood-brain barrier permeability in type II diabetes demonstrated by gadolinium magnetic resonance imaging. *Journal of Neurology, Neurosurgery, and Psychiatry, 74*(1), 70–76. https://doi.org/10.1136/jnnp.74.1.70.

45. Stewart, W. F., Van Rooyen, J. B., Cundiff, G. W., Abrams, P., & Herzog, A. R. (2003). Prevalence and burden of overactive bladder in the United States. *World Journal of Urology, 20*, 327–336. https://doi.org/10.1007/s00345-002-0270-8.

46. Van de Waterbeemd, H., Camenisch, G., Folkers, G., et al. (1998). Estimation of blood-brain barrier crossing of drugs using molecular size and shape, and H-bonding descriptors. *Journal of Drug Targeting, 6*(3), 151–155. https://doi.org/10.3109/10611869808997480.

47. Vanova, N., Pejchal, J., Herman, D., Dlabkova, A., & Jun, D. (2018). Oxidative stress in organophosphate poisoning: Role of standard antidotal therapy. *Journal of Applied Toxicology, 38*(8), 1058–1070. https://doi.org/10.1002/jat.3625.

48. Volpicelli, L. A., & Levey, A. I. (2004). Muscarinic acetylcholine receptor subtypes in cerebral cortex and hippocampus. *Progress in Brain Research, 145*, 59–66. https://doi.org/10.1016/S0079-6123(03)45005-0.

49. Wiercinski, A., & Jackson, J. P. (2022). Nerve agents. In *StatPearls* [Internet]. StatPearls Publishing. Retrieved from: https://www.statpearls.com (accessed on 30 July 2024).

Chapter 3

CARDIOVASCULAR-RENAL DRUGS

Contents

Introduction

Cardiovascular diseases were once thought to be serious health issues, mostly in Western countries. Nevertheless, developing nations like Ethiopia are also experiencing a rise in the prevalence of cardiovascular diseases. Heart arrhythmias, angina pectoris, congestive heart failure, and hypertension are the most common cardiovascular conditions. This chapter covers the pharmacology of the majority of medications currently on the market since they can lower the morbidity and mortality caused by these disorders.

Orientation and Directional Terms

Term	Definition	Illustration
Cardiovascular diseases (CVDs)	Cardiovascular diseases (CVDs) are the leading cause of death globally, taking an estimated 17.9 million lives each year. CVDs are a group of disorders of the heart and blood vessels and include coronary heart disease, cerebrovascular disease, rheumatic heart disease and other conditions.	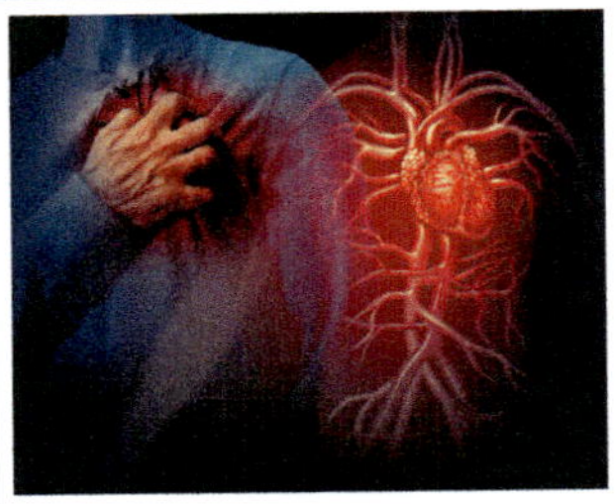
Hypertension	Hypertension (high blood pressure) is when the pressure in your blood vessels is too high (140/90 mmHg or higher). It is common but can be serious if not treated. People with high blood pressure may not feel symptoms.	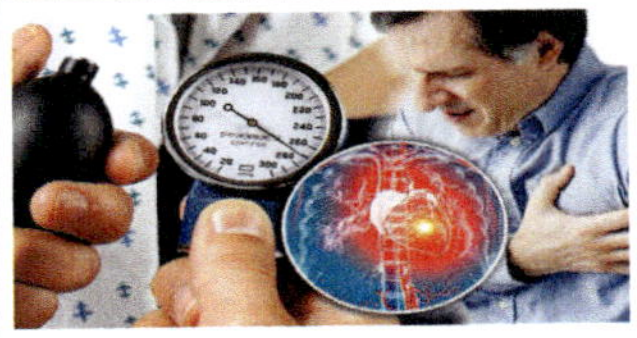
Angiotensin-converting enzyme	Angiotensin-converting enzyme is a central component of the renin–angiotensin system (RAS), which controls blood pressure by regulating the volume of fluids in the body. It converts the hormone angiotensin I to the active vasoconstrictor angiotensin II. Therefore, ACE indirectly increases blood pressure by causing blood vessels to constrict. ACE inhibitors are widely used as pharmaceutical drugs for treatment of cardiovascular diseases.	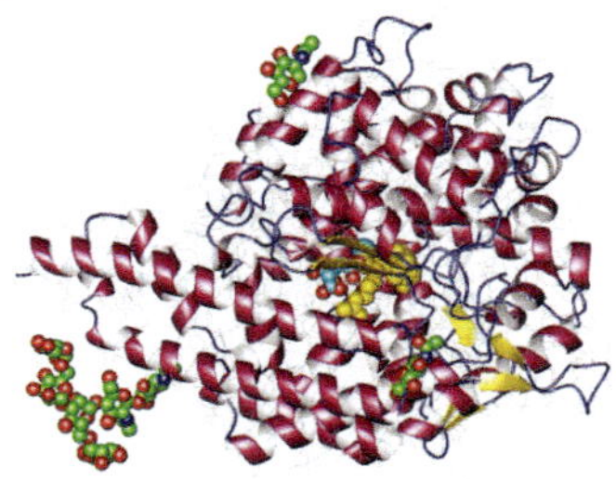
Hydrochlorothiazide	Hydrochlorothiazide is a medication approved by the U.S. Food and Drug Administration (FDA) to treat hypertension and peripheral edema. Hydrochlorothiazide is a thiazide-type diuretic that inhibits sodium resorption in the distal convoluted tubules of the kidney.	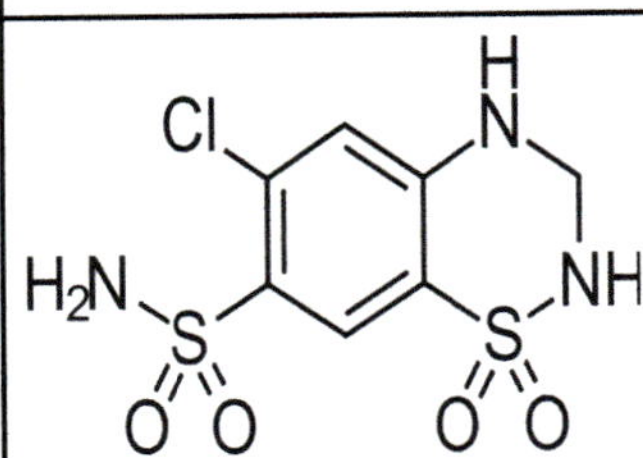
Body mass index	Body mass index is a value derived from the mass and height of a person. The BMI is defined as the body mass divided by the square of the body height, and is expressed in units of kg/m^2, resulting from mass in kilograms and height in metres	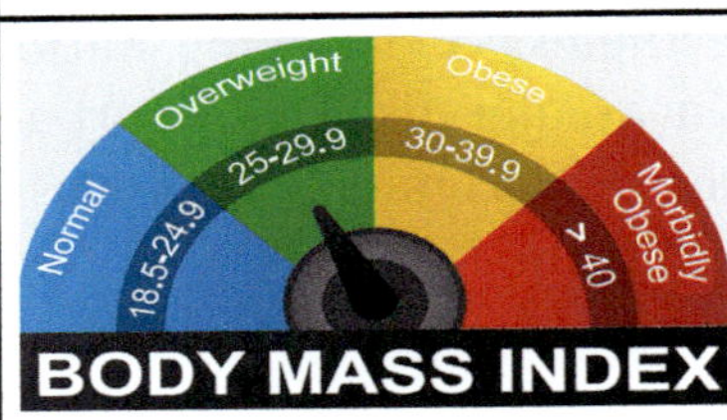

3.1. Antihypertensive Drugs

A class of medications known as antihypertensives is used to treat hypertension or high blood pressure. The goal of antihypertensive medication is to avert high blood pressure-related problems like myocardial infarction, heart failure, stroke, and kidney failure. Research indicates that a 5 mmHg drop in blood pressure can lower the risk of stroke by 34% and ischemic heart disease by 21%. It can also lessen the chance of heart failure, dementia, and cardiovascular disease-related death. Antihypertensives come in a variety of classes and reduce blood pressure in various ways. Angiotensin II receptor antagonists (ARBs), calcium channel blockers, ACE inhibitors, beta-blockers, and thiazide diuretics are some of the most significant and commonly used drugs.

Numerous extensive studies have been conducted on the best initial medication for hypertension, leading to national guidelines. Preventing the major endpoints of hypertension, such as heart attacks, strokes, and heart failure, should be the main objective of treatment. The age of the patient, any coexisting medical conditions, and end-organ damage all influence the kind and dosage of medication that is given. The various classes of antihypertensives vary in price, capacity to prevent endpoints, and adverse effect profiles. The decision to use more costly agents when less expensive ones would be just as effective could have a detrimental effect on the country's healthcare budget. As of 2018, when medication is required to treat high blood pressure, low-dose thiazide diuretics are the preferred first-line treatment. Clinical evidence suggests that thiazide-type diuretics and calcium channel blockers are the most effective initial treatments for the majority of patients, both in terms of cost and efficacy. However, NICE in the UK recommends ACE inhibitors for patients under the age of 55.

3.1.1. Indications

One of the main factors contributing to an increase in cardiovascular disease is thought to be hypertension (HTN).

HTN stages are defined as follows by the American College of Cardiology (ACC) and the American Heart Association (AHA) in 2017:

- Normal blood pressure (BP): systolic BP is less than 120, and diastolic BP is less than 80.
- Elevated BP: systolic BP is 120 to 130, and diastolic BP is less than 80.
- Stage 1 HTN: systolic BP 130 to 139 or diastolic BP 80 to 89.
- Stage 2 HTN: systolic BP at least 140 or diastolic at least 90.
- Hypertensive crises: systolic BP over 180 and/or diastolic BP over 120

According to the 2019 ACC/AHA Guideline on the Primary Prevention of Cardiovascular Disease, lifestyle changes such as weight loss, a diet low in sodium, increased physical activity, and moderation in alcohol consumption should be the first line of treatment for all patients with elevated blood pressure. Low carbohydrate diets are also effective at lowering blood pressure, especially in overweight or obese adults with hypertension.

- To prevent cardiovascular events in patients with stage 1 HTN, antihypertensive medication should be started if the patient has a 10-year atherosclerotic cardiovascular disease (ASCVD) risk of 10% or higher and a target blood pressure of less than 130/80. Patients with stage 1 hypertension and a risk of less than 10% for ASCVD over the next 10 years are advised to adopt lifestyle modification strategies.

- Even if the 10-year ASCVD risk is less than 10%, all patients with stage 2 HTN should begin taking antihypertensive medications to lower their blood pressure to a target lower than 130/80 mm Hg.
- In patients with chronic kidney disease, the target BP is 130/80.
- Antihypertensive drugs should be started for patients with type 2 diabetes mellitus (T2DM) if their blood pressure is higher than 130/80 mm Hg, with the end goal of lowering blood pressure below 130/80 mm Hg.
- Treatment for hypertension with antihypertensive medications typically begins with monotherapy when conservative management with lifestyle modification fails. When patients do not respond to monotherapy, combination therapy is frequently used.
- It has been demonstrated that keeping a systolic blood pressure of less than 130 mm Hg can prevent complications in patients with heart failure, diabetes, coronary artery disease, stroke, and other cardiovascular diseases. Lowering blood pressure does reduce the risks associated with cardiovascular disease. Age and race have an impact on the response to initial monotherapy.

There are multiple classes of antihypertensive medications used for the treatment of HTN; the most recommended classes used as first-line for treatment are:

- Thiazide-type diuretics
- Calcium channel blockers
- Angiotensin-converting enzyme (ACE) inhibitors and angiotensin II receptor blockers (ARBs)

3.1.1.1. Thiazide Diuretics

In JNC8 guidelines, thiazide diuretics can be used as the first-line treatment for hypertension (either alone or in combination with other antihypertensives) in all age groups, regardless of race, unless the patient has evidence of chronic kidney disease, in which case an angiotensin-converting enzyme inhibitor or angiotensin II receptor blocker is indicated. Thiazide and thiazide-like diuretics are typically the first line of treatment for hypertension.

Unless there are contraindications, the Antihypertensive and Lipid-Lowering Treatment to Prevent Heart Attack Trial ALLHAT study advised thiazide diuretics as the first line of treatment for hypertension.

There was no indication that the use of hydrochlorothiazide as a single agent, at a dose of 12.5mg or 25mg would reduce morbidity or death.

Studies reveal that thiazide-type diuretics, such as indapamide and chlorthalidone, are more effective and less expensive in preventing heart disease. They should be used as the first line of treatment for hypertension. Chlorthalidone and indapamide, thiazide-like diuretics, are more effective than hydrochlorothiazide in treating hypertension, according to numerous studies. When compared to hydrochlorothiazide, they are more effective at lowering the risk of cardiovascular disease.

The recommended medication to begin treating hypertension as a monotherapy is chlorthalidone. According to studies, it's the best diuretic for lowering blood pressure, preventing death, and reducing morbidity. When researchers tracked 24-hour ambulatory blood pressure, it proved to be more effective than hydrochlorothiazide in lowering blood pressure. In a study comparing 24-hour ambulatory blood pressure readings with office blood pressure readings, the effects of hydrochlorothiazide were found to be shorter during the day. When transferring from hydrochlorothiazide to chlorthalidone, systolic blood pressure drops by 7 to 8 mm Hg. According to the Antihypertensive and Lipid-Lowering Treatment to Prevent Heart Attack Trial (ALLHAT), lisinopril and amlodipine led to more cardiovascular problems than chlorthalidone at doses of 12–25 mg/day.

When compared to amlodipine and lisinopril, chlorthalidone has been shown to have a lower incidence of pelvic fractures, making it the first choice for older patients with osteoporosis. Chlorthalidone was more effective in preventing cardiovascular disease, including strokes and incidence, when compared to doxazosin mesylate and lisinopril. It was also more effective in preventing heart failure when compared to amlodipine (Engberink et al, 2015).

3.1.1.2. Calcium Channel Blockers CCBs

Similar to thiazide-type diuretics, CCBs are advised by JNC8 guidelines to be used as a first-line treatment in all patients with HTN, regardless of age or race, either alone or in combination with other antihypertensives; patients with chronic kidney disease, on the other hand, should use ACE inhibitors or ARBs as recommended as the first-line treatment.

Like thiazide diuretics, CCBs have been demonstrated to reduce all cardiovascular events except heart failure. When thiazides are intolerable to a patient, they are the most effective substitute. Dihydropyridines and non-dihydropyridines are the two categories into which CCBs fall.

Dihydropyridines are more frequently used to treat hypertension because they are stronger vasodilators. Their impact on heart conduction and contractility is minimal. They are therefore more frequently utilized in the treatment of HTN. In this group, amlodipine and nifedipine are the most commonly used drugs. Non-dihydropyridines have a greater impact on cardiac conduction and contractility but are less effective as vasodilators. They are less frequently used to treat HTN and more often as antiarrhythmic drugs.

When treating hypertension in patients of African descent who do not exhibit signs of heart failure or chronic kidney disease, CCB or a thiazide diuretic should be the first line of treatment. Compared to amlodipine, long-acting nifedipine exhibits a stronger antihypertensive effect. Dihydropyridines are a safe supplemental treatment for angina pectoris or better blood pressure control in patients with congestive heart failure (CHF), but they shouldn't be used as the main course of treatment for the condition. In patients with sick sinus syndrome, second and third-degree heart blocks, and CHF with reduced ejection fraction, non-dihydropyridines are generally contraindicated.

In one study, amlodipine was found to have better control over 24-hour ambulatory blood pressure than valsartan. Amlodipine was found to be more effective than atenolol in the ASCOT trial at reducing the risk of cardiovascular disease and is linked to a lower risk of developing diabetes. Amlodipine was more effective than thiazide diuretics in lowering the risk of cardiovascular disease, regardless of the patient's weight, whereas thiazides are less effective in patients with normal body mass index (BMI) than in those who are obese.

3.1.1.3. ACE Inhibitors and ARBs

For individuals suffering from chronic kidney disease and heart failure, the preferred antihypertensives are ARBs and CE inhibitors. For individuals with chronic kidney disease who exhibit proteinuria, they are recommended as the initial line of treatment. Along with thiazides and CCBs, these two classes of antihypertensive drugs are listed in JNC8 guidelines as the first-line treatment for HTN in non-Black patients.

They have been shown to have a cardioprotective effect in patients at high risk of cardiovascular disease, independent of their antihypertensive action.

Both classes are advised as first-line treatments for patients with left ventricular dysfunction and either ST-elevation MI or non-ST elevation MI combined with diabetes, systolic dysfunction, or anterior infarct. They also have comparable efficacies and treatment indications.

When it comes to lowering blood pressure, preventing stroke, and preventing heart failure, thiazide is superior to ACE inhibitors; conversely, CCBs are superior to ACE inhibitors in these areas.

It has been demonstrated that using ramipril in patients with symptomatic heart failure or asymptomatic patients with low ejection fraction reduces mortality, the incidence of stroke, and MIs. According to the study, perindopril reduces cardiovascular events in patients with normal systolic dysfunction and stable coronary artery disease. It was discovered that losartan was superior to atenolol in terms of lowering blood pressure and reducing morbidity and mortality.

When comparing the effects of telmisartan and ramipril in patients with diabetes or heart failure, telmisartan was associated with less angioedema.

3.1.1.4. Beta-Blockers

It is not recommended to use beta-blockers as the sole treatment for hypertension unless there is a clear indication of myocardial infarction and heart failure. When used in younger patients, beta-blockers are linked to lower cardiovascular morbidity and mortality; however, in older patients, they are less protective and have been linked to an increased risk of strokes.

3.1.1.5. Combination Therapy

When a patient with HTN is not responding to monotherapy, a combination should be taken into account. For patients with stage 2 hypertension, combining two antihypertensive drugs should be a therapeutic option. According to a study, combining medications from two different classes lowers blood pressure by an estimated five times more than doubling the dose of a single medication.

The beta-blocker-diuretic combination is not as good as the ARB-diuretic or ACE inhibitor-CBB combinations. Combining beta-blockers and diuretics is linked to an increased risk of developing diabetes. Combinations containing beta-blockers should be used by clinicians in patients with heart failure, tachycardia, or those who have had an MI. When compared to hydrochlorothiazide monotherapy, thiazide plus a potassium-sparing diuretic combination is just as effective at managing hypertension (HTTN) and has a lower incidence of hypokalemia.

When a combination is needed, ARBs or ACE inhibitor-based formulations are favored over CCB and diuretic combination formulations. Patients with CKD should be treated with these kinds of combinations (ACE inhibitors or ARB-based combinations).

In patients at high risk, the benazepril-amlodipine combination reduces the incidence of cardiovascular events and slows the progression of nephropathy better than the benazepril-hydrochlorothiazide combination. It is not advised to combine ACE inhibitors and ARBs as this combination has more side effects than advantages. A third agent should be added when the combination of two medications is unable to meet the desired course of treatment. This is typically accomplished by adding a third agent from the first-line group of medications, which includes thiazide-like diuretics, CCBs, ACE inhibitors, and ARBs. The doctor should think about treating resistant hypertension by adding a fourth antihypertensive medication from any other class if the patient does not respond to the three-drug regimen.

- **Potassium Sparing Diuretics:** First-line treatment rarely involves the use of mineralocorticoid receptor antagonists. When added to other antihypertensive drugs in resistant HTN, spironolactone and eplerenone are thought to be beneficial in the treatment of hypertension. This combination of drugs works well when added to a triple hypertension medication regimen, but because of the increased risk of hyperkalemia, it should be used with caution when combined with ACE inhibitors or ARBs. They have been shown to lower mortality rates and aid in lowering rates of hypokalemia, making them an effective treatment for heart failure. In the treatment of resistant hypertension, spironolactone is more effective at lowering blood pressure than doxazosin and bisoprolol when added to first-line antihypertensive medications.
- **Hydralazine:** If you have heart failure, you can add hydralazine to your regimen to treat resistant hypertension, either by itself or in conjunction with nitrates. Hydralazine is linked to elevated sodium avidity and sympathetic tone; these effects can be mitigated by taking a beta-blocker and loop diuretics together.
- **Clonidine:** A central alpha-2 agonist, clonidine is not recommended as a first line of treatment but may be added if combination therapy is not successful for the patient. The preferred method is transdermal.
- **Minoxidil:** When hydralazine treatment is not successful, minoxidil is typically considered as a treatment option. Although it typically controls blood pressure well, it is linked to fluid retention, which can be helped by taking a loop diuretic. It elevates the sympathetic tone, which might necessitate the addition of a beta-blocker.
- **Alpha-blockers:** Since alpha-blockers are less effective than other first-line medications in preventing cardiovascular disease, they should not be used as the primary treatment for hypertension.

3.1.2. Mechanism of Action

1) **Thiazide and Thiazide-like diuretics**: The exact mechanism of action of diuretics of the thiazide class is unknown. Through the blocking of the Na/Cl channels, thiazides prevent the distal tubule from carrying sodium. Thiazides primarily affect the distal tubule, though they can also slightly affect the proximal tube by obstructing sodium transport. An ACE inhibitor or an ARB can improve blood pressure control. Thiazide diuretics can acutely activate the renin-angiotensin system and cause systemic vascular resistance, which prevents a good response to the diuretic treatment. This increase in renin-angiotensin activity may resolve

with chronic thiazide treatment. Thiazides cause initial volume depletion associated with decreased cardiac output, which recovers within 6 to 8 weeks of starting the treatment in a reverse autoregulation mechanism while the blood pressure remains controlled. Moreover, the mechanism underlying the slight vasodilation effect of thiazide-type diuretics is still unknown.

2) **Calcium channel blockers**: CCBs inhibit Ca^{2+} entry into cells by binding to L-type voltage-gated calcium channels found in the heart muscle. This is the mechanism of action of CCBs. In non-dihydropyridines, this effect can be detrimental inotropic, inhibiting the sinoatrial and atrioventricular nodes, resulting in slow cardiac contractility and conduction. In dihydropyridines, this effect primarily causes peripheral vasodilation.

3) **ACE inhibitors**: By blocking the angiotensin-converting enzyme, ACE inhibitors lower blood pressure by reducing the synthesis of angiotensin II. They also raise bradykinin levels by preventing its degeneration, which results in vasodilation.

4) **ARBs**:To prevent the angiotensin II effect, angiotensin II is bound to the angiotensin 1 AT1 receptors, which is how ARBs function. ARBs do not alter the levels of kinin, in contrast to ACE inhibitors.

5) **Beta-blockers**: The mechanism of action of beta-blockers is to prevent catecholamines from attaching to the Beta 1, 2, and 3 receptors. The beta-1 receptor is mainly present in the heart muscle, the beta-2 receptor is found in the smooth muscles of the bronchi and peripheral arteries, and the beta-3 receptor is present in the adipose tissue of the heart. Beta-blockers with cardioselectivity (e.g., metoprolol tartrate, atenolol, betaxolol, and acebutolol) only inhibit beta-1 receptors, which results in a reduction in bronchospasms. Beta-blockers have a negative inotropic effect, which lowers heart rate and contributes to less oxygen consumption by preventing catecholamines from binding to beta receptors.

6) **Loop diuretics**: The mechanism of action of loop diuretics is to raise the sodium exertion at the cortical and medullary levels of the thick ascending limb. This action results in a drop in volume, which in turn lowers blood pressure.

7) **Potassium Sparing Diuretics:** Impact the primary cells in the collecting duct and late distal tubule; they impede the absorption of sodium at this stage, resulting in a reduction in the excretion of hydrogen and potassium ions. As antagonists of the mineralocorticoid receptor, spirolactone and eplerenone block the mineralocorticoid receptor.

8) **Hydralazine**: As an arteriolar vasodilator, hydralazine reduces the cytoplasmic concentration of Ca^{2+}, thereby inhibiting its release in the smooth muscles of the vessels.

9) **Clonidine**: The rostral ventrolateral medulla's alpha-2 receptors are stimulated by clonidine, which lowers plasma norepinephrine levels and the sympathetic outflow from the central nervous system, ultimately resulting in a decrease in cardiac output.

10) **Minoxidil**: As an arteriolar vasodilator, minoxidil opens the smooth muscle of the vessels' adenosine triphosphate-sensitive potassium channels.

11) **Alpha-blockers**: Vasodilation results

from the inhibition of alpha-1 receptors, which is how alpha-blockers work. This inhibits the contraction of vascular smooth muscle.

3.1.3. Administration

Diuretics of the thiazide type are only administered orally. Tablets containing 12 mg and 25 mg of hydrochlorothiazide are available, however, the daily dose can reach 50 mg. Tablets containing 25 and 50 mg of chlorthalidone are available, however, a daily dose of up to 100 mg is possible.

Calcium channel blockers containing dihydropyridine are taken orally. The maximum daily dose of amlodipine is 10 mg. The maximum daily dose of nifedipine extended-release is 120 mg. Both oral and intravenous forms of non-dihydropyridine CCBs are available; the intravenous form of diltiazem is helpful for controlling heart rate in cardiac arrhythmias. Diltiazem has a maximum oral dosage of 480 mg per day. There are oral and intravenous forms of verapamil available. For tachyarrhythmias, particularly atrial fibrillation, the IV form is utilized. The maximum daily dosage of oral verapamil is 480 mg.

All ACE inhibitors are given orally, except enalapril, which is also given intravenously. However, all ARBs are only available in oral dosage forms. There are oral and IV forms of beta-blockers. While potassium-sparing diuretics are primarily used orally, loop diuretics can be obtained via IV or oral means. Oral or intravenous administration of hydralazine is possible. The daily maximum oral dose of hydralazine is 300 mg.

Since oral forms of clonidine can raise the risk of rebound hypertension, transdermal clonidine administration is the recommended method. The maximum dose of clonidine in oral immediate-release form is0.8mg three times a day, while the maximum transdermal dose is 0.3mg/24hrs patch applied

once a week. Oral minoxidil is used to treat hypertension. Alpha-blockers can only be taken orally to treat hypertension.

3.1.4. Adverse Effects

1) Thiazides Side Effects

There are several side effects linked to thiazide and thiazide-like diuretics. The majority of these adverse effects are directly linked to the dosage of the diuretic; the most frequent metabolic side effects are hypokalemia and hyponatremia, which are followed by hyperuricemia, hypomagnesemia, hyperlipidemia, and elevated glucose levels. According to a study, older adults taking chlorthalidone had a higher chance of being hospitalized for severe hypokalemia. Sleep disturbance and sexual dysfunction are other non-dose related side effects.

2) CCB Side Effects

Peripheral edema and dihydropyridine CCB therapy are frequently linked. Compared to amlodipine, long-acting nifedipine is linked to a higher incidence of edema; the edema is correlated with the CCB dosage. It has nothing to do with accumulating salt, staying hydrated, or getting heart failure. Diuretic therapy has no effect on CCB-induced edema because it is not caused by a volume increase; however, a reduced risk of peripheral edema development was observed when ACE inhibitors or ARBs were combined with CCBs, albeit to a lesser extent. Dihydropyridines may result in gingival hyperplasia, headaches, flushing, and dizziness.

Non-dihydropyridines can cause constipation in 25% of patients and are linked to bradycardia. When prescribing CCBs to elderly patients or patients who have a high risk of bleeding, care must be taken because these agents inhibit platelet aggregation and are linked to an increased risk of gastrointestinal bleeding.

3) ACE Inhibitors and ARBs Side Effects

Cough, hypotension, fatigue, and azotemia are the most frequent side effects associated with ACE inhibitors. Reversible renal impairment is also a common side effect, particularly if the patient experiences volume depletion from vomiting or diarrhea.

Up to 20% of ACE inhibitor users may experience cough. The cough can go away after stopping for up to 14 to 28 days. Cough is less common when taking ARBs; when losartan and hydrochlorothiazide are compared, the incidence of cough is similar in both cases. Patients with asthma can safely use ARBs; when compared to CCBs, candesartan did not show a correlation with a higher incidence of cough in asthma patients. Compared to telmisartan, ramipril showed a greater incidence of cough.

Treatment with ACE inhibitors is frequently linked to mild hyperkalemia. Patients with renal failure, diabetes, or CHF are more likely to experience hyperkalemia, even in those with normal renal function. The incidence of developing syncope, acute kidney injury, and hyperkalemia is comparable between telmisartan and ramipril. There is a higher incidence of symptomatic hypotension when using telmisartan.

Angioedema is an uncommon ACE inhibitor side effect that affects 0.3% of ramipril users. Compared to ACE inhibitors, ARBs have a lower correlation with angioedema.

3.1.5. Contraindications

Patients with sulfonamide allergies and those who are anuric should not take thiazide-type diuretics. Patients who have a history of drug hypersensitivity should not take CCBs. Patients with heart failure, reduced ejection fraction, sick sinus syndrome, and second or third-degree AV blockade are among the non-dihydropyridine contraindications. When dihydropyridine is helpful for patients with impaired liver function, extra caution is required. Dihydropyridine should be avoided in patients with cardiogenic shock, severe aortic stenosis, and unstable angina.

Patients with a history of ACE inhibitor hypersensitivity, ACE inhibitor-related angioedema, other types of angioedema, pregnancy, or aliskiren use should not take ACE inhibitors. Patients with aortic valve stenosis, abnormal renal function, and volume depletion are considered relative contraindications. It is not advised to use ARBs while pregnant. Combining ARBs with ACE inhibitors is generally not advised. Patients with volume depletion, patients taking other medications that cause hyperkalemia, and patients with abnormal renal function are other relative contraindications for ARB treatment.

Patients with asthma should not take beta-blockers, especially nonselective beta-blockers. Bradycardia and hypotension are relative contraindications. Some believe that patients experiencing coronary artery spasms brought on by cocaine should not take them. Patients with a history of sulfonamide hypersensitivity, anuria, or hepatic coma should not use loop diuretics. Patients with hyperkalemia or chronic kidney disease should not take potassium-sparing diuretics; caution should be exercised when taking them with ACE inhibitors, ARBs, or aliskiren. Patients who have a hypersensitivity to this class should not use them.

Patients who have recently experienced myocardial infarctions or who have a history of depression should not take clonidine as it is contraindicated in those who are hypersensitive to alpha-2 agonists. If a patient has ever experienced hydralazine allergy, hydralazine should not be administered. Hydralazine has been shown to activate the sympathetic nervous system in patients with coronary artery disease. Hydralazine treatment may cause pulmonary artery pressure to rise in patients with rheumatic mitral valve disease. Patients who are hypersensitive to minoxidil as well as women who are pregnant or nursing should not use minoxidil. Patients using phosphodiesterase inhibitors or those with a history of orthostatic hypotension should not take alpha-blockers.

3.1.6. Monitoring

Potassium-sparing diuretics induce hyperkalemia, whereas thiazides and loop diuretics can induce hypokalemia. Patients taking thiazides and loop diuretics should also have their electrolyte levels and uric acid levels checked. Patients using loop diuretics should be monitored for ototoxicity and deafness.

Treatment with ACE inhibitors and ARBs frequently results in hyperkalemia, so extra care must be taken when taking these medications with potassium-sparing diuretics. When using ACE inhibitors, ARBs, or potassium-sparing diuretics, patients with chronic kidney disease should have their potassium levels regularly monitored. Renal function needs to be monitored because ACE inhibitors and ARBs have the potential to cause acute kidney injury.

Patients taking dihydropyridine CCBs need to be watched for hypotension and edema. Since beta-blockers and non-dihydropyridine CCBs can induce bradycardia, heart rate needs to be watched, particularly when these two drugs are taken together. Patients taking sotalol need to have their QTc interval monitored. It is advised to keep an eye out for orthostatic hypotension and tachyarrhythmias in patients taking alpha-blockers. It is recommended to monitor the patient's ANA levels and complete blood count while they are receiving hydralazine treatment. Patients who experience fever, arthralgia, or other systemic symptoms should exercise extra caution.

3.1.7. Toxicity

Toxicology from thiazides and loop diuretics can result in metabolic acidosis (hypochloremic) and electrolyte imbalances, primarily hypokalemia and hyponatremia, as well as dehydration, which can be severe. These diuretics have no known antidote; volume and electrolyte replacement are the mainstays of treatment.

The main treatment for potassium-sparing diuretics toxicity is to discontinue all medications that cause hyperkalemia, and add IV hydration, calcium gluconate, insulin with glucose, sodium bicarbonate, and potassium binding resins.

The reduced ionotropy effect on the heart muscle causes non-dihydropyridine CCB toxicity, which results in bradycardia and hypotension. It is possible to experience idioventricular rhythm and total heart block. Dihydropyridine CCBs have minimal effect on heart rate but cause severe hypotension and peripheral vasodilation. For hypotension, intravenous hydration is advised; for bradycardia, an external pacemaker is advised. If intravenous hydration is ineffective at raising blood pressure, intravenous calcium chloride or calcium gluconate can help hypotension. If the blood pressure does not get better, IV vasopressors may be an option.

ARB and ACE inhibitor toxicity can result in hyponatremia, hyperkalemia, and severe hypotension. Since there are no known counteragents, intravenous hydration and hyperkalemia management are advised.

Similar to CCBs, beta-blockers can result in second or third-degree AV blocks, bradycardia, and hypotension. The first line of defense is IV glucagon; if there is no improvement, IV hydration and an external pacemaker may be needed.

Severe hypotension, tachycardia, and skin flushing are possible side effects of hydralazine toxicity; in extreme situations, patients may experience myocardial ischemia or cardiac shock. There is no known cure; in severe cases, IV hydration and IV vasopressors are the interventions of choice. Severe tachycardia may be treated with beta-blockers.

Bradycardia, hypotension, miosis, and lethargy are some of the symptoms of clonidine toxicity. Respiratory depression may arise in extreme situations. Vasopressors and hydration are part of the supportive care protocol. In this case, dopamine and norepinephrine are typical options. For severe bradycardia, IV atropine is a treatment option; external pacemakers are saved for situations where atropine treatment is ineffective.

Hypotension and tachycardia can be symptoms of minoxidil poisoning. Vasopressors and IV hydration are used in supportive care. The main treatments for alpha-blocker toxicity include IV hydration and vasopressors, which can result in severe hypotension.

3.1.8. Enhancing Healthcare Team Outcomes

Healthcare professionals are advised to exercise extra caution when monitoring adherence to and potential side effects from antihypertensives, a broad class of medications. The prevention of cardiovascular disease depends on treating hypertension (HTN), and selecting the right medication class will help you achieve the right level of control with the least amount of side effects.

Patients taking these medications need to be closely monitored by an interprofessional team consisting of clinicians, nurses, and pharmacists. The antihypertensive regimen is initiated by the clinician; the pharmacies should then pay close attention to monitoring drug-drug interactions, treatment compliance, and medication reconciliation. In addition to keeping an eye on the patient's diet and activity levels and assessing the home environment, the nurse is crucial in identifying obstacles to the patient's good response to the treatment. To detect any early adverse reactions, home-visiting nurses will keep an eye on patients' blood pressure and heart rate responses to the treatment. Any potential issues with adherence, adverse reactions, or modifications to the home environment should be communicated to the clinician by the pharmacist and the nurse. This thorough interprofessional team effort contributes to maximizing the regimen's benefits and providing the patient and family with the best possible care.

3.2. Drugs Used in Heart Failure

When the heart cannot sustain a cardiac output high enough to meet the needs of the metabolizing tissues, congestive heart failure results.

Heart failure is usually caused by one of the following:

- Ischemic heart disease;
- Hypertension;
- Heart muscle disorders; and
- Valvular heart disease.

Drugs used to treat heart failure can be broadly divided into:

- Drugs with a positive inotropic effect.
- Drugs without a positive inotropic effect.

3.2.1. Drugs with Positive Inotropic Effect

Drugs with a positive inotropic effect increase the force of contraction of the heart muscle.

These include:

- Cardiac glycosides;
- Bipyridine derivatives;
- Sympathomimetics; and
- Methylxanthines.

1. **Cardiac Glycosides:** A class of steroid compounds known as cardiac glycosides can modify electrical functions and raise cardiac output. Digoxin and digitoxin are cardiac glycosides that are frequently used. The inhibition of membrane-bound Na^+/K^+ ATPase, also known as the "sodium pump," is the mechanism by which cardiac glycosides exert their inotropic action. As a result, there is an increase in the movement of sodium within cells and an accumulation of sodium within the cells. The increased intracellular sodium will cause a decrease in the transmembrane exchange of calcium and sodium, which will raise the intracellular calcium that interacts with contractile proteins. While their pharmacokinetic characteristics vary, all cardiac glycosides have comparable pharmacodynamic characteristics. Digitoxin, for instance, has a longer half-life and is more lipid-soluble than digoxin.

Therapeutic uses of cardiac glycosides include:

- Congestive heart failure
- Atrial fibrillation;
- Atrial flutter; and
- Paroxysmal atrial tachycardia.

Toxicity of cardiac glycosides include:

- Gastrointestinal effects such as anorexia, nausea, vomiting, diarrhea
- Cardiac effects such as bradycardia, heart block, arrhythmias
- CNS effects such as headache, malaise, hallucinations, delirium, visual disturbances (yellow vision)

One way to manage mild toxicities like gastrointestinal and visual disturbances is to lower the drug's dosage. To treat arrhythmias or severe toxicity, potassium supplementation, anti-arrhythmic medication administration (e.g. lidocaine), as well as the administration of antibodies against digoxin.

2. **Bipyridine Derivatives, e.g., Amrinone, Milrinone:** These medications have both vasodilator and positive inotropic effects. The inhibition of phophodiesterase, an enzyme that causes cyclic AMP to become inactive, is the proposed mechanism of action. When these enzymes are inhibited, cAMP levels rise. When cardiac glycosides and vasodilators fail to treat heart failure, bipyridine derivatives are used.
3. **Beta-Adrenergic Stimulants, e.g., Dobutamine, Dopamine:** Beta-adrenergic stimulants such as dobutamine and dopamine directly stimulate the β_1 receptor on the heart, and dopamine also causes a release of norepinephrine. They increase heart rate and contractility and are used in the short term in cardiac decompensation as in severe heart failure, and to correct hemodynamic imbalances that occur during sepsis, trauma, myocardial infaction or renal failure."

3.2.2. Drugs Without Positive Inotropic Effect

Positive inotropic drugs are those that strengthen the heart muscle's contraction. They are frequently used to treat illnesses where the heart's capacity to pump blood is impaired, such as heart failure. Not all medications used to treat cardiovascular diseases, nevertheless, have beneficial inotropic effects.

These include:

- Diuretics, e.g. hydrochlorothiazide, furosemide
- Vasodilators, e.g. hydralazine, sodium nitroprusside
- Angiotensin-converting enzyme inhibitors e.g. captopril, enalapril

1. Diuretics

Heart failure is associated with fluid overload. Therefore, first-line medication for treating patients with heart failure is diuretics. A thiazide may be adequate in cases of mild failure, but they are ineffective at low glomerular filtration rates. Loop diuretics are necessary for moderate or severe failure. Diuretics are useful in acute failure because they lower ventricular preload. The management of acute symptoms of fluid overload associated with heart failure may require the administration of loop diuretics intravenously. Once symptoms are under control, they can be used orally.

2. Vasodilators

Because they reduce preload (via venous dilatation), afterload (through arteriolar dilatation), or both, the vasodilators are useful in treating acute heart failure. Only the arterial bed is affected directly by hydralazine's vasodilator action. A significant increase in cardiac output results from a decrease in systemic vascular resistance. " Sodium nitroprusside produces both venous and arterial vasodilation. It is used for rapid lowering of blood pressure during hypertensive crises, or to rapidly lower peripheral resistance in the management of acute heart failure"

3. Angiotensin-converting enzyme (ACE) inhibitors

Reduction of angiotensin II has a beneficial impact on the course of the disease because of its widespread involvement in the undesired compensatory responses to heart failure.

These medications lessen preload by decreasing salt and water retention through a decrease in aldosterone secretion, and they also lessen afterload by decreasing peripheral resistance. "ACE-inhibitors are consired to be the drugs of choice for the management of chronic heart failure.

The following are essential for long-term management of chronic heart failure:

- Modify cardiovascular risk factor profile, e.g. cigarette smoking, obesity, salt intake Underlying causes should be treated, e.g. anemia, hypertension, valvular disease. If this proves inadequate, diuretics should be given.
- Give ACE inhibitor and digitalis (ACE inhibitors are used before digitalis). In patients with persisting symptoms give vasodilators besides increasing the dose of diuretics and ACE inhibitors.

3.3. Pharmacological Treatment of Chronic Stable Angina Pectoris

The term "angina pectoris" refers to William Heberden's 1768 report to the Royal College of Physicians, which is considered the classic description of the clinical symptoms of angina. Angina pectoris is a term used to describe both the typical chest pain associated with myocardial ischemia and the syndrome that is characterized by myocardial ischemia, obstructive atherosclerotic coronary artery disease, and chest pain. Currently, there is no systematically agreed definition for angina pectoris. In this context, the term "angina" refers to the typical central chest pain that is linked to myocardial ischemia, regardless of the existence or non-existence of organic coronary artery stenosis, which limits blood flow.

An imbalance between the myocardium's oxygen supply and demand leads to the development of angina pectoris. It is a sign of ischemia in the heart. Angina appears when the increased oxygen demand cannot be met by the increased coronary blood flow. It is now clear that the development of angina is significantly influenced by coronary artery spasm.

When angina attacks don't change in intensity, nature, or precipitating factors and last for at least two months, they are deemed "chronic" and "stable."

The most prevalent clinical sign of ischemic heart disease, stable angina affects 58% of patients with CAD. In England, its prevalence rises with age, from about 8% in men and 3% in women between the ages of 55 and 64 to 14% in men and 8% in women between the ages of 65 and 74. For patients with stable angina, the annual mortality rate from coronary heart disease is between 1.5%.

An imbalance between myocardial oxygen demand and coronary blood supply causes stable angina. This imbalance is frequently, but not always, linked to the presence of obstructive coronary artery disease. Because transient myocardial ischemia activates mechano- and chemosensitive myocardial receptors, it usually causes "constrictive" chest pain. Individuals with diabetes mellitus and the elderly may have "silent" myocardial ischemia, and patients with stable angina may or may not exhibit the usual symptoms.

Presently available treatment approaches for chronic stable angina attempt to slow the progression of atherosclerotic coronary artery disease (CAD) and its aftereffects, control symptoms, lessen the ischemic burden, and enhance prognosis. The best course of action for treating angina should be customized for each patient, taking into account the features and intensity of symptoms, the location, severity, and functional importance of coronary artery stenoses, the presence of co-morbidities, and the patient's preferences. The effectiveness of the medication, any side effects, and patient compliance all play a significant role in determining whether a particular treatment plan is successful or unsuccessful for any given patient.

3.3.1. Pathophysiological and Pathogenic Mechanisms: Determinants of Clinical Presentation

Angina frequently has a multifactorial etiology. An imbalance in the supply and demand of oxygen in the heart is the fundamental cause of angina. This is commonly caused by flow-limiting CAD, but there are many other possible contributing factors as well, such as coronary microvascular dysfunction, coronary artery spasm that restricts blood supply, and/or other factors. Angina that is induced by effort, mixed angina, or angina that occurs while at rest is largely determined by the underlying pathogenic mechanism.

1. Effort-induced Angina

Angina is brought on by a fixed restriction in coronary blood flow caused by long-standing obstructive epicardial CAD. This prevents the coronary blood supply from physiologically matching increases in myocardial metabolic demand brought on by exercise. "Obstructive" stenosis is defined as a stenosis of 50% or more in the left main coronary artery or 70% or more in another major epicardial artery. The symptoms of flow-limiting coronary stenoses-induced stable angina are frequently triggered by physical activity and/or emotional stress, and they manifest at a consistent and repeatable threshold. Exercise stress testing is evaluated using the Canadian Cardiovascular Society (CCS) grading of angina, a functional classification of exercise tolerance that can be linked to metabolic equivalent units (METs).

2. 'Mixed' angina

Combination mechanisms can also lead to an imbalance in the supply and demand of oxygen in the heart during angina. Patients with "mixed angina pectoris," which is defined as variable-threshold effort angina and occasionally angina at rest, present with clinical manifestations of excessive coronary artery vasoconstriction at the site of organic stenoses. (Lindholm et al, 2005; Kones et al, 2010; Ettehad et al, 2016)

3. Microvascular Angina

The primary factor influencing coronary flow reserve—defined as the ratio of maximally induced myocardial flow to resting coronary blood flow—is coronary microvascular resistance. Angina related to exertion may be brought on by abnormal coronary microcirculation vasodilatory responses (microvascular angina). It is noteworthy that a mere 38% of patients undergoing elective diagnostic coronary angiography who did not have a history of heart disease are discovered to have obstructive CAD. Exercise-induced myocardial ischemia in many of these patients with classic angina symptoms is due to coronary microvascular dysfunction. Cardiac syndrome X patients have transient myocardial ischemia due to impaired endothelial function, which causes abnormal coronary microvascular vasodilatation, increased coronary vasoconstriction, or both. Typical exertional angina, positive stress test responses, and normal coronary angiograms are characteristics of this condition.

About two-thirds of patients without significant epicardial CAD in the ACOVA (Abnormal Coronary Vasomotion in Patients with Stable Angina and Unobstructed Coronary Arteries) study had positive intra-coronary acetylcholine tests for distal epicardial or microvascular spasm. It is recommended that clinicians consider the potential diagnosis of microvascular dysfunction or coronary microvascular spasm in patients with angiographically normal coronary arteries but typical angina.

4. Other contributing mechanisms

After a brief period of myocardial ischemia, the activation of late inward sodium currents exacerbates the oxygen imbalance and prolongs the angina episode. This is due to impaired diastolic relaxation and increased wall tension brought on by calcium overload, which is the result of intracellular acidosis. Pathogenesis may also be aided by additional metabolic disruption, such as aberrant substrate supply and utilization, enzymatic activity, and mitochondrial function. Other possible contributing factors that can exacerbate myocardial ischemia include aortic stenosis, hypertrophic cardiomyopathy, severe anemia, and thyrotoxicosis (if present).

3.3.2. Diagnosis and Management

- **Importance of the clinical history for diagnosis and management of stable angina pectoris:** A thorough clinical history is essential for the diagnosis of chronic stable angina as well as the identification of potential underlying pathogenic mechanisms. The amount of underlying CAD does not always correspond with the severity of chest pain, but the type and degree of anti-anginal treatments used for a given patient will depend on the severity of their symptoms.

For the purpose of patient management, the CCS classification of angina can offer clinically significant diagnostic and prognostic hints. Angina can only be triggered by intense or prolonged exertion in CCS grade I patients. On the other hand, angina can be triggered by mild exertion or even while at rest in CCS grade IV patients. It's critical to keep in mind that CAD severity is not always reflected in CCS grade. In contrast, chest pain that is gradually more frequent and/or severe (referred to as "crescendo" angina) in comparison to the typical chronic stable symptoms may indicate acute coronary syndrome, which includes unstable angina and myocardial infarction. In such cases, careful monitoring and prompt investigation are necessary.

- Ø **Diagnostic Investigation:** The National Institute for Health and Clinical Excellence's (NICE) guideline on chest pain describes a risk stratification that is based on pre-test probability, which is derived from age, sex, the nature of symptoms, and cardiovascular risk factors.

This guidance informs future research. NICE suggests CT coronary calcium scoring as the first-line investigation for patients (10–29%) with stable symptoms who are at low risk for coronary artery disease. Although there are good reasons for this recommendation, cardiologists frequently turn to alternative diagnostic testing such as exercise stress testing or stress echocardiography because it is not always easy or practical to implement this strategy in practice. Patients with moderate cardiovascular risk (30–60%) are recommended to undergo functional imaging with stress echocardiography, nuclear myocardial perfusion scanning, or first-pass cardiac magnetic resonance scanning. In patients who fall into the high-risk category (61–90%), NICE suggests moving straight to invasive coronary angiography. Exercise tolerance testing with an ECG is not advised for the diagnosis of CAD, although it is still a useful diagnostic tool in practice and can provide valuable functional information in many cases.

3.3.3. Pharmacological Management of Angina Pectoris

While the general guidelines for treatment apply to all angina patients, it is best to tailor the course of care for each patient. Reducing or reversing the underlying pathophysiological mechanisms, alleviating symptoms, and enhancing cardiovascular risk profiles are the goals. Key interventions include lifestyle changes (e.g. smoking cessation, dietary modification and increased physical exercise), management of hypertension, diabetes and obesity, and other secondary cardiovascular disease prevention measures, such as the use of anti-platelet and lipid-lowering agents, pharmacological anti-anginal therapies and percutaneous and/or surgical revascularization when appropriate.

Based on recently updated NICE guidelines, Figure 3.1 offers a suggested workable therapeutic algorithm.

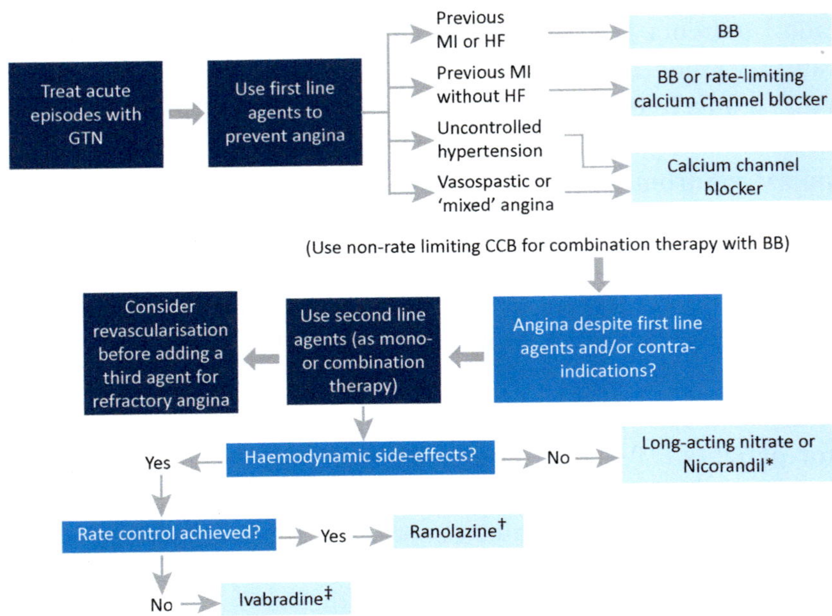

Figure 3.1. *Proposed practical algorithm for pharmacological treatment of chronic stable angina based on NICE guidance.*

B = beta-blocker; CCB = calcium channel blocker; DM = diabetes mellitus; GTN = glyceryltrinitrate; HF = heart failure; MI = myocardial infarction. *Added cardio-protective properties; †improves HbA1c in DM; ‡prognostic benefit in HF.

Source: https://www.ncbi.nlm.nih.gov/pmc/articles/PMC5873712/.

3.3.3.1. Treatment of Chest Pain Episodes

The most effective treatment for angina episodes is sublingual glyceryltrinitrate (GTN). GTN causes systemic and coronary vasodilatation by acting as a donor of nitric oxide. The sublingual mucosae quickly absorb GTN, and its effects typically manifest in a matter of 2 to 10 minutes. When taking sublingual nitrate, headaches, nausea, dizziness, and hot flushes are common side effects. The use of GTN is not recommended in cases of aortic stenosis, hypertrophic cardiomyopathy, systemic hypotension, or when phosphodiesterase-5 inhibitors (sildenafil). Unless it is contraindicated, GTN is advised for all patients with stable angina. Patients should be advised about the proper usage of GTN, including when to take it and any possible side effects. They should be advised to them to let their doctor know if the symptoms don't go away. When taken before engaging in physical exertion, GTN can also be helpful in preventing episodes of exertional angina.

3.3.3.2. First-line Anti-Anginal Drugs

Studies have demonstrated that first-line anti-anginal medications, such as beta-adrenergic receptor blockers and calcium channel blockers, can prevent myocardial ischemia and angina. According to the results of the TIBET (Total Ischemic Burden European Trial), atenolol and slow-release nifedipine had comparable anti-anginal effects; the two drugs did not significantly enhance each other's effects. Similar rates of cardiovascular events and mortality were observed in patients with stable angina treated with metoprolol or verapamil in the APSIS (Angina Prognosis Study in Stockholm) study. The presence of co-morbidities, patient preference, and contraindications typically influence the decision between these two medication classes. One of these agents can be substituted for the other if the first is not well tolerated. If combination therapy is required, the use of a non-heart-rate limiting dihydropyridine calcium channel blocker (e.g. amlodipine or slow-release nifedipine) is recommended. Beta-blockers have anti-anginal effects because they lower blood pressure, heart rate, and contractility, which lower the amount of oxygen that the heart needs to function. Additionally, lowering heart rate prolongs the diastolic phase of the cardiac cycle, which enhances myocardial flow.

Long-acting, cardioselective beta-blockers without intrinsic sympathomimetic activity are preferred for maximum efficacy. It is necessary to titrate the dose to reach the desired resting heart rate of 50–60 beats per minute. Although it hasn't been proven instable angina, the prognostic benefit of beta-blockers in angina has been extrapolated from studies of post-myocardial infarction.

The adverse effects and contraindications of beta-blocker therapy frequently limit its potential benefits. The most frequent adverse effects of beta-blockers include depression, erectile dysfunction, fatigue, dizziness, syncope, bronchospasm, and hyperglycemia. Patients with sick sinus syndrome, acute heart failure, severe bradycardia, second or third-degree heart block, hypotension, reactive airway diseases, and peripheral vascular disease should not use these agents. Because unopposed α-adrenergic receptors may have unwanted effects, beta-blockers are generally not used in patients with vasospastic angina. Rebound myocardial ischemia may occur from the abrupt withdrawal of beta-blockers.

Calcium channel blockers target L-type Ca^{2+} receptors to cause vasodilation in both the systemic and coronary arteries, leading to a decrease in afterload and better blood flow to the heart muscle. Non-dihydropyridines like verapamil and diltiazem also have anti-anginal effects by reducing heart rate and contractility. It is recommended to use long-acting versions of these medications. Common side effects may include dizziness, headache, fatigue, flushing, abdominal pain, nausea, and peripheral edema. Just like beta-blockers, non-dihydropyridine calcium channel blockers should not be used in patients with severe bradycardia, 2nd or 3rd-degree heart block, sick sinus syndrome, hypotension, or acute heart failure. (Lindholm et al, 2005; Kones et al, 2010; Ettehad et al, 2016)

3.3.3.3. Second-Line Anti-Angina Therapies

For patients who do not respond well to beta-blockers and calcium-channel blockers, or if they cannot take these medications, there are alternative options recommended by NICE guidelines. These include vasodilators like long-acting nitrates and nicorandil, a medication that slows the heart rate selectively; ivabradine; and ranolazine, which improves cardiac metabolism by acting on the fast sodium current. The choice and sequence of these second-line treatments depend on factors such as the underlying causes of the condition, the patient's individual characteristics and other health conditions, potential drug interactions, and patient preferences.

3.3.3.4. Long-Acting Nitrates

Long-acting nitrates (such as isosorbide mononitrate or isosorbide dinitrate) have been demonstrated to lessen the frequency and severity of angina attacks in patients with stable angina when administered alone or in conjunction with first-line anti-anginal medications, despite the lack of evidence that nitrates improve patient prognosis. These medications' modes of action, adverse reactions, and contraindications resemble those discussed above for sublingual nitrates. Before these medications are prescribed for a particular patient, it is important to take into account the development of nitrate tolerance and the recently reported negative effects of long-acting nitrates.

3.3.3.5. Nicorandil

In addition to being a nitric oxide donor, nicoterandil also opens sarcolemmal K^+-adenosine triphosphate (K-ATP) channels, which results in K^+ efflux, hyperpolarization, and inhibition of L-type Ca^{2+} channels, which in turn causes systemic and coronary vasodilatation. Nicorandil monotherapy has advantages akin to those of amlodipine, diltiazem, metoprolol, and nitrates. Patients taking nicorandil in addition to other conventional anti-anginal therapies showed a lower rate of both fatal and non-fatal myocardial infarction as well as a lower rate of admission for cardiac chest pain in the IONA (Impact of Nicorandil in Angina) study. Nicorandil's cardio-protective effects may be the result of ischemic preconditioning brought on by the opening of mitochondrial K-ATP channels. Frequent adverse reactions to nicorandil include flushing, headaches, nausea, dizziness, and vomiting. Metformin may counteract nicorandil's effects by blocking K-ATP channels. Those taking nicorandil should avoid using phosphodiesterase-5 inhibitors and nitrates due to the possibility of severe systemic hypotension.

3.3.3.6. Ivabradine

Ivabradine is a novel anti-anginal medication that selectively lowers heart rate. Ivabradine affects the intrinsic pacemaker cells of the sino-atrial node by inhibiting I_f channels. Myocytes in the sino-atrial node spontaneously depolarize when the I_f channel is activated by hyperpolarization in diastolic range voltages and by adrenergically induced increases in cyclic adenosine monophosphate. This results in an inward Na^+/K^+ ionic current across the sarcolemma. The heart rate is lowered by inhibiting the I_f current. In patients with elevated I_f channel activity, ivabradine is more beneficial. It has no effect on contractility, atrioventricular node conduction, or blood pressure. Ivabradine lowers resting heart rate by 10 beats per minute on average. Heart rate reduction is dose dependant, with a stronger effect in patients with higher baseline heart rates. The effect plateaus at 20mg twice daily.

Large-scale trials have demonstrated that ivabradine's anti-anginal efficacy is comparable to that of atenolol and amlodipine. Patients with stable angina and heart rates ≥70 beats per minute saw lower rates of hospital admission for fatal and non-fatal myocardial infarction and coronary revascularization with ivabradine compared to placebo in the BEAUTIFUL (morbidity-mortality Evaluation of the I_f inhibitor ivabradine in patients with coronary disease and left ventricular dysfunction) trial.

Patients with stable angina who are in sinus rhythm, cannot tolerate conventional heart-rate-lowering medications (beta-blockers and non-dihydropyridine calcium channel blockers), or whose resting heart rate is not optimal while on conventional monotherapy should be prescribed ivabradine. Common side effects include headache, dizziness, blurred vision, first-degree heart block, ventricular extra-systoles, and visually apparent "flashing lights," which are frequently mild and temporary. Bradycardia, sick sinus syndrome, atrial fibrillation, heart block, acute myocardial infarction, acute heart failure, hypotension, and renal and hepatic failure are contraindications. The CYP3A4 liver enzymes are responsible for the metabolism of ivabradine, and there may be substantial interactions with medications that disrupt these enzymes (such as azole antifungals, diltiazem, verapamil, macrolide antibiotics, and grapefruit juice). Patients with asthma and chronic obstructive pulmonary disease can safely use ivabradine.

3.3.3.7. Ranolazine

A derivative of piperazine, ranolazine is believed to reduce diastolic wall tension and extrinsic coronary artery compression, inhibit late inward Na+ currents induced by ischemia, and avoid Ca^{2+} overload. Additionally, it may enhance coronary vasodilatation mediated by endothelial cells. Although the concentration needed to inhibit myocardial fatty-acid oxidation is significantly higher than the therapeutic levels used to treat angina, it was originally believed to have anti-metabolic properties. Ranolazine has the benefit of not significantly altering hemodynamics; on average, heart rate and systolic blood pressure are reduced by less than 2 beats per minute and less than 3 mmHg, respectively. However, it is linked to an increase in QT interval that is dose-dependent.

The MARISA (Monotherapy Assessment of Ranolazine in Stable Angina), CARISA (Combination Assessment of Ranolazine in Stable Angina), and ERICA (Efficacy of Ranolazine in Chronic Angina) trials have demonstrated the clinical efficacy of ranolazine in treating chronic stable angina both as monotherapy and in combination with other anti-anginal medications. The MERLIN-TIMI 36 (Metabolic Efficiency with Ranolazine for Less Ischemia in Non-ST-elevation acute coronary syndromes) trial found no reduction in cardiovascular death, acute myocardial infarction, or recurrent ischemia when ranolazine was administered in place of a placebo.

Headaches, nausea, constipation, dizziness, and abdominal pain are typical ranolazine side effects. Prolonged QT intervals, concurrent use of other QT-prolonging medications, a history of ventricular tachycardia, moderate to severe renal impairment, and severe hepatic failure are contraindications to ranolazine. There is a chance for drug interactions because CYP3A4 in the liver and CYP2D6 to a lesser extent metabolize ranolazine. Since ranolazine also weakly inhibits cytochrome p450 enzymes, patients on ranolazine may need to take lower doses of P-glycoprotein substrates (such as digoxin and simvastatin).

3.3.3.8. Other Anti-Anginal Drugs

There are numerous other anti-anginal medications. Although they are not covered by NICE guidelines at this time, they might be used in the UK in the future. Many European countries use trimetazidine as a metabolic modulator because it is an effective thiolase that inhibits the beta-oxidation of fatty acids in the myocardium and shifts cardiac metabolism towards more efficient pathways. Although angiotensin-converting enzyme inhibitors aren't technically anti-anginal medications, they have been demonstrated to enhance prognosis in individuals with diabetes, heart failure, and after myocardial infarction. They are therefore recommended in those situations, and more research is needed to fully understand their function instable angina pectoris.

Phase II clinical trials are presently evaluating F 15845 (3-(R)-[3-(2-methoxyphenylthio-2-(S)-methylpropyl] amino-3,4-dihydro-2H-1,5-benzoxathiepine bromhydrate), a recently identified selective inhibitor of the persistent Na^{+} current that has demonstrated anti-ischemic qualities and the capacity to avert ischemia-induced arrhythmias in animal models.

3.3.4. Individual Approach to Anti-Anginal Drug Selection

For many patients, effective symptom control may require the use of multiple medications with various modes of action. However, a large number of patients—particularly those who experience hemodynamic side effects—are unable to tolerate traditional angina therapies. According to the NICE guideline, patients who are awaiting revascularization or for whom revascularization is not appropriate should only add a third medication if two anti-anginal medications are unable to adequately control their symptoms.

Due to their established prognostic value, beta-blockers are the first-choice medication for patients who have experienced a previous myocardial infarction or heart failure. Rate-limiting calcium channel blockers have the potential to enhance prognosis in individuals recovering from myocardial infarction who do not exhibit heart failure. Calcium channel blockers are the recommended treatment for angina patients who need to have well-controlled hypertension. For patients who tolerate short-acting nitrates but whose symptoms still worsen even after taking beta-blockers or calcium channel blockers, long-acting nitrates make sense. Nitrates do not improve prognosis; however, nicorandil may have additional cardio-protective benefits in addition to its anti-anginal effects.

Ivabradine and ranolazine are good choices since they don't have vasoactive effects, making them suitable for patients who experience hypotension or other hemodynamic side effects from traditional anti-anginal therapies. Ivabradine can be used safely by patients with obstructive airways disease because it effectively lowers heart rate without having a significant impact on hemodynamic effects. Beta-blockers and ivabradine can also be taken together. The combination of ivabradine and atenolol was found to be effective and well-tolerated in patients with stable angina in the ASSOCIATE (Antianginal efficacy and Safety of the association of the if current Inhibitor ivabradine with a beta-blocker) trial. Additionally, the combination was not linked to any adverse effects. In patients with systolic heart failure, ivabradine has also been demonstrated to lower cardiovascular death and hospital admission. Ranolazine has been linked to a significant decrease in HbA1c concentrations, which is an additional metabolic benefit for diabetic patients.

It is crucial to keep in mind that angina is not exclusively caused by the presence of obstructive epicardial CAD; rather, it is the result of the interaction of several intricate vascular and metabolic mechanisms. Anti-anginal regimens ought to the greatest extent feasible, target the patient's specific underlying pathophysiological mechanisms. This is especially crucial for patients with angiographically "normal" coronary arteries, objectively documented myocardial ischemia, and chest pain, as these conditions frequently involve distal epicardial vasoconstriction and coronary microvascular dysfunction. For these people, vasodilators such as calcium channel blockers are beneficial. When someone has genuine vasospastic angina, i.e. for long-term symptom management of Prinzmetal's variant angina, calcium channel blockers (typically at high doses) are the best treatment option; however, nitrates, especially sublingual GTN, can also be very helpful. (Lindholm et al, 2005; Kones et al, 2010; Ettehad et al, 2016)

3.4. Antiarrhythmic Medications

3.4.1. Indications

Traditionally, antiarrhythmic drugs have been arranged using the Vaughan-Williams (VW) classification scheme. The primary mechanism of action is used by the system to categorize the medications (although some agents maintain characteristics from multiple classes). There are four primary categories in the VW classification, and some references include a fifth.

3.4.1.1. Class I: Sodium channel blockers

1. Class Ia

Fast sodium channel blockage of a moderate degree is caused by class Ia. Procainamide, disopyramide, and quinidine are among the medications. Because Replace with: "they prolong the QTc interval", these sodium channel blockers have the highest pro-arrhythmic potential; therefore, their use is restricted. Quinidine is used as an alternative to a rare genetic disorder that causes potentially fatal cardiac arrhythmias an implanted cardioverter-defibrillator (ICD) in certain patients with Brugada a rare genetic disorder that causes potentially fatal cardiac arrhythmias. Patients with recurrent ventricular arrhythmias (VA) and short QT syndrome may benefit from quinidine treatment. Patients with short QT syndrome who have had ICD placement may experience fewer shocks when on quinidine therapy. Disopyramide is still occasionally used to treat hypertrophic obstructive cardiomyopathy (HOCM), especially when combined with verapamil or beta-blockers to treat symptoms like dyspnea or angina in patients with HOCM who do not respond well to these treatments alone. For those who are suspected of having Brugada syndrome but do not yet have a confirmed diagnosis, procainamide can be a useful diagnostic tool. When atrial fibrillation (AF) occurs in patients with Wolff-Parkinson-White (WPW) and is accompanied by a wide QRS complex or a rapid pre-excited ventricular response, procainamide is advised as a medication to restore sinus rhythm. Moreover, it may be helpful in trying to stop ventricular arrhythmia and tachycardia.

2. Class Ib

Class Ib antiarrhythmic drugs cause a slight sodium channel blockage. Mexiletine and lidocaine are examples of such. These medications shorten the QTc interval, are only effective for VA (particularly VA following myocardial infarction), and have no bearing on atrial arrhythmias. Mediletine shortens the QTc interval in long QT syndrome and has been used to lessen ICD and recurrent arrhythmias.

3. Class Ic

Class Ic antiarrhythmic drugs cause a significant degree of sodium blockage without changing the QT interval. Among the drugs are propafenone and flecainide. When a patient has symptomatic supraventricular tachycardia (SVT) and neither structural heart disease nor ischemic heart disease is present, these medications are appropriate for continued treatment. As well as for patients who cannot or choose not to undergo catheter ablation. These agents are also useful for pharmacological cardioversion of atrial fibrillation (AF). Some patients may use the "pill in pocket" strategy. The pill in the pocket refers to a treatment strategy where the patient with paroxysmal AF does not take a regularly scheduled maintenance dose of the medication but instead carries a loading dose of the agent.

Let's say the patient believes an AF episode has begun. In that scenario, they try chemical cardioversion to return to a more regular rhythm and take a loading dose of the appropriate treatment medication as a one-time dose. Propafenone and flecainide shouldn't be administered to patients who have structural heart disease. In an attempt to lower the frequency of premature ventricular contractions (PVCs), patients who had a prior myocardial infarction and were treated with class Ic agents (flecainide, encainide, moricizine) exhibited higher mortality compared to placebo in the Cardiac Arrhythmia Suppression Trials (CAST I and II). This trial means that patients with left ventricular dysfunction will not usually be prescribed class Ic agents. Based on this data, most ventricular arrhythmias are essentially ruled out for class Ic agent treatment.

3.4.1.2. Class II : Beta-blockers

For rate control in patients with atrial flutter and paroxysmal, persistent, or permanent AF, beta-blockers (BB) are recommended. When treating patients with symptomatic supraventricular tachycardia (SVT), oral beta-blockers are helpful for continued care. Because of their superior safety profile and efficacy in treating ventricular arrhythmias, beta-blockers are frequently used as first-line antiarrhythmic care. When treating long QT syndrome and catecholaminergic polymorphic ventricular tachycardia, beta-blocker therapy lowers adverse cardiac events. Beta-blocker therapy helps patients with symptomatic (PVCs) in otherwise healthy hearts by lowering recurrent arrhythmias and improving symptoms.

3.4.1.3. Class III : Potassium channel blockers

Potassium channel blockers lengthen the QTc interval and reduce potassium efflux out of the cell.

- Amiodarone inhibits the conduction of the AV and sinus nodes through sympatholytic, sodium, and calcium antagonistic actions. To maintain sinus rhythm in AF patients, particularly in those with left ventricular systolic dysfunction, this medication is advised. It makes sense in pharmacological cardioversion as well. Although it is less effective than non-dihydropyridine calcium channel blockers, this agent can be used to achieve ventricular rate control in critically ill patients without the need for pre-excitation. The most often prescribed antiarrhythmic drug for VA suppression is amiodarone. Intravenous amiodarone should be given to patients with hemodynamically unstable persistent VA following defibrillation to establish a stable rhythm. Additionally, it has demonstrated efficacy in VA suppression in ischemic heart disease patients receiving continuous beta-blocker therapy.
- Dronedarone lowers the hospitalization rate for AF in patients with sinus rhythm who have a history of non-permanent AF. However, in patients with AF that cannot be brought back to a normal sinus rhythm, the doctor should not prescribe dronedarone (permanent AF). The FDA review claims that in these patients, the risk of heart failure, stroke, and cardiovascular death doubles.
- The only indication for dofetilide is atrial arrhythmias. For patients with atrial fibrillation or atrial flutter, oral dofetilide is helpful for acute pharmacological cardioversion.
- The effects of potassium channel blockers and class II non-cardioselective beta-blockers are shared by sotalol. Consequently, it can be used by medical professionals to treat supraventricular and ventricular arrhythmias. While preventing recurrent AF, it is ineffective in converting AF to sinus rhythm. Sotalol demonstrated effectiveness in inhibiting VA as well.
- Ibutilide is indicated for AF or atrial flutter only

3.4.1.4. Class IV

Diltiazem and verapamil, two non-dihydropyridine calcium channel blockers, slow conduction through the AV node and reduce conduction velocity. They help with atrial flutter and ventricular rate control in both acute and chronic AF. For the acute management of hemodynamically stable patients with SVT, focal, and multifocal atrial tachycardias, there are two options: diltiazem and verapamil.

3.4.2. Mechanism of Action

The cycle of ion movement known as the cardiac action potential causes the cardiac myocyte to successively depolarize and repolarize, which in turn causes muscle contraction. The baseline resting membrane potential of a cardiac myocyte is between negative 80 and negative 90 mV. The following is a breakdown of how antiarrhythmic drugs work: they slow ion movement at different stages of the cardiac action potential:

- **Phase 0:** "the depolarization" phase of the action potential; occurs by the rapid movement of sodium ions (Na^+) into the cell along an electrochemical gradient, which leads to a membrane potential of approximately positive 30 mV.
- **Phase 1:** "The notch,"; the initial or early repolarization phase of the action potential, involves the efflux of potassium (K^+) ions.
- **Phase 2:** "The plateau" phase – this phase is a balance of inward calcium ion movement that offsets the outward K^+ movement.
- **Phase 3**: "The repolarization" phase of the action potential; this phase is primarily caused by the movement of K^+ ions along their electrochemical gradient out of the cell, essentially taking the positive charge of the K^+ ion out of the cell. It restores the negative potential of the cardiac myocyte.
- **Phase 4:** Restoration of the Na/K-ATPase, which restores the resting membrane potential of the cardiac myocyte.

3.4.3. Administration

The majority of antiarrhythmic drugs can be taken orally or intravenously, depending on how serious the condition is. Procainamide and lidocaine are two examples of class I antiarrhythmics that are given intravenously because their main application is for acute treatment. An oral analog of lidocaine is mediletine. Quinidine comes as an oral and intravenous formulation. Both capsules and controlled-release capsules are used to administer disopyramide. It is possible, safe, and effective to convert recent-onset atrial fibrillation to sinus rhythm by oral administration of flecainide or propafenone. A saline flush should come after the quick bolus infusion of adenosine via proximal IV. Digoxin can be injected intramuscularly or administered orally, intravenously, or by mouth. When administering antiarrhythmic medications to patients who have a known risk of TdP, such as amiodarone, disopyramide, dofetilide, ibutilide, and sotalol, continuous cardiac monitoring is necessary.

3.4.3.1. Hepatic Impairment

Lowering the dosage of many antiarrhythmics is advised due to hepatic impairment, particularly in cirrhosis patients. There has been evidence of a reduction in systemic clearance and a significant extension of the elimination half-life for medications like carvedilol, lidocaine, propafenone, and verapamil. As a result, it is advised that patients with moderate to severe liver cirrhosis reduce their dosage by two to three times. Since the renal route is the primary route of elimination for disopyramide, sotalol, and procainamide, dosage reductions for those medications are likely not necessary in patients with liver disease, provided that renal function is normal. If ascites, hepatomegaly, jaundice, or other clinical signs of hepatic injury are present, or if serum aminotransferase activities are regularly elevated above five times the upper limit of normal, amiodarone therapy should be discontinued.

3.4.3.2. Renal Impairment

Hypokalemia, hypomagnesemia, and reduced renal function all raise the risk of digoxin toxicity. Digoxin should therefore be administered with caution to patients who already have renal disease. If eGFR is less than 35 ml/min/1.73 m, flecainide therapy requires dose modification. Patients with a creatinine clearance of less than 40 milliliters per minute should not take sotalol. It is advised to modify the dosage of dofetilide based on the initial measurement of creatine clearance. Kidney Disease Improving Global Outcomes guidelines state that the drug should not be administered to patients whose creatinine clearance is less than 20 milliliters per minute.

3.4.3.3. Pregnancy Considerations

Recurrence during pregnancy in women with preexisting cardiac arrhythmias is a cause for concern. Clinicians should select antiarrhythmic therapy at the lowest effective dose possible due to the potential for teratogenicity. Since 2015, a new rule that explains the possible risks and benefits for the mother and fetus has replaced the FDA's pregnancy letter category system (A, B, C, D, and X). Quinidine's ease of placental transfer has made it a useful treatment for supraventricular and ventricular arrhythmias in both mothers and fetuses. According to reports, procainamide use during pregnancy does not appear to cause any problems for the developing fetus.

Disopyramide should be avoided due to the possible increased risk of preterm labor and the paucity of information regarding the drug's safety during pregnancy. Intravenous lidocaine works well during pregnancy as long as there are no obvious fetal problems. Moreover, it is commonly employed as an anesthetic in the postpartum period. Intravenous lidocaine treatment for ventricular arrhythmias is a viable option. Although there isn't enough information, mexiletine use during pregnancy may be safe, but caution should be exercised. Since flecainide has more clinical experience with propafenone than propafenone, flecainide is preferred over propafenone in pregnant patients without structural heart disease.

In pregnancy, beta-blockers are frequently used to treat tachycardia and hypertension. Reduced birth weight is a concern related to β-blockers. More specifically, atenolol raises the risk of low birth weight. Except for atenolol (category D) and pindolol (category B), all β-blockers were previously classified as FDA category C. Fetal hypothyroidism is the side effect of amiodarone that is most frequently reported. Nonetheless, the majority of hypothyroidism is transient and goes away with replacement medication. Amiodarone has been linked to rare congenital abnormalities and cases of symptomatic fetal bradycardia. Therefore, amiodarone should be used when other therapies are either ineffective or contraindicated and treatment is required for life-threatening arrhythmias. As usual, medical professionals need to weigh the advantages of amiodarone against its drawbacks (category D).

3.4.3.4. Breastfeeding Considerations

Physicians ought to talk about the risks vs. benefits of jointly deciding on specific medications to take during pregnancy and lactation with the patient. Antiarrhythmic medications such as lidocaine, procainamide, adenosine, digoxin, verapamil, diltiazem, atenolol, and esmolol are presumed to be compatible with breastfeeding, per the guidelines of the American College of Obstetricians and Gynecologists (ACOG). Sotalol and amiodarone may be harmful to nursing mothers.

3.4.4. Adverse Effects

The use of antiarrhythmic drugs raises many issues. Primarily, the majority of agents possess some degree of pro-arrhythmic potential. In actuality, the drugs themselves can cause other arrhythmias, some of which may be more dangerous, even while they are intended to suppress the original arrhythmia. Quinidine, procainamide, and disopyramide, for instance, are class Ia sodium channel blockers that effectively lengthen the QTc interval and raise the risk of ventricular tachycardia (torsades de pointes).

More medication-specific side effects are associated with class Ia antiarrhythmics. Procainamide may cause lupus erythematosus, which is reversible if the offending medication is stopped. Cinchononism is a side effect of quinine therapy that includes headache, tinnitus, nausea, dizziness, and vision changes. Due to its anticholinergic properties, disopyramide can cause many negative side effects, including dry and flushed skin, thirst, hyperthermia, mydriasis, confusion, agitation, and retention of urine. Patients who have had a myocardial infarction should not take class Ic antiarrhythmics due to their potential for arrhythmogenic effects.

Bradycardia and AV block are two cardiovascular side effects of beta-blocker therapy. Lethargy, dyslipidemia, and an aggravation of asthma and COPD are among the noncardiac side effects of beta-blockers. This possible adverse effect is common to all K^+ channel blockers. If the action potential phases and the ECG are compared, it becomes clear why this is happening. Ventricular repolarization is represented by the T wave on the ECG. The action potential's third phase is known as repolarization. Phase 3 of the action potential is prolonged if a K^+ channel blocker is administered because of the sluggish efflux of K^+ ions. A prolonged QTc interval results from a prolonged action potential repolarization phase, which also prolongs the T-wave on the corresponding ECG. Based on extracted safety data from eight clinical trials, dronedarone should not be used in patients with severe heart failure, decompensated heart failure, or permanent atrial fibrillation. Amiodarone can cause a variety of side effects, such as corneal microdeposits, myopathy, elevated liver function tests, hypo- or hyperthyroidism, pulmonary fibrosis, and nausea.

Unwanted side effects from verapamil include bradycardia, constipation, and AV block. Headaches, vertigo, and edema are the side effects of diltiazem that are most commonly reported. Common side effects of calcium channel blockers (CCBs), such as verapamil and diltiazem, include i.e. peripheral edema. When peripheral edema is misdiagnosed as a new medical condition and a diuretic is prescribed to treat it, this can lead to a prescribing cascade.

Sweating, flushing, and a feeling of impending doom are minor side effects of adenosine that are typically temporary because of the drug's short half-life. Asystole, AV block, hypotension, and chest pain are examples of more serious side effects. Patients with asthma should not receive adenosine as it can trigger bronchospasm.. Due to the possibility of tachycardia exacerbation, clinicians should refrain from administering adenosine to patients with SVT involving accessory pathways (WPW, antidromic AVRT).

Digoxin toxicity-specific arrhythmia is atrial tachycardia with AV block. The symptoms of digoxin toxicity include nausea, vomiting, abdominal pain, exhaustion, disorientation, and changes in color vision.

Ivabradine therapy was linked to a higher incidence of atrial fibrillation, according to a recent meta-analysis, and the effect was more pronounced in patients with LVEF >40%. In another meta-analysis, visual abnormalities and asymptomatic bradycardia were also noted.

3.4.5. Contraindications

One of the most widely used antiarrhythmic medications, amiodarone, has boxed warnings for cardiac, hepatic, and pulmonary toxicity. In cases of cardiogenic shock, sick sinus syndrome, second- or third-degree atrioventricular block, and documented hypersensitivity to amiodarone or iodine, amiodarone should not be used. In cases of acute decompensated heart failure, sick sinus syndrome, sinoatrial block, severe hepatic impairment, and significant bradycardia, ivabradine is contraindicated. Patients who have previously experienced amide-type anesthetic hypersensitivity should not use lidocaine. Procainamide should not be used in cases of complete heart block, idiosyncratic hypersensitivity, or systemic lupus erythematosus with a confirmed diagnosis. Quinidine should not be used in individuals with a history of immune thrombocytopenia or those with complete AV block, who rely on a pacemaker to regulate their heartbeat.

Likewise, individuals with second- or third-degree AV block who do not have a working pacemaker should not take mexiletine. A boxed warning regarding proarrhythmias in patients with structural heart disease applies to propafenone. Additionally, propafenone should not be used in cases of Brugada syndrome, sick sinus node syndrome/AV block without an artificial pacemaker, or cardiogenic shock. Encainide or flecainide treatment was associated with higher mortality rates in the CAST trial patients with asymptomatic non-life-threatening ventricular arrhythmias who had a MI more than six days but less than two years prior.

In patients with bronchial asthma, sinus bradycardia, greater than first-degree AV block, cardiogenic shock, and acute decompensated heart failure, non-selective beta-blockers should not be used. Furthermore, there's a chance that abruptly stopping beta-blockers could exacerbate ischemic heart disease. Patients with second and third-degree heart block, bradycardia, and decompensated heart failure should not receive IV metoprolol. Patients with second- or third-degree AV block, cardiogenic shock, decompensated heart failure, severe sinus bradycardia, and hypersensitivity reactions should not take esmolol. Patients with liver cirrhosis and CYP3A4 inhibitors or inducers should not take ranolazine. Higher doses may also be linked to syncope, QTc prolongation, and renal dysfunction.

3.4.6. Monitoring

All antiarrhythmic medications have the potential to worsen arrhythmias, so they should only be given intravenously while the patient is being monitored for cardiac issues. Each medication in the Vaughn-Williams classification has its own unique side effects that must be considered before use. For instance, procainamide can cause a lupus-like condition, while quinidine can lead to cinchonism. The classification system is helpful because it outlines the main way each medication works and the general side effects it typically causes. For example, class III K^+ channel blockers, referred to as "repolarization" blockers, prolong phase 3 of the action potential and also cause a longer QT interval on an EKG. It is worth noting that using Bazett's formula to calculate QTc during atrial fibrillation can result in an overestimation, leading to lower doses of antiarrhythmic medication and potentially reducing its effectiveness.

Beta-blockers administration is best monitored with an electrocardiogram and heart rate monitoring rather than TDM. Amiodarone, while effective as an antiarrhythmic agent, can lead to complications like corneal opacities, thyroid issues, and lung problems with long-term use, making it less ideal for geriatric patients compared to young adults. Digoxin has a narrow therapeutic range of 0.5 to 2 ng/mL, with close monitoring required to prevent toxicity. Other medications like amiodarone, verapamil, quinidine, and diltiazem can increase digoxin levels and lead to toxicity, necessitating a reduction in dosage and frequent monitoring. Healthcare providers should also monitor electrolytes to prevent hypokalemia and reduce the morbidity associated with antiarrhythmic drugs by recognizing adverse reactions and monitoring therapeutic drug levels closely.

3.4.7. Toxicity

If an individual overdoses on antiarrhythmic drugs, healthcare providers must ensure an open airway, assist with breathing, and provide circulatory support. Severe hypotension may also require vasopressor support.

Symptoms of digoxin toxicity include vomiting, nausea, arrhythmias that are fatal, and neurological symptoms. For ventricular tachyarrhythmias caused by digoxin toxicity, lidocaine can be used, and for bradyarrhythmias, atropine. Furthermore, in cases of severe toxicity, antibody fragments specific to digoxin are effective. TdP is treated with dosage reduction or stopping medication altogether when dofetilide is used excessively or therapeutically. Guidelines suggest using activated charcoal for management if the arrhythmia does not go away if ingestion occurs within 15 minutes. This should be followed by giving IV magnesium and taking care of any electrolyte imbalance. On the other hand, isoproterenol/dopamine is administered as a bridge to pacing if the arrhythmia persists.

Vasopressors, high-dose insulin euglycemic treatment, and catecholamines are given in cases of beta-blocker poisoning. There is evidence linking glucagon to improved hemodynamics. For CCB overdose, intravenous calcium, dopamine, and norepinephrine are used. High-dose insulin is linked to a decreased death rate from calcium channel blocker toxicity. Patients experiencing severe shock or cardiac arrest are treated with extracorporeal life support. According to the case report, amiodarone and flecainide overdoses have been effectively treated with lipid emulsion therapy.

3.5. Diuretics

A diuretic is a substance that helps increase the production of urine, including forced diuresis. Diuretics are commonly referred to as "water tablets" and come in various categories. They work by increasing the excretion of water through the kidneys. On the other hand, an antidiuretic like vasopressin inhibits the excretion of water in urine.

3.5.1. Medical Uses

Diuretics are prescribed to treat a variety of conditions in medicine, including kidney disease edema, hypertension, liver cirrhosis, heart failure, and water poisoning. In cases of overdose or poisoning, some diuretics, like acetazolamide, help to increase the excretion of substances like aspirin and help to make the urine more alkaline. Sometimes, individuals with eating disorders—particularly those suffering from bulimia nervosa—abuse diuretics in an attempt to reduce their body weight.

Certain diuretics, such as thiazides and loop diuretics, have antihypertensive properties that are unrelated to their diuretic effect. That is to say, the drop in blood pressure happens through different mechanisms and at lower doses than those needed to cause diuresis, rather than because of a decrease in blood volume brought on by an increase in urine production. Compared to most other diuretics, indapamide has a wider therapeutic window for hypertension (without a noticeable diuresis) because it was created with this in mind.

3.5.2. Types

3.5.2.1. High-Ceiling/Loop Diuretics

Diuretics with high ceilings have the potential to significantly reduce filtered water and salt content by up to 20%. Compared to normal renal sodium reabsorption, which leaves only approximately 0.4% of filtered sodium in the urine, this is a significant amount. Because of this feature, loop diuretics are frequently used interchangeably with high-ceiling diuretics. Water is excreted in the urine by loop diuretics, like furosemide, because they prevent the body from reabsorbing sodium at the ascending loop in the nephron. Normally, water follows sodium back into the extracellular fluid. Examples of other high-ceiling loop diuretics are torsemide and ethacrynic acid.

3.5.2.2. Thiazides

Water normally follows penetrating solutes, so thiazide-type diuretics like hydrochlorothiazide act on the distal convoluted tubule and inhibit the sodium-chloride symporter, causing water to be retained in the urine. Due to a concurrent relationship with sodium loss from the convoluted tubule, there is an increased loss of water from the body that has not been retained, which causes frequent urination. Thiazides lower preload, which lowers blood pressure, which is the basis for their short-term anti-hypertensive effect. However, the long-term impact is brought on by an unidentified vasodilator effect that lowers blood pressure by reducing resistance (Engberink et al, 2015).

3.5.2.3. Carbonic Anhydrase Inhibitors

The proximal convoluted tubule contains the enzyme carbonic anhydrase, which is inhibited by carbonic anhydrase inhibitors. This has many effects, such as decreased sodium absorption and bicarbonate buildup in the urine. Methazolamide and acetazolamide are two medications in this class.

3.5.2.4. Potassium-Sparing Diuretics

Potassium is retained and not lost as much as with other diuretics because these diuretics do not encourage the secretion of potassium into the urine. The term "potassium-sparing" refers to an effect rather than a mechanism or location; nonetheless, the term almost always refers to two specific classes that have their effect at similar locations:

- Aldosterone antagonists: spironolactone, which is a competitive antagonist of aldosterone. Aldosterone normally adds sodium channels in the principal cells of the collecting duct and late distal tubule of the nephron. Spironolactone prevents aldosterone from entering the principal cells, preventing sodium reabsorption. Similar agents are eplerenone and potassium canreonate.
- Epithelial sodium channel blockers: amiloride and triamterene.

3.5.2.5. Calcium-Sparing Diuretics

Agents causing a relatively low rate of excretion of calcium are sometimes referred to as "calcium-sparing diuretics."

An elevated rate of calcium in serum may result from a decreased calcium concentration in the urine. In hypocalcemia, the calcium sparing effect may be advantageous; in hypercalcemia, it may be detrimental.

The thiazides and potassium-sparing diuretics are considered to be calcium-sparing diuretics.

- The thiazides cause a net decrease in calcium lost in urine.
- Although there is a net increase in calcium lost in urine as a result of potassium-sparing diuretics, this increase is far less than that of other diuretic classes.

On the other hand, loop diuretics encourage a notable rise in the excretion of calcium. This may raise the chance of decreased bone mass.

3.5.2.6. Osmotic Diuretics

Substances that raise osmolarity but have restricted tubular epithelial cell permeability are known as osmotic diuretics, such as mannitol. They mainly function by increasing the volume of extracellular fluid and plasma, which increases blood flow to the kidney and especially to the peritubular capillaries. This decreases medullary osmolality, which affects urine concentration in the loop of Henle (which typically transports solutes and water using the high osmotic and solute gradient). Additionally, the filtrate's osmolality and water retention are increased by the restricted tubular epithelial cell permeability.

It was once thought that the main way osmotic diuretics, like mannitol, work was by filtering them in the glomerulus so they couldn't be reabsorbed. As a result, the filtrate becomes more osmolar due to their presence, and water is held in the urine to preserve osmotic balance.

Similar to mannitol, glucose can act as an osmotic diuretic. Contrary to mannitol, blood often contains glucose. However, in some diseases, like diabetes mellitus, the blood's concentration of glucose (hyperglycemia) surpasses the kidney's maximum capacity for reabsorption. This results in the osmotic retention of water in the urine because glucose is still present in the filtrate. Hypotonic water and Na^+ are lost due to glucosuria, which results in a hypertonic state with volume depletion symptoms like dry mucosa, hypotension, tachycardia, and a decrease in skin turgor. Certain medications, particularly stimulants, can raise blood sugar levels, which can lead to increased urination.

3.5.2.6. Low-Ceiling Diuretics

A diuretic with a fast flattening dose effect curve is referred to as low-ceiling (as opposed to high-ceiling, where the relationship is almost linear). This group includes some diuretic classes, like the thiazides.

3.5.3. Mechanism of Action of Diuretics

Diuretics increase the volume of urine that the kidneys can process (i.e., encourage diuresis). This is accomplished by altering the kidneys' sodium processing mechanism. Water excretion will rise in tandem with an increase in sodium excretion by the kidneys. Most diuretics work by preventing sodium from being reabsorbed in various tubular system segments, which increases renal diuresis.

Furthermore, when two diuretics are taken together, their synergistic effects can result in a significant increase in effectiveness compared to using either medication alone. Diuretics work by compensating for altered sodium reabsorption in one nephron segment in another nephron segment. As a result, blocking multiple nephron sites greatly increases efficiency.

The sodium-potassium-chloride co-transporter in the ascending loop of Henle is inhibited by loop diuretics. Because this transporter typically reabsorbs about 25% of the sodium, inhibiting this pump may cause the distal tubule's sodium concentration to rise significantly, the surrounding septum to become less hypertonic, and the collecting duct to absorb less water. Both increased water loss and increased sodium loss are the results of this modified sodium and water treatment. Loop diuretics are categorized as extremely potent diuretics because they significantly reduce sodium reabsorption by acting in the loop of Henle. These particular diuretics also cause the production of renal prostaglandins, which support renal function by increasing renal blood flow and redistributing blood flow to the cortex.

The most widely used diuretics are thiazide diuretics, which work by blocking the sodium-chloride transporter in the distal tubule. These diuretics are not as effective in producing diuresis and sodium diuresis as loop diuretics are because this transporter typically reabsorbs only approximately 5% of filtered sodium. But thiazide diuretics are also strong enough to satisfy the diuretic's therapeutic need.

Potassium-sparing diuretics are the third class of diuretics. This class of diuretics functions as an antagonist to aldosterone at the receptor site in the distal tubule, in contrast to loop diuretics and thiazides, which act directly on sodium transport. More water and sodium enter the collecting duct as a result, and are expelled in the urine. Since they do not induce hypokalemia like loop diuretics and thiazides do, they are known as hyperkalemic diuretics. Additionally, this class of diuretics is frequently used in conjunction with thiazides or loop diuretics to help prevent hypokalemia due to their relatively weak effect on overall sodium balance.

Carbonic anhydrase inhibitors are another class of diuretics. They prevent bicarbonate from being transported from the proximal tubule into the renal interstitium, which reduces sodium reabsorption at this location and consequently sodium loss, bicarbonate, and increased urine volume. Since it is the weakest diuretic, cardiovascular disease rarely uses it. The primary application for them is glaucoma therapy.

The last category is that of osmotic diuretics. By raising the osmolality of the blood and renal filtrate, osmotic diuretics block the reabsorption of water and salt. This diuretic mechanism is responsible for their effects. Isosorbide and mannitol are two examples of medications in this class that can be used to lower intracranial pressure.

3.5.4. Side Effects

Diuretics are generally safe. Side effects include:

- Urinating more often.
- Too little sodium in the blood.
- Too little potassium in the blood.

Hypokalemia is the term for extremely low potassium levels brought on by thiazide diuretics. Hypokalemia can result in potentially fatal irregular heartbeats. Potassium levels need to be monitored, and potassium-sparing diuretics can be added to other diuretics in order to prevent hypokalemia. Other side effects of diuretics can include:

- Dizziness.
- Headaches.
- Dehydration.
- Muscle cramps.
- A type of arthritis called gout, which causes severe joint pain, usually in the big toe.
- Trouble getting erections, also called erectile dysfunction or impotence.

3.6. Drugs Used in Hypotensive States and Shock

Antihypotensive medications, which can be categorized as follows, are used to raise low blood pressure.

I. Agents intended to increase the volume of blood in active circulation

These include intravenous fluids such as whole blood, plasma components, plasma substitutes and solution of crystalloids

II. Vasoconstrictor drugs include

Direct and sympathomimetic medications are two categories of peripherally acting vasoconstrictors.

Ephedrine, adrenaline, noradrenaline, phenylephrine, are sympathomimetics that are used to raise blood pressure.

Two examples of direct vasoconstrictors are angiotensin and vasopressin.

3.6.1. Treatment of Shock

A clinical syndrome known as shock is typified by a reduction in tissue blood flow. Oliguria, heart failure, disorientation, mental confusion, seizures, cold extremities, and coma are typical warning signs and symptoms.

The majority of shock victims are hypotensive, but not always. The type of shock determines the treatment. The pathophysiology of the condition is the primary determinant of the drug selection.

- Dopamine or another cardiotonic medication is recommended for cardiogenic shock and reduced cardiac output. Cardiotonic medication may be administered in conjunction with vasodilator medications (nitropruside, nitroglycerine) in cases of severe CHF, which is defined by decreased CO and elevated PVR. In the unlikely event that pulmonary congestion develops, diuretics may also be recommended.
- The first choice drug for anaphylactic shock or neurogenic shock, which is identified by intense vasodilation and reduced peripheral vascular resistance, is a vasoconstrictor such as which is a precursor for norepinephrine.
- Intravenous fluids that replenish the lost fluid type should be administered in cases of hypovolemic shock.
- appropriate antibiotic therapy in addition to other therapeutic interventions for septic shock. (Lindholm et al, 2005; Kones et al, 2010; Ettehad et al, 2016)

A Closer Look

Pharmacologic Management of the Cardio-renal Syndrome

Kidney disease progression and a decline in function are frequently preceded by cardiac dysfunction. On the other hand, renal dysfunction is a significant co-morbidity of heart failure and a strong indicator of mortality and cardiovascular problems. Cardio-renal syndrome is the term used to describe the codependent relationship between heart failure and kidney failure (CRS). In an effort to better understand CRS and its underlying causes, a revised definition and classification of the syndrome have recently been put forth.

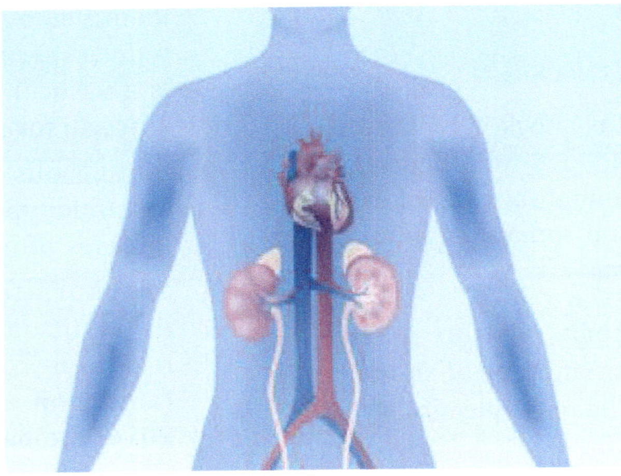

Source: https://ckdexplained.co.uk/why-do-heart-and-kidney-disease-go-together-cardiorenal-syndrome/

Given their similar pathophysiology, cardiac and renal dysfunctions frequently occur concurrently. The sympathetic nervous system, inflammation, renin-angiotensin-aldosterone system (RAAS) activation, and an imbalance between nitric oxide and reactive oxygen species have all been suggested as mediators of this relationship.

There is no agreement on how to treat patients with cardio-renal and/or reno-cardiac syndrome, despite the fact there are clinical guidelines for managing acute and chronic heart failure as well as renal dysfunction separately. Patients with largely normal kidney function were recruited for the majority of heart failure clinical trials. Trials specifically designed for populations with concomitant cardiac and renal dysfunction have not been conducted, so it is impossible to evaluate the safety and efficacy of CRS therapies or provide evidence-based treatment recommendations. For this reason, managing CRS patients pharmacologically continues to be extremely difficult.

Novel therapeutic approaches, however, have recently been researched to preserve or enhance renal and cardiac function. Furthermore, current treatments are being altered to provide more positive effects for kidney and heart function than those previously offered by conventional treatments, as a result of the rising incidence and significance of CRS in the current clinical setting. A comprehensive consensus statement about CRS, including management strategies, was recently published by the International Acute Dialysis Quality Initiative Panel.

Ø Management of Acute Cardio-renal Syndrome

A specific course of treatment for acute CRS aims to mitigate increased serum creatinine, decreased glomerular filtration rate, decreased urine output, and prevent weight loss. Most of the time, inotropic agents and vasodilators are used in conjunction with neurohormonal antagonists and diuretics in modern pharmacologic management. Although the outcomes of clinical trials employing kidney-targeting medications, such as vasopressin antagonists, adenosine antagonists, and natriuretic peptides, have been underwhelming thus far, these drugs may still have therapeutic value.

- **Inotropic Agents and Low-dose Dopamine**

Patients with low cardiac output and low blood pressure are frequently treated with inotropic drugs. Medication like milrinone and dobutamine raise cardiac index in proportion to renal blood flow, but there is no conclusive evidence linking these increases to improved clinical outcomes or lower mortality.

- **Diuretics and Vasodilators**

In addition to providing CRS patients with temporary symptom relief, diuretics and vasodilators are crucial in the early management of CRS and its side effects, such as venous hypertension, elevated intra-abdominal pressure, and renal congestion. Diuretics, however, can worsen electrolyte imbalances, reduce effective circulating volume, throw off neurohormonal balance, and impair renal function when taken in excess. Since high-dose diuretics are frequently needed to treat both heart failure and renal dysfunction, the dosage that is given must be carefully calculated to enhance fluid balance and relieve symptoms without inducing unfavorable physiological effects.

Vasodilators rapidly lower ventricular filling pressure and central venous pressure, which can reduce myocardial oxygen consumption and alleviate pulmonary congestion. Nitroglycerine, commonly used for treating acute decompensated heart failure (ADHF), may also lower trans-renal perfusion pressure by decreasing venous pressure. It is unclear if nitroglycerine improves kidney function or long-term survival. Sodium nitroprusside, another vasodilator, acts on cyclic guanosine monophosphate in vascular smooth muscle to produce significant arterial and venous dilation. In a nonrandomized trial, ADHF patients treated with sodium nitroprusside had positive long-term outcomes, regardless of inotropic support or kidney dysfunction. However, thiocyanate accumulation is a potential dangerous side effect in patients with impaired kidney function.

- **Vasopressin and Adenosine Antagonists**

Tolvaptan and conivaptan are examples of selective vasopressin V2 antagonists that can promote free water clearance and raise serum sodium levels without affecting plasma potassium and magnesium levels. 4,133 patients with ADHF were included in the Efficacy of Vasopressin Antagonist in Heart Failure Outcome Study with Tolvaptan (EVEREST) trial, which discovered that early tolvaptan administration was linked to a reduction in mean body weight and an improvement in dyspnea. Vasopressin antagonists have been shown to alleviate symptoms in a subset of patients with hyponatremia and oliguria, however, there was no improvement in mortality compared to placebo. Renal dysfunction in heart failure may be made worse by elevated adenosine levels. Urine output can be increased while kidney function is preserved by medications that specifically block adenosine A1-receptors while maintaining adenosine A2-receptor activity. Patients treated with the selective A1 receptor antagonist rolofylline in one study experienced a continuous rise in urine production without a deterioration in renal function. The PROTECT trial, however, was unable to show any improvement in outcomes, such as death or re-hospitalization due to renal or cardiovascular disease, or any functional benefit. Similarly, there was no discernible improvement in the clinical status and recent or acute worsening of renal function with rolofylline in the multicenter, international, randomized, double-blind, placebo-controlled REACH-UP trial.

Ø ***Management of Chronic Cardio-renal Syndrome***

- **RAAS blockade**

It has been demonstrated that RAAS inhibitors lower mortality in heart failure patients; however, most of these studies did not include patients with severe renal impairment. These medications not only increase the prognosis for heart failure patients but also stop the development of renal insufficiency in diabetic nephropathy and other types of chronic kidney disease. All patients with renal dysfunction whose serum creatinine concentration was less than 3 points per milliliter were included in the Cooperative North Scandinavian Enalapril Survival Study (CONSENSUS) of patients with severe heart failure. Treatment with an angiotensin-converting enzyme (ACE) inhibitor improved the outcomes for the subgroup of patients whose serum creatinine levels were greater than 2 mg/dL. When treating patients with CRS, ACE inhibitors or angiotensin II-receptor blockers (ARB) should be used with caution due to the possibility of hyperkalemia and a brief rise in creatinine levels. To lower the risk of renal deterioration, patients should begin RAAS blockers at the lowest possible dose, and kidney function should be regularly monitored both during the initiation and uptitration phases of treatment. This is particularly crucial for patients who are dehydrated. Additionally, concurrent NSAID use needs to be avoided.

In patients who develop heart failure following an acute myocardial infarction, the mineralocorticoid receptor antagonists" spironolactone and and eplerenone reduce morbidity and mortality. The RALES and EPHESUS trials showed that adding low-dose spironolactone or eplerenone to patients already receiving standard heart failure medications significantly improved the outcome. Patients with renal dysfunction are more likely to experience hyperkalemia, even though numerous studies have demonstrated that mineralocorticoid receptor antagonists have organ-protective benefits. Therefore, more research is needed to determine the long-term effects of mineralocorticoid receptor antagonists on renal outcome, mortality, and safety in patients with CRS.

- **β-blockers**

In both cardiac and renal failure, sympathetic nervous system activation is frequently observed. It is crucial to stop the progression of renal and cardiovascular disease by interfering with this response. The β-blocker carvedilol may be more advantageous than previous β-blocker formulations because it has positive effects on renal function in certain patients with heart and kidney disease. However, patients with severe renal dysfunction were excluded from large randomized clinical trials on β-blocker treatment for heart failure, and their effects on renal outcome were not taken into account.

- **Antithrombotic therapy**

Aspirin has long been thought to be safe for use in patients with kidney disease, even though it may affect GFR through its effects on renal prostaglandins and cyclooxygenase. This was corroborated by the first UK Heart and Renal Protection Study, which demonstrated that even in patients with risk factors for minor bleeding, low-dose aspirin (100 mg/d) did not significantly increase the risk for major bleeding or renalmpairment. Additional research is necessary to determine the effectiveness of other antithrombotic medications, such as clopidogrel and low-molecular weight heparins, in patients with reduced renal function.

- **Anemia management**

More than one-third of CRS patients have anemia. The term "cardio-renal anemia syndrome" (CRAS) describes a pathologic triad that negatively affects morbidity and mortality when anemia, heart failure, and renal failure occur simultaneously. Regarding the definition, importance, and managemen of CRAS, there is no agreement. Particularly debatable is the use of erythropoiesis-stimulating agents (ESAs) in the management of CRAS. In heart failure, elevated serum erythropoietin is a poor indicator of morbidity and mortality. Nonetheless, erythropoietin receptor activation in the heart may offer protection against inflammation, fibrosis, and apoptosis, which justifies the use of ESAs in heart failure patients. In comparison to oral iron therapy alone, a randomized, double-blind, controlled study revealed that correcting anemia with erythropoietin and oral iron over the course of a year improved cardiac function, left ventricular remodeling, and B-type natriuretic peptide levels. Parenteral iron therapy is becoming more and more popular as a means of treating anemia in congestive heart failure patients. Independent of the effects on hemoglobin level, two recent trials, FERRIC-HF and FAIR-HF, showed that patients treated with intravenous iron showed improved symptomatology and increased capacity for exercise. According to these findings, intravenous iron therapy may be used to treat CRAS.

Summary

- Antihypertensives are a class of drugs that are used to treat hypertension (high blood pressure). Antihypertensive therapy seeks to prevent the complications of high blood pressure, such as stroke, heart failure, kidney failure and myocardial infarction.
- Hypertension (HTN) is considered one of the leading causes of increased cardiovascular disease.
- Chlorthalidone is the first choice for older patients with osteoporosis, as it was associated with a lower incidence of pelvic fractures when compared to amlodipine and lisinopril.
- Antihypertensives are a broad group of medications, and healthcare workers are recommended to have special caution in monitoring adherence and possible adverse reactions to these medications.
- Congestive heart failure occurs when there is an inability of the heart to maintain cardiac output sufficient to meet the requirements of the metabolizing tissues.
- Angina pectoris develops as a result of an imbalance between the oxygen supply and the oxygen demand of the myocardium. It is a symptom of myocardial ischemia.
- The pathogenesis of angina is often multi-factorial. The basic underlying mechanism that leads to angina is an imbalance of myocardial oxygen supply and demand.
- The antiarrhythmic medications have typically been categorized according to the Vaughan-Williams (VW) classification system. The system classifies the medications according to the primary mechanism of action (although several agents retain properties from multiple classes).
- A diuretic is any substance that promotes diuresis, the increased production of urine. This includes forced diuresis. A diuretic tablet is sometimes colloquially called a water tablet. There are several categories of diuretics.

References

1. Armstrong, C. (2014). JNC8 guidelines for the management of hypertension in adults. *American Family Physician, 90*(7), 503–504.
2. Beaty, R. S., Moffett, B. S., Hall, S., & Kim, J. (2015). Evaluating the safety of intraoperative antiarrhythmics in pediatric cardiac surgery patients. *Pediatric Cardiology, 36*(7), 1465–1469. https://doi.org/10.1007/s00246-015-1148-3.
3. Chockalingam, A., Gnanavelu, G., Subramaniam, T., et al. (2004). Canadian Cardiovascular Society classification of effort angina: An angiographic correlation. *Coronary Artery Disease, 15*(2), 111–114. https://doi.org/10.1097/00019501-200403000-00010.
4. Crosby, J., Bhopalwala, H., Kharawala, A., Dewaswala, N., Ganti, S. S., & Bhopalwala, A. (2021). Refractory Torsades de Pointes due to Dofetilide overdose. *Journal of Investigative Medicine High Impact Case Reports, 9*, 23247096211056492. https://doi.org/10.1177/23247096211056492.
5. Di Somma, S., Liguori, V., Petitto, M., et al. (1993). A double-blind comparison of nicorandil and metoprolol in stable effort angina pectoris. *Cardiovascular Drugs and Therapy, 7*(1), 119–123. https://doi.org/10.1007/BF00705833.

6. Ernst, M. E., Carter, B. L., Goerdt, C. J., Steffensmeier, J. J., Phillips, B. B., Zimmerman, M. B., & Bergus, G. R. (2006). Comparative antihypertensive effects of hydrochlorothiazide and chlorthalidone on ambulatory and office blood pressure. *Hypertension, 47*(3), 352–358. https://doi.org/10.1161/01.HYP.0000200557.04719.4d.

7. Ettehad, D., Emdin, C. A., Kiran, A., Anderson, S. G., Callender, T., Emberson, J., Chalmers, J., Rodgers, A., & Rahimi, K. (2016). Blood pressure lowering for prevention of cardiovascular disease and death: A systematic review and meta-analysis. *The Lancet, 387*(10022), 957–967. https://doi.org/10.1016/S0140-6736(15)00805-3.

8. Finkielman, J. D., Schwartz, G. L., Chapman, A. B., Boerwinkle, E., & Turner, S. T. (2005). Lack of agreement between office and ambulatory blood pressure responses to hydrochlorothiazide. *American Journal of Hypertension, 18*(3), 398–402. https://doi.org/10.1016/j.amjhyper.2004.09.012.

9. Fox, K., Garcia, M. A., Ardissino, D., et al. (2006). Guidelines on the management of stable angina pectoris: Executive summary: The Task Force on the Management of Stable Angina Pectoris of the European Society of Cardiology. *European Heart Journal, 27*(13), 1341–1381. https://doi.org/10.1093/eurheartj/ehl014.

10. Guermonprez, J. L., Blin, P., & Peterlongo, F. (1993). A double-blind comparison of the long-term efficacy of a potassium channel opener and a calcium antagonist instable angina pectoris. *European Heart Journal, 14*(Suppl B), 30–34. https://doi.org/10.1093/eurheartj/14.suppl_B.30.

11. Hendriks, J. M., & Heidbüchel, H. (2019). The management of atrial fibrillation: An integrated team approach - Insights of the 2016 European Society of Cardiology guidelines for the management of atrial fibrillation for nurses and allied health professionals. *European Journal of Cardiovascular Nursing, 18*(2), 88–95. https://doi.org/10.1177/1474515118770598.

12. Huang, K. Y., Tseng, P. T., Wu, Y. C., Tu, Y. K., Stubbs, B., Su, K. P., Matsuoka, Y. J., Hsu, C. W., Lin, C. H., Chen, Y. W., & Lin, P. Y. (2021). Do beta-adrenergic blocking agents increase asthma exacerbation? A network meta-analysis of randomized controlled trials. *Scientific Reports, 11*(1), 452. https://doi.org/10.1038/s41598-020-80345-3.

13. Kandler, M. R., Mah, G. T., Tejani, A. M., Stabler, S. N., & Salzwedel, D. M. (2011). Hydralazine for essential hypertension. *Cochrane Database of Systematic Reviews,* (11), CD004934. https://doi.org/10.1002/14651858.CD004934.pub2.

14. Kaplan, N. M. (2011). Chlorthalidone versus hydrochlorothiazide: A tale of tortoises and a hare. *Hypertension, 58*(6), 994–995. https://doi.org/10.1161/HYPERTENSIONAHA.111.179477.

15. Kaski, J. C. (2004). Pathophysiology and management of patients with chest pain and normal coronary arteriograms (cardiac syndrome X). *Circulation, 109*(5), 568–572. https://doi.org/10.1161/01.CIR.0000119658.85621.6C.

16. Kaski, J. C., Arrebola-Moreno, A., & Dungu, J. (2011). Treatment strategies for chronic stable angina. *Expert Opinion on Pharmacotherapy, 12*(18), 2833–2844. https://doi.org/10.1517/14656566.2011.629155.

17. Khan, N., & McAlister, F. A. (2006). Re-examining the efficacy of beta-blockers for the treatment of hypertension: A meta-analysis. *Canadian Medical Association Journal, 174*(12), 1737–1742. https://doi.org/10.1503/cmaj.060174.

18. Kones, R. (2010). Recent advances in the management of chronic stable angina I: Approach to the patient, diagnosis, pathophysiology, risk stratification and gender disparities. *Vascular Health and Risk Management, 6*(1), 635–656. https://doi.org/10.2147/VHRM.S7513.

19. Lindholm, L. H., Carlberg, B., & Samuelsson, O. (2005). Should beta-blockers remain first choice in the treatment of primary hypertension? A meta-analysis. *The Lancet, 366*(9496), 1545–1553. https://doi.org/10.1016/S0140-6736(05)67578-6.

20. LiverTox: Clinical and Research Information on Drug-Induced Liver Injury [Internet]. (2018). National institute of diabetes and digestive and kidney diseases; Bethesda (MD): May 20, 2018. *Ranolazine.* Retrieved from: https://www.ncbi.nlm.nih.gov/books/NBK548514/ (accessed on 30 July 2024).

21. Lloyd-Jones, D. M., Hong, Y., Labarthe, D., Mozaffarian, D., et al. (2010). Defining and setting national goals for cardiovascular health promotion and disease reduction: The American Heart Association's strategic impact goal through 2020 and beyond. *Circulation, 121*(4), 586–613. https://doi.org/10.1161/CIRCULATIONAHA.109.192703.

22. MacIntyre, C. J., & Sapp, J. L. (2017). Treatment of persistent ventricular tachycardia: Drugs or ablation? *Trends in Cardiovascular Medicine, 27*(7), 506–513. https://doi.org/10.1016/j.tcm.2017.05.002.

23. Maseri, A., Chierchia, S., & Kaski, J. C. (1985). Mixed angina pectoris. *American Journal of Cardiology, 56*(9), 30E–33E. https://doi.org/10.1016/0002-9149(85)90282-8.

24. Messerli, F. H., & Bangalore, S. (2009). Antihypertensive efficacy of aliskiren: Is hydrochlorothiazide an appropriate benchmark? *Circulation, 119*(3), 371–373. https://doi.org/10.1161/CIRCULATIONAHA.108.837865.

25. Musat, D. L., Adhaduk, M., Preminger, M. W., Arshad, A., Sichrovsky, T., Steinberg, J. S., & Mittal, S. (2013). Correlation of QT interval correction methods during atrial fibrillation and sinus rhythm. *American Journal of Cardiology, 112*(9), 1379–1383. https://doi.org/10.1016/j.amjcard.2013.06.028.

26. Olde Engberink, R. H., Frenkel, W. J., van den Bogaard, B., Brewster, L. M., Vogt, L., & van den Born, B. J. (2015). Effects of thiazide-type and thiazide-like diuretics on cardiovascular events and mortality: Systematic review and meta-analysis. *Hypertension, 65*(5), 1033–1040. https://doi.org/10.1161/HYPERTENSIONAHA.115.05365.

27. Ong, P., Athanasiadis, A., Borgulya, G., et al. (2012). High prevalence of a pathological response to acetylcholine testing in patients with stable angina pectoris and unobstructed coronary arteries: The ACOVA Study (Abnormal Coronary Vasomotion in patients with stable angina and unobstructed coronary arteries). *Journal of the American College of Cardiology, 59*(8), 655–656. https://doi.org/10.1016/j.jacc.2011.10.852.

28. Ong, P., Athanasiadis, A., Mahrholdt, H., et al. (2012). Increased coronary vasoconstrictor response to acetylcholine in women with chest pain and normal coronary arteriograms (cardiac syndrome X). *Clinical Research in Cardiology, 101*(10), 673–681. https://doi.org/10.1007/s00392-012-0474-2.

29. Patel, M. R., Peterson, E. D., Dai, D., et al. (2010). Low diagnostic yield of elective coronary angiography. *New England Journal of Medicine, 362*(10), 886–895. https://doi.org/10.1056/NEJMoa0907114.

30. Pincus, M. (2016). Management of digoxin toxicity. *Australian Prescriber, 39*(1), 18–20. https://doi.org/10.18773/austprescr.2016.005.

31. Rotella, J. A., Greene, S. L., Koutsogiannis, Z., Graudins, A., Hung Leang, Y., Kuan, K., Baxter, H., Bourke, E., & Wong, A. (2020). Treatment for beta-blocker poisoning: A systematic review. *Clinical Toxicology, 58*(10), 943–983. https://doi.org/10.1080/15563650.2020.1779410.

32. Add: Saslow LR, Jones LM, Sen A, Wolfson JA, Diez HL, O'Brien A, Leung CW, Bayandorian H, Daubenmier J, Missel AL, Richardson C. Comparing Very Low-Carbohydrate vs DASH Diets for Overweight or Obese Adults With Hypertension and Prediabetes or Type 2 Diabetes: A Randomized Trial. Ann Fam Med. 2023 May-Jun;21(3):256-263. doi: 10.1370/afm.2968. PMID: 37217318; PMCID: PMC10202504.

33. Silverman, M. E. (1987). William Heberden and some account of a disorder of the breast. *Clinical Cardiology, 10*(3), 211–213. https://doi.org/10.1002/clc.4960100316.

34. St-Onge, M., Dubé, P. A., Gosselin, S., Guimont, C., Godwin, J., Archambault, P. M., Chauny, J. M., Frenette, A. J., Darveau, M., Le Sage, N., Poitras, J., Provencher, J., Juurlink, D. N., & Blais, R. (2014). Treatment for calcium channel blocker poisoning: A systematic review. *Clinical Toxicology, 52*(9), 926–944. https://doi.org/10.3109/15563650.2014.964094.

35. Thomopoulos, C., Parati, G., & Zanchetti, A. (2018). Effects of blood pressure-lowering treatment on cardiovascular outcomes and mortality: 14–Effects of different classes of antihypertensive drugs in older and younger patients: Overview and meta-analysis. *Journal of Hypertension, 36*(8), 1637–1647. https://doi.org/10.1097/HJH.0000000000001798.

36. Wald, D. S., Law, M., Morris, J. K., Bestwick, J. P., & Wald, N. J. (2009). Combination therapy versus monotherapy in reducing blood pressure: Meta-analysis on 11,000 participants from 42 trials. *American Journal of Medicine, 122*(3), 290–300. https://doi.org/10.1016/j.amjmed.2008.09.038.

Chapter

4

DRUGS ACTING ON THE RESPIRATORY SYSTEM

Contents

Introduction

The upper airway passages, nasal cavities, pharynx, trachea, bronchi, and bronchioles are all part of the respiratory system. The exchange of gases between the body's tissues and the external environment occurs during respiration. It includes inhaling air through the respiratory system, taking in oxygen from the lungs, transferring oxygen throughout the body through the bloodstream, using oxygen for metabolic processes in cells, and exhaling carbon dioxide.

The goal of drug therapy for pulmonary disorders is typically to change a particular physiological function. The medications used to treat some of the more prevalent respiratory system disorders—in particular, asthma, allergies, and congestions linked to specific respiratory disorders—will be the main topic of this chapter..

Orientation and Directional Terms

Term	Definition	Illustration
Asthma exacerbations	Asthma exacerbations are progressive increases in asthma symptoms, including coughing, shortness of breath, or wheezing. These increases are significant enough that the individual needs to change their treatment methods or current asthma action plan.	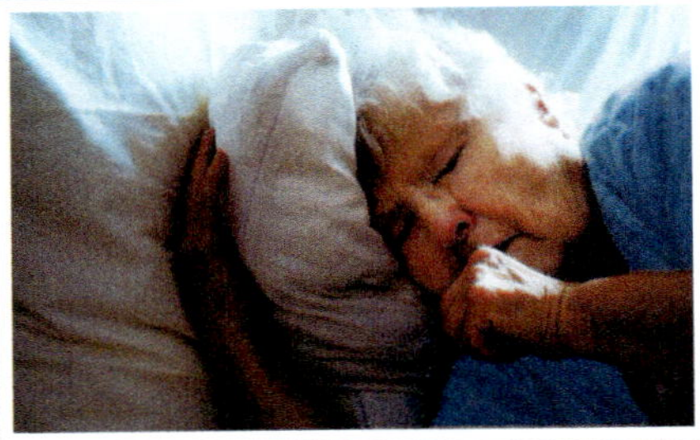
Spirometry	Spirometry is the most common of the pulmonary function tests. It measures lung function, specifically the amount and/or speed of air that can be inhaled and exhaled. Spirometry is helpful in assessing breathing patterns that identify conditions	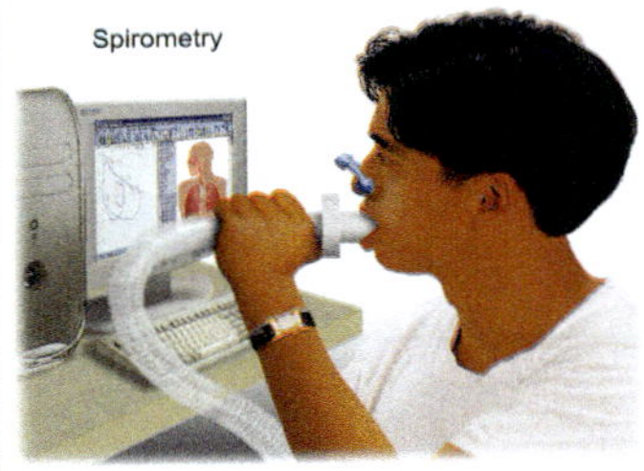
Mast cells	Mast cells are a type of white blood cell that are part of the body's immune system and are found in connective tissues throughout the body. They are especially found in the skin, near blood vessels and lymph vessels, in nerves, in the lungs, and in the intestines	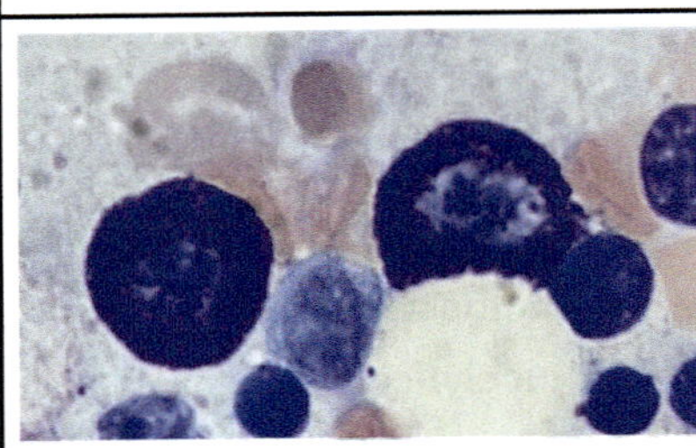
Respiratory tract infection (RTI)	Respiratory tract infection (RTI) is defined as any infectious disease of the upper or lower respiratory tract. Upper respiratory tract infections (URTIs) include the common cold, laryngitis, pharyngitis/tonsillitis, acute rhinitis, acute rhinosinusitis and acute otitis media.	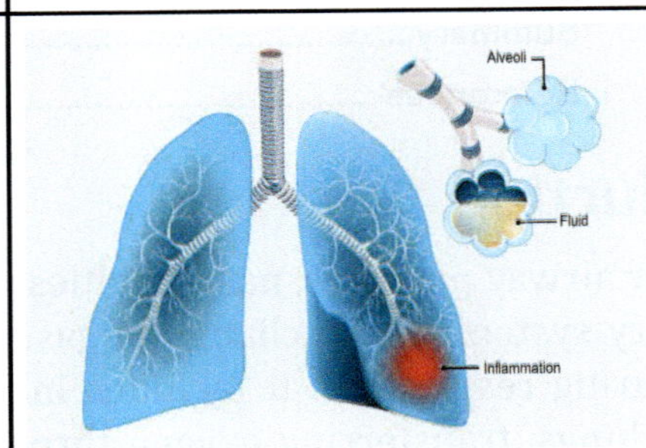
Dextromethorphan	Dextromethorphan is used to temporarily relieve cough caused by the common cold, the flu, or other conditions. Dextromethorphan will relieve a cough but will not treat the cause of the cough or speed recovery. Dextromethorphan is in a class of medications called antitussives.	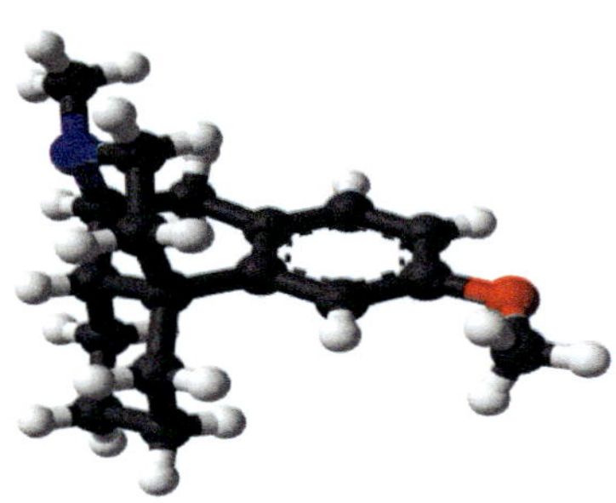

4.1. Pathophysiology of Asthma

The prevalence of asthma has increased since the early 1990s. Asthma prevalence increased from 34.7 per thousand between 1982 and 1992. In the United States, the prevalence of asthma is approximately 8%. Additionally, there have been some contradictory global trends, with some nations experiencing a rise in cases or a stagnation in cases. Asthma typically affects boys more than girls until the age of twenty, at which point both sexes are equally affected. Disparities in childhood may result from atopy or from the smaller airways of boys in comparison to girls. Additionally, asthma has a family history component. But the genes that cause asthma to be inherited are still unknown. Although there is a strong correlation between the phenotype of asthma and inheritance, the mechanism underlying this correlation is more intricate because asthma does not follow a Mendelian pattern. It is highly probable that multiple genes contribute to the transmission of asthma, with various forms of locus heterogeneity and polygenic inheritance resulting in the multifaceted expression of asthma. Certain antigens or pollutants are targeted by atopy or IgE antibodies, potentially exacerbating the condition. Studies have indicated a strong correlation between the total IgE level in the serum and asthma. Higher IgE response to environmental allergens from animals, mold, dust mites in the home, and farm animals has sensitized asthma, aggravating symptoms and raising airway reactivity. The underlying cause is a rise in exposure to these allergens, but the causal relationship is not well established. There is a correlation between smoking and an increased risk of developing asthma, but the exact relationship between air pollution and asthma is also unclear. It's interesting to note that obesity demonstrated a positive linear correlation between elevated BMI and asthma. To gain a more comprehensive understanding of the multifactorial disease, further research is necessary.

4.1.1. Organ Systems Involved

The lungs are the organ system that is impacted by asthma. The lungs are made up of segments and lobes; the left lung has eight or nine segments depending on how the lobe is divided, and the right lung has 10 segments. The respiratory system is divided into two anatomical zones: the conducting zone and the respiratory zone. The respiratory zone, which is where gas exchange occurs, is from the alveolar duct to the alveoli, while the conducting zone runs from the nose to the bronchioles. The main function of breathing is to move air through the lungs and into the alveolar sacs. The trachea splits into the left and right bronchi. The left bronchus is smaller and more horizontally oriented, whereas the right bronchus is larger and more vertically oriented. Following that, the bronchi split into secondary and tertiary bronchi. Smooth muscle and elastic fibers, which respond to" inflammatory mediators inflammatory mediators, bronchoconstrictors, or bronchodilators, are present in the bronchi to preserve the integrity of their walls. There are significantly more smooth muscle fibers as one moves from the bronchi to the alveoli. Lung compliance in normal respiratory physiology refers to the lungs' propensity to expand, whereas lung elastance refers to their capacity to revert to their resting position. The physiologic mechanism alters in asthmatic patients as a result of inflammation, narrowing the airway's radius. When combined, these mechanisms cause a slight change in the lungs' compliance, which makes breathing more difficult.

4.1.2. Mechanism

An asthma exacerbation occurs in two stages: the early phase and the late phase. IgE antibodies that are released and sensitized by plasma cells start the early phase. These antigens are among the environmental triggers that these antibodies react to. IgE antibodies then attach to basophils and mast cells with a high affinity. The mast cells release cytokines and ultimately degranulate in response to an inhaled pollutant or risk factor. Prostaglandins, leukotrienes, and histamine are released from mast cells. The smooth muscle is then contracted, tightening the airway. Th2 lymphocytes generate GM-CSF and a range of interleukins (IL-4, IL-5, and IL-13) that promote inflammation and facilitate cell-to-cell communication. IL-3 and IL-5 aid in the survival of basophils and eosinophils. Fibrosis, hyperplasia, and remodeling are all promoted by IL-13. The late phase, which lasts for a few hours, is characterized by the localization of helper and memory T-cells, neutrophils, eosinophils, and basophils to the lungs, which results in inflammation and bronchoconstriction. In addition, mast cells are crucial for transporting the late-phase reactants to the sites of inflammation. Depending on the severity of the disease, it is imperative to identify both of these mechanisms to target therapy and relieve both inflammation and bronchoconstriction. It's interesting to note that people who gradually develop a thicker airway have a narrower airway and a longer disease duration. Breathing becomes more difficult due to an intermittent airflow obstruction caused by inflammation and bronchoconstriction.

One of the most important characteristics of asthma is "airway hyperresponsiveness," which is an excessive bronchoconstrictor response, typically to distinct stimuli. The mechanisms causing airway hyperresponsiveness are diverse. Increasing the mass of smooth muscle in the airways or the production of more histamine by mast cells are two possible causes. Airway smooth muscle cell contractility progresses further by elevated intracellular free calcium and vagal tone. Bronchial provocation tests are used to measure the severity of airway hyperresponsiveness. Because airway hyperresponsiveness is linked to a higher risk of lung function decline and the onset and exacerbation of asthma from childhood to adulthood, this feature is clinically significant. As a result, asthma and hyperresponsiveness can be prevented early on by using targeted treatment. When combined, these mechanisms cause a slight change in the lungs' compliance, which makes breathing more difficult. It can get harder for someone to breathe normally when they have inflammation, mucus in the bronchiolar trees, granular white blood cells, and exudate. The smooth muscle layer and lamina reticularis will narrow due to an increase in the epithelium brought on by the proliferation of myofibroblasts, which produce collagen. Consequently, the basement membrane thickens more than usual. An individual may experience permanent airflow obstruction, which is thought to be brought on by airway remodeling.

Smooth muscle content increases as a result of epithelial cells changing into mesenchymal cells during remodeling. With tight junctions, epithelial cells lose their functional polarity and adhesion, rearranging themselves to become mesenchymal cells. Furthermore, through their interactions with mast cells, eosinophils can release TGF-B and other cytokines that worsen airway remodeling. If these mechanisms of airway remodeling are not appropriately treated and managed over time, they may exacerbate asthma and worsen inflammation.

4.1.3. Related Testing

A range of tests can be performed by clinicians to diagnose asthma. Expiratory airflow limitation, reversible obstruction documentation, and the exclusion of any other diagnosis must all be determined by tests. Spirometry assessment of the patient's obstruction and observation of a reversible change following bronchodilator therapy are suggestive of an asthma diagnosis. Spirometry is used to confirm the diagnosis of"asthma and determine the degree of obstruction. Spirometry with a FEV1 (forced vital capacity) of less than 0.8 and a

FEV1(forced vital capacity) ratio of less than 0.7 is used to define an air obstruction. The FEV1 and FEV1/FVC ratios decrease in proportion to the severity of asthma. If spirometry is normal, bronchoprovocation testing using methacholine is an additional testing technique. As a muscarinic agonist, methacholine constricts smooth muscle in the lungs by binding to M1, M2, and M3 receptors. One can assess the degree of bronchoconstriction with methacholine. Allergy testing can help identify specific triggers that exacerbate asthma, but it is not always helpful in diagnosing the condition.

4.1.4. Clinical Significance

Clinicians need to recognize the slightly different clinical picture that asthma can present. Wheezing, dyspnea, and coughing, which is frequently worse at night, are common symptoms of asthma. There are several things that aggravate asthma. These include exercise, cold air, and the pollutants mentioned above. Additional non-specific symptoms, such as tachypnea, tachycardia, or a patient seated in a tripod position, may indicate a severe obstruction. If asthma is not properly managed and treated, it can become a serious illness. Given that asthma manifests in two stages, it is imperative to focus on and reduce inflammation, bronchoconstriction, and airway remodeling. Different stages of asthma are identified based on spirometry results and/or clinical indications. Asthma can be classified into four severity levels: intermittent, mild, moderate, and severe. Treatment and management of asthma vary depending on the individual stage of the condition. Less than two days per week of symptoms and fewer than two nighttime awakenings per month are indicative of intermittent asthma. In mild asthma, awakenings during the night occur three to four times per month, and episodes occur more than twice a week (though not every day). When a patient has moderate asthma, they experience nighttime awakenings more frequently than once a week but not every night. When a patient has severe asthma, they frequently wake up during the night more than seven times in a week and experience symptoms all day long. These parameters allow for the proper treatment to be given to lessen the patient's symptoms. The most often prescribed drugs include; inhaled and systemic glucocorticoids, long- and short-acting beta-agonists, and muscarinic antagonists. When an asthma attack occurs, the goal of a beta-agonist is to attempt to bronchodilate the patient's lungs. The G protein receptors that beta-agonists bind to and activate cAMP is their mechanism of action. Then, through a mechanism that is still unclear, cAMP triggers smooth muscle relaxation. Moreover, glucocorticoids can be used to lessen lung remodeling and inflammation. Increasing IL-10 production is a glucocorticoid's main mechanism of action. T-cell activation, inflammatory cytokines, and various white blood cells like mast cells and eosinophils are all inhibited by IL-10. Short- and long-term improvements in breathing are brought about by these effects, which also reduce inflammation. Muscarinic antagonists reduce the attraction and viability of inflammatory cells, which reduces the release of cytokines and blocks the inflammatory effect. For a synergistic effect, muscarinic antagonists can be combined with glucocorticoids or beta-agonists.

4.1.5. Natural History of Asthma

An important question to consider is whether early administration of anti-inflammatory medication during the course of asthma could stop the progression of airway inflammation, remodeling, and eventual irreversible airway obstruction that is associated with the persistence and severity of asthma. This would help to prevent lung function from permanently declining. Two conditions must be met for early ICS initiation to be more advantageous than delayed initiation: (1) individuals with mild to moderate persistent asthma as a group experience a progressive decline in lung function that is measurable and clinically significant; and (2) ICS treatment not only provides long-term asthma control but also prevents or slows this decline.

4.1.5.1. Natural History of Persistent Asthma

1. Children

The fact that asthma is a variable illness is widely known. The course and symptoms of asthma can differ from person to person and over time within an individual's experience. The term "natural history" refers to how asthma develops over time, either in remission or with escalating severity. It has been suggested that a progressive deterioration in lung function occurs concurrently with the persistence or exacerbation of asthma symptoms over time. It appears from recent research that this might not be the case. Instead, the course of asthma can differ significantly amongst younger children, older kids and teens, and adults; this variance is most likely influenced by age rather than symptoms.

According to a prospective cohort study whose follow-up started at birth, children whose asthma-like symptoms started before the age of three had asthma-related lung growth deficiencies by the time they were six years old. Further follow-up on lung function measures taken between the ages of 11 and 16 revealed that the group of children whose asthma symptoms started before the age of three had significantly worsened lung function between the ages of 11 and 16 compared to the group of children who did not have asthma symptoms for the first six years of life; however, there was no additional loss in forced expiratory volume in 1 second (FEV1) when compared to the children who did not have asthma. The group whose symptoms of asthma started after the age of three did not show signs of lung function deficiencies.

In a long-term study involving children aged 8 to 10, it was discovered that bronchial hyperresponsiveness was linked to reductions in lung function growth in both children with and without active asthma symptoms. Therefore, in this age group, symptoms did not predict or determine deficits in lung function.

In a study conducted on nearly 1,000 children from a birth cohort in Dunedin, New Zealand, Sears and colleagues measured lung function on multiple occasions between the ages of 9 and 26. During the follow-up, they discovered that children with asthma consistently had lower FEV1/forced vital capacity (FVC) ratios. But regardless of how severe their symptoms were, their lung function levels matched those of kids without asthma, and after age nine, no more lung function losses were seen.

Data from the Childhood Asthma Management Program (CAMP) study suggests that the age at which an individual develops asthma can impact their lung function growth. During the enrollment of children aged 5–12 with mild or moderate persistent asthma, a negative relationship between lung function and duration of asthma was observed. While the analysis did not differentiate between age of onset and duration of asthma, it is likely that children with a longer duration of asthma had symptoms starting before 3 years of age, resulting in poorer lung function. After 4–6 years of follow-up, most children in the CAMP study did not show deficits in lung growth. However, a subset of children experienced a decline in lung growth, with predictors at baseline being male gender and younger age.

Together, these studies indicate that the majority of lung function growth deficits seen in asthmatic children happen in those whose symptoms start within the first three years of life, and that symptoms that start after that age are typically not linked to appreciable lung function growth deficits. Therefore, children who experience symptoms before the age of three and appear destined to develop persistent asthma would be a promising target for interventions aimed at preventing deficits in lung function, and possibly the development of more severe symptoms later in life. It's crucial to differentiate this group from the vast majority of kids who stop having symptoms after the age of six and start wheezing before the age of three. Until recently, it was impossible to determine which children, among those who displayed early asthma-like symptoms, would develop persistent asthma without the use of validated algorithms. Such a predictive index has been created using information from long-term longitudinal studies of children who were enrolled from birth.

First, among children under three who had more than three wheezing episodes in the preceding year, the studies identified an index of risk factors for the development of persistent asthma symptoms. After that, the index was used on a birth cohort that was tracked until the age of 13. In comparison, 97% of children who did not have asthma after the age of 6 had a negative asthma predictive index before the age of 3 years, while 76% of children who were diagnosed with asthma after the age of 6 had a positive asthma predictive index before the age of 3. After that, the index was improved and put to the test in a clinical trial to see if treating kids with a positive asthma predictive index could stop them from developing persistent wheezing. The asthma predictive index generated by these studies identifies the following risk factors for developing persistent asthma among children younger than 3 years of age who had four or more episodes of wheezing during the previous year: either (1) one of the following: parental history of asthma, a physician diagnosis of atopic dermatitis, or evidence of sensitization to aeroallergens, or (2) two of the following: evidence of sensitization to foods, ≥4% peripheral blood eosinophilia, or wheezing apart from colds.

2. Adults

Adult asthmatic patients appear to experience an accelerated loss of lung function. The degree of persistent airflow obstruction correlated with both the severity and duration of the subjects' asthma in a study of adults with asthma who received two weeks of high-dose prednisone if airflow obstruction persisted after two weeks of bronchodilator therapy.

Two extensive, prospective epidemiological studies assessed the pace at which adults with asthma experienced a decline in their lung function. Spirometry was done every three years in an 18-year prospective study involving 186 control participants without asthma, 26 smokers with asthma, and 66 nonsmokers with asthma (Peat et al. 1987). In the study group, 73% of participants had at least six spirometric assessments. The individuals with asthma had a decline in lung function (FEV1) that was about 40% steeper than the participants without asthma. Less than 25% of participants with asthma had a slope less steep than the mean for those without asthma, suggesting that this was not the result of extreme measurements made by a small number of participants. In a different study, 13,689 adults were evaluated using spirometry three times over a 15-year period (778 of whom had asthma, and 12,911 did not). Individuals with asthma experienced an average annual decline in FEV1 of 38 mL, compared to 22 mL for those without asthma. The researchers noted that even though the study's definition of asthma was limited to patient reports, it is likely that the subjects who reported having asthma actually had asthma rather than chronic obstructive pulmonary disease (COPD) because the cohort's 6% prevalence rate for asthma did not rise with age. These studies do not allow us to determine whether people with mild, moderate, or severe asthma were the only ones who experienced a loss of pulmonary function. However, the evidence points to the possibility of an accelerated loss of lung function in adult asthmatics.

After including a new survey in 1994–1995 to the study on the decline in lung function from Busselton, Australia, James and colleagues reanalyzed the data. The subjects (N = 9,317) had taken part in the follow-up study from 1994 to 1995, or they had been adults (19 years of age or older) in one or more of the cross-sectional Busselton Health Surveys conducted between 1966 and 1981. James and colleagues used the complete data sample and discovered that subjects with asthma had significantly lower lung function over the course of the follow-up period; however, the majority of the differences were caused by lung function deficits that existed at the start of the follow-up (when subjects were 19 years old). After accounting for the impact of smoking, the excess FEV1 decline linked to asthma was 3 points78 mL for women and 3 points69 mL for men annually. The clinical significance of these results is questionable despite their statistical significance. The data from the Tucson Epidemiologic Study of Airway Obstructive Disease were reanalyzed by Sherrill and colleagues. With longitudinal data for lung function measured in up to 12 surveys over a maximum of 20 years, a total of 2,926 subjects were included. They discovered that FEV1 did not decrease more quickly than usual in individuals with a diagnosis of long-term asthma, in contrast to those with a diagnosis of COPD. This also applied to participants with COPD and asthma. Griffith and associates examined the deterioration in lung function in 5,242 individuals over 65 who were enrolled in the Cardiovascular Health Study. Over the course of seven years, each participant had up to three lung function tests. The FEV1 levels of subjects with asthma were lower than those of subjects without asthma. However, there were no appreciable increases in the rate of FEV1 decline in individuals with asthma after emphysema and chronic bronchitis were taken into account. (Barnes, 2002; Bateman et al, 2004; Sun et al, 2010)

4.2. Antitussive Drugs

Traditionally, medications that suppress cough by acting on the central nervous system have been referred to as centrally-acting antitussives. This classification, by definition, acknowledges the presence of components of the central nervous system that are both sensitive to antitussive medications and play a significant role in the development of cough. Peripherally-acting antitussives, which are believed to act selectively on components of the peripheral nervous system that are crucial in the production of coughing, are thought to be distinct from this class of antitussive medications.

4.2.1. Cough as an Unmet Clinical Problem

Although a cough is a common symptom of health and an essential defensive mechanism, when it persists, it is the primary cause of medical attention seeking for patients. According to epidemiologic studies, up to 40% of people can experience coughing at any given time. The most frequent causes of cough are upper respiratory tract infections (URTIs) or the common cold, but other common causes include postinfectious cough, chronic cough that doesn't go away, and cough brought on by pulmonary conditions like lung cancer, idiopathic pulmonary fibrosis, asthma, and chronic obstructive pulmonary disease (COPD), or a side effect of ACE inhibitors. The causes of cough in children are different from those in adults; prolonged bacterial bronchitis, viral URTIs, and asthma are common causes of cough in children. However, even in cases where an underlying cause has been found, clinicians are well aware that a considerable portion of patients experience cough that is resistant to particular therapies. Whether it is acute or chronic, a cough is linked to a markedly lower health-related quality of life. Frequent symptoms of chronic cough include sleep disturbance, nausea, chest pains, and lethargy. Patients also frequently experience low mood, urine incontinence, and social embarrassment. When a cough causes missed work and decreased productivity, it has a substantial financial impact on both the person suffering from the condition and society as a whole.

The enormous sales of nonspecific antitussive medications—$3 billion annually in the United States alone, and growing in recent years—reflect the clinical need for these medications. Many people purchase over-the-counter (OTC) antitussive drugs for their kids or themselves. The American College of Chest Physicians (ACCP) actually advises against the use of antitussive medications for URTIs due to recent challenges to the efficacy of most antitussive medications, particularly those for URTIs. The most popular antitussive medication is dextromethorphan, which has been offered over-the-counter (OTC) in the US since 1958. The U.S. approved it. S. Food and Drug Administration (FDA) after examining research that included a small number of clinical trials showing some degree of benefit. The absence of placebo arms in the trials, the inclusion of hospitalized patients with tuberculosis and other respiratory diseases, the use of unvalidated outcome measures, and the dubious clinical benefit all constituted limitations to these studies. Since then, a small placebo-controlled trial that addressed many of these limitations has been conducted, but the results did not corroborate previous findings of clinical benefit. However, a different clinical study did find a noteworthy effect on cough (see below). Moreover, some researchers have asked the FDA to examine the safety and effectiveness of over-the-counter antitussive medications that contain dextromethorphan due to the possibility of accidental overdose and abuse, especially in children where there are few studies on the subject. As this chapter will demonstrate, the evidence currently available does not clearly indicate the effectiveness of dextromethorphan or many other licensed antitussive medications. Consequently, more research is required to identify more effective antitussive medications. Still, a great deal of progress has been made in our knowledge of the pathophysiology of cough, and this has led to the identification of several possible targets for the creation of novel drug classes. The majority of cough types are characterized by cough reflex hypersensitivity, so one of the main challenges is to create peripherally acting medications that restore the cough reflex sensitivity to physiological levels while avoiding the side effects of many cough medications that affect the central nervous system (CNS). The assessment of antitussive drugs should be made easier by the recent development of objective cough frequency monitors and validated health status tools.

4.2.2. Basic Physiology of the Cough Reflex

Vagal afferent nerves that terminate in the larynx, trachea, and bronchi are activated when a cough is produced. The lungs and airways are innervated by several subtypes of vagal afferent nerves. By contrasting their action potential conduction velocities, sites of termination, cell body locations, embryologic origins, neurochemistry, and reactions to chemical and mechanical stimuli, these subtypes can be distinguished from one another. These investigations provide solid proof that the onset of cough is related to subtypes of bronchopulmonary C- and A-delta fibers. The A-delta fibers exhibit rapid adaptation in response to acid environments and punctate mechanical stimulation. These A-delta fibers can cause coughing even in unconscious animals, and they may serve as a protective mechanism for the airways against aspiration. A-delta fibers have a conduction velocity that is roughly three to five times faster than C-fibers. However, bradykinin and agonists of the ionotropic receptors, transient receptor potential vanilloid 1 (TRPV1) (capsaicin, resiniferatoxin, protons), and transient receptor potential A1 (TRPA1) (allyl isothiocyanate, acrolein, cinnamaldehyde) activate the C-fibers involved in the cough reflex, which are comparatively insensitive to mechanical stimuli and lung stretch. It has been demonstrated that both humans and animals will cough in response to these chemical cues. TRPV1 has been localized to nerve terminals in human airways, and single cell polymerase chain reaction analyzes verify the expression of TRPV1 and TRPA1 in the neurons projecting these bronchopulmonary C-fibers in animal lungs. The A-delta fibers that control cough are highly responsive to protons and punctate mechanical stimulation, but they are insensitive to agonists of either TRPA1 or TRPV1. The gating of acid-sensitive ion channels is most likely responsible for the proton-evoked activation of A-delta fibers. The A-delta fibers controlling cough, however, terminate only in the extrapulmonary airways, in contrast to the C-fibers controlling cough, which terminate throughout the intrapulmonary and extrapulmonary airways.

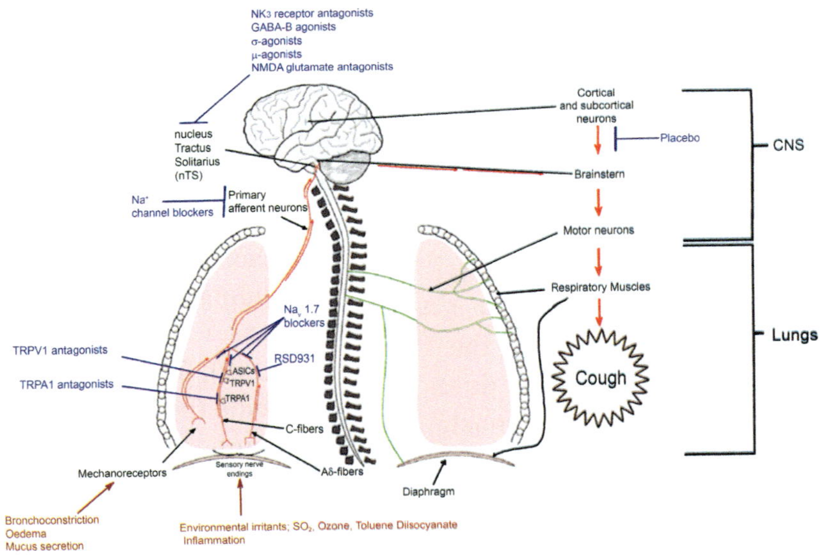

Figure 4.1. *Multiple vagal afferent nerve subtypes innervate the airways and lungs.*

Source: https://www.researchgate.net/figure/Multiple-vagal-afferent-nerve-subtypes-innervate-the-airways-and-lungs_fig1_261138942.

It is also possible that other vagal afferent nerves modulate the cough reflex; these pathways may promote or prevent coughing that is inadvertently evoked. For example, highly sensitive to mechanical stimuli, especially those that cause bronchospasm, are receptors that adapt quickly. Several experimental and clinical studies indicate that bronchospasm may enhance cough reflex sensitivity or evoke coughing in susceptible individuals, such as subjects with asthma, despite the fact that it is usually a poor stimulus for coughing. In contrast, animals' coughing is acutely inhibited by a subtype of bronchopulmonary C-fibers that innervate the lungs and intrapulmonary airways (Figure 4.1).

One of the few distinct reflexes that needs to be initiated by a sustained, high-frequency activation of afferent nerves is the cough. The necessity of prolonged activation of high-frequency sensory nerves in coughing has significant therapeutic implications. Cough may be significantly affected by medications that reduce the peak frequencies of the action potentials of vagal afferent nerves or decrease the effectiveness of synaptic transmission at the primary termination sites of these afferent nerves. On the other hand, stimuli that promote central synaptic transmission (such as convergent afferent input from esophageal afferent nerves in patients with reflux disease) or increase the excitability of these vagal afferent nerves (such as airway inflammation) may increase sensitivity to tussive stimuli.

The nucleus tractus solitarius is where vagal afferent nerves terminate centrally (nTS). The nTS can receive direct or indirect inputs from afferent nerves innervating the nasal mucosa and esophagus. This anatomic basis enables the association between cough and upper airway diseases, including gastroesophageal reflux disease (GERD). N-methyl-D-aspartate (NMDA)-type glutamate receptors play a distinct and significant role in controlling cough at the central synapses of the vagal afferent nerves, according to pharmacological and physiological analyzes. This finding may help to explain why dextromethorphan has an antitussive effect on patients and raise the possibility that new NMDA antagonists could be effective antitussive medications.

4.2.3. Drugs in Current Use for the Treatment of Cough

4.2.3.1. H_1-Receptor Antagonists

In many cases, H_1-Antihistamines, also known as Histamine H_1-Receptor Antagonists, can also function as Inverse Agonists, joining forces with the inactive form of the H_1-receptor to stabilize it and tip the balance in favor of the inactive state. Furthermore, certain muscarinic, alpha-adrenergic, and serotonin receptors, as well as certain ion channels, can be inhibited by certain H_1-antihistamines. Six chemical types have historically been used to categorize H_1-antihistamines: ethanolamines, ethylenediamines, alkylamines, piperazines, piperidines, and phenothiazines. However, more recently, the classification of first-generation H_1-antihistamines based on their function has become more popular. These first-generation antihistamines are lipophilic, penetrate the central nervous system, and are therefore sedating agents. In contrast, second-generation H_1-antihistamines are lipophobic, penetrate the central nervous system less, and are therefore comparatively nonsedating.

H1-antihistamines have been shown in numerous animal studies to have antitussive properties. The first-generation agent chlorpheniramine, the second-generation H_1-receptor antagonist loratadine, and the muscarinic receptor antagonist ipratropium bromide all inhibited the guinea pigs' ability to cough up allergens or capsaicin. These results suggest that histamine H_1-receptors and cholinergic mechanisms are involved in the model's induction of coughing. It's worth noting that a subsequent set of experiments using conscious guinea pigs to assess the effects of oral administration of an example of one of each of the six chemical classes came to the conclusion that several H_1-receptor antagonists did not prevent capsaicin-induced cough, suggesting that the antitussive effects of these drugs are not directly linked to histamine H_1-receptor blockade. Moreover, the older H_1-receptor antagonists' antitussive effects were unrelated to their sedative and minute ventilation effects. Additional research has shown that oxatomide has an antitussive effect on unanesthetized guinea pigs challenged with citric acid, that epinastine can enhance the antitussive effect of dihydrocodeine against mice that have a capsaicin-induced cough, and that azelastine can suppress the cough caused by capsaicin in conscious guinea pigs, possibly in part by inhibiting substance P release from sensory nerves.

A more recent study using human embryonic kidney (HEK) cells expressing $TRPV_1$ showed that the first-generation H_1-antihistamine dexbrompheniramine inhibited $TRPV_1$ receptor activation, pointing to a possible additional mechanism for the antitussive effect of H_1-receptor antagonists. This discovery is especially noteworthy in light of the recent hypothesis regarding the possible significance of $TRPV_1$ receptors in human cough.

Induced cough tests on human volunteers in good health have produced contradictory findings. In a placebo-controlled crossover study, diphenhydramine given orally at a dose of 25 mg was found to inhibit the production of cough due to citric acid, while terfenadine given orally at a dose of 120 mg did not prevent the production of cough due to capsaicin. When given in oral dosages of 180 mg, the second-generation medication fexofenadine failed to prevent subjects' acute viral upper respiratory tract infections (URTIs) or capsaicin-induced cough in both healthy volunteers and subjects. Another small study, however, showed that nonasthmatic patients with chronic cough could not induce cough with ultrasonically nebulized distilled water (UNDW) when treated with loratadine, a second-generation agent.

The ACCP guidelines for the clinical management of adult cough suggest that the best course of treatment for both acute cough from the common cold and chronic cough from upper airway cough syndrome (previously known as postnasal drip syndrome) is to combine a decongestant with a first-generation H1-antihistamine. In the lack of suitably powered prospective, randomized, controlled clinical trials, this recommendation is primarily based on a substantial body of clinical experience and expert opinion. Nonetheless, a prospective evaluation of 45 adult patients with chronic cough who were treated with a first-generation H1-antihistamine/decongestant combination as the initial step of a therapeutic algorithm showed improvement in 39 patients' cough, and this was the only therapy required by 16 patients. This supports the recommendation. (Barnes, 2002; Bateman et al, 2004; Sun et al, 2010)

4.2.3.2. Dextromethorphan

Dextromethorphan hydrobromide (dextromethorphan) was initially discovered in 1953 as an effective cough treatment that does not cause the unpleasant side effects commonly associated with codeine, such as drowsiness, nausea, dependency, and constipation. It has since become a key ingredient in numerous over-the-counter medications.

The dextro-isomer (D-isomer) of levorphanol methyl ether is dextromethorphan HBr [(+)-3-methoxy-17-methylmorphinan hydrobromide monohydrate]. It is believed to bind to high- and low-affinity brain sites that are different from opioid and other neurotransmitter binding sites. The (O) methylated (+) form of racemorphan (dextromethorphan) may obstruct binding to the analgesic/addictive receptors in the medulla, thereby mitigating the side effects of narcotics, through a steric hindrance mechanism.

The full mechanism of action of dextromethorphan is not fully known. Studies have indicated that it interacts with various receptors, such as N-methyl-D-aspartate (NMDA) glutamate receptors, σ-1 receptors, nicotinic receptors, and serotonergic receptors. This intricate process is thought to reduce coughing by changing the threshold for initiating cough mainly through its role as an NMDA antagonist, which blocks glutamate receptors in the brainstem's nTS.

The gastrointestinal tract absorbs dextromethorphan well; in people who metabolize it well, maximum plasma concentrations of the drug occur ~1–4 hours after oral administration, whereas in people who metabolize it poorly, they occur 4–6 hours after oral administration. The plasma elimination half-life of dextromethorphan is approximately 1–4 hours for individuals with extensive metabolisms and 17–42 hours for those with poor metabolisms. The primary metabolite dextromethorphan has a half-life of plasma elimination of one to three hours in extensive metabolizers and five to thirteen hours in poor metabolizers.

By means of O-demethylation, cytochrome P450 converts dextromethorphan to dextrorphan, and to a lesser extent, N-demethylation converts it to 3-methoxymorphinan. 3-Methoxymorphinan undergoes additional metabolism to yield 3-hydroxymorphinan (through N-demethylation). It has also been demonstrated that dextromethorphan is metabolized via the CYP2D6-mediated O-demethylation pathway through the use of immunoinhibition and quinidine, a known inhibitor of this pathway.

After long-term daily oral dosing of 120 mg, peak plasma concentrations of dextromethorphan were found to range from 0.5 to 5.9 ng/ml in extensive metabolizers and 182 to 231 ng/ml in poor metabolizers. The main metabolite, dextorphan, has been shown to have antitussive properties and is believed to be responsible for the main pharmacological effect at therapeutic doses. Animal studies have shown that dextorphan possesses antitussive activity that is approximately three quarters of that of dextromethorphan at a dose of 2.0 mg/kg.

4.2.3.3. Opiates: Codeine and Morphine

Codeine is a natural alkaloid derived from the poppy plant, specifically Papaver bractreatum. It is chemically similar to morphine but with a methyl group attached at the 3 position. When used in cough medications, codeine is often synthesized from its parent molecule. Codeine is considered a mild opioid, with its main therapeutic effect occurring when it is broken down in the liver by cytochrome P450 2D6 into morphine. Another enzyme, CYP3A4, also plays a role in converting codeine into its active form, norcodeine. After being metabolized, codeine and its byproducts are further processed by UGT 2B7 to form glucuronides, which are responsible for the drug's antitussive properties. Because of its complex metabolic process, codeine is considered a prodrug and can exhibit genetic variability and interactions with other drugs that are metabolized by the cytochrome system. One significant interaction to note is with dextromethorphan, another common antitussive, which competes with codeine for metabolism by cytochromes, ultimately affecting the way both drugs work in the body (Figure 4.2).

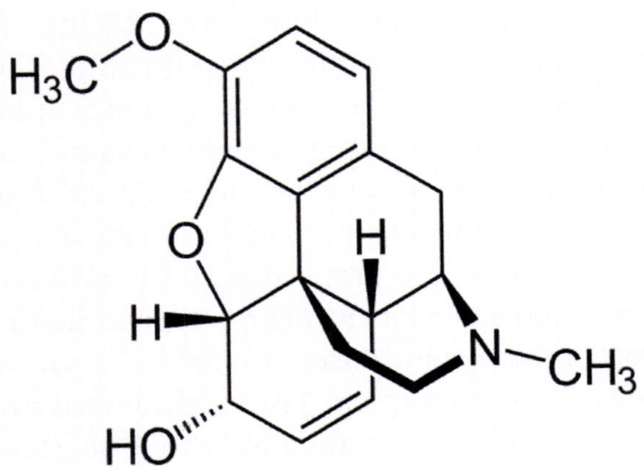

Figure 4.2. *Chemical structure of codeine.*

Source: https://upload.wikimedia.org/wikipedia/commons/thumb/5/5c/Codein_-_Codeine.svg/800px-Codein_-_Codeine.svg.png.

Although opium and its ethanolic extract laudanum are no longer used medicinally, there is still debate regarding the relative contributions of the different exogenous and endogenous alkaloids to the antitussive effects of opiates. Opium has a long history of use in suppressing coughs. A codeine intravertebral artery injection prevents the anesthetized cat from coughing when the brain stem is electrically stimulated, indicating that codeine is an effective antitussive on its own.

Supporting the use of codeine as an antitussive in humans, a small study in patients with persistent cough found that oral dosing with 60 mg of syrup was superior to a placebo, and that cough suppression was correlated with log plasma concentrations of codeine.

In summary, well-conducted studies in humans do not back the use of codeine as an effective cough suppressant. Its common use as a comparison in studies of new cough medications has caused confusion. However, research has shown inhaled codeine to be effective in animals. It is worth noting that opioids' effects on cough were first observed over 200 years ago using an inhaler. This hints that using codeine directly in the airways may be the best way to enhance its effectiveness.

The antitussive properties of morphine have long been known, especially in the context of palliative care. However, the realization that codeine's primary therapeutic effect came from its breakdown into morphine prompted research into the potential benefits of morphine alone for treating persistent cough. A significant reduction of more than one third in the median cough recorded on the diary record card was observed in patients receiving 5 mg of morphine sulfate twice daily for one month in a placebo-controlled, double-blind crossover study involving 27 patients with chronic intractable cough. Analyzing each patient's response separately revealed a difference between those who had a great response and those who had no benefit. Despite this pronounced clinical response, the citric acid cough challenge showed no improvement. Dosage escalation to 10 mg twice daily was allowed in an open label extension of the study, and six more patients reported improvement. The only significant adverse event was constipation.

Because morphine is classified as a controlled substance in some jurisdictions, its use as a regular therapy for chronic cough has been hindered. Clinical experience indicates that, in contrast to pain, the daily dose of 20 mg is the ceiling of therapeutic response. Considering the quick (within hours) action, individual drug efficacy assessments should be acceptable. Given the significant individual variation in response, none of the opiate medications should be considered the "gold standard" antitussive agent as a comparator in clinical studies. Morphine is the preferred opioid of choice in the clinic due to its more consistent bioavailability.

4.2.3.4. Local Anesthetics

Given that sensory nerves are involved in the cough reflex, it is perhaps not surprising that local anesthetics can inhibit both experimentally induced cough and cough in a variety of clinical circumstances. Local anesthetics have been reported to have antitussive effects. This antitussive effect is most likely brought on by local anesthetics' capacity to block NaV+ channels in sensory nerves. The majority of the information relates to the use of lidocaine/ lignocaine. For instance, it has been demonstrated that inhaled lignocaine (20 mg) can suppress cough in nonsmoking volunteers that is brought on by inhaled capsaicin. Hansson and colleagues found no evidence that combining adrenaline with lignocaine affected the antitussive effect of lignocaine or the plasma levels of this local anesthetic after inhalation, despite the fact that local anesthetics are frequently used in combination with adrenaline to prolong their activity. Another treatment option for the coughing that comes with tracheal intubation is intravenous lidocaine. Numerous randomized double-blind placebo-controlled studies have supported the widespread use of topical lidocaine to suppress coughing related to bronchoscopy. The study by Antoniades and Worsnop, which showed noticeably reduced cough rates following the administration of 2% lidocaine versus normal saline when applied through a flexible bronchoscope, is a good example of this. In addition, these authors discovered that when compared to placebo treatment, lidocaine usage allowed for a lower use of sedatives like fentanyl or midazolam. On the other hand, after using lidocaine jelly and aerosolized lidocaine, more researchers observed a higher rate of postoperative cough. Though not as much as that caused by betamethasone gel, a more recent study did find a decrease in postoperative coughing following the application of lidocaine jelly over the tracheal tube during elective surgery performed under general orotracheal anesthesia. Nebulized lidocaine has also been demonstrated to be beneficial in treating a man with an intractable cough who is 52 years old, four patients who have a chronic intractable cough, and cough that is nearing the end of life. Epifivicaine aerosols have also been found to be beneficial in treating refractory cough. Nebulized lidocaine has also been shown to be beneficial in treating COPD patients' coughs. Fascinatingly, studies have indicated that oral mexiletine lessens the cough reaction to capsaicin and tartaric acid.

4.2.3.4. Caramiphen

Caramiphen edisylate's anticholinergic properties led to its initial development as a muscle relaxant. Caramiphen appears to work centrally as an antitussive agent, but some have argued that it should be categorized as a peripherally acting medication. Domenjoz discovered that it had the same cough-suppressive effects as codeine when applied to rats' tracheas mechanically stimulated. Although caramiphen was largely ineffective when administered orally, subsequent animal experiments confirmed this antitussive effect when administered intravenously. When taken orally, it does, however, occasionally, reduce coughing in people.

4.2.3.5. Carbetapentane

Cough suppressants like carbetapentane [2-[2-(diethylamino)ethoxy]ethyl 1-phenylcyclopentanecarboxylate] are used to treat coughs brought on by sinusitis, bronchitis, common colds, and influenza. It is taken orally, frequently in conjunction with H1-receptor antagonists and guaifenesin. Although the precise mechanism of action of carbetapentane's antitussive effects is unknown, it is believed to primarily act on the central nervous system (CNS), where it may have relevance at the sigma, kappa, and mu-opioid receptors in addition to its antimuscarinic and local anesthetic properties (at least when applied topically). When electrical stimulation of the trachea causes cough in anesthetized cats, antitussive activity has been demonstrated. Similarly, in conscious guinea pigs, it has been shown to prevent cough induced by inhaled citric acid.

Maximum plasma concentrations in humans are reached 1.2 hours after oral carbetapentane dosage, and the half-life is 2.3 hours. However, the FDA determined that carbetapentane should not be made available as an over-the-counter cough treatment in the United States due to the dearth of published clinical data indicating clinical efficacy with this medication.

4.2.3.6. Chlophedianol

It was first demonstrated that clophedianol, or 1-phenyl-1-(o-chlorophenyl)-3-dimethylamino-propranol-1 hydrochloride, exhibited antitussive properties against coughs induced in a variety of species through experimentation. It was first made available as an over-the-counter oral medication (OTC) in Germany in the 1950s as an antitussive. It is commonly taken in combination with decongestants and H_1-receptor antagonists to treat upper respiratory tract infections. Clophedianol has been reported to possess antitussive, antihistamine, and local anesthetic properties. It is also believed that clophedianol suppresses coughs centrally, though its exact mode of action is unknown. Very few clinical studies have been published, and there is little information available on the pharmacokinetics of chlophedianol. One clinical study found that chlophedianol was equally effective as isoaminilie citrate at suppressing experimentally induced cough in healthy subjects and at lowering cough counts in patients with a range of chest diseases in a double-blind randomized controlled trial.

4.2.3.7. Levodropropizine

Levodropropizine has been shown in several studies to have antitussive effects on both adults and children. Levodropropizine is a peripherally acting, nonopioid antitussive that is prescribed for adults and children over the age of two to treat mild cases of coughing. Levodropropizine's exact mode of action is unknown, however at doses that lessen coughing brought on by allergens or UNDW, it does not prevent asthmatic subjects' methacholine-induced bronchoconstriction, indicating that it does not function as an antitussive secondary to muscarinic receptor antagonism. Levodropropizine's mechanism of action has been the subject of one of the few studies that has looked into it; at least in experimental animals, it appears that the drug can affect the firing of sensory C-fibers.

Peak plasma levels were reached 40–60 minutes following levodropropizine administration, suggesting a fast gastrointestinal absorption in healthy adults. Furthermore, levodropropizine's pharmacokinetics were shown to be linear over a dose range of 30 to 90 mg, meaning that neither elderly patients nor pediatric patients require a change in levodropropizine dosage.

Levododropropizine has been used in several studies involving subjects whose cough was brought on by chemical or mechanical stimulation. In a double-blind study involving 10 individuals with allergic asthma or chronic bronchitis, Bariffi induced coughing by inhaling nebulized distilled water before and after seven days of treatment with 60 mg of levodropropizine three times daily or placebo. Cough was considerably lessened in the levodropropizine group after 7 days of treatment, but not in the placebo group. Levodropropizine (30, 60, or 90 mg) was tested in a crossover trial against citric acid-induced cough in 11 healthy volunteers. Two hours after levodropropizine injection of 30 mg and an hour after levodropropizine administration of either 60 or 90 mg showed a significant reduction in cough frequency. Six bronchitis patients were included in the same study, and their level of cough was assessed both before and after taking 60 mg of levodropropizine. Levodropropizine treatment resulted in an overall reduction in the severity of the cough. Levodropropizine treatment had no negative effects on respiratory function or airway clearance mechanisms in the 22 additional patients with chronic bronchitis who received 60 mg of the medication three times a day for one week. However, one patient experienced drowsiness following the administration of 90 mg of levodropropizine. Once more, levodropropizine showed a significant suppression of citric acid-induced cough at 1, 2, and 6 hours post-administration in a double-blind trial with eight healthy volunteers.

In a separate double-blind trial, 40 patients received a single 120 mg dose of levodropropizine or a placebo one hour before fiber optic bronchoscopy. Levodropropizine group patients experienced a significant reduction in the severity of their cough and required fewer additional doses of local anesthetic. This study supported the findings of a previous trial that included 8 patients receiving levodropropizine and 8 receiving a placebo. Twice before fiber optic bronchoscopy, 60 mg of levodropropizine was given in this double-blind trial, i.e., two doses: one the night before and one forty minutes before the test. Mistretta assessed levodropropizine's effectiveness in treating coughs brought on by capsaicin. Twelve patients with allergic rhinitis received treatment for eight days in a double-blind crossover trial using 60 mg of levodropropizine three times a day in addition to a placebo, with a minimum one-week wash-out period. Before each treatment session and on the final day of each treatment cycle, the capsaicin challenge test was conducted. When compared to baseline and placebo, the total number of coughs caused by capsaicin in the 10 patients under evaluation was significantly lower following levodropropizine treatment. Furthermore, levodropropizine significantly raised the threshold concentration of capsaicin needed to cause two and five coughs, but a placebo did not. Schönffeldt also employed capsaicin-induced cough in a double-blind crossover study that included a three-day wash-out period after treatment with 60 mg of levodropropizine three times a day and a placebo. Twenty healthy participants were recruited for the trial; however, two participants were dropped due to unrelated illnesses. The levodropropizine treatment resulted in a significant increase in cough threshold, whereas the placebo did not. Six double-blind clinical trials involving 60 mg of levodropropizine three times a day were conducted by Allegra and Bossi against two active controls and a placebo. The study's participants were hospitalized patients suffering from different types of coughs. The trial lasted for three days. Forty patients received levodropropizine treatment and another forty received a placebo in the two trials compared to placebo. Levodropropizine proved to be significantly more effective than a placebo in these trials. Levodropropizine and morclofone were used to treat a total of 28 patients in two studies. Levodropropizine's impact was statistically significant, while morclofone did not result in a discernible improvement. The last two trials showed similar significant efficacy for both drugs, but against cloperastine. Levodropropizine was administered to 22 patients and cloperastine to 23 patients in these trials.

The majority of levodropropizine clinical trials lack validated objective end points and do not include a placebo control. Thus, for five days, 60 mg of levodropropizine and 15 mg of dextromethorphan were compared in a clinical trial conducted by Catena and Daffonchio. A total of 110 patients received treatment with levodropropizine and 99 patients received treatment with dextromethorphan in this double-blind study. Regardless of the severity of the initial cough, statistically significant improvements were already observed by the second day of levodropropizine treatment. Only three days into the dextromethorphan treatment did there appear to be a noticeable improvement. Both medications considerably decreased the number of night awakenings brought on by coughing (92% for levodropropizine and 72% for dextromethorphan); however, levodropropizine demonstrated a noticeably greater improvement than dextromethorphan.

Luporini investigated the impact of levodropropizine on cough related to lung cancer. 75 mg of levodropropizine and 10 mg of dihydrocodeine were given three times a day for seven days to 66 and 69 patients, respectively, in a double-blind, comparative trial. While somnolence was reported in significantly more patients treated with dihydrocodeine (15 patients; 22%) than with levodropropizine (5 patients; 8%), both medications resulted in a similar and significant decrease in cough score and night awakenings. Levodropropizine's effectiveness was assessed in 25 lung cancer patients in an open study based on patient and physician satisfaction. Physicians rated the drug as sufficient in 12% of cases, good in 48%, and optimal in 40% after patients received 60 mg of levodropropizine three times a day for an average of nine to thirteen days of treatment. In 16% of the cases, the patients rated the drug's efficacy as sufficient, in 32% as good, and in 48% as optimal. Additionally, the drug was well tolerated.

The study examined the effectiveness and tolerability of levodropropizine and clobutinol (both 60 mg three times a day) in elderly patients over 60 years of age. The patients' mean age was 71.4 years. The study was double-blind, with 95 patients receiving levodropropizine treatment and 96 receiving clobutinol treatment. On the first day of treatment with both medications, there was an improvement in the frequency and intensity of cough, and after three days of treatment, the cough was even less frequent and severe. Dyspnea was also looked into before and during the study, and both medications significantly improved dyspnea.

Levodropropizine 60 mg three times a day was given for an average of 7.5 days to 25 tuberculosis patients. After just one day, the treatment was successful, and 96% of the cases showed good or ideal results at the conclusion of the course of treatment. In a five-day, double-blind, controlled trial, 24 adults took oral dextromethorphan three times a day and 26 adults took levodropropizine three times a day. Overall, levodropropizine was 70% effective, while dextromethorphan was 62% effective. Levodropropizine's (93%) efficacy rate in treating severe cough was noticeably higher than that of dextromethorphan (70%) in this regard.

From a clinical standpoint, levodropropizine's effectiveness and tolerability in pediatric and elderly patients are comparable to those in adults. Fiocchi examined 70 kids with acute UTRI who ranged in age from 2 months to 14 years, with a mean of 4 points 6 years. Three mild and transient adverse events related to levodropropizine were recorded. Levodropropizine (2 mg/kg per day), divided into three dose administrations for five days or more, was reported to show a clinical improvement in 69 of 70 patients.

Ninety-four percent of patients in a larger clinical trial with 180 participants between the ages of 0 and 12 (mean age of 5 years and treated for one week) reported good or very good efficacy. Eight (4.4%) adverse events that happened during treatment were most likely or unquestionably connected to levodropropizine. In a double-blind, comparative clinical trial, 128 patients receiving levodropropizine and 122 receiving dropropizine were treated for nonproductive coughs resulting from different causes in children aged 2–14 years. On the first day of treatment, both medications significantly decreased the frequency of coughing and the number of cough-related nighttime awakenings. For the two days following treatment, improvement persisted. Around 11 patients receiving levodropropizine and sixteen receiving dropropizine reported adverse events.

In one study, 77 pediatric patients with acute or chronic bronchitis received injections of levodropropizine or dextromethorphan for three days. Levodropropizine was much more successful than dextromethorphan on days two and three, with an improvement already evident on the first day. Overall, the tolerability was quite good.

4.2.4. Other Drugs Having an Effect on Cough

Numerous other drug classes have also been demonstrated to have a clinically meaningful effect in reducing cough, frequently as a result of their action on an underlying disease mechanism that causes cough as a symptom (e.g., antibiotics, glucocorticosteroids, and other medications) and are therefore presumably not strictly antitussive medications; however, we included them because they are frequently used clinically for this indication.

4.2.4.1. Menthol and TRPM8 Agonists

The secretory gland of the peppermint plant, Mentha x piperita, specifically Mentha avrensis, is the source of menthol, a monoterpene, which is used to extract the majority of peppermint oil found in nature. It is believed that l-menthol, the most prevalent and physiologically active isomer, is the active antitussive ingredient.

The initial demonstration of menthol's pharmacological action was its specific binding to lung cell membranes. Later, a seminal study from the David Julius laboratory disclosed the molecular mechanism underlying the action of menthol. They demonstrated that menthol activates TRPM8, a nociceptor belonging to the TRP family. The cooling sensation that is felt when inhaling menthol is caused by activation of the menthol receptor, which is mainly found on afferent sensory neurons. This activation allows calcium to enter the cell and release it intracellularly, which leads to depolarization. Additionally, menthol may have a more central action by increasing glutamate release at the presynaptic level, which would improve neurotransmission. Antinociception is another TRPM8-mediated menthol response that is thought to be mediated by blocking the neuronal voltage-gated sodium channels Nav1.8 and Nav1.9. Whether or not this action plays a role in the menthol's antitussive properties is still unknown. Higher concentrations of menthol also activate L-type calcium channels and nicotinic acetylcholine receptors, among other pharmacological effects; however, it is unclear how much of these actions contribute to menthol's antitussive properties.

With a long history, menthol is now a common ingredient in many over-the-counter preparations, ranging from food flavorings to dental care. The commercialization of menthol's antitussive properties occurred in 1890 when Lumsford Richardson created a topical rub. Many syrups, lozenges, and inhalers have joined the multimillion dollar "vaporub" product line (Figure 4.3).

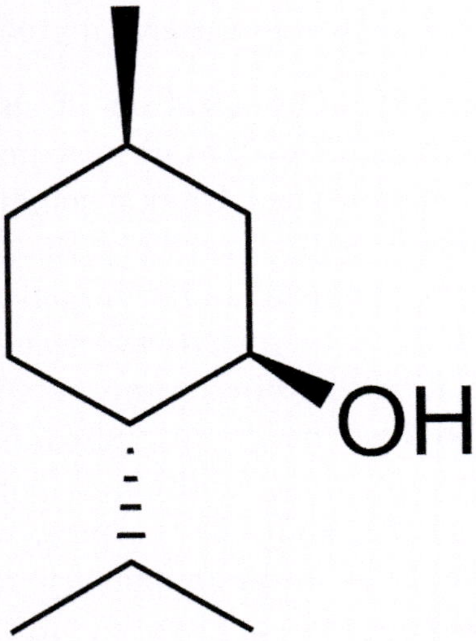

Figure 4.3. *Chemical structure of menthol.*

Source: By Daveryan at en.wikipedia - Own work, Public Domain, https://commons.wikimedia.org/w/index.php?curid=11903118.

4.2.4.2. Erdosteine

A homocysteine analog called erectase is sold in several nations as an expectorant and antioxidant for the management of COPD and bronchitis. Erdosteine exhibits a variety of intriguing pharmacological characteristics that are relevant to the management of respiratory disorders, such as antioxidant activity, some anti-inflammatory effects, and effects on the mucociliary escalator and mucous properties. These have already been examined somewhere. A recent meta-analysis provided convincing proof of the efficacy of erdosteine in treating patients with COPD and bronchitis based on several controlled clinical trials. Metabolite 1 appears to be the primary metabolite responsible for most of the actions of erdosteine. Additionally, there is some evidence supporting the potential antitussive effects of erdosteine. Therefore, it is unclear whether erdosteine has a direct antitussive effect or whether its effects are secondary to anti-inflammatory activity or effects on mucous. In the guinea pig, erdosteine has been shown to inhibit citric acid-induced cough. However, in the same study, these authors also showed other effects in the airways. To determine whether erdosteine possesses clinically relevant antitussive activity, well-controlled clinical trials must be conducted as there is currently very little, frequently anecdotal, evidence of the drug's antitussive effect.

4.2.4.3. Antibiotics

Despite international guidelines' recommendations against their use, antibiotics are frequently used to treat acute coughs. The United States and the United Kingdom are among the countries that use antibiotics the most, although there are significant cultural differences in this regard. Acute bronchitis, whooping cough, and URTI, or the common cold, are among the clinical conditions that fall under the umbrella of acute cough. Clinical assessment alone frequently makes it impossible to distinguish between them. Antibiotics are not advised for viral infections, which are by far the most common cause of cough. However, severe bacterial respiratory tract infections and the early stages of whooping cough should be treated with antibiotics. However, it can be challenging to distinguish between these conditions and viral illnesses, so clinical judgment is needed in each case. Many placebo-controlled trials have been conducted on antibiotics for the treatment of acute cough, with erythromycin, amoxicillin, and doxycycline being the most frequently investigated drugs. The majority of clinical trials have evaluated overall health and the degree to which the acute illness has resolved. Because cough outcomes are frequently unreported or scarce, it is challenging to assess their clinical significance. Seldom has the sensitivity of the cough reflex been investigated in antibiotic placebo-controlled trials. Cough reflex sensitivity is elevated in acute cough, but it's unclear if antibiotics hasten the decrease that occurs when the illness resolves.

4.2.4.4. Glucocorticosteroids

Some patients with cough have shown evidence of airway inflammation, which has shed light on several common causes of cough as well as some of the peripheral mechanisms underlying cough reflex sensitization. One way to differentiate asthmatic from nonasthmatic cough and identify patients who are likely to benefit from corticosteroid therapy is through the measurement of particular cellular and mediator profiles within the airway.

4.2.4.5. β_2-Agonists

Research on humans and experimental animals has shown that β_2-agonists, such as salbutamol (albuterol), can suppress coughing. However, there is disagreement over whether these medications' antitussive properties are solely attributable to their bronchodilator action or stem from other mechanisms. Different β_2-agonists given in different ways to guinea pigs have been demonstrated to suppress cough produced by methacholine, citric acid, capsaicin, and both allergic and capsaicin-induced cough. However, in one study, isoproterenol perfusion of the extra thoracic trachea beforehand did not prevent animals under anesthesia from coughing up citric acid.

Research utilizing artificially induced cough in human volunteers in good health has produced inconsistent findings regarding the antitussive properties of β_2-agonists. Several studies have shown that these agents can suppress cough. For example, fenoterol has been shown to suppress cough induced by add ultrasonically nebulized distilled water (UNDW), albuterol to suppress cough induced by citric acid, and procaterol to suppress cough induced by substance P in volunteers with acute urinary tract infections. Though it causes significant bronchodilation, inhaled procaterol has been shown to have no effect on subjects with asthma or chronic bronchitis, or on cough reflex sensitivity to inhaled capsaicin in normal volunteers. Moreover, it has been demonstrated that albuterol does not prevent normal volunteers from coughing up citric acid or capsaicin. However, albuterol provided a good degree of protection against cough related to smoking.

Numerous studies have assessed the impact of β_2-agonists on pathologic cough in cough variant asthma (CVA) patients. Based on clinical experience, the majority of CVA patients will see an improvement in their cough after just one week of β_2-agonist therapy; however, it may take up to eight weeks of treatment, including an ICS, to fully resolve their cough. On the other hand, it has been demonstrated that in asthmatic subjects, leukotriene receptor antagonists (LTRAs) are more effective than β_2-agonists and ICS asthmatic cough. (Barnes, 2002; Bateman et al, 2004; Sun et al, 2010)

4.2.4.5. Muscarinic Receptor Antagonists

The parasympathetic nervous system controls mucus release into the airways and bronchomotor tone. The lung's muscarinic (M) receptors mediate these effects. The lungs contain three different types of M receptors (M_1, M_2, and M_3), which are the targets of muscarinic receptor antagonists that are currently on the market. Relatively little research has been done to assess how muscarinic receptor antagonists affect different types of pathologic cough, despite the abundance of basic and clinical data regarding these agents' effects on pulmonary function and airway tone.

Muscarinic receptor antagonists have been shown to have an antitussive effect in numerous animal studies. Ipratropium bromide inhibited the induction of cough in guinea pigs that were awake, while atropine reduced the sensitivity of the cough reflex to inhaled capsaicin. Atropine potently suppressed electrically induced cough in conscious dogs. However, in conscious guinea pigs, ipratropium bromide was found to inhibit citric acid-induced bronchoconstriction but not cough, and in guinea pigs under anesthesia, atropine was not found to inhibit citric acid-induced cough. Since muscarinic receptors are absent from airway afferent nerves, any antitussive effect of muscarinic receptor antagonists is unlikely to be a direct airway effect on the cough reflex.

4.2.4.6. Mucolytics and Expectorants

Medications known as expectorants and mucolytics, which affect the airway mucociliary apparatus, are frequently prescribed to treat productive cough. Mucolytics lower mucus viscosity and expectorants are thought to increase mucus volume, which helps ciliary transport and coughing clear airway secretions. It is believed that encouraging an efficient cough will lessen the frequency of coughs.

For both adults and children, guaifenesin—previously marketed as glyceryl guaicolate—is the only expectorant with FDA approval. Veterinarians also employ it as a muscle relaxant. Because of its expectorant properties, guaifenesin has been extracted from the guaiac tree's bark for many centuries. Guaifenesin is a white, crystalline powder that is taken orally and soluble in both water and alcohol. It is eliminated through urine and has a brief half-life of one hour. There are twice-daily modified release preparations available. Although guaifenesin's exact mode of action is unknown, it is believed to affect the cholinergic innervation of the mucous glands that line the airways. Guaifenesin is widely used, but there is little proof that it affects mucociliary clearance or ciliary motility *in vivo* or *in vitro*. Moreover, there is conflicting clinical evidence regarding its expectorant and antitussive efficacy. In patients with URTIs, Kuhn did not find a statistically significant decrease in the frequency or subjectively reported severity of coughing. Sputum viscosity did, however, decrease in patients with productive coughs, though it's unclear if they thought this was clinically helpful. Robinson's larger study, which used a lower dose of guaifenesin, on the other hand, found a significant reduction in the patients' subjective cough severity; after therapy, 75% of patients reported a reduced cough severity, compared to 31% in the placebo group. According to a more recent study, guaifenesin reduces the sensitivity of the cough reflex in URTI patients. Nonetheless, the current data does not allow for the establishment or rejection of guaifenesin's or other expectorants' definitive antitussive effect. More research is required, ideally with patients who have acute cough, suitable sample sizes, and validated endpoints like objective cough monitoring and health status questionnaires. Research is also needed to determine how guaifenesin interacts with antitussive medications like dextromethorphan, as this combination of medications is commercially available despite having little proof of its effectiveness.

Even less evidence supports mucolytics' antitussive effects. The amino acid L-cysteine is the source of carbocisteine, also known as S-carboxymethyl L-cysteine. It is extensively utilized in the treatment of COPD patients, where it has been demonstrated to lessen exacerbations, and is extensively accessible in Europe and South America. Carbocisteine is eliminated through urine and has a half-life of one and a third of an hour. The evidence supporting this medication's mucolytic action is contradictory: while Edwards and colleagues observed a decrease in mucus viscosity, Goodman and colleagues and Thomson and colleagues found no effect of carbocisteine on mucus clearance. Resetting the balance between sialomucins and fucomucins is thought to be the mechanism of action, as it increases the former, which is a crucial component of mucus and restores viscoelastic properties. Carbocisteine may possess several antitussive properties, such as the capacity to elevate the chloride content in respiratory secretions, diminish airway tachykinins, and lessen hypersensitivity to cough reflex. Overall, though, there is little clinical evidence of carbocisteine's antitussive effects because the majority of studies on the drug's effects on mucolytic activity in patients with chronic bronchitis. There has never been any evidence of an impact when cough severity is reported as an outcome measure in placebo-controlled trials. Similarly, most studies reporting the severity of coughs did not report a significant effect from N-acetylcysteine, another commonly used mucolytic drug.

4.2.4.7. Antacids/Proton Pump Inhibitors and Gastrointestinal Motility Drugs

It seems surprising at first that medications that affect the gastrointestinal tract could be helpful in treating coughing. This claim is predicated on the theory that one of the main physiological roles of the cough reflex, if not the primary one, is to reduce aspiration into the airway. Therefore, conditions affecting the upper gastrointestinal tract may induce cough directly or by making the afferent airway sensory nerves more sensitive.

Food aspiration has long been known to cause coughing, but until 50 years ago, reflux and aspiration-related gastroesophageal diseases were not frequently linked to persistent coughing. To this day, there is much disagreement over the type of gastrointestinal illness that is linked to cough and the underlying mechanisms—in particular, the induction of airway inflammation and afferent neuronal hypersensitivity.

It was soon discovered that GERD, along with its classic symptoms of dyspepsia and heartburn, was frequently associated with certain patients who had persistent cough. Because of this, the first suggested therapeutic target for medications acting on the gastrointestinal tract and used to treat cough was GERD with esophagitis caused by reflux of acid stomach contents. In fact, blocking the production of acid with H_2-receptor antagonists and proton pump inhibitors has become the standard treatment advised in guidelines from both European and American institutions. Early uncontrolled and open-label research indicated a high rate of response.

Other non-respiratory symptoms like dysphonia and rhinitis suggest that non-acid reflux and aspiration may be the cause of cough. The phrase "silent reflux" was actually coined due to the patient's loss of voice and absence of typical peptic symptoms—it is hardly a fitting moniker for a disease that causes coughing. The use of promotility agents as antitussives resulted from these observations as well as the understanding that dysmotility of the upper gastrointestinal tract may cause coughing. The lack of effective medications for this common symptom has led to the promotion of a wide range of agents in addition to those with approved indications for gastrointestinal motility disorders for the treatment of cough.

In a single, double-blind crossover study, the effects of 150 mg of ranitidine, an H2-receptor antagonist, taken twice daily for two weeks on the reported cough scores of 25 patients were compared with a placebo. While both groups showed some response to treatment, the ranitidine arm showed noticeably more improvement. Proton pump inhibitor therapy has been supported by the addition of ranitidine at night because nocturnal acid secretion is controlled by the vagal nerve through a histaminergic mechanism and because an increase in gastric pH may lessen the typical morning cough.

Several uncontrolled trials found that patients with persistent cough responded well, and sometimes completely, to "aggressive" antacid therapy combined with PPIs. Due to these reports, PPIs are now prescribed twice daily for reflux cough in many centers and have been included in national and international guidelines. However, placebo-controlled trials have yielded far less encouraging results, which led to the conclusion in a recent Cochrane review that "there is insufficient evidence to conclude that treatment with PPI for cough associated with GERD is beneficial in adults." (Barnes, 2002; Bateman et al, 2004; Sun et al, 2010)

4.2.4.8. Xanthines

In addition to being a popular bronchodilator, theophylline has been proven to have definite anti-inflammatory effects in individuals with COPD and asthma. Theophylline, however, has also been demonstrated to have antitussive properties. For instance, theobromine and theophylline have both been shown to suppress citric acid-induced cough in both healthy and allergic guinea pigs. Some patients have also reported that theophylline suppresses cough brought on by the consumption of ACE inhibitors. More recently, it has been shown that theobromine inhibits human coughing and sensory nerve activation. Currently, a large multicenter trial is assessing theobromine's clinical effects on chronic cough. It has recently been shown that theophylline inhibits the cough reflex by affecting BK K^+ channels.

4.2.4.9. Cromones

Since the initial discovery of sodium cromoglycate (DSCG) and its related medication, nedocromil sodium, these medications have been used as antiallergic medications. Although the mechanism of action of these medications has been widely reported as the stabilization of mast cells, it has been recognized that the cromones also affect the function of sensory nerves. Therefore, it has been reported that DSCG and nedocromil sodium affect sensory nerve fibers. According to reports, nedocromil sodium causes a prolonged, chloride-dependent depolarization; this feature could account for DSCG's capacity to suppress cough in both clinical and experimental settings. For instance, nedocromil has been shown to suppress the cough that dogs experience when they ingest citric acid, and DSCG has been shown to suppress the cough that some patients experience when they ingest ACE inhibitors. Furthermore, it has been demonstrated that DSCG and nedocromil sodium both suppress the cough linked to asthma. Cromones' exact mode of action on sensory nerves is unknown, but DSCG and nedocromil sodium have both recently been proposed to function as agonists at G-coupled receptor 35, while DSCG may also function as a tachykinin antagonist, in addition to their action on Cl^2 channels.

4.2.5. Clinical Trial Design for Evaluation of Antitussive Drugs

The selection of patients is a critical step in any trial. Individuals who have an inexplicable persistent cough are a good model for researching antitussive medications because their cough frequency is high and consistent over time, which makes these studies effective in illustrating the effects of treatment. It is crucial to recognize that the mechanisms underlying chronic cough are unknown, so an agent's failure in this patient group may not rule out its substantial activity in other conditions. Studies on acute cough are effective in identifying the effects of medications with anticipated quick onset of action because acute cough has a comparable high frequency of coughing and, while coughing rapidly improves, cough measures are very repeatable. Although viral URTIs have also been linked to sub-acute cough, only one study that focused on this population found it difficult to find and enlist participants.

The gold standard is, of course, double-blind, randomized, placebo-controlled clinical trials. For patients with chronic cough, crossover and parallel group designs are both feasible; the specific design to be used should be determined by the properties and mode of action of the agent to be evaluated. Whether to use an active comparator or an inert placebo depends on how frequently and how severe side effects from the medication occur. Cough frequency monitors are the perfect tool for objective primary outcome measurement in proof of concept studies. However, a placebo arm would seem to be essential in determining the likely antitussive action of any drug—new or old—given the significant placebo response observed in many clinical trials evaluating cough. In later phase studies, subjective outcome measures—such as visual analog scales and health-related quality of life—are crucial for capturing the patients' perception of their symptoms and determining whether reductions in cough frequency have a meaningful clinical benefit. When the tussive agent activates a relevant pathway (e.g., capsaicin challenge in TRPV1 antagonist testing), measurements of the cough reflex sensitivity may offer valuable pharmacodynamic evidence of target engagement. It is yet unknown, though, if improvements in cough frequency are inevitably predicted by changes in cough reflex sensitivity. More information about the design of clinical trials, sample size, and minimally significant differences in outcome tools has been covered elsewhere. To accurately assess treatments that are currently on the market and those that are being developed, carefully planned clinical trials using validated endpoints are required. (Barnes, 2002; Bateman et al, 2004; Sun et al, 2010)

4.3. Mucolytics

Drugs called mucolytics are used to treat patients with COPD, cystic fibrosis, and bronchiectasis who have hypersecretion of mucus and its side effects, such as recurrent infections. They are members of the class of agents known as mucoactive agents. The various options and their corresponding mechanisms of action, indications, and contraindications are discussed in this activity. These are important tools for managing and treating productive cough and related muco-obstructive respiratory disorders, so healthcare team members should take note of them.

4.3.1. Indications

Medications classified as mucolytics are members of the mucoactive agent class. They work to improve the mucus layer that lines the respiratory tract by exerting their influence on it. The various epithelia inside our bodies use mucus as their first line of defense against harmful pathogens. Its duties also include shielding the epithelium from irritating substances that cause excoriation in the digestive system. It contains a variety of proteins, including glycoproteins, immunoglobulins, and even some antimicrobial enzymes like lysozyme. The biophysical characteristics of mucus are primarily determined by the cross-bridging of polymeric gel-forming mucins. By preventing the formation of biofilms and inhibiting bacterial growth, this layer provides excellent bacterial protection. In addition to preventing fluid loss, the mucus layer serves as a physical barrier against respiratory irritants. Sputum is expectorated mucus.

The mucus-secreting cells and the mucociliary escalator are the two main mechanisms that control the amount of mucus in our bodies. Mucus is secreted by goblet cells of the mucous membranes and submucosal glands of the respiratory, GI, and reproductive systems. Mucus is cleared towards the pharynx by the mucociliary escalator, and the cough reflex eventually expectorates it out. There are, nevertheless, some circumstances in which this rule is violated.

Mucus hypersecretion results from long-term airway irritation in diseases like asthma and COPD. The accumulation of excess mucus occurs when mucociliary clearance mechanisms are overloaded by excessive mucus production. Mucus plugs are created as a result, further reducing the clearance. The airways react by releasing an excessive amount of inflammatory mediators in an effort to remove the blockage. Unfortunately, this simply makes things worse because it causes the mucus viscosity to rise, which further reduces clearance and triggers the onset of inflammation and fibrosis. This condition is made worse by the invasion of bacteria such as Staphylococcus aureus and Pseudomonas aeruginosa in the static mucus. This sets off a vicious cycle that always culminates in a severe escalation of the illness. In these circumstances, traditional mucolytics such as N-acetylcysteine are recommended because they improve mucus clearance by reducing viscosity and enhancing flowability.

Because mucus secretion is compromised in diseases such as cystic fibrosis, filamentous actin polymers and DNA derived from inflammatory cells are the predominant components of airway secretions. Additionally thick and viscous, these secretions are a common target for bacteria. Another class of mucolytics that targets DNA polymers is useful in this situation.

4.3.2. Mechanism of Action

Mucolytics are divided into two subgroups:

1. **Classic Mucolytics:** Mucus is one of the many complex proteins made up of disulfide bonds. The class's prototype medication, N-acetyl L-cysteine (NAC), functions through the thiol-disulfide interchange mechanism and retains a reducing ability. Cysteine residues can be found throughout the structure of the mucin polymers. These residues serve as anchors for the disulfide bonds, which cause the polymer to crosslink. The disulfide bonds affixed to cysteine residues are hydrolyzed by the free thiol group present in the structure of NAC. The S-S bond is reduced to an S-H (sulfhydryl) bond in this reaction, disrupting the three-dimensional structure of mucus and making it unable to anchor the complex protein structure.

This subgroup includes:

- **N – Acetylcysteine:** This possesses anti-inflammatory and antioxidative qualities in addition to the mucolytic action described previously. These substances aid in lowering the inflammatory mediators and reactive oxygen species that irritate respiratory airways.
- **Carbocysteine:** It has an additional expectorant effect by increasing the volume of sputum. Because it doesn't irritate the respiratory tract, it is extremely safe and effective for asthmatics. Because it greatly lowers the bacterial load in these patients' airways, it may be indicated for reducing AECOPD (acute exacerbation of chronic obstructive pulmonary disease). Up to 70% of cases of AECOPD have been linked to pulmonary infections.
- **Erdosteine and Fudosteine:** These are more recent medications with extra anti-oxidant and anti-tussive properties. They are thiol derivatives. Their active metabolite, Met-1, contains a sulfhydryl group that functions during the neutrophils' respiratory burst. Additionally, ergosteine has demonstrated a strong antibiotic-potentiating effect. Additionally, reports have suggested that it protects against alpha-1 antitrypsin.

2. **Peptide Mucolytics:** This, as opposed to traditional mucolytics, maintain the protective mucins. DNA polymers and F-actin linkages that tend to proliferate in purulent secretions are the targets of peptide mucolytics. Peptide mucolytics are therefore very helpful in conditions like cystic fibrosis because they work by depolymerizing the DNA polymers or F-actin network that are frequently present in purulent secretions, thereby reducing mucus viscosity.
   - **Dornase Alfa:** Dornase alfa breaks down DNA polymers to produce a mucolytic effect. In patients with cystic fibrosis, it results in a slight increase in FEV1 (forced expiratory volume after one second).
   - **Thymosin β_4:** Thymosin β_4 produces its mucolytic effect by acting on F-actin. Purulent secretions produce large amounts of F-actin, which is filamentous and increases viscosity. Therefore, by depolymerizing these filaments, thymosin may be useful in dissolving airway pus.

4.3.3. Administration

Nebulized N-acetylcysteine can be applied topically, intravenously, or orally. The oral route is much more tolerable, even though the topical route had the benefit of inducing a cough reflex and activating the mucociliary clearance mechanism. This topic is covered in more detail under adverse reactions. It is advised to take 200–600 mg orally every day to treat muco-obstructive disorders. Pregnant women and children are safe, as has been established.

For patients with cystic fibrosis, a recommended dose of dornase alfa is 2.5 mg given in nebulized form once or twice daily. Research indicates that FVC and FEV1 can improve as soon as three days after starting treatment. Along with the medication, patients with cystic fibrosis should continue receiving standard therapies such as chest physical therapy and antibiotics. For children of all ages and adolescents, the recommended dosage and method of administration are the same. Early administration has been shown to be beneficial in infants and young children with cystic fibrosis, even in the absence of any clinical signs or symptoms of the illness. While there is little information available about the safety of dornase alfa during pregnancy, doses significantly higher than the maximum recommended human dose in animal models did not appear to have any effect on fetal outcome.

Oral preparations of carbopime are used to treat patients. Doses range from 750 mg twice day to 4.5 g once daily. There is evidence to suggest that administering the medication at night resulted in a higher concentration of active compounds.

Oral administration of ethosteine is possible, with dosages ranging from 600 to 900 mg. Elderly patients with chronic liver disease should, however, have their dose carefully titrated due to the possibility of an increased plasma concentration and elimination half-life in these patients.

4.3.4. Adverse Effects

- Vomiting and diarrhea are the side effects of oral N-acetylcysteine that are most commonly reported. The incidence of vomiting and diarrhea increased by 50% and 43.5%, respectively, after 16 to 18 days of taking N-acetylcysteine. Less than 5% of cases are reported to have elevated blood pressure, respiratory distress, chest pain, fever, rectal bleeding, headache, hypotension, lethargy, and skin allergy. Because aerosolized N-acetylcysteine has an irritating effect and a strong odor that can make vomiting occur, it is not well tolerated. Patients receiving intravenous N-acetylcysteine have a high rate of anaphylactic reactions.

- When comparing Dornase alfa to a placebo, laryngitis, voice changes, and rash are the most frequently reported adverse reactions. Chest pain, conjunctivitis, and pharyngitis were other less serious side effects. The majority of these side effects were temporary, and it wasn't stated that they were bad enough to necessitate stopping the medication or changing the dosage. As of yet, dornase alfa-related anaphylactic reactions have not been documented. The clinical significance of the serum antibodies to dornase alfa that developed in 2–4% of patients treated with the medication across all studies has not yet been determined.
- With carbocisteine, reports of mild stomach discomfort, gastric ulceration, and fixed drug eruptions have been made.
- Patients receiving erdosteine have reported experiencing headache, nausea, erythema, and epigastralgia; the latter two of these symptoms resulted in the patient stopping their medication.

4.3.5. Monitoring

It took 30 minutes to reach the maximum plasma concentration of 3.47 mg/L after an oral dose of 400 mg of N-acetylcysteine. N-acetylcysteine has a volume of distribution that ranges from 0.33 to 0.47 L/kg. Half of the medication was discovered to be bound to plasma proteins four hours after an intravenous dose. When taken orally, N-acetylcysteine is extensively metabolized in the gut wall and liver, resulting in a bioavailability of approximately 6–10%. Only 30% of this medication is eliminated by the kidneys; the majority is eliminated non-renally.

Dornase alfa aerosol inhalation results in a negligible systemic absorption, according to animal research. Even extremely high dosages (10 mg three times a day) did not cause a discernible rise in the blood DNase concentration. The minimal amount of systemic absorption that does happen is thought to be protein-bound and leaves the body without accumulating significantly in the tissues. This suggests that patients taking this medication require little to no monitoring. After inhaling a dose of 2 points5 mg of dornase alfa, the mean sputum concentration was found to be 2 µg/mL within the first 15 minutes, and two hours later, it decreased to 0 points6 µg/mL. In animal models, the disappearance half-life from the lungs was estimated to be approximately 11 hours. The bioavailability was less than 2% in primates.

Following absorption, carbocisteine exhibits one-compartment open model kinetics and reaches its peak plasma concentration in one to one and a half hours. The medication is partially metabolized in the liver and excreted unchanged by the kidneys in amounts as high as 60%.

Erdosteine has a comparable elimination half-life after oral administration and takes 1.4 hours to reach its peak plasma concentration. It has two blocked sulfhydryl groups in it. These have the advantageous quality of not affecting the mucus lining the stomach because they are only released after its hepatic metabolism. Reports of notable drug accumulation are nonexistent.

4.3.5.1. Drug Interactions

- Activated charcoal should not be administered with oral N-acetylcysteine because a 3 g preparation will absorb 54.6% of the medication, while a 6 g preparation will absorb 96.2%, significantly decreasing the medication's effectiveness.

- When taken orally in conjunction with intravenous cyclophosphamide, N-acetylcysteine protects the kidneys, urethra, bladder, and ureters from the harmful metabolites of the drug.
- When given together, N-acetylcysteine may be able to prevent doxorubicin-induced cardiomyopathy in animal models.
- It has been demonstrated that dornase alfa significantly increases the antibiotic activity of amikacin and tobramycin against a variety of strains of Staphylococcus aureus and Pseudomonas aeruginosa.
- When erdosteine and amoxicillin were administered to patients experiencing an acute infective exacerbation of chronic bronchitis, the antibiotic's concentration in the sputum increased. This, in contrast to placebo, led to a more marked and early improvement in clinical symptoms.
- When amoxicillin and erdosteine are given together, there is a documented increase in the amount of amoxicillin in the sputum of patients experiencing an acute infective exacerbation of chronic bronchitis.

4.3.6. Toxicity

There is a broad therapeutic index for N-acetylcysteine. Nonetheless, toxicities have occasionally resulted from dosing mistakes. These occur more frequently when the medication is administered intravenously. A reported incident involved the administration of 10 times the recommended loading dose to a female patient, age 23. This dosage resulted in hemolysis, acute renal failure, thrombocytopenia, and finally death. However, another study demonstrated that oral N-acetylcysteine administration, which is frequently used in patients with muco-obstructive disorders, is safer than intravenous administration and significantly less likely to result in dosage errors. Studies have indicated that orally administered doses up to 30g/day for three days were well tolerated, with only mild side effects such as diarrhea and vomiting.

Dornase alfa is a relatively well-tolerated medication because of its short half-life and poor systemic absorption. In single-dose inhalational studies, animal models exposed to doses as high as 180 times the maximum recommended human dose did not develop toxicity to dornase alfa. (Barnes, 2002; Bateman et al, 2004; Sun et al, 2010)

4.3.6.1. Enhancing Healthcare Team Outcomes

According to WHO estimates, approximately 250 million people worldwide have COPD, and the disease claims 3 million lives annually. Regretfully, it is anticipated that this number will increase in the upcoming years, which will have a significant socioeconomic impact. Thus, it is critical to focus on treatments that could enhance lifestyle and lower acute exacerbations, hospital stays, and mortality in such patients while research for a conclusive COPD treatment continues. Mucolytics have enormous promise in this field.

To manage a case of COPD, a well-coordinated interprofessional team comprising pulmonologists, physiotherapists, nurses, pharmacists, and family clinicians (MDs, DOs, NPs, PAs) is needed. The patient needs to be counseled on the significance of making lifestyle changes first. The patient needs to be fully instructed by the doctor on the advantages of the medications they are prescribed, how to use a nebulizer correctly, the right dosage, and any potential side effects. This strategy will maximize patient adherence. Additionally, patients need to be informed about the significance of routine follow-up appointments. Clinical psychologists, support groups, and de-addiction centers also play a critical role in helping patients who smoke postpone the progression of their disease. When used appropriately, this interprofessional approach to patient care with mucolytics can lead to better outcomes and fewer adverse events.

The treatment of cystic fibrosis has advanced significantly over the past 30 years. The average patient survival age nowadays is close to 40 years old. This is partially explained by the development of treatments like mucolytics. Using an interprofessional team that is well-organized to manage this endeavor can help it go farther. While physician-prescribed mucolytics play a significant role in this, other key players include nurses, chest physiotherapists, dieticians, and child psychiatrists.

Large-scale studies for N-acetylcysteine, dornase alfa, carbocisteine, and erdosteine provide evidence that mucolytics are effective, despite recent challenges to this theory. (Barnes, 2002; Bateman et al, 2004; Sun et al, 2010)

4.4. Expectorants

A kind of cough medication called an expectorant thins and loosens mucus. These drugs are usually used to treat chest congestion, particularly in cases where high mucus production is the cause of the symptoms. Drugs in the mucoactive class, expectorants, help clear the airways of mucus.

The most widely used expectorant is guaifenesin. It is the active component of Robitussin and Mucinex 404. Expectorants are available as liquids, tablets, and over-the-counter (OTC) pills.

4.4.1. Uses

Expectorants are frequently prescribed for the treatment of acute (short-term) respiratory tract infections, which include bronchitis, pneumonia, and the common cold. Phlegm accumulation in the throat or lungs may be brought on by these infections. This thick mucus is often difficult to cough up, and when it accumulates, it can cause a persistent cough and chest pain.

Expectorants help you cough up more mucus more efficiently by thinned respiratory secretions in your airways. These drugs function by lubricating the passageways of the airways.

Congestion in the chest is less painful when mucus is coughed up. The risk of infection may also be decreased by coughing up debris and infectious materials like viruses and bacteria.

4.4.2. Different Types of Expectorants

Expectorants fall into one of two categories: natural or medicinal. The primary component of prescription expectorants thins the secretions in your respiratory tract. It increases the productivity of your cough by thinning those secretions. Medicinal expectorants are available over-the-counter in liquid, pill and tablet forms. Medicinal expectorants include:

1. **Guaifenesin**: Guaifenesin is the expectorant that is most frequently used. It is the active component of several medications, such as Robitussin® and Mucinex®. Guaifenesin is a common ingredient in cough, cold, and flu remedies. Furthermore, guaifenesin is an active component of over-the-counter decongestants, fever reducers, cough suppressants, and antihistamines. As of right now, the only expectorant authorized by the U.S. Food and Drug Organization. To make your mucus less

sticky, guaifenesin hydrates it.

2. **Potassium iodide:** Potassium iodide is an expectorant with prescription strength. If you have a long-term lung condition, your doctor might recommend potassium iodide. Excessive mucus production is a potential complication of chronic lung diseases. These illnesses consist of pulmonary emphysema, bronchitis, and asthma. Potassium iodide facilitates coughing and helps to release mucus.

Natural expectorants are another option if you're trying to loosen up mucus and relieve chest congestion. Natural expectorants include:

- **Menthol:** Plants in the mint family naturally produce this chemical. Cough drops, also known as throat lozenges, and cough syrups frequently contain menthol. In addition to providing a cooling sensation, menthol occasionally relieves sore throats. According to one study, menthol may help to relax your airway muscles. This helps your cough by letting more air into your respiratory system.
- **Ivy leaf extract**: Known for its effects on mucus production, ivy leaf extract is a natural expectorant. Any medication containing dry ivy extract may be useful in treating coughs, according to one study.
- **Oral hydration:** Staying hydrated is crucial when using expectorants of any kind. Increase your fluid intake by making a cup of tea or drinking more water. Steer clear of caffeine and alcohol as much as you can.
- **Steam:** Breathing in warm, humid air can help relieve a chronic cough. The mucus in your airway may be loosened by the steam. To help your lungs retain more moisture, consider taking a long shower or using a humidifier.
- **Honey:** Honey has the potential to ease coughing and break up mucus. Honey can be mixed with warm milk or added to a cup of tea. However, infants under the age of 12 months should not be given honey due to the increased risk of botulism.

4.4.3. Side Effects of Expectorants

In most cases, expectorants don't have harmful side effects. However, expectorants come with a range of possible side effects. As long as guaifenesin is taken as prescribed, it's usually safe to use. Potential side effects of guaifenesin can include:

- Dizziness.
- Constipation.
- Headache.
- Tiredness (fatigue).
- Rash.
- Nausea and vomiting (if taken in high doses).

Side effects with potassium iodide are more likely and possibly more severe. The side effects of potassium iodide can include:

- Abdominal pain.
- Nausea and vomiting.
- Acid reflux.
- Diarrhea.
- Skin rash.
- Numbness in hands or feet.
- Swelling or tenderness in your salivary glands.
- Excess salivation.
- Sore gums.
- Brassy, metallic taste in your mouth.
- Confusion.
- Headache.
- Tiredness (fatigue).

- Irregular heartbeat (arrhythmia).

Menthol is usually safe unless you're allergic to it. If you're having an allergic reaction to menthol, the possible side effects can include:

- Hives.
- Difficulty breathing.
- Wheezing.
- Swelling of your face or throat.

The possible side effects of ivy leaf extract can include:

- Nausea and vomiting.
- Diarrhea.
- Hives.
- Skin rash.

Expectorants combined with other medications, such as all-in-one cold or flu medication, are more likely to cause side effects. These side effects can include:

- Tiredness (fatigue).
- Dizziness.
- Nervousness.
- Restlessness.
- Nausea and vomiting. (Barnes, 2002; Bateman et al, 2004; Sun et al, 2010)

A Closer Look

New Drug Targets for Chronic Cough

Coughing is a necessary neurally mediated reflex that has developed to clear out chemical and mechanical irritants and shield the upper airways from blockage. However, cough poses a clinically challenging source of significant physical and psychological morbidity when it is heightened or persistent. Cough is still the most common symptom in the United States that prompts people to visit a doctor. A persistent cough, which is defined as a cough that lasts longer than eight weeks, is also common throughout the world and is the reason for 10% of respiratory referrals to secondary care.

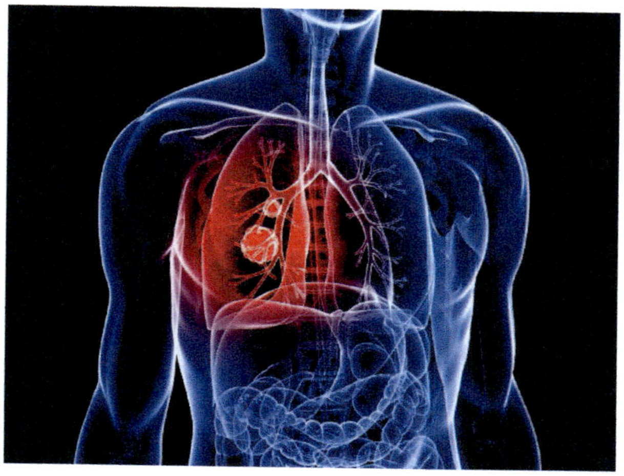

Source: https://asiamd.com/tag/chronic-cough/

Coughing has enormous social and medical costs associated with it. Around 34 million working days are lost in the UK each year due to minor illnesses caused by acute cough, and over £100 million is spent annually on over-the-counter antitussive medications. In 12–42% of cases, chronic cough remains unexplained or refractory despite thorough and sometimes time-consuming diagnostic protocols. As a result, patients are often put through a series of antitussive trials that have limited clinical efficacy and/or undesirable side effects. In a recent online study spanning 29 European nations, the majority of participants with persistent cough reported that the cough medications they had tried were ineffective or had no effect at all (57% and 36%, respectively). Only 7% of respondents said that the cough medications they had tried were successful. Our inadequate comprehension of the mechanistic underpinnings of cough is reflected in the lack of efficacious treatments. In fact, it's becoming more widely acknowledged that treating cough syndromes effectively requires looking beyond the existence—or absence—of underlying disease processes in favor of a deeper comprehension of the physiological mechanisms governing the cough reflex itself.

The recent diagnosis of the "cough hypersensitivity syndrome" (CHS) by a task force of the European Respiratory Society signaled a paradigm shift. Cough is the primary symptom of community-onset asthma (CHS), a clinical entity that is frequently brought on by minimal exposure to heat, mechanical stress, or chemicals. Numerous observations support the theory that dysregulated sensory neural pathways and central processing in cough reflex regulation are the primary mechanisms underlying CHS. First of all, CHS shares symptoms with neuropathic disorders, including pain. Exaggerated coughing in response to known tussive stimuli, such as strong odors and smoke (hypertussia), non-tussive stimuli, such as talking and laughing (allotussia), and abnormal sensations, such as laryngeal paraesthesia, is a common complaint among CHS patients. Second, patients with persistent coughs have higher concentrations of neuropeptides in their airways. These are released from sensory nerves and can function as neurotransmitters and trigger local inflammatory responses. Animal models of bronchopulmonary C-fiber activation leading to an increase in Aδ-mediated cough reflex sensitivity suggest that central sensitization to respiratory sensations involves convergence of sensory bronchopulmonary C-fibers with low threshold Aδ-fibers onto second-order neurons in the brainstem. Functional neuroimaging studies are starting to shed light on the neurobiology of chronic cough. These studies have shown that regions previously linked to voluntary cough suppression are also more activated in the cortical and subcortical brain centers that integrate the location and intensity of the cough stimulus. In certain patients, centrally acting neuromodulatory medications like morphine, amitriptyline, and gabapentin, as well as speech and physical therapy techniques, are also beneficial. However, there is a lack of direct evidence for neural dysfunction because human neural tissues are extremely difficult to obtain, except peripheral lung tissues. As a result, CHS remains a conceptual entity at this time.

The primary CHS regulator is still a mystery. Numerous stimuli can activate the ion channels on the respiratory vagal afferent nerve termini, causing coughing and other reflexes. Transient receptor potential (TRP) channels are the primary ion channel family implicated in the initiation of sensory reflexes. The majority of data relevant to cough physiology has been obtained for transient receptor potential vanilloid (TRPV) 1, transient receptor potential ankyrin (TRPA) 1, TRPV4, and transient receptor potential melastatin (TRPM) 8. Chilli peppers' main ingredient, capsaicin, is one of the most powerful tussigens used in inhalation cough challenge tests because it binds TRPV1 receptors, causing pain, burning sensation, coughing, and the urge to cough. The vagal afferent C- and Aδ-nociceptive fibers that innervate the airways express TRPV1, and the airway nerves of patients with chronic cough express more TRPV1 receptors. However, in a recent clinical trial, the potent TRPV1 receptor antagonist XEN-D0501 failed to significantly alter objective 24-hour cough frequency or subjective urge-to-cough in patients with refractory chronic cough, despite efficacy being predicted in preclinical guinea pig and human *in vitro* vagal models. Additionally found on vagal sensory afferents, TRPA1 receptors bind a variety of irritants, including cigarette smoke and other tussigenic environmental pollutants, but not capsaicin. They also serve as cold thermosensors. However, a TRPA1 antagonist did not demonstrate appreciable antitussive effects in humans, in spite of the preclinical promise of TRPA1 receptors as efficient antitussive targets. Neurokinin antagonists are another instance where preclinical models of cough have not consistently translated to clinical efficacy. and the recently developed GSK2339345 voltage-gated sodium channel blocker.

Summary

- The respiratory system includes the upper airway passages, the nasal cavities, the pharynx and the trachea as well as the bronchi and bronchioles.
- The organ system affected by asthma is the lungs. The lungs consist of lobes and segments, with the right lung having 10 segments and the left lung having eight or nine, depending on the division of the lobe.
- Drugs that act in the central nervous system to suppress cough have classically been designated as centrally acting antitussives.
- Cough is an important protective reflex and a universal symptom in health, but when persistent, it is the most common reason why patients seek medical attention. In epidemiologic studies, up to 40% of the population at any one-time report cough.
- Upper respiratory tract infection (URTI) or the common cold is by far the most common cause of cough, but postinfectious cough, unexplained chronic cough, and cough due to pulmonary disorders such as asthma, chronic obstructive pulmonary disease (COPD), idiopathic pulmonary fibrosis, and lung cancer are also common.
- Mucolytics are drugs used to manage mucus hypersecretion and its sequelae like recurrent infections in patients of COPD, cystic fibrosis, and bronchiectasis.
- Mucolytics are drugs belonging to the class of mucoactive agents. They exert their effect on the mucus layer lining the respiratory tract with the motive of enhancing its clearance.
- An expectorant is a type of cough medicine that thins and loosens mucus. These medications are typically used for managing chest congestion, especially when symptoms are caused by a lot of mucus

References

1. Abelmann, W. H., Gaensler, E. A., & Badger, T. L. (1954). Clinical evaluation of toryn, a new synthetic cough depressant. *Diseases of the Chest, 25*(6), 532–541. https://doi.org/10.1378/chest.25.6.532.
2. Adcock, J. J., Douglas, G. J., Garabette, M., Gascoigne, M., Beatch, G., Walker, M., & Page, C. P. (2003). RSD931, a novel anti-tussive agent acting on airway sensory nerves. *British Journal of Pharmacology, 138*(3), 407–416. https://doi.org/10.1038/sj.bjp.0705156.
3. Adcock, J. J., Schneider, C., & Smith, T. W. (1988). Effects of codeine, morphine and a novel opioid pentapeptide BW443C, on cough, nociception and ventilation in the unanesthetized guinea-pig. *British Journal of Pharmacology, 93*(1), 93–100. https://doi.org/10.1111/j.1476-5381.1988.tb12058.x.
4. Agertoft, L., & Pedersen, S. (1994). Effects of long-term treatment with an inhaled corticosteroid on growth and pulmonary function in asthmatic children. *Respiratory Medicine, 88*(5), 373–381. https://doi.org/10.1016/S0954-6111(05)80051-4.
5. Akbari, O., Faul, J. L., Hoyte, E. G., Berry, G. J., Wahlstrom, J., Kronenberg, M., DeKruyff, R. H., & Umetsu, D. T. (2006). CD4+ invariant T-cell-receptor+ natural killer T cells in bronchial asthma. *New England Journal of Medicine, 354*(11), 1117–1129. https://doi.org/10.1056/NEJMoa052981.

6. Albert, R. K., Connett, J., Bailey, W. C., Casaburi, R., Cooper, J. A. D. Jr, Criner, G. J., Curtis, J. L., Dransfield, M. T., Han, M. K., Lazarus, S. C., et al.; COPD Clinical Research Network. (2011). Azithromycin for prevention of exacerbations of COPD. *New England Journal of Medicine, 365*(7), 689–698. https://doi.org/10.1056/NEJMoa1104623.

7. Aliprandi, P., Castelli, C., Bernorio, S., Dell'Abate, E., & Carrara, M. (2004). Levocloperastine in the treatment of chronic nonproductive cough: Comparative efficacy versus standard antitussive agents. *Drugs in Experimental and Clinical Research, 30*(4), 133–141.

8. Allegra, L., & Bossi, R. (1988). Clinical trials with the new antitussive levodropropizine in adult bronchitic patients. *Arzneimittelforschung, 38*(8), 1163–1166.

9. American Thoracic Society. (2000). What constitutes an adverse health effect of air pollution? Official statement of the American Thoracic Society. *American Journal of Respiratory and Critical Care Medicine, 161*(2 Pt 1), 665–673. https://doi.org/10.1164/ajrccm.161.2.ats5-00.

10. Barnes, P. J. (2002). Cytokine modulators as novel therapies for asthma. *Annual Review of Pharmacology and Toxicology, 42*, 81–98. https://doi.org/10.1146/annurev.pharmtox.42.091001.153545.

11. Bateman, E. D., Boushey, H. A., Bousquet, J., Busse, W. W., Clark, T. J., Pauwels, R. A., & Pedersen, S. E. (2004). Can guideline-defined asthma control be achieved? The gaining optimal asthma controL study. *American Journal of Respiratory and Critical Care Medicine, 170*(8), 836–844. https://doi.org/10.1164/rccm.200310-1442OC.

12. Boyce, J. A. (2003). Mast cells: Beyond IgE. *Journal of Allergy and Clinical Immunology, 111*(1), 24–32. https://doi.org/10.1067/mai.2003.12.

13. Brightling, C. E., Bradding, P., Symon, F. A., Holgate, S. T., Wardlaw, A. J., & Pavord, I. D. (2002). Mast-cell infiltration of airway smooth muscle in asthma. *New England Journal of Medicine, 346*(22), 1699–1705. https://doi.org/10.1056/NEJMoa012948.

14. Busse, W. W. (1996). The role of leukotrienes in asthma and allergic rhinitis. *Clinical and Experimental Allergy, 26*(8), 868–879. https://doi.org/10.1111/j.1365-2222.1996.tb01391.x.

15. Busse, W., Corren, J., Lanier, B. Q., McAlary, M., Fowler-Taylor, A., Cioppa, G. D., van As, A., & Gupta, N. (2001). Omalizumab, anti-IgE recombinant humanized monoclonal antibody, for the treatment of severe allergic asthma. *Journal of Allergy and Clinical Immunology, 108*(2), 184–190. https://doi.org/10.1067/mai.2001.118299.

16. Covar, R. A., Spahn, J. D., Murphy, J. R., & Szefler, S. J. (2004). Progression of asthma measured by lung function in the childhood asthma management program. *American Journal of Respiratory and Critical Care Medicine, 170*(3), 234–241. https://doi.org/10.1164/rccm.200312-1690OC.

17. Covar RA, Fuhlbrigge AL, Williams P, Kelly HW; the Childhood Asthma Management Program Research Group. The Childhood Asthma Management Program (CAMP): Contributions to the Understanding of Therapy and the Natural History of Childhood Asthma. Curr Respir Care Rep. 2012 Dec;1(4):243-250. doi: 10.1007/s13665-012-0026-9. PMID: 23336093; PMCID: PMC3546823.

18. Hooper, C., & Calvert, J. (2008). The role for S-carboxymethylcysteine (carbocisteine) in the management of chronic obstructive pulmonary disease. *International Journal of Chronic Obstructive Pulmonary Disease, 3*(4), 659–669. https://doi.org/10.2147/copd.s3994.

19. Nasr, S. Z., Kuhns, L. R., Brown, R. W., Hurwitz, M. E., Sanders, G. M., & Strouse, P. J. (2001). Use of computerized tomography and chest x-rays in evaluating efficacy of aerosolized recombinant human DNase in cystic fibrosis patients younger than age 5 years: A preliminary study. *Pediatric Pulmonology, 31*(5), 377–382. https://doi.org/10.1002/ppul.1125.

20. Sadowska, A. M., Verbraecken, J., Darquennes, K., & De Backer, W. A. (2006). Role of N-acetylcysteine in the management of COPD. *International Journal of Chronic Obstructive Pulmonary Disease, 1*(4), 425–434. https://doi.org/10.2147/copd.2006.1.4.425.

21. Sun, L., Tang, L., Xu, Y., Wang, S., Li, Y., & Kang, J. (2010). The effect and mechanism of action of carbocysteine on airway bacterial load in rats chronically exposed to cigarette smoke. *Respirology, 15*(7), 1064–1071. https://doi.org/10.1111/j.1440-1843.2010.01862.x.

Chapter

DRUGS USED IN GASTROINTESTINAL DISEASES

5

Contents

Introduction

The term "gastrointestinal diseases" describes conditions that affect the esophagus, stomach, small, large, and rectum as well as the liver, gallbladder, and pancreas, which are the digestive system's accessory organs.

The disorders of impaired normal motility, digestion, absorption, and secretions of the gastrointestinal tract that can be treated with pharmaceuticals include reflux esophagitis, gastroparesis, peptic ulcer, gastroparesis, diarrhea, constipation, and infections. The gastrointestinal system's medications are intended to treat and care for diseases that may impact the pancreas, liver, and biliary tract, among other digestive system organs.

Orientation and Directional Terms

Term	Definition	Illustration
Peptic ulcer disease (PUD)	Peptic ulcer disease (PUD) is a condition that causes a break in the lining of the stomach, small intestine, or lower esophagus. The break is caused by gastric acid or pepsin, and can extend into the muscularis propria layer of the gastric epithelium.	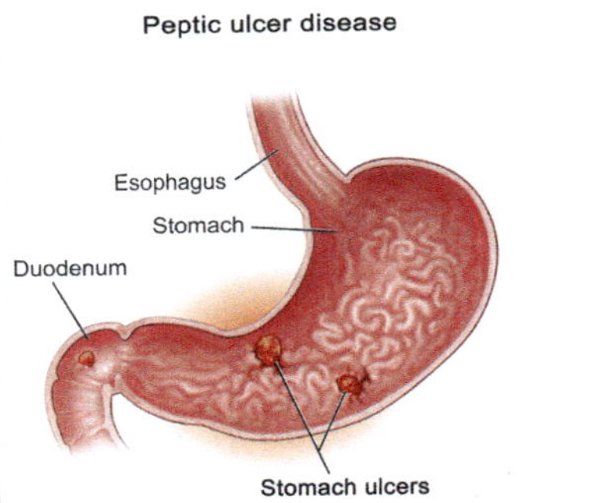
Vasoactive intestinal peptide	Vasoactive intestinal peptide, also known as vasoactive intestinal polypeptide or VIP, is a peptide hormone that is vasoactive in the intestine. VIP is a peptide of 28 amino acid residues that belongs to a glucagon/secretin superfamily, the ligand of class II G protein–coupled receptors.	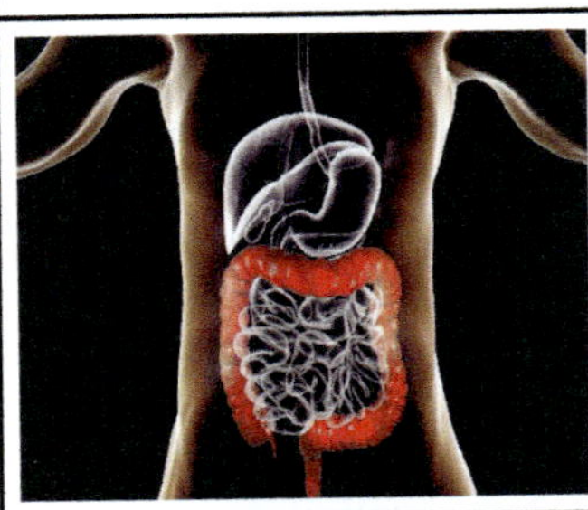
Gastrin-releasing peptide	Gastrin-releasing peptide (GRP) is a neuropeptide, a regulatory molecule encoded in the human by the GRP gene. GRP has been implicated in a number of physiological and pathophysiological processes. Most notably, GRP stimulates the release of gastrin from the G cells of the stomach.	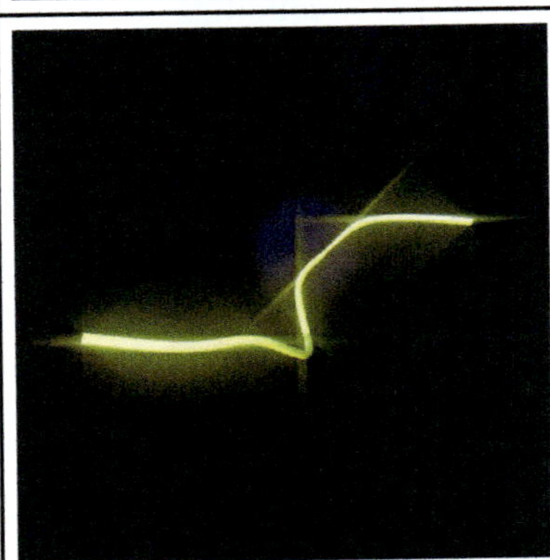
Histidine decarboxylase	Histidine decarboxylase is the sole member of the histamine synthesis pathway, producing histamine in a one-step reaction. Histamine cannot be generated by any other known enzyme. HDC is therefore the primary source of histamine in most mammals and eukaryotes. The enzyme employs a pyridoxal 5'-phosphate (PLP) cofactor, in similarity to many amino acid decarboxylases.	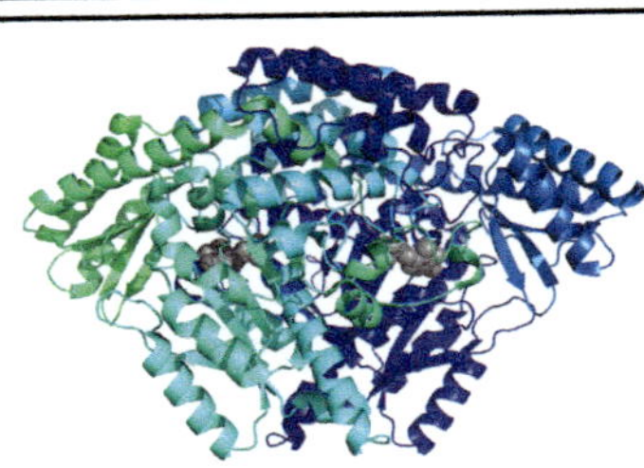

5.1. Acid Peptic Diseases: Pharmacological Approach to Treatment

The pathogenic mechanisms underlying acid peptic diseases are distinct but overlap, usually involving the effects of acid on compromised mucosal defense. Acid reflux is one of those conditions that harms the mucosa of the esophagus and may also cause injury to the larynx, leading to the development of pulmonary symptoms. According to histology, a peptic ulcer is characterized by a mucosal defect that reaches or surpasses the muscularis mucosa and mucosal damage brought on by the secretion of gastric acid and pepsin. Less frequently, ulcers develop in the jejunum, lower esophagus, or distal duodenum, but most often in the stomach and proximal duodenum.

Acid-related disorders are common and significant causes of morbidity and mortality, and they have an impact on the productivity and quality of life of those who suffer from them. In the USA, about 40% of adults report monthly heartburn, 20% report weekly heartburn, and 7% report daily heartburn. As a result, gastroesophageal reflux disease (GERD) is one of the most prevalent gastrointestinal (GI) disorders, with annual costs exceeding $10 billion. Peptic ulcer disease (PUD) affects several million people annually in the United States of America, despite a decreasing incidence due to increased application of eradication therapy against Helicobacter pylori.

In general, the creation of effective and secure medications based on physiological targets has been a remarkable accomplishment in contemporary medicine. The management of stomach acid has been a crucial component of this achievement. Peptic acid diseases are caused by different but related pathogenic mechanisms, but they all share the final mechanism of acid-induced tissue damage. The activation of enzymes on the surface of parietal cells and the stimulation of receptors on the basolateral membrane by hormones and neurones regulate the secretion of gastric hydrochloric acid. These physiological targets are the focus of modern therapy.

The objectives of treatment include symptom relief, improving the mucosa(esophagus, stomach and duodenum) affected by the ulcer's healing process, and preventing recurrence.

Milestones in the treatment of these diseases have included:

- The discovery of the histamine H2-receptor and its functional antagonists
- Identification of the H^+ K^+-adenosine triphosphatase (H^+K^+-ATPase) enzyme and the development of proton-pump inhibitors (PPIs)
- Confirmation of *H. pylori* as a peptic ulcer causative agent with the subsequent development of effective antibiotic eradication regimens

5.1.1. Physiology of Acid Secretion

The epithelium of the stomach is composed of glands and pits. The oxyntic gland area, which makes up about 80% of the organ, and the pyloric gland area, which makes up the remaining 20%, are the two main functional zones. Hydrochloric acid and intrinsic factor are secreted by parietal cells, which are primarily found in the oxyntic glands. They are mostly restricted to the fundic area of the stomach and are found in the lower two-thirds of the oxyntic glands. Chief cells secrete pepsinogen, the precursor of the digestive enzyme, and are found at the base of the oxyntic glands. Within the glands are neuroendocrine cells that contain hormonal and paracrine signaling molecules that control the activity of the parietal cell. D cells, A-like cells, enterochromaffin (EC) cells, and enterochromaffin-like (ECL) cells are a few of these.

5.1.1.1. Regulation of Acid Secretion

Parietal cell acid secretion is triggered by many food-related variables. Cellular, peripheral, and central mechanisms are used for regulation. Acid is produced when H^+ and HCO_3^-.are formed through the catalysis of CO_2 and H_2O by carbonic anhydrase. The H^+K^+-ATPase pump then converts H+ ions into $K^{+,}$ and subsequently couples with CL^- ions that enter the parietal cell from the blood to exchange for HCO_3^-.

The majority of the vagal fibers that supply the stomach are afferent, meaning they communicate with the brain about changes in the stomach's chemistry and mechanics. The efferent fibers are preganglionic neurons that synapse with postganglionic neurons in the stomach wall instead of innervating the parietal cells directly. Neurotransmitters such as substance P, acetylcholine, pituitary adenylate cyclase-activating polypeptide (PACAP), vasoactive intestinal peptide (VIP), and gastrin-releasing peptide (GRP) are found in these neurons. Postganglionic neurons can control acid secretion directly by affecting the parietal cell or indirectly by modifying the secretion of hormonal and paracrine ligands through these messengers. The smooth muscle layer contains unmyelinated nerve endings that make up the stomach's sympathetic receptors. These are more sensitive to chemical stimuli than mechanical ones, and they are involved in the transmission of pain perception in inflammatory conditions like gastritis.

Histamine, gastrin, and acetylcholine are the main stimulants for acid secretion in the stomach. When released from postganglionic enteric neurons, these substances increase levels of adenosine 3′,5′-cyclic monophosphate (cAMP), inositol triphosphate (IP3), diacylglycerol, and calcium inside the cells. This triggers a series of events that cause H^+K^+-ATPase-rich tubulovesicles to merge with the apical plasma membrane, allowing the H^+K^+-ATPase to release protons directly into the lumen of the canaliculus of the parietal cell and then into the lumen of the gastric gland.

1. Histamine

Histamine is synthesized by ECL cells in the oxyntic mucosa and is a significant regulator of acid secretion as a paracrine stimulator. The production of histamine in ECL cells involves the conversion of L-histidine via histidine decarboxylase (HDC). In the gastrointestinal tract, H_2 receptors on parietal cells enhance adenylate cyclase activity, leading to the production of cAMP. The expression of HDC is influenced by factors like gastrin, *H. pylori*, and PACAP. Studies involving the knockout of HDC and the H_2 receptor have highlighted the crucial role of hormonal regulation in gastric acid secretion. HDC-deficient mice exhibit reduced histamine production, which impairs acid secretion and response to gastrin. Conversely, H_2 receptor antagonists have a limited impact on acid secretion compared to cholinergic stimuli. H_2 receptors are present in smooth muscle and cardiac myocytes, potentially contributing to cardiac arrhythmias following rapid administration of intravenous H_2 antagonists. Furthermore, H_3 agonists indirectly promote acid secretion by inhibiting somatostatin-induced histamine release. Presently, there are no approved medications specifically targeting the H_3 receptor.

2. Gastrin

During meal stimulation, gastrin is the main driver of acid secretion, produced in response to dietary amino acids in the digestive system. Gastrin starts off as a larger molecule that is later broken down into peptides that stimulate acid production, including gastrin-17 and gastrin-34. It also produces fragments like progastrin 1–35 and progastrin 1–19. Gastrin is a powerful stimulant for stomach acid production by promoting the release of histamine from ECL cells.

Gastrin and cholecystokinin (CCK) are similar in that they share the same C-terminal pentapeptide sequence. CCK-1 and CCK-2 are the two primary classes of gastrin/CCK receptors that have been identified. While CCK-2 receptors can detect both gastrin and CCK, CCK-1 receptors are specific to CCK. Phospholipase C is activated and intracellular calcium is released when CCK-2 receptors in parietal and ECL cells are stimulated. Gastrin is believed to control histamine secretion by promoting the release of histamine that has been stored as well as by activating the HDC gene transcription. Additionally, glutathione can cause hyperplasia, hypertrophia, and carcinoids in rats, as well as have a trophic effect on the oxyntic mucosa, specifically on ECL cells. Many neoplasms, such as gastric carcinoids and cancers of the stomach, colon, pancreas, and lung, are sensitive to gastrin. This finding sparked worries about the possibility of human carcinogenesis due to chronic hypergastrinemia brought on by PPIs. Prolonged retrospective observation in humans hasn't shown any evidence of a rise in cancer incidence, though.

Gastrin primarily acts through the CCK-2 receptor in the stomach. The release of gastrin is regulated by both central and peripheral pathways. Neural signals to G cells can either inhibit or stimulate gastrin release. Food in the stomach triggers peripheral pathways through mechanical distension, pH levels, and the presence of certain substances. A decrease in gastric pH below 3 triggers a feedback mechanism involving calcitonin-gene related peptide to inhibit gastrin release. Hydrogen ions can also prevent amino acid uptake by G cells. Luminal pH activates sensory nerve cells, leading to the release of somatostatin which suppresses gastrin secretion.

3. Acetylcholine

Acetylcholine released by parasympathetic vagal efferents controls basal acid secretion in the body. It binds to muscarinic (M_3) receptors on parietal cells, directly stimulating acid secretion. It can also indirectly stimulate acid secretion by inhibiting somatostatin release through activation of M_2 and M_4 receptors on D cells. Targeting acetylcholine with anticholinergic drugs is common in treating peptic ulcers, but the necessary doses often come with unwanted side effects like dry mouth, blurred vision, and urinary retention.

4. Somatostatin

The primary physiological inhibitor of acid secretion is somatostatin. Two releases are available for it. While somatostatin 28 is the predominant form found in the small intestine, somatostatin 14 is primarily found in the stomach, pancreas, and enteric neurons. Somatostatin inhibits parietal cells to a tonic degree; however, its main effects come from blocking the release of histamine and gastrin from G and ECL cells. Both gastrin and stomach acid stimulate the secretion of somatostatin. It is elevated by vasoactive intestinal peptide activation and suppressed by cholinergic activation. Although the somatostatin analog octreotide has not been conclusively shown to be effective in treating acute ulcer bleeding in the age of modern acid suppression agents, it may have some use in this regard.

Ghrelin has been investigated as an acid secretion stimulant that involves the vagus nerve and histamine release, among other regulators of acid secretion. The neuropeptide GRP is one neurotransmitter that has been connected to meal-stimulated acid secretion. The GRP antagonist BIM26226 has been shown to block vagally mediated acid secretion in humans in a manner similar to that of atropine, indicating that GRP may be a significant neurotransmitter in the vagal–cholinergic pathway in addition to mediating its effects through gastrin release. In addition, CCK may act as a physiological inhibitor brought on by the intestines' nutrient content. Additional somatostatin-stimulating agents that inhibit acid secretion include leptin, amylin, glucagon-like peptide, CCK, VIP, and EGF.

5.1.1.2. H^+K^+-ATPase (The Proton Pump)

The proton pump, also known as H^+K^+-ATPase, is the molecular mechanism that drives the secretion of gastric acid and is exclusively in charge of releasing hydrogen ions into the stomach and gastric gland lumen. This is the final stage of the stomach acid secretion process. Through ATP hydrolysis, the proton pump facilitates the exchange of luminal K+ for cytoplasmic H+. It is made up of two subunits: a glycosylated β-subunit and an α-subunit. The α-subunit performs the catalytic and transport roles of the enzyme, interacts with ATP, establishes the characteristics of cation binding, breaks down ATP, and serves as the location where PPIs bind. The smaller glycosylated β-subunit is crucial for the structural and functional stability of ATPase, as it shields the enzyme from degradation. Furthermore, it seems to be crucial for the apical membrane pump's targeting, the oxyntic mucosa's development, and the pump's recycling from the "active" secretory canaliculi back to the tubulovesicular membranes when the cell enters a "resting" state. It's interesting to note that since mice develop achlorhydria when either the α- or β-subunits are deleted, each subunit is essential for enzyme activity.

H^+K^+-ATPase is an enzyme that is exclusively present on the secretory membranes of parietal cells. These cells are rich in H^+K^+-ATPase membranous structures in the form of microtubules, vesicles, and tubulovesicles when they are at rest and not under stimulation. The stimulation of gastric HCl secretion results in a morphological change that causes the tubulovesicles to migrate into the apical plasma membrane. This allows the H^+K^+-ATPase to secrete protons straight into the gastric gland lumen. The tubulovesicular compartment is restored and the pumps are removed from the apical membrane when secretion stops.

5.1.2. Drugs Modulating Gastric Acid

5.1.2.1. Antacids

Although antacids are no longer the first line of treatment for most acid-peptic disorders, histamine 2 antagonists and proton pump inhibitors (PPIs) still have a place in treatment because they are widely accessible, affordable, and safe for most people. Antacids are useful for the quick relief of mild or intermittent symptoms because they start working almost instantly. Antacids primarily affect the stomach by inhibiting the proteolytic enzyme pepsin and partially neutralizing gastric hydrochloric acid. The medication does not need to be absorbed systemically when it is neutralized by acid in the gut lumen. They are all taken orally, and the amount of acid that an antacid dose neutralizes is typically used to determine how potent an antacid is. Antacids work very quickly to lessen stomach acidity when taken empty; however, if food is consumed first, this time can be extended to one to three hours.

Sodium bicarbonate, calcium carbonate, magnesium hydroxide, and aluminum hydroxide are ingredients found in many commonly used antacids. Solid tablets or liquid suspensions are the typical formulations. Initially widely used as an antacid, sodium bicarbonate is still used now and then as part of a self-prescribed regimen of "baking soda" mixed with water or in combination products with aspirin. Sodium bicarbonate is soluble, which has made it less desirable because higher doses can cause systemic alkalosis and a high sodium load, which can be harmful to patients who have renal insufficiency or systolic heart failure. Less soluble agents can be found in most widely used antacids, either by themselves or in combination. For instance, the solubility of calcium carbonate is limited. Soluble calcium chloride is produced by reaction with HCl and subsequently transformed back into calcium carbonate in the small intestine's alkaline environment. This reduces absorption as it precipitates out into the stool. The insoluble antacids magnesium hydroxide and aluminum hydroxide are other frequently used agents. Products containing calcium and aluminum may make you constipated. These medications are frequently used in conjunction with magnesium hydroxide to counteract this, as magnesium hydroxide alone can result in loose stools and diarrhea.

Another factor influencing antacid efficacy has been compliance, which seems to be restricted by the requirement for frequent dosage and the weak relationship between ulcer healing and symptomatic relief. Antacids have a limited ability to heal peptic ulcers and are not currently used to treat PUD. A meta-analysis indicates that it is ineffective for nonulcer dyspepsia. Given the paucity of research in the era of powerful acid-suppressing medications and the tenuous connection between acidity and symptoms in nonulcer dyspepsia, this is not surprising. In comparison, antacids show a small (10%) improvement in GERD symptoms when compared to a placebo. Although antacids are useful in treating critically ill patients for stress-ulcer prophylaxis, their current main use is in the management of mild symptomatic reflux and dyspepsia.

Antacid-related adverse events are dose-related. Excessive dosages of antacids containing calcium can result in the milk-alkali syndrome, a condition marked by metabolic alkalosis, hypercalcemia, and renal insufficiency. When taken by itself, magnesium-containing antacids can result in diarrhea and cause hypermagnesemia in people with impaired renal function. In end-stage renal patients, calcium carbonate is the recommended antacid because aluminum-containing antacids can cause encephalology and osteomalacia. All antacids have the potential to cause drug interactions, even though specific drug interactions are uncommon. This is because they can alter the pH of the stomach or urine, change the rates of absorption, bioavailability, renal elimination, and drug dissolution, or decrease the amount of time that drugs are hydrolyzed by gastric acid.

5.1.2.2. H_2-Receptor Antagonists

In 1972, functional antagonists of the H_2 receptor were first reported. Since then, the development of PPIs has surpassed this class of agents' primacy in treating acid-related diseases, having revolutionized PUD treatment. The four H_2-receptor antagonists (H2RAs) that are readily accessible are nizatidine, ranitidine, famotidine, and cimetidine. They're all H_2 receptor-active. The H2RAs function as inverse agonists with a functional antagonistic relationship to histamine activity because they are reversible structural analogs of histamine that reduce the tonic activation rate of the receptor.

During nonfeeding periods, the basal rate of acid release is primarily mediated by histamine. This is especially crucial during the nighttime fasting periods, which is why H2RA dosage at bedtime is recommended. With a pH of over 3 for duodenal ulcers and over 4 for GERD, models based on 24-hour pH monitoring and data from clinical trials have shown that ulcer healing depends on the degree of acid suppression as well as the length of the 24-hour cycle with decreased acidity.

With the exception of their heterocyclic ring, metronidines, ranitidines, famotidines, and nizatidines all share structural and pharmacokinetic traits. Following oral dosage, H2RAs are well absorbed in the small intestine and reach peak concentrations in 1–3 hours. Ingesting food may rarely affect this rate, but concurrent antacid therapy use may. All medications have linear pharmacokinetics and are mainly removed by the kidneys, excreting between 30 and 60% of the drug in its unaltered form in the urine. Patients with renal impairment require dose adjustments; patients with liver disease do not.

With a few common dose-dependent adverse events reported in about 15% of treated patients, H2RAs have a long history of use. To maximize the effect on nocturnal basal acid secretion, the H2RAs are typically given once a day before bedtime. Even in patients with a history of nocturnal acid breakthrough, the additional benefit of incorporating H2RA at night into a pre-existing PPI regimen remains questionable. With time, the effects on acid secretion usually diminish. This is not typical tolerance; rather, it is likely an exaggerated first-dose response. Rebound acid secretion upon drug cessation may be a clinical manifestation of decreased H_2-receptor degradation brought on by H2RA use. These qualities, along with the H2RAs' quicker start of action in comparison to PPIs, make them more appropriate for symptom-driven on-demand usage than for use as main acid controllers.

Excellent safety data for the H2RAs supports their widespread use as over-the-counter drugs. Cimetidine has a slight antiandrogenic effect that has been linked to impotence and gynecomastia. Anemia, thrombocytopenia, myelosuppression, and neutropenia are examples of hematological abnormalities. Confusion, restlessness, headaches, and mental status changes are examples of CNS symptoms. These are more prevalent in older patients with hepatic and renal complications in the intensive care unit (ICU). Rarely, after fast intravenous delivery or high-dose treatment—especially in patients with low physiologic reserve—cardiac effects are observed. Cimetidine may interact with other medications because it inhibits cytochrome P450 (CYP) enzymes, especially CYP3A4 and 2D6. Additionally, some medications' tubular secretion is inhibited by cimetidine, and it is through this mechanism that the medication can also slightly raise serum creatinine.

H2RA is useful in treating acid reflux disease and appears to be beneficial in treating heartburn symptoms when taken as needed, but it is ineffective in treating erosive esophagitis. The doses of over-the-counter H2RAs (famotidine 10 mg and ranitidine 75 mg) are lower than those found in the prescription product insert; nonetheless, at these levels, they effectively lessen the food-stimulated gastric response and reduce overnight gastric acidity for 12 hours. They work well for treating GERD symptoms as well.

In nonulcer dyspepsia, histamine receptor antagonists are somewhat helpful, but not as helpful as proton pump inhibitors. H2RAs are better than a placebo, but not as effective as PPIs in treating esophageal reflux disease. In the same way that PPIs are better than H2RAs at treating ulcer symptoms and promoting healing, they also prevent an acute peptic ulcer from rebleeding. Standard doses of H2RAs are effective in preventing duodenal but not gastric ulcers in the prevention of NSAID-induced injury, while double-dose H2RAs were effective in preventing both duodenal and gastric ulcers as seen by endoscopy.

5.1.2.2. Proton Pump Inhibitors

Since the gastric H^+K^+-ATPase was found to be the common pathway for acid production, treating GI tract disorders has completely changed when this step in the process is inhibited. As far as gastric acid secretion inhibitors go, the PPIs are the strongest. Oral options include the recently approved dexlansoprazole as well as five commonly used PPIs (omeprazole, esomeprazole, lansoprazole, pantoprazole, and rabeprazole). While lansoprazole, esomeprazole, and pantoprazole intravenous formulations are available in the United States, omeprazole is administered intravenously in other nations. PPIs are prodrugs that function as weak bases and require an acidic environment to inhibit H^+K^+-ATPase. The structure of all these compounds is the same: they are substituted pyridylmethylsulfinyl benzimidazoles, with substitutions occurring on either the pyridine or the benzimidazole rings. Their acid dissociation constant (pKa) causes them to accumulate in the parietal cell's secretory canaliculus, where they reach greater concentrations than in plasma. After protonation, the PPI transforms into the active sulfenamide species, which joins forces with cysteine residues in the H^+K^+-ATPase α-subunit to create disulfide bonds. This leads to an inhibitory mechanism that is independent of histamine, acetylcholine, or gastrin stimulus for acid secretion, as well as an action duration that surpasses plasma half-life. In contrast, PPIs lessen mucosal damage by reducing pepsin secretion, just like H2RAs do.

Furthermore, PPI dosing in the morning is linked to noticeably better acid suppression than H2RA dosing, which is best done at night. PPIs should be taken before breakfast because eating will mobilize H^+K^+-ATPase to become active and responsive to medication action, and the amount of H^+K^+-ATPase in the parietal cells is highest following a prolonged fast. The effects of the PPIs get stronger with each administration, and by the third day, most people reach a steady state where about 70% of the pumps are inhibited for two hours. Furthermore, as more enzymes are recruited, acid suppression gets better over time. As such, intermittent use of a PPI taken "as needed" does not consistently result in adequate acid inhibition or a clinical response that is satisfactory.

Hepatic CYP2C19 is involved in the metabolism of proton-pump inhibitors. Rabeprazole is distinct among PPIs because the CYP system is only involved in 15–20% of its metabolism. Pharmacogenetic variation causes individual differences in metabolism. Approximately 2.6% of Caucasian people and 15–20% of Asian people are poor metabolizers. They are known to have higher plasma drug levels, more profound acid inhibition, and higher healing rates in *H. pylori* patients with PPIs treatment plans. Pharmacogenetic testing of patients is not recommended, though, as it has not been shown to consistently improve outcomes.

All proton pump inhibitors (PPIs) are considered safe based on both clinical trials and post marketing pharmacovigilance. Long-term safety concerns for this class of drugs include prolonged hypergastrinemia, potential links to gastric atrophy and chronic hypochlorhydria. Gastrin is a hormone that may promote cancer growth. Initially, PPIs came with a black box warning about this issue, but it was later removed because studies showed no evidence of mutagenic effects or increased risk of colon cancer or gastric carcinoids. There have been some associations between PPI use and hip fractures, renal complications, community-acquired pneumonia, and increased risk of enteric infections, including Clostridium difficile. However, the data on these associations are varied, and a clear cause-and-effect relationship has not been proven.

Since high levels of gastric acid normally inhibit gastrin secretion, PPI suppression of gastric acid disrupts the negative-feedback mechanisms that regulate gastrin secretion. As a result, prolonged PPI treatment results in hypergastrinemia. Rebound acid hypersecretion (RAHS) is a phenomenon that has been shown in both humans and animals using omeprazole. It was initially observed in animals receiving the medication. A potential mechanism that could explain RAHS after proton-pump inhibition ends is that PPIs may cause hyperplasia or even neoplasia of ECL cells, as Gastrin has a trophic effect on these cells. Nevertheless, research has not revealed any conclusive evidence that the hyperplasia seen in PPI therapy patients advances to the higher grades of hyperplasia that may be the precursor to gastric ECL cell tumors, despite established strong associations between elevated serum gastrin concentration and ECL cell hyperplasia. Nonetheless, this factor's clinical significance translates into a possible exacerbation of GERD symptoms, which appears to be more significant in *H.pylori* patients without. This clinical consideration may shorten the time that patients with dyspepsia or GERD receive treatment, putting them at risk for long-term side effects from PPI use. However, there needs to be more research done in this field because issues like this have only been sparsely documented in the literature.

Drugs with acid-dependent absorption may have less bioavailability when taken with proton-pump inhibitors. These include ampicillin, digoxin, iron, and the HIV-protease inhibitor atazanavir. Omeprazole inhibits CYP2C19, which raises the concentrations of substrates like phenytoin and diazepam. It has been observed that omeprazole reduces the platelet inhibitory effect of clopidogrel, but not pantoprazole or esomeprazole. However, there is insufficient evidence to demonstrate adverse clinical outcomes based on this pharmacodynamic interaction. PPIs should not be used in conjunction with prostaglandins, H_2-antagonists, or other antisecretory agents because doing so significantly reduces their acid-inhibiting effects. If concurrent therapy is necessary, it is advised to wait a suitable amount of time between administering the PPI and the H_2 antagonist.

5.1.3. Mucosal Protective Agents

5.1.3.1. Sucralfate

The fundamental ingredients of sucralfate are aluminum hydroxide and sulfated sucrose as an aluminum salt. It is a medication that binds to ulcerated tissue and the gastric mucosa and is not absorbed. These characteristics have cytoprotective and healing effects. The sulfate ions in gastric acid stimulate angiogenesis, growth factor delivery, and granulation tissue formation by binding to proteins in the damaged gastric tissue of ulcer craters. It is recommended to use this binding, which is favored by a low pH, 30 to 60 minutes before meals. Because sucralfate is excreted in feces and has only been shown to slightly raise serum and urine aluminum levels, it is best to avoid it in patients who have renal failure.

When compared to H2RAs, sucralfate is equally effective in healing gastric and duodenal ulcers. The main use is in the prevention of stress ulcers in patients who are very sick. Although there is a lack of clinical trial data, sucralfate and H2RAs seem to be equally effective in preventing critical care stress ulceration and hemorrhage. Sucralfate preserves the sterilizing effects of an acidic stomach and keeps the intragastric pH lower than H2RAs and possibly PPIs, which may give it an advantage over these medications for the prevention of stress-related mucosal damage. Because of this, compared to antacids and H2RAs, it has been reported to have a lower incidence of nosocomial pneumonia. Studies have not, however, shown a discernible difference between sucralfate and acid-suppression therapy in terms of the incidence of nosocomial pneumonia in critically ill patients.

5.1.3.2. Bismuth

Bismuth salicylate, a salicylic acid salt that is frequently used, has antacid qualities. Bismuth inhibits *H. pylori* and has been given the green light by the US FDA to be used in conjunction with other medications to eradicate it. Other processes that could aid in ulcer healing include mucus and bicarbonate secretion, mucosal prostaglandin synthesis, and inhibition of pepsin activity. It is mostly excreted in feces after being unabsorbed. It combines with hydrogen sulfide in the colon to produce bismuth sulfide, which darkens the stools. It is now used in *H. pylori* and has a modest efficacy in nonulcer dyspepsia infections.

5.1.3.3. Prostaglandins Analogs

The goal of prostaglandin therapy is to improve epithelial cell growth and repair while balancing the systemic effects of NSAIDs. Early research resulted in the creation of arbaprostil, rioprostil, enprostil, and misoprostol. The only prostaglandin E_2 that has been approved by the FDA for the prevention of NSAID-related ulcers is analog, which is intended to help address the prostaglandin deficiency caused by NSAIDs in the gastric mucosa. It is typically taken orally and has a good absorption rate, reaching a peak plasma concentration in 30 minutes and a half-life of 1.5 hours. The drug's metabolites are eliminated in the urine, and it has no effect on the CYP system. The only prostaglandin analog that has been shown to lessen severe gastroenterologic side effects from NSAID therapy is misoprostol, which has also been shown to be more effective than H2RAs at preventing stomach ulcers but not duodenal ulcers. However, due to common side effects such as diarrhea and cramping in the abdomen that lead to therapy discontinuation and problems with adherence associated with multiple daily doses, misoprostol only makes up 2% of medical co-therapy prescriptions for NSAID users.

5.1.4. Acid-Related Diseases

Acid reflux disease (GERD) is a broad category of disorders affecting the stomach, duodenum, and esophagus. In the USA, the prevalence of chronic acid-related disorders is about 23%; of these, GERD accounts for over half of the disease burden. According to some reports, up to 44.9% of patients have one or more upper gastrointestinal symptoms. One of the most prevalent gastrointestinal conditions, GERD affects over 60 million Americans, with up to 20% of those affected experiencing symptoms at least twice a week. Another GI condition caused by acid reflux, PUD affects 500,000 people annually in the USA and is most common in people between the ages of 25 and 64. These illnesses lower patients' quality of life, raise their medical expenses, and may eventually lead to more serious illnesses like adenocarcinoma.

1. Gastroesophageal Reflux Disease

The esophageal mucosa is exposed to acidic stomach contents, pepsin, and bile acids, which causes gastroesophageal reflux disease. Reflux is caused by interactions between the stomach, lower esophageal sphincter, gastroesophageal junction, and nervous system, both anatomically and functionally. Changes in reflux result in modifications to the esophageal protective and clearance mechanisms. The esophageal mucosa may be damaged by GERD, a chronic condition that typically manifests as erosive esophagitis. Nevertheless, it is thought that between 50 and 70% of GERD patients never experience esophagitis; these individuals are known as having nonerosive gastroesophageal reflux disease (NERD). The typical symptoms of GERD patients are regurgitation of acid and heartburn. A clinical diagnosis can be made with 90% accuracy when both of these are present. However, the degree of esophageal damage is not predicted by the frequency or intensity of heartburn. Other possible GERD presentations that may or may not lead to a diagnosis include coughing, dysphagia, and chest pain.

Considering the different pathogenic mechanisms, the treatment of this entity has concentrated on reducing the amount of acid produced by the stomach and limiting its exposure. Since GERD is a chronic illness, treatment must be ongoing. Over 80% of patients need to take acid-suppressive drugs to manage their symptoms. Due to these factors, the general consensus is that a symptom-based strategy, as opposed to one based on pathogenesis, should be used for the first round of GERD treatment. PPIs are the drug of choice for an empirical therapeutic trial, even though a response to such a strategy does not fully establish the diagnosis of GERD. PPIs have demonstrated superior results when compared with H2RAs for treating heartburn and healing erosive esophagitis.

The cornerstone of GERD treatment is acid suppression. Antacids are mainly used as a symptomatic breakthrough adjunct in PPI or H2RA regimens, or as a self-initiated treatment by patients. H2RA formulations that are sold over-the-counter offer a low-cost initial treatment. Furthermore, up to 60% of patients can anticipate symptomatic relief, and roughly 50% of patients treated with H2RAs can expect to heal; in contrast, PPI rates are 78% and 83%, respectively, making PPIs more effective when used empirically to treat heartburn. PPI treatment of endoscopically confirmed symptomatic GERD shows better efficacy in achieving clinical remission and healing rates in this context.

When it comes to GERD patients, symptom relief can be harder to achieve than mucosal healing. In these situations, additional PPI dosages or a longer course of treatment may be required. When compared to patients with erosive GERD, who experience relief rates of about 80%, most NERD patients in omeprazole 20 mg trials experienced less symptomatic relief. After four weeks of therapy with omeprazole (20 mg/day), only 46–57% of NERD patients showed improvement in their heartburn symptoms. Furthermore, only 45 and 39% of NERD patients, respectively, reported feeling better after taking lansoprazole 15 or 30 mg/day. This means that prolonging therapy or raising doses for patients who are labeled as "nonresponders" won't always result in a better outcome. This implies that the etiology of at least some NERD symptoms is nonacid.

Full-dose PPIs are superior to half-dose PPIs in terms of preventing relapse; however, relapse of symptoms can happen in as many as 70–80% of patients with NERD and esophagitis, especially in more severe cases of esophagitis. As a result, maintenance therapy is frequently needed to control symptoms, which drives up prescription costs for GERD sufferers.

Sometimes a twice-daily PPI is insufficient to completely stop stomach acid secretion overnight. Roughly 70% of patients with gastroesophageal reflux disease and normal volunteers experience nocturnal gastric acid breakthrough (NAB), which is defined as an intragastric pH of less than 4 for more than one continuous hour over the course of the night. Furthermore, in patients with severe erosive esophagitis, Barrett's esophagus, and extraesophageal manifestations of GERD, esophageal acid exposure may be sufficient to cause nocturnal symptoms and mucosal injury during the nocturnal gastric acid breakthrough period (30–50%). This pharmacologic phenomenon was shown in both healthy individuals and GERD patients, and it has been documented with comparable frequency in relation to omeprazole, lansoprazole, rabeprazole, and pantoprazole. Furthermore, NAB happens in the early evening for patients who take a PPI once daily before breakfast, and the phenomenon happens 6–7 hours after this dose for patients who take their PPI before dinner. Many tactics have been used to try and manage nighttime acids, such as taking a PPI once at night, taking it twice a day, or combining H2RAs with a PPI regimen. Notwithstanding high-dose acid suppression with omeprazole or additional ranitidine at night, patients with chronic conditions like systemic sclerosis may still experience esophageal acid exposure without improvement in NAB, GERD, or quality of life. However, the evidence supporting any one of these approaches is weak.

Moreover, there is greater debate regarding the clinical utility of NAB in patients with mild GERD and healthy volunteers. In a report, 17 patients with symptomatic NAB had their esophageal pH and nocturnal acid breakthrough examined. Acid-suppressive drug regimens varied for each participant, with the PPI being increased to twice daily, administered early in the morning or right before bed, an H2RA added at night, or the PPI increased to three times daily. The researchers concluded that nocturnal acid breakthrough is an isolated gastric phenomenon and that esophageal acid suppression and symptom control are independent of the degree of nocturnal acid elimination. They found that the treatment regimens resulted in NAB elimination of 9–41% and that the majority of these patients, at least 60%, did not have their nocturnal acid breakthrough controlled by any of these methods. These findings imply that there might be a discrepancy between symptom control and NAB. NAB is described as an intragastric phenomenon that isn't always connected to GERD symptoms or exposure to intraesophageal acid at night. Therefore, it appears that no specific approach may be successful in controlling nocturnal acidity, and that not all cases of symptomatic reflux disease will necessarily resolve with the complete removal of NAB.

Certain formulations, like omeprazole with immediate release (IR-OME), when taken at night have demonstrated encouraging outcomes for a quicker and more effective management of acid production during the night. Randomized controlled clinical trials demonstrated that this novel formulation provides better control of pH at night than delayed-release proton pump inhibitors (PPIs). This is based on the theory that the sodium bicarbonate portion of the formulation will rapidly alkalinize the stomach contents, leading to the rapid activation of proton pumps, which will be better inhibited by the peak plasma concentrations achieved by the omeprazole moiety. Furthermore, the median percentage time of intragastric pH of greater than 4 at night for IR-OME (55%) was higher than for pantoprazole (27%).

Up to 15% of GERD patients experience Barrett's esophagus, a serious complication that increases the risk of esophageal adenocarcinoma by 0.5% annually. When compared to H2RAs or no therapy at all, acid suppression becomes significant for patients with Barrett's esophagus because it may slow the progression of dysplasia. Approximately 50–80% of patients after a lengthy and aggressive therapy have esophageal squamous islands formed as a result of these pharmaceutical agents when used twice daily or at higher doses; regrettably, there is no concrete proof that these agents cause Barrett's esophagus to regress or that cancer is prevented in the long run.

Patients with symptoms not typical of GERD are referred to as having extraesophageal manifestations of the disease. These comprise signs and symptoms like sore throats, asthma attacks, persistent coughs, and non-cardiac chest pain. Prolonged coughing is caused by GERD in 10–40% of cases, as indicated by endoscopy, barium x-ray, pH monitoring, and therapeutic response to acid suppression. When analyzing the data from clinical trials, it is evident that patients' responses to empirical PPIs vary, and there are no established recommendations for medical treatment for GERD-induced cough, regardless of the method used to diagnose the condition. Similarly, Cochrane reviews showed that although certain patients with laryngitis and asthma responded better to treatment, it is difficult to identify these patients and overall GERD therapy is not linked to statistically significant improvements in outcome. One major area of debate and uncertainty is the efficacy of PPIs in treating extraesophageal GERD symptoms. The connection between *H. pylori* and GERD is still unknown. Research indicates that eliminating *H. pylori* has no effect on esophageal acid exposure or GERD relapse. checking for and eliminating *H. pylori* has not been demonstrated to be helpful for GERD sufferers. Actually, the eradication of *H. pylori* may be linked to a slight exacerbation of pan-gastritis patients' GERD symptoms.

2. Peptic ulcer disease

The incidence of peptic ulcer disease is declining, but it is still a relatively common disorder. The cornerstone of treatment for individuals with PUD is antisecretory therapy. Indeed, there has been a significant improvement in healing and cure rates since the introduction of PPIs. Elimination of *H.pylori*. The infection has transformed the way PUD is treated and is currently the cornerstone of care for this illness. This has led to a reduction in the recurrence of ulcers and a high rate of ulcer healing, particularly in those with duodenal ulcers. 34 studies involving patients with duodenal ulcers were meta-analyzed by *H.pylori*. With a number needed to treat of 14, eradication combined with antisecretory therapy was more effective at healing ulcers than antisecretory medication alone. *H. pylori* is still a significant factor that is also connected to the emergence of stomach cancer and dyspeptic symptoms, eliminating *H.pylori* Considering these dangers, infection makes logical.

The first treatment strategy for PUD was the use of antacids. These days, they are hardly ever used for PUD due to side effects, poor patient compliance, and low cure rates. With the discovery of cimetidine, the first H2RA, the surgical approach to treating peptic ulcers was replaced with a medical one. After four weeks of therapy, all currently available H2RAs cause 70–80% of duodenal ulcers to heal, and after eight weeks, 87–94% do so. Continuous daily nighttime H2RA dosing has been shown to not only heal duodenal ulcers but also to stop ulcer recurrence. PPIs are currently the recommended medications due to their superior efficacy and ease of use, even though H2RAs are also effective in treating PUD. PPIs have been demonstrated to have antimicrobial activity against H and to treat peptic ulcers that may be resistant to high-dose H2RAs. pylori in a lab setting.

3. Duodenal ulcers

H. pylori is the cause of the majority of duodenal ulcers. The biological mechanism involves elevated acid production and potential downregulation of somatostatin. In humans, eradication encourages ulcer healing. All PPIs do is suppress *H. pylori* without its eradication, and the effective eradication of *H. pylori* requires a combination of appropriate acid suppression and antibiotic therapy. The ability of omeprazole and lansoprazole to raise intragastric pH, which maximizes the antimicrobial activity of concurrently administered medications like amoxicillin, is most likely the reason for their long-lasting suppression of gastric acid secretion. After two weeks, PPI-based triple therapies for PUD produce a significantly lower ulcer recurrence rate of 12–14%.

FDA-approved treatments typically involve a combination of currently available PPIs and either metronidazole or clarithromycin-amoxicillin. Omeprazole, lansoprazole, and esomeprazole are among those that are authorized for use in a 10- to 14-day regimen. Based on trial data showing comparable outcomes when compared with control regimens using omeprazole for 10 days, rabeprazole can be used in a 7-day regimen. Studies conducted in Europe have shown that triple therapy based on PPIs can effectively eradicate *H. pylori* in as little as 4–5 days, and that these quick eradication treatments improve patient adherence and lower the possibility of medication side effects. PPI therapy is better when administered twice daily as opposed to once daily. First-line treatments have a 70–95% success rate for eradication, and 10- and 14-day regimens are typically 7–9% more effective than the most popular 7-day regimens. The American College of Gastroenterology suggests a 14-day course of clarithromycin triple therapy, taking into account multiple results of different meta-analyzes. This recommendation is especially relevant in the USA, where eradication rates have traditionally been 80% or less with shorter therapy durations.

4. Gastric Ulcers and NSAID-induced mucosal injury

Numerous tactics have been created to stop NSAID-induced gastropathy, and some of them are frequently used in medical settings. These tactics include the creation of COX-2-specific inhibitors (coxibs), cotherapy with gastroprotective drugs, PPIs, and H2RAs. It's interesting to note that people who have gastric ulcers typically have normal or reduced basal and stimulated acid production. Due to changes in mucosal defenses, NSAID-induced stomach ulcers happen more frequently. The primary treatment for this illness is still acid suppression because, after 8 weeks of therapy, most gastric ulcers heal when the stomach pH stays above 3 for 18 to 20 hours each day. Rather than being correlated with the level of acid suppression during the day or night, these therapeutic outcomes are related to the length of acid inhibitory therapy.

It is well known that using NSAIDs increases the risk of gastroduodenal injury. Patients taking these medications have a 15–25% chance of developing endoscopically visible ulcers. Ages over 60, a history of GI ulcers, high NSAID dosages, steroid use, or anticoagulation therapy use are all linked to an increased risk of developing GI complications.

The 2008 ACCF/ACG/AHA practice guidelines advise choosing an NSAID in accordance with a personal risk assessment. The strategies used include starting at the lowest effective doses for the shortest amount of time and, in patients who are considered to be at high risk, using a PPI or misoprostol in addition to an NSAID or a selective COX-2 inhibitor, either with or without a PPI. Although mucosal protective agents like misoprostol are approved for such purposes, the best course of action for patients who must continue using NSAIDs is still up for debate. Diarrhea, even at low doses, limits the use of these agents. PPIs seem to promote healing more quickly than H2RAs, misoprostol, or sucralfate; however, a Cochrane review indicated that the only treatment that has been demonstrated to lessen perforation, hemorrhage, or obstruction complications is high dose misoprostol (800 mg). If there are any real efficacious benefits to misoprostol, they are negligible, and its unpleasant side effect profile has few applications.

Trials and meta-analysis demonstrated that among those patients requiring long-term aspirin therapy, the recurrence of a prior GI bleeding episode is less common when using concomitant PPIs and that omeprazole is superior to *H. pylori*-eradication therapy in preventing recurrent bleeding in NSAID users. Despite this consistent evidence, there are substantial recurrence rates further along the treatment course of these patients. At 12-weeks duration, *H. pylori*-negative patients have been shown to have relapse of their disease of up to 20% despite the use of lansoprazole, with relapse rates of 3 and 13% for duodenal and gastric ulcer patients, respectively, after using omeprazole for 24 weeks. As most NSAIDs are dosed twice daily or are designed to provide 24 h activity, and current PPIs dosed once daily are only able to keep intragastric pH above 4 for only up to 70% of a 24 h period, patients may not be fully protected in a 24 h period against the deleterious effects of NSAIDs.

5. PPI Therapy for Bleeding Ulcers

In the United States, there are 160 hospital admissions for acute upper gastrointestinal hemorrhage for every 100,000 people, or over 400,000 hospital admissions annually, due to upper GI bleeding, a common medical condition. The incidence rises with age and is greater in men. Consensus statements show that, after initial endoscopic control of the bleeding, the use of PPIs reduces rebleeding rates and the need for surgery, even though there are no appreciable changes in overall mortality. Control of intragastric pH promotes platelet aggregation and pepsin inhibition. This latter parameter is especially significant because it will become the more significant predictor of death in patients with bleeding ulcers, necessitating early endoscopy. The odds ratios for mortality and rebleeding following endoscopic treatment only reached 0.55 (95% CI: 0.40–0.76) and 0.38 (95% CI: 0.32–0.45) in a meta-analysis of endoscopic therapy for bleeding peptic ulcers, highlighting the significance of this procedure in the management of these ulcers.

High-dose omeprazole therapy reduces the risk of additional bleeding and surgical requirements in patients with bleeding peptic ulcers and recent bleeding indicators. This strategy suggests that because oral formulations provide prolonged, effective acid suppression, using high-dose oral PPIs twice daily may reduce the risk of rebleeding. However, when treating acute ulcer bleeding or ulcers with high-risk stigmata for bleeding, the use of intravenous formulations of PPIs at doses that include an initial bolus of 80 mg followed by a continuous infusion of 8 mg/h of intravenous omeprazole or pantoprazole has become the standard.

6. Stress-related Mucosal Disease

In an ICU setting, ulcers or mucosal erosions that frequently occur in the fundus and stomach body, as well as in the antrum, duodenum, or distal esophagus, are referred to as stress-related mucosal disease. They put ICU patients at risk for 1 in 5 to 15% bleeding, which can result in an increase in mortality. For ICU patients who have a high risk of stress ulceration, prophylaxis is recommended. Clinical trials have shown that when compared to placebo or no prophylaxis, H2RAs, PPIs, and antacids decrease the frequency of overt GI bleeding in ICU patients.

Although proton-pump inhibitors are now used in intensive care units to prevent bleeding, their clinical effectiveness has not been thoroughly evaluated in comparison to that of H2RAs and sucralfate. In comparison to prophylactic agents that do not change gastric pH, like sucralfate, multiple randomized trials and meta-analyzes indicate that prophylactics that raise stomach pH may raise the incidence of nosocomial pneumonia. In the prevention of stress-induced ulcer bleeding, PPIs seem to have an advantage over H2RAs, despite the lack of conclusive evidence. (Baker, 2006; Malfertheiner et al, 2006; DeCamp et al, 2008; Liu et al, 2011)

5.2. Laxatives

Laxatives are drugs that induce more frequent bowel movements and loosen stools. Constipation is treated and prevented with them. The mechanisms of action and potential adverse effects of laxatives differ. To clear the colon for rectal and bowel exams, specific stimulants, lubricants, and saline laxatives are used; in some cases, enemas may be added. Diarrhea may result from laxative dosages that are too high. Certain laxatives can be taken orally or rectally and contain multiple active ingredients.

5.2.1. Indications

A class of drugs known as laxatives is widely prescribed to treat constipation and other gastrointestinal disorders. Their principal mode of action is to facilitate the process of bodily excretion by improving digestion and encouraging bowel movements. When treating constipation, osmotic or stimulant laxatives are usually the first choice. The next course of action may be to use prokinetics or secretagogues if they are ineffective in treating constipation.

Patients with opioid-induced constipation, chronic idiopathic constipation (CIC), and irritable bowel syndrome (IBS) can all benefit from laxatives. To prevent constipation, Yasser Masri et al. have documented the prophylactic use of laxatives in intensive care unit (ICU) patients. Furthermore, O'Brien et al. have recommended laxatives be used in conjunction with opioid therapy for sickle cell disease patients, especially those who have recently undergone surgery and small children.

Constipation is a common diagnosis that needs to be properly assessed and treated. Notably, there are other options for treating constipation besides laxative therapy. The first line of treatment should be a change in lifestyle, with more fluid intake and a diet high in fiber-rich foods like spinach, cabbage, Brussels sprouts, asparagus, and broccoli. When lifestyle changes are made but constipation still occurs, laxative use becomes an option. Treatment for chronic constipation is a multimodal approach that includes dietary modifications, behavior modification, patient education, and laxative therapy if needed.

Laxatives are sometimes used to relieve constipation and also help clear the colon in preparation for procedures like colonoscopies. The 2023 guidelines published by the American Gastroenterological Association state that CIC is a common clinical condition that affects 8–12% of US adults. When it comes to pharmacological interventions, the treatment options include a variety of prescription and over-the-counter medications, including lactulose, bisacodyl, magnesium oxide, and polyethylene glycol (PEG). Treatment options for CIC that is not responding include plecanatide, linaclotide, lubiprostone, and prokinetic agents.

5.2.2. Mechanism of Action

Laxatives are categorized based on the mechanism of action they exert, as mentioned below:

- ***Laxatives that form bulk***: These substances hold onto fluid in the stool, giving it more weight and consistency. Typical examples include methylcellulose, dietary fiber, and psyllium. Water intake must be sufficient for bulk-forming agents to function. In turn, dehydration can result in bloating and intestinal blockage.
- ***Osmotic agents***: Osmotic agents: These medications pull water into the intestinal lumen and have a low absorption rate. Common examples include PEG, sorbitol, lactulose, and milk of magnesia.
- ***Prokinetic agents***: Tegaserod and cisapride function as 5-hydroxytryptamine receptor agonists. By acting on intrinsic neurons, they stimulate mucosal secretion and release acetylcholine. However, because of severe cardiovascular adverse effects, cisapride has been taken off the market. Tegaserod is accessible through novel experimental drug procedures. Prucalopride is a 5-HT4 agonist with high affinity and selectivity. Additionally, agents ATI-7505 and Velusetrag are being looked into.
- ***Lubricants***: Mineral oil aids the passage of stools by its lubricating action throughout the intestines.
- ***Stimulants***: Stimulate the myenteric plexus and the Auerbach plexus, increasing intestinal secretions and motility. They also decrease the absorption of water from the lumen of the bowel. Examples include Bisacodyl, senna, cascara, and sodium picosulfate (SPS). Senna and cascara are present in herbal teas or remedies.
- ***Surface active agents***: Docusate lowers the surface tension, which leads to water and fats penetrating the stool.
- ***Guanylate cyclase agonist***: Linaclotide induces cGMP, leading to cystic fibrosis transmembrane conductance regulator (CFTR), which, in turn, causes water and electrolyte secretion into the lumen. Plecanatide is also an intestinal secretagogue acting through a similar mechanism.
- ***Chloride channel activator***: Lubiprostone, a chloride channel activator, leads to water and chloride secretion into the stool and softer stool consistency.
- ***Peripherally acting mu-opioid receptor antagonists***: By blocking mu-opioid receptors in the gastrointestinal tract, these medications treat opioid-induced constipation while maintaining enteric nervous system function and avoiding central nervous system penetration. This class of drugs includes methylnaltrexone, naloxegol, and naldemedine. In cases where escalation of therapy is necessary, the American Gastroenterological Association supports peripherally acting mu-opioid receptor antagonists (PAMORAs) in addition to conventional laxatives as first-line agents.

5.2.3. Adverse Effects

While most laxatives are generally safe when used appropriately, they can have adverse effects, as mentioned below.

- Osmotic agents like lactulose can have adverse effects like bloating, nausea, vomiting, and diarrhea.

- Stimulant laxatives are known to cause abdominal pain.
- Cisapride was withdrawn from the market after cardiovascular adverse effects, including prolonged QT interval that increases the risk for Torsades de Pointes.
- Mineral oil can cause aspiration and lipoid pneumonia.
- Osmotic agents like magnesium can cause metabolic disturbances, especially in the presence of renal impairment. Magnesium excretion depends on renal function and requires caution in chronic kidney disease.
- Osmotic agents result in volume load and should be used with caution in renal or cardiac dysfunction.
- With prokinetic agents, adverse effects like headache, nausea, and diarrhea have been described.
- Secretagogues like linaclotide can occasionally cause diarrhea.
- Long-term stimulant laxative use is correlated with the loss of haustral folds in the colon; this could indicate neuronal or muscular injury caused by these agents.
- *In vitro* studies have described stimulant laxatives like senna and bisacodyl as having neoplastic potential, but data are lacking in human studies so far.
- Naloxegol may lead to severe abdominal pain and diarrhea, necessitating hospitalization. Reported cases include gastrointestinal perforation. However, according to the literature, Naloxegol has a low level of causality with adverse events, including gastrointestinal perforation, seizures, stroke, cardiovascular mortality, and ventricular arrhythmia.
- A cohort study utilized UK Biobank data to explore the relationship between regular laxative use and dementia incidence in adults aged 40 to 69 without prior dementia history. The study revealed that regular use of laxatives increases the risk of all-cause dementia. Increased risk was notably observed among those using multiple or osmotic laxatives.

5.2.4. Contraindications

The contraindications involved with laxatives are provided below.

- Generally, patients with hypersensitivity reactions to any active drug or excipients should avoid a particular medicine.
- Patients should avoid laxatives during pregnancy, and bulk laxatives are considered safe during pregnancy. Stimulant laxatives are considered second-line.
- Contraindications to bulk-forming agents include bedridden patients and those with altered cognition.
- Psyllium agents are contraindicated in those with allergic reactions.
- Use lactulose cautiously in pediatric patients, debilitated patients with hepatic impairment, and older patients.
- Sorbitol should be used with caution in patients with renal impairment.
- The use of Tegaserod is contraindicated in severe renal and hepatic impairment.
- Prucalopride is contraindicated in patients with intestinal obstruction or perforation, ulcerative colitis, Crohn's disease, and toxic megacolon.
- Lubiprostone is contraindicated in patients with intestinal obstruction and patients with severe hepatic impairment.

- The FDA has released a boxed warning for plecanatide. Avoid plecanatide in patients aged 6 or younger due to potential dehydration-related fatalities.

5.2.5. Monitoring

It is crucial to routinely assess the therapeutic efficacy and potential failures in patients receiving laxative therapy as part of their ongoing care. Furthermore, it's critical to keep a close eye out for hemorrhoids or fissures, which are frequently linked to persistent constipation. Patients, especially those with conditions that make them more susceptible to electrolyte abnormalities, should have their serum electrolyte levels continuously monitored. This is especially important when using osmotic laxatives for an extended length of time.

When patients experience constipation brought on by opioids, the American Gastroenterological Association advises keeping an eye on their Bowel Function Index. By identifying patients who have not sufficiently responded to first laxative treatments for opioid-induced constipation, this scoring system helps to indicate when therapy needs to be escalated.

5.2.6. Toxicity

Abuse of laxatives is not unusual and is observed in individuals with bulimia nervosa or anorexia nervosa as well as elderly patients who use laxatives for constipation but then stop using them. Patients with surreptitious diarrhea are also included. Patients who abuse laxatives typically experience constipation, vomiting, and diarrhea that alternates.

Dehydration and electrolyte abnormalities such as hyponatremia, hypokalemia, hyperuricemia, and hyperaldosteronism may be present in these patients. Together, hypokalemia and dehydration can result in renal insufficiency. Potassium and volume depletion in diarrhea exacerbate hypokalemia by increasing aldosterone secretion.

Giving up the causing agent is the treatment for laxative abuse. The primary obstacles are rebound symptoms, which are extremely upsetting for the patient and include weight gain, edema, and constipation. Edema results from water retention in the kidneys. When a patient stops using laxatives, diuretics should be used cautiously to help with edema and constipation and to increase patient tolerance. Careful monitoring of electrolytes and renal function is necessary. The tapering of diuretics can take three months.

5.2.7. Enhancing Healthcare Team Outcomes

While laxatives are useful in treating many illnesses, they can also have unfavorable side effects like nausea, abdominal pain, and urine retention. Since constipation is a common condition in outpatient care and necessitates appropriate patient education, prescribing guidelines for laxative use are essential for clinicians. When older patients are admitted as inpatients, constipation is common and often results in longer hospital stays.

To effectively manage patients' use of laxatives, interprofessional healthcare providers such as clinicians, nurses, pharmacists, dieticians, and care staff should collaborate. To maintain functional bowel movements during hospitalization, several interventions are used, such as medication compliance, stool chart maintenance, and medication review. In addition, pharmacists review medication administration and let clinicians know about any issues they find. Pharmacists, nurses, gastroenterologists, and clinicians working together in an interprofessional setting can improve patient outcomes and lower the risk of adverse drug reactions. (Baker, 2006; Malfertheiner et al, 2006; DeCamp et al, 2008; Liu et al, 2011)

5.3. Antiemetic Medications

In the medical field, nausea is a frequently observed symptom that can be challenging for any patient to manage. Causes can range from a straightforward defense mechanism of the body against an ingested toxin to a complex network of signals triggered by anesthesia, motion, stress, pregnancy, psychiatric disorders, position, and/or fear. There could be one or more neurohumoral pathways at play. The treating physician must carefully consider the indications before treating a patient's symptoms. Treatment for postoperative nausea—a rather common side effect of general anesthesia—and vomiting will differ from treatment for chronic nausea resulting from chemotherapeutic agents and doses. Treatment for acute onset nausea/emesis may be minimal or brief, and it is more likely associated with a specific insult or issue. Prolonged therapy is required for chronic nausea, which is likely to be multifactorial and potentially more difficult to treat. There's no hard-and-fast rule when it comes to treating nausea. When there is no definitive diagnosis, empirical treatment for nausea is usually well tolerated and can be very beneficial to the patient. Among other surgical emergencies, practitioners should be cautious not to ignore small bowel obstructions, perforated viscus, and acute appendicitis. Pregnant women of childbearing age should give pregnancy some thought.

5.3.1. Classes of Antiemetics

To reduce nausea and vomiting, different classes of antiemetics focus on distinct pro-emetic pathways. Some focus on multiple pathways. Antagonists of dopamine, serotonin, neurokinin, histamine, and acetylcholine are among the classes of antiemetics. Benzodiazepines, corticosteroids, and cannabinoid agonists all have antiemetic properties (Table 5.1).

Table 5.1. *Antiemetics*

Class	Mechanisms of Action
Dopamine antagonists Benzamides – metoclopramide Benzimidazoles – domperidone Phenothiazines – prochlorperazine, * chlorpromazine* Butyrophenones – droperidol, * haloperidol* Atypical antipsychotics – olanzapine*	Block dopamine type 2 (D2) receptors centrally in the chemoreceptor trigger zone and peripherally in the gastrointestinal tract. Domperidone blocks peripheral D2 receptors only. At higher doses, effects on other receptors are seen. These include blockade of serotonin, histamine, adrenergic and muscarinic receptors.

Class	Mechanisms of Action
Serotonin antagonists Ondansetron Granisetron Palonosetron Tropisetron	Block 5-HT3 receptors in the chemoreceptor trigger zone and gastrointestinal tract.
Neurokinin antagonists Aprepitant Fosaprepitant Netupitant Netupitant/palonosetron fixed-dose combination	Block neurokinin type 1 receptors in the central and peripheral nervous system.
Antihistamines Doxylamine Cyclizine Pheniramine Promethazine	Block H1 receptors Cyclizine, doxylamine, promethazine and pheniramine all block muscarinic receptors. Promethazine also blocks dopamine D2 receptors.
Anticholinergics Hyoscine	Block muscarinic receptors in vestibular nuclei, vomiting centre and higher brain centres.
Corticosteroids Dexamethasone	Central inhibition of prostaglandin synthesis and encephalin release. When combined with 5-HT3 antagonists there are reduced serotonin concentrations in the gut and increased sensitivity of 5-HT3 receptors to antiemetics.
Benzodiazepines Lorazepam	Agonist action at the GABAA receptor provides anxiolysis. Action at the chemoreceptor trigger zone to suppress the activity of dopamine.
Cannabinoids Tetrahydrocannabinol Nabilone Dronabinol Nabiximols	Activate cannabinoid CB1 (inhibitory) receptors in the central nervous system and peripheral nervous system to modulate release of neurotransmitters.

* Also block serotonin, histamine, adrenergic and muscarinic receptors

Source: https://www.ncbi.nlm.nih.gov/pmc/articles/PMC7186277/.

5.3.2. Mechanism of Action

Nausea and vomiting can have a variety of routes and causes. The nucleus tractus solitarius in the medulla, the area postrema in the floor of the fourth ventricle, and the different motor nuclei that comprise a central pattern generator are examples of specific brain regions. The perception of nausea by the brain is also influenced by a complex interplay between vagal afferents and efferents to the cortex, hypothalamus, and limbic regions. These pathways involve several chemoreceptors, such as histamine H_1, muscarinic M_1, dopaminergic D_2, serotonin 5-HT3, neurokinin-1, and neurokinin.

As such, most of the anti-emetics can broadly fit into the following classes based on the mechanism of action:

- Serotonin-receptor antagonists
- Glucocorticoids
- Anticholinergics
- Neurokinin-receptor antagonists (substance-P)
- Dopamine receptor antagonists
- Cannabinoids
- Antihistamines
- Other

5.3.3. Treatment of Specific Causes of Nausea and Vomiting

While many antiemetics can be used to treat nausea and vomiting caused by a variety of conditions, there are some situations in which one medication may be better than another (Table 5.2).

Table 5.2. *Indications and Scheduling for Antiemetic Drugs*

Indication	Therapeutic Options (Scheduling)
Gastroenteritis	Dopamine antagonists
	Serotonin antagonists
Opioid-induced nausea and vomiting	Serotonin antagonists
	Dopamine antagonists • droperidol
Migraine-related nausea and vomiting	Dopamine antagonists • metoclopramide with paracetamol • metoclopramide • prochlorperazine

Vestibular causes of nausea and vomiting	Antihistamines
	Anticholinergics
	Dopamine antagonists
Chemotherapy-induced nausea and vomiting	Serotonin antagonists
	Neurokinin-1 antagonists
	Corticosteroids • dexamethasone
	Dopamine antagonists • olanzapine, haloperidol
	Benzodiazepines • lorazepam
Radiation-induced nausea and vomiting	Serotonin antagonists
	Corticosteroids • dexamethasone
	Dopamine antagonists
Postoperative nausea and vomiting	Dopamine antagonists
	Serotonin antagonists
	Antihistamines
	Corticosteroids • dexamethasone
	Neurokinin-1 antagonists
	Benzodiazepines • lorazepam

Source: https://www.ncbi.nlm.nih.gov/pmc/articles/PMC7186277/table/t2/?report=objectonly.

5.3.3.1. Gastroenteritis

Infections with bacteria, viruses, or protozoa can result in acute gastroenteritis. Adults experiencing vomiting due to gastroenteritis have access to serotonin antagonists like ondansetron and dopamine antagonists like prochlorperazine or metoclopramide as treatment options.

Children who suffer from acute gastroenteritis often struggle with nausea and vomiting. Antiemetics such as promethazine, metoclopramide, and prochlorperazine were commonly used in children until the early 2000s. However, because of reports of side effects like sedation and extrapyramidal reactions, their use is currently controversial. Guidelines like the ones released by the Royal Children's Hospital Melborne now suggest serotonin antagonists like ondansetron when an antiemetic medication is necessary. According to these guidelines, oral ondansetron should only be taken once based on weight. Kids between the weights of 8 and 15 kg should get 2 mg, kids between the weights of 15 and 30 kg should get 4 mg, and kids over 30 kg should get 8 mg. For children under six months of age or under eight kilograms in weight, ondansetron is not advised.

According to a systematic review, oral ondansetron was found to decrease vomiting, hospitalization, and the need for intravenous rehydration in children with acute gastroenteritis. Intravenous ondansetron or metoclopramide also had positive effects on reducing vomiting and hospitalization. Additionally, one study in the review indicated that rectal dimenhydrinate was successful in decreasing vomiting.

5.3.3.2. Opioid-induced

The effectiveness of antiemetics in treating nausea and vomiting caused by opioids is not well understood. There is a lack of clear evidence due to studies primarily focused on postoperative nausea and vomiting, which involved the use of opioids and anesthesia. Therefore, the selection of an antiemetic for opioid-induced nausea and vomiting will vary depending on factors such as medical conditions, drug side effects, cost, and the clinician's experience with the medication.

Low-dose droperidol (less than 4 mg daily) was found to be effective in reducing opioid-induced nausea and vomiting, according to a systematic review. At 8 or 16 mg per day, ondansetron was effective; however, metoclopramide is not better than a placebo. Since opioid-induced nausea and vomiting is not currently covered by the Pharmaceutical Benefits Scheme (PBS), the role of serotonin antagonists may be restricted.

5.3.3.3. Migraine-related

Migraines are often linked to symptoms such as nausea, vomiting, and decreased gastrointestinal movement. Because of this issue with movement and slowed absorption of medication, alternative methods of administering antiemetics may be necessary, such as injecting the medication.

In migraineurs, the prokinetic antiemetic metoclopramide shortens the time it takes for non-steroidal anti-inflammatory medications and oral aspirin to be absorbed. In one study, it shortened the time needed for tolfenamic acid to reach a maximum plasma concentration from two hours fifty-one minutes to eighteen minutes, and it shortened the time needed for aspirin to do the same. Furthermore, administering metoclopramide along with paracetamol led to a shorter time to peak plasma concentration and a higher peak plasma concentration of paracetamol in healthy volunteers. It took 48 minutes instead of 120 minutes on average to reach the peak plasma concentration of paracetamol. Because metoclopramide may help reduce nausea while increasing the effectiveness of concurrent analgesics, it has been included in many guidelines.

Prochlorperazine and chlorpromazine, two dopamine antagonists, are useful in managing nausea and vomiting. Research on serotonin antagonists' effectiveness in treating migraines is lacking.

5.3.3.4. Pregnancy

Up to 90% of women experience nausea and vomiting during the first trimester of pregnancy. Antihistamines such as doxylamine and diphenhydramine are effective if medication treatment is required, and there is no higher risk of congenital malformations with them. Metoclopramide is likewise useful and does not raise the risk of birthweight reduction, spontaneous abortion, or congenital malformation. There is insufficient evidence to recommend the safety of other dopamine antagonists during pregnancy. Serotonin antagonists, like ondansetron, are increasingly being used during pregnancy. Ondansetron, however, has little safety information. A 2018 study found that there was a marginally higher risk of oral clefts but no increased risk of cardiac malformation. As a result, ondansetron is not advised as a first-line therapy.

5.3.3.5. Vestibular Disorders Including Motion Sickness

The vomiting center is stimulated by the vestibular nuclei in disorders like benign paroxysmal positional vertigo and motion sickness, which can cause nausea and vomiting. Histamine receptors and acetylcholine muscarinic receptors are the main neurotransmitters in this pathway. Therefore, antihistamines like promethazine, anticholinergics like hyoscine, and dopamine antagonists like prochlorperazine are the main treatments.

5.3.3.6. Palliative Care

The causes of nausea and vomiting in palliative care can broadly be divided into:

- disease state-related (e.g. cancer burden, ileus, uremia in kidney disease or gastrointestinal edema in heart failure)
- treatment-related (e.g. chemotherapy-induced or opioid-induced)
- biochemical (e.g. hypercalcemia)
- toxin-mediated (secondary to anorexia-cachexia syndrome).

There is insufficient data to inform the selection of antiemetics in palliative care. In as many as 40% of cases, metoclopramide 10 mg three times a day proves to be effective. In approximately 47% of cases, haloperidol 12.5–5 mg daily is effective, while up to 70% of cases respond well to chlorpromazine 25 mg four times a day. Olanzapine, 2–7 mg/day, is also thought to be beneficial, though it's unclear how exactly it works. Dopamine antagonists may have limited utility due to adverse reactions, including sedation and anticholinergic effects, especially with olanzapine and chlorpromazine.

The use of serotonin antagonists in palliative care for refractory nausea and vomiting has been the subject of conflicting data. Tropisetron outperformed metoclopramide or chlorpromazine in a single randomized trial, even when dexamethasone was added. The most successful combination was tropisetron, dexamethasone, and chlorpromazine. Ondansetron, metoclopramide, or a placebo proved to be equally effective in preventing opioid-induced nausea and vomiting in palliative care, according to a different trial. Antihistamine effectiveness has not been the subject of any randomized trials; however, cyclizine may be effective, according to an uncontrolled study based on patient reports.

In palliative care, anticholinergics like hyoscine are used, but not primarily for nausea. They are frequently recommended for terminal bowel obstruction and excessive stomach secretions.

Bowel obstruction, increased intracranial pressure, and nausea and vomiting brought on by chemotherapy can all be effectively treated with corticosteroids like dexamethasone (4–8 mg daily). Dexamethasone, when combined with tropisetron and either metoclopramide or chlorpromazine, improves the management of nausea and vomiting at as little as 2 mg per day.

5.3.3.7. Chemotherapy-Induced

Different chemotherapy drugs have different emetogenic potentials. For instance, a serotonin antagonist can be used to treat nausea and vomiting brought on by low-emetogenic chemotherapy, like paclitaxel, whereas a combination of a serotonin antagonist, neurokinin antagonist, and dexamethasone is needed to treat highly-emetogenic chemotherapy, like cisplatin.

Olanzapine and haloperidol work well for treating chemotherapy-induced nausea and vomiting. As part of the first-line management of highly emetogenic chemotherapy, olanzapine is now advised.

Metoclopramide, prochlorperazine, and antihistamines are less effective in treating nausea and vomiting brought on by chemotherapy. As an adjuvant therapy, benzodiazepines like lorazepam may be utilized. They serve to lessen nervousness as well as dread of nausea and vomiting. Data on the usage of anticholinergics are lacking.

Cannabinoid products have been tried for chemotherapy-induced nausea and vomiting, despite not being registered in Australia. According to a systematic review, prochlorperazine was not as effective as cannabinoids when used as a placebo. The efficacy in comparison to metoclopramide, domperidone, or chlorpromazine could not be determined from the available data. There is no comparison between cannabinoids and more recent antiemetics like neurokinin antagonists or serotonin. They might be useful for patients whose nausea and vomiting brought on by chemotherapy don't go away with first-line therapy. Cannabinoids, on the other hand, are only accessible via the Special Access Scheme.

5.3.3.8. Radiation-Induced

The body area exposed to radiation affects how severe the nausea and vomiting are. For instance, combination treatment with a serotonin antagonist and dexamethasone is necessary for total body irradiation, which carries a significant risk of nausea and vomiting. Head and neck radiation carries a reduced risk and is treatable with a serotonin antagonist on its own.

When used alone or in conjunction with dexamethasone, serotonin antagonists are more efficacious than dopamine antagonists. Radiation-induced nausea and vomiting can be further minimized by combining dexamethasone with a serotonin antagonist.

5.3.3.9. Postoperative

A systematic review discovered that the following treatments for postoperative nausea and vomiting were more successful than placebo: dexamethasone, droperidol, cyclizine, and serotonin antagonists (ondansetron, granisetron, and tropisetron). Avoiding specific antiemetics may be necessary, contingent on the clinical circumstances. For instance, because serotonin antagonists cause constipation, patients who are already at high risk of intestinal obstruction should either avoid using them or use them carefully, as they may exacerbate or conceal a progressive ileus.

At the recommended dosage of 10 mg, metopramide is no more effective than a placebo and less effective than serotonin antagonists. Metoclopramide doses above 25 mg may be more effective, but their use is restricted due to the higher risk of side effects like dystonia.

According to a recent study, benzodiazepines like lorazepam may help lessen postoperative nausea and vomiting. One milligram of lorazepam taken orally 60 minutes before general anesthesia, as compared to a placebo, significantly decreased postoperative nausea and vomiting as well as the need for antiemetic medication during the recovery phase.

Additionally, research has shown that neurokinin antagonists, like aprepitant, are useful in lowering post-operative nausea and vomiting. For this indication, they are not currently PBS subsidized, though.

5.3.4. Adverse Effects

The mechanisms of action of antiemetics, such as antagonizing neurotransmitters, contribute to some of their adverse effects.

5.3.4.1. QT Prolongation

When prescribing antiemetic medications, it's crucial to take the possibility of lengthening the QT interval on the ECG into account. Even though the effect might not be substantial on its own, other risk factors that affect the QT interval, such as medications, hypokalemia, and hypocalcemia, raise the possibility of dysrhythmia.

The QT interval is reversibly prolonged in a dose-dependent manner by serotonin antagonists. Although this is a class effect, each drug has a different risk. When given intravenously, ondansetron and granisetron both prolong the QT interval at doses greater than 8 mg and 10 micrograms/kg, respectively. On the other hand, no reports of QT prolongation after oral administration exist. Tropisetron and palonosetron have no connection to QT prolongation.

There were no significant side effects associated with the use of serotonin antagonists like ondansetron in children, according to a systematic review. It is crucial to remember that repeated parenteral ondansetron injections have been linked to several instances of cardiac arrhythmia or even death in children.

The US Food and Drug Administration (FDA) has issued "black box" warnings for haloperidol and droperidol because dopamine antagonists cause QT prolongation. However, parenteral droperidol 10 mg did not cause an increased rate of QT prolongation when compared to midazolam, according to the Australian DORM52 and DORM-253 studies. Higher droperidol dosages, up to 20–30 mg, may not always be linked to QT prolongation, according to new research. Moreover, the risk is negligible because less than 4 mg/day is required to produce an antiemetic effect. Although the typical antiemetic dose of haloperidol is 1 mg, it can prolong the QT interval at cumulative intravenous doses as low as 2 mg.

QT prolongation is linked to other dopamine antagonists, such as prochlorperazine, metoclopramide, and chlorpromazine; however, it is unknown at what dosage ECG abnormalities can occur. Although dopamine causes QT prolongation, doses up to 80 mg per day had no effect on QT interval in a recent randomized controlled trial involving healthy volunteers. However, since an elderly patient may be more susceptible to side effects than a healthy volunteer, it is necessary to stick to the recommended dosage and proceed with extra caution. At therapeutic dosages, olanzapine has no effect on the QT interval.

5.3.4.2. Extrapyramidal Symptoms

A variety of extrapyramidal side effects, such as dystonia, akathisia, and parkinsonism, are possible; the risk increases with quick intravenous injection. They are carried out by blocking dopamine receptors in the striatum and substantia nigra. Extrapyramidal symptoms are 4–25% common in patients treated with metoclopramide and 25–67% common in patients treated with prochlorperazine, with the latter's incidence rising with higher doses. These wildly fluctuating rates are indicative of a broad spectrum of antiemetic dosages, as well as different administration routes and rates (e.g., intravenous infusion versus bolus injection). Patients on metoclopramide for longer than 12 weeks are more likely to experience tardive dyskinesia.

Regarding haloperidol and droperidol, the FDA has issued warnings due to the possibility of extrapyramidal symptoms. A report of 1–4% is known to occur following acute droperidol administration; however, the DORM-2 study did not report this incidence. Extrapyramidal symptoms are more common with haloperidol, even at doses less than 4 mg. At doses ranging from 5 to 20 mg, olanzapine has also been linked to symptoms of extrapyramidal seizures.

Serotonin antagonists, such as ondansetron, have been linked to extrapyramidal symptoms in case reports. These happened after receiving repeated intravenous doses of ondansetron ranging from 7 to 37 milligrams per day. Although there has been inconsistent evidence, it has been suggested that intravenous doses as low as 4 mg may be sufficient to trigger extrapyramidal symptoms.

Care must be taken when administering dopamine antagonists to elderly patients, especially those with Parkinson's disease, due to the possibility of extrapyramidal symptoms, especially at higher dosages. Domperidone, a peripherally acting dopamine antagonist that does not cross the blood–brain barrier, is a possible treatment option for these patients. Children should not take dopamine antagonists because of the high frequency of extrapyramidal symptoms, especially dystonic reactions.

5.3.4.3. Sedation

Dopamine antagonists are frequently linked to drowsiness. Although sedation may be a desired effect in some situations, this can limit the antiemetic efficacy of these medications. Droperidol is more sedating in psychosis than olanzapine and haloperidol combined, but at higher doses than those needed for antiemetic use. In as many as 17% of cases, droperidol at dosages of 0.25–1.25 mg produced sedation. While haloperidol at doses of 1–4 mg daily is reported to cause sedation in up to 21% of cases, low-dose olanzapine (2.5–7.5 mg) is linked to sedation in 20% of cases.

There is uncertainty regarding the exact rate of sedation associated with metoclopramide, prochlorperazine, and chlorpromazine. Sedation is also linked to antihistamines like promethazine, cyclizine, and doxylamine. Promethazine has a greater sedative effect than prochlorperazine or metoclopramide.

Although ondansetron may be less sedating than promethazine but as sedating as metoclopramide, according to a randomized trial, serotonin antagonists are generally believed to be non-sedating. The profound sedation that benzodiazepines and cannabinoids produce may restrict their application as antiemetic drugs.

5.3.4.4. Anticholinergic Effects

Anticholinergic side effects of many antiemetic medications include delirium, confusion, hallucinations, visual disturbance, constipation, urine retention, and tachycardia. Adverse effects of anticholinergic medications are linked to an increased risk of falls, cognitive impairment, and all-cause mortality in elderly patients. It is known that dopamine antagonists, hyoscine, and antihistamines have anticholinergic properties. The drugs most likely to cause the most harm are dopamine antagonists, like chlorpromazine and olanzapine, and antihistamines, like promethazine and doxylamine.

5.3.4.5. Constipation

One well-known side effect of anticholinergic medications like hyoscine and serotonin antagonists like ondansetron is constipation. Patients experiencing constipation may benefit more from the prokinetic nature of dopamine antagonists like domperidone and metoclopramide. (Baker, 2006; Malfertheiner et al, 2006; DeCamp et al, 2008; Liu et al, 2011)

5.4. Treatment of Hemorrhoids

The enlargement and/or distal displacement of anal cushions, which are prominences of the anal mucosa formed by loose connective tissue, smooth muscle, and venous and arterial vessels, are the symptoms of a very common anorectal disease known as hemorrhoids. Although the actual prevalence of hemorrhoids is unknown, new research indicates that the condition is becoming more common over time. An epidemiologic study conducted in the United States in 1990 found that 4.4% of adults had hemorrhoids, while reports from South Korea and Austria in the 21st century found that the prevalence was 144% and 38.9%, respectively. Hemorrhoids are thought to affect 25% of Britons and 75% of Americans at some point in their lives, with pregnant women and older adults most likely to suffer from them.

According to Google's 2012 annual roundup, hemorrhoids were the top trending health issue in the United States, surpassing gastroesophageal reflux disease and sexually transmitted diseases. Many individuals with hemorrhoids, or incorrectly believed to have hemorrhoids, often opted for self-medication instead of seeking professional medical help. It was found that nearly half of the information available on the internet regarding hemorrhoid treatment was of poor quality. Clinicians are advised to treat patients with hemorrhoids using evidence-based medicine and standard care practices. In most cases, low-graded hemorrhoids can be effectively treated with non-operative procedures by primary care physicians, gastroenterologists, or general surgeons in an outpatient setting. Surgery is recommended for high-graded hemorrhoids, when non-operative methods are unsuccessful, or when complications arise.

5.4.1. Contemporary Pathophysiology of Hemorrhoids

The precise pathophysiology is not well understood. The pathologic term for the symptomatic and abnormally downward displacement of normal anal cushions is currently hemorrhoids. The hemorrhoid plexus is abnormally distorted and dilated in the sliding anal cushions due to abnormal blood circulation and destructive alterations in the supporting connective tissue. In patients with hemorrhoids, a recent study examining the morphology and hemodynamics of the arterial supply to the anal canal showed a hyperperfusion state of the hemorrhoidal plexus, indicating the dysregulation of vascular tone within hemorrhoid tissue. Furthermore, it was clear that some inflammatory cells and recently formed microvessels were present in the hemorrhoidal tissue. Hemorrhoids that prolapse circumferentially may be caused by an internal rectal prolapse. Conclusion: Although the exact pathophysiology of hemorrhoid development is unknown, many factors, such as internal rectal prolapse (rectal redundancy), vascular abnormality, hyperperfusion of the hemorrhoid plexus, sliding anal cushion, and tissue inflammation, are likely to play a role. Different theories regarding the development of hemorrhoids may result in various methods for treating them.

5.4.2. Risk Factors for Hemorrhoids

It has been suggested that many risk factors, such as pregnancy, aging, obesity, especially abdominal obesity, and depressed mood, are the causes of hemorrhoids. In the meantime, it is generally accepted that certain circumstances involving elevated intraabdominal pressure, like prolonged straining and constipation, result in hemorrhoids due to impaired venous drainage of the hemorrhoid plexus. There is evidence linking certain dietary and lifestyle choices, such as consuming high-fiber foods, spicy foods, and alcohol, to the development of hemorrhoids and the exacerbation of acute hemorrhoid symptoms.

5.4.3. Diagnosis and Classification of Hemorrhoids

The most typical sign of hemorrhoids is painless bleeding from the rectal area during bowel movements, either with or without prolapsing anal tissue. Normally, blood is not mixed with stool; rather, it is coated on the stool's outer surface or visible when cleaning up after a bowel movement. Because the hemorrhoid plexus has direct arteriovenous communication, the blood is usually bright red. Anal pain and a lump at the anal verge may be present in patients with complicated hemorrhoids, such as acutely thrombosed external hemorrhoids and strangulated internal hemorrhoids. Patients with simple hemorrhoids rarely experience any kind of anal pain. In actuality, an anal fissure and anorectal abscess are more likely to be the cause of severe anal pain in patients with hemorrhoids.

Hemorrhoids must be diagnosed with a precise history and a comprehensive physical examination that includes anoscopy and a digital rectal examination. Patients experiencing rectal bleeding, particularly those who may be at risk of colorectal cancer, should be scheduled for a flexible sigmoidoscopy or colonoscopy unless bright red blood is clearly visible from hemorrhoids.

Hemorrhoids are generally classified by their location; internal (originates above the dentate line and covered by anal mucosa), external (originates below the dentate line and covered by anoderm) and mixed type. Internal hemorrhoids are further graded based on their appearance and degree of prolapse:

- Grade I: non-prolapsing hemorrhoids;
- Grade II: prolapsing hemorrhoids on straining but reduce spontaneously;
- Grade III: prolapsing hemorrhoids requiring manual reduction; and
- Grade IV: non-reducible prolapsing hemorrhoids which include acutely thrombosed, incarcerated hemorrhoids.

5.4.4. Management of Hemorrhoids

Options for treatment are primarily determined by the kind and severity of hemorrhoids, the patient's preferences, and the medical professionals' experience.

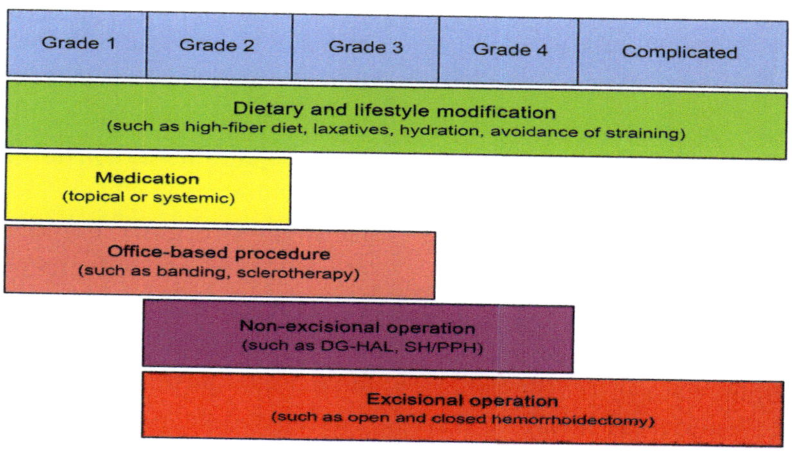

Figure 5.1. *Current treatment of internal hemorrhoids based on their severity and degree of prolapse.*

Source: https://www.ncbi.nlm.nih.gov/pmc/articles/PMC4541377/#:~:text=Medical%20treatment,-The%20main%20goal&text=For%20an%20oral%20preparation%2C%20flavonoids,%2Dinflammatory%20effects%5B2%5D.

Treatment for low-grade internal hemorrhoids can include medical intervention, dietary and lifestyle changes, and/or office-based procedures like sclerotherapy and rubber band ligation. High-graded hemorrhoids, strangulated hemorrhoids, and low-graded hemorrhoids that are not responsive to non-surgical treatment typically call for surgery. In the meantime, unless an external hemorrhoid becomes acutely thrombosed or causes discomfort to the patient, it does not require special treatment (Figure 5.1).

5.4.4.1. Dietary and Lifestyle Modification

A meta-analysis of 7 clinical trials with 378 hemorrhoidal patients revealed that taking a fiber supplement consistently reduced the risk of bleeding by about 50% and relieved symptoms. While the effectiveness of dietary and lifestyle modifications in treating hemorrhoids is still largely unknown, many doctors recommend them as a preventative and conservative measure in their conservative hemorrhoid treatment plans. Increasing dietary fiber and oral fluid intake, exercising frequently, avoiding drugs that cause constipation or diarrhea, and avoiding straining and reading on the toilet are some of the common recommendations.

5.4.4.2. Medical Treatment

Instead of curing the underlying hemorrhoids, the primary objective of medical treatment is to manage the acute symptoms. Both contemporary and conventional medications are used; they come in a range of forms, such as pills, suppositories, creams, and wipes. But there isn't enough solid data in the literature to conclude that topical treatment for symptomatic hemorrhoids is actually effective. The most popular phlebotonic agent for treating hemorrhoids in an oral preparation is flavonoids. It is clear that flavonoids have anti-inflammatory properties, can decrease capillary permeability, lower venous capacity, promote lymphatic drainage, and increase vascular tone. In 2012, a comprehensive meta-analysis on the use of phlebotonics for hemorrhoids revealed that the treatment significantly improved symptoms related to bleeding, pruritus, discharge, and overall symptom improvement. Additionally, phlebotonics reduced symptoms following a hemorrhoidectomy.

5.4.4.3. Operative Treatment

In cases of high-grade symptomatic hemorrhoids, low-grade hemorrhoids not responding to non-surgical treatment, and hemorrhoids resulting in complications like thrombosis and strangulation, surgery is typically necessary. If the patient has other concurrent anorectal conditions that necessitate surgery, or if the patient prefers, an operation for hemorrhoids may be performed.

Hemorrhoids should be completely removed from both the internal and external components, the procedure should be simple to learn and execute, have little pain or complications following the procedure, and show minimal recurrence. The process might also be inexpensive and economical. Regretfully, none of the operations that are currently in place manage to attain all the perfect circumstances. For grade III–IV hemorrhoids and complex hemorrhoids, excisional hemorrhoidectomy remains the standard procedure. It is noteworthy that while both closed (Ferguson) and open (Milligan-Morgan) hemorrhoidsemies were equally safe and effective, long-term patient satisfaction and continence were better with the Ferguson technique. Both methods, however, have the potential to cause excruciating postoperative pain. More modern methods, such as Ligasure hemorrhoidectomy, doppler-guided hemorrhoidal artery ligation, and stapled hemorrhoidopexy, have been incorporated into the surgical treatment of hemorrhoids in an effort to reduce or eliminate post-hemorrhoidectomy pain. Furthermore, perioperative hemorrhoid care has improved dramatically.

Hemorrhoids can be surgically excised using a range of tools, including scalpels, scissors, cautery devices, and, more recently, LigasureTM, a vessel sealing device. Comparing Ligasure hemorrhoidectomy to conventional hemorrhoidectomy, a recent Cochrane Review shows that the former led to a shorter convalescence period, less postoperative pain, and a shorter operating time. In the meantime, there was no discernible difference between the two methods in terms of long-term results or postoperative complications. On a day-case basis, excisional hemorrhoidectomy can be safely carried out with perianal infiltration of local anesthetics, regional anesthetics, or general anesthesia. It is clear that some medications, such as topical metronidazole or sucralfate administration, postoperative phlebotonic drug administration, and perioperative analgesia using oral non-steroidal anti-inflammatory drugs and gabapentin, could reduce pain following a hemorrhoidectomy (Figure 5.2).

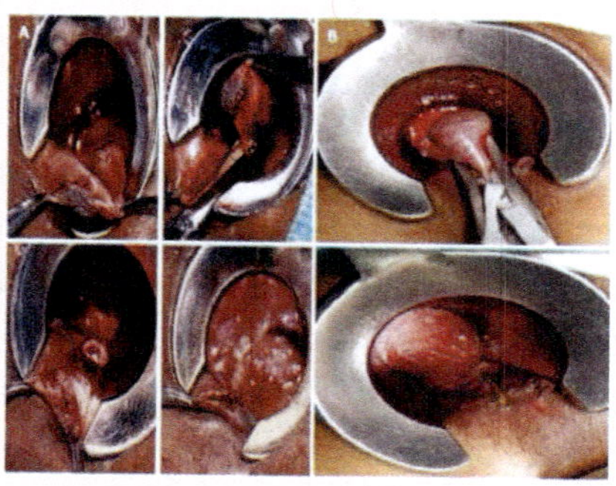

Figure 5.2. *Hemorrhoidectomy by (A) scissors and (B) Ligasure – a vessel sealing device.*

Source: https://www.ncbi.nlm.nih.gov/pmc/articles/PMC4541377/#:~:text=Medical%20treatment,-The%20main%20goal&text=For%20an%20oral%20preparation%2C%20flavonoids,%2Dinflammatory%20effects%5B2%5D.

Hemorrhoidal plication (also called ligation anopexy or mucopexy) and doppler-guided hemorrhoidal artery ligation (DG-HAL), also known as transanal hemorrhoidal dearterialization (THD), are examples of non-excisional hemorrhoidal procedures. The use of DG-HAL in surgery has made it possible to stop hemorrhoids' blood supply without having to remove the hemorrhoid. Hemorrhoid bundles shrink as a result of the surgical ligation of the superior hemorrhoidal artery's terminal branches. Hemorrhoid plication is frequently carried out using DG-HAL to better control prolapse. For grade IV hemorrhoids, however, the recurrence rate after DG-HAL was as high as 60%. Because of this, DG-HAL is only thought to be one of the most successful procedures for grade II–III hemorrhoids, with a 10% prolapse and 10% bleeding recurrence rate after a year. It should be noted that DG-HAL is not a completely painless procedure; about 20% of patients reported experiencing postoperative pain, particularly during the defecation. For grade II–III hemorrhoids, a ligation anopexy or mucopexy has also been shown to be a good substitute for excisional hemorrhoidectomy, with a shorter recovery period and less pain following surgery. More research on the long-term effects of non-excisional procedures for hemorrhoids is required because there is a chance of revascularization and recurrent prolapse.

Treating advanced internal hemorrhoids can also be accomplished with stapled hemorrhoidopexy, sometimes referred to as a prolapse and hemorrhoids (PPH) procedure. Not hemorrhoids per se, but a ring of superfluous rectal mucosa immediately above hemorrhoid bundles is excised using a circular staple device. This will cause prolapsing hemorrhoids to shrink (due to a partial interruption of blood supply to the hemorrhoid plexus) and reposition (hemorrhoidopexy). Stapled hemorrhoidopexy had a significantly higher rate of prolapse and reintervention for prolapse, but it also had less pain, a shorter operative time, and a quicker patient recovery than conventional hemorrhoidectomy, according to a recent systematic review of 27 randomized controlled trials. Fascinatingly, the most recent meta-analysis comparing the surgical outcomes of Ligasure hemorrhoidectomy and stapled hemorrhoidopexy in 2013 found that both surgical techniques were practically equivalent, with Ligasure hemorrhoidectomy having technical advantages and a slightly better immediate postoperative result.

Stapled hemorrhoidopexy should only be used for patients with circumferential prolapsing hemorrhoids and should only be performed by a skilled surgeon. This is because it is a relatively expensive procedure that has no discernible benefits over Ligasure hemorrhoidectomy and can result in serious postoperative complications like rectal stricture and rectal perforation as well as excruciating chronic anal pain.

5.5. Medications for Inflammatory Bowel Disease

Crohn's disease and ulcerative colitis are included in the category of inflammatory bowel disease (IBD), a relapsing-remitting illness marked by chronic inflammation at multiple sites in the gastrointestinal tract that causes diarrhea and pain in the abdomen.

A cell-mediated immune response in the mucosa of the gastrointestinal tract causes inflammation. Although the exact cause of inflammatory bowel disease is unknown, evidence points to patients with a complex genetic predisposition having normal intestinal flora that mistakenly trigger an immune response (possibly involving aberrant epithelial barriers and mucosal immune defenses). There are no known dietary, environmental, or infectious causes. Tumor necrosis factor, interleukins, and cytokines are among the inflammatory mediators released during the immune response.

Despite some similarities, Crohn's disease and ulcerative colitis can usually be differentiated (see table Differentiating Crohn Disease and Ulcerative Colitis). Indeterminate colitis is the term used when a surgical pathologic specimen cannot be classified, which applies to about 10% of colitis cases that are initially unclassified. Only inflammatory colon diseases (e.g., ulcerative, granulomatous, ischemic, radiation-induced, infectious) are referred to as colitis. Sometimes, irritable bowel syndrome, a functional disorder, is mislabeled as spastic (mucous) colitis.

5.5.1. 5-Aminosalicylic Acid (5-ASA, Mesalamine)

5-ASA has additional positive effects on the inflammatory cascade in addition to blocking the synthesis of prostaglandins and leukotrienes. Oral administration of 5-ASA requires formulation for delayed absorption due to its rapid absorption by the proximal small bowel and its limited intraluminal activity.

The original agent in this class, sulfasalazine, complexes 5-ASA with sulfapyridine, a sulfa moiety, delaying absorption. Bacterial flora in the colon and lower ileum cleaves the complex, releasing the 5-ASA. On the other hand, the sulfa moiety hinders the absorption of folate (folic acid), leading to many unfavorable effects such as headaches, nausea, and dyspepsia. It also can cause serious adverse reactions such as hemolytic anemia or agranulocytosis, and in rare cases, hepatitis, pneumonitis, or myocarditis. In up to 80% of men, reversible declines in sperm motility and count occur. Sulfasalazine should be taken with food if it is to be used. The dosage and frequency should be gradually increased over several days to 1 to 1.5 g four times a day, starting at a low level (e.g., 0.5 g orally twice a day). Patients should get liver tests every six to twelve months, as well as daily oral folate supplements (1 mg). Rarely, mesalamine-induced acute interstitial nephritis occurs; regular renal function monitoring is advised because most cases are treatable with early detection.

Drugs that complex 5-ASA with other vehicles appear to be nearly as effective as they are less harmful. Bacterial azoreductases cleave olsalazine (5-ASA dimer) and balsalazide (5-ASA conjugated to an inactive compound) as well as sulfasalazine. These medications are less effective for proximal small-bowel disease because they are primarily activated in the colon. Clinical studies on female patients have not demonstrated the efficacy of balsalazide in tablet form. Diarrhea can occasionally be brought on by osalazine, particularly in pancolitis patients. By administering the medication with meals and gradually increasing the dose, this issue is reduced.

Delay-release and/or extended-release coatings are used in other 5-ASA formulations to postpone the drug's release until it enters the distal ileum and colon. Combination delayed-release and extended-release formulations can be administered once daily; the patient may take them more consistently due to their less frequent dosage. From a therapeutic standpoint, all of these 5-ASA formulations are essentially equivalent.

5-ASA is also offered as an enema or suppository to treat left-sided colon disease and proctitis. When combined with oral 5-ASA, these rectal preparations provide additional benefits for proctitis and proctosigmoiditis. They are useful for both acute treatment and long-term maintenance. 5-ASA foam should be administered to patients whose rectal irritation prevents them from enduring enemas.

5.5.2. Corticosteroids

When 5-ASA compounds are insufficient, corticosteroids, starting at high doses, are helpful for acute flare-ups of the majority of IBD forms. Corticosteroids, however, are inappropriate for maintenance.

For severe illness, intravenous hydrocortisone or methylprednisolone are used; oral prednisone or prednisolone may be used for moderate to severe illness. After the course of treatment, which typically lasts seven to twenty-eight days, the dosage is lowered every week to 20 mg once daily. Following that, treatment is further tapered by 2.5 to 5 mg per week, depending on the clinical response, and maintenance therapy with 5-ASA or immunomodulators is started. When short-term corticosteroids are taken in large doses, side effects can include acute psychotic episodes, hyperglycemia, hypertension, insomnia, and hyperactivity.

Proctitis and left-sided colon disease can be treated with hydrocortisone enemas or foam; an enema solution is administered once or twice daily. For optimal results, the enema should be kept in the colon for as long as possible. This can be achieved by instilling the medication at night while the patient is sleeping on their left side and has their hips elevated. If the treatment works, it should be taken every day for two to four weeks, then every other day for one to two weeks, and finally stopped gradually over the course of one to two weeks.

As a corticosteroid with a high (>90%) first-pass liver metabolism, budesonide may significantly affect gastrointestinal tract disorders but minimally suppress adrenal function when taken orally. Compared to prednisolone, oral budesonide causes fewer side effects, but it acts more slowly and is usually prescribed for milder conditions. Budesonide has not yet shown to be useful for long-term maintenance, but it may be useful in sustaining remission for eight weeks. The medication is available for ulcerative colitis and small-bowel Crohn's disease. It also comes in an enteric-coated, delayed-release form. Outside of the US, it can also be purchased as an enema.

Oral vitamin D 400 to 800 units/day and calcium 1200 mg/day should be administered to all patients started on corticosteroids, including budesonide. Patients with cirrhosis or other chronic liver diseases should use corticosteroids with caution as their bioavailability and clinical effects may be amplified. (Baker, 2006; Malfertheiner et al, 2006; DeCamp et al, 2008; Liu et al, 2011)

5.5.3. Immunomodulating Medications

In combination therapy with biologic agents, the antimetabolites methotrexate, 6-mercaptopurine, and azathioprine are also utilized.

5.5.3.1. Azathioprine and 6-Mercaptopurine

T-cell function is inhibited by azathioprine and its metabolite 6-mercaptopurine, which may also cause T-cell apoptosis. They may reduce the need for corticosteroids and keep remission for years, and they are long-term effective. Since these medications frequently take one to three months to show clinical benefits, corticosteroids cannot be totally stopped until at least the second month. The dosage varies according to each person's metabolism. In patients who are intermediate metabolizers, the dose of azathioprine or 6-mercaptopurine should be lowered by 50% and modified based on clinical response and hematologic monitoring.

The most frequent side effects include malaise, vomiting, and nausea. White blood cell counts should be performed on a regular basis (biweekly for the first month, then every one to two months) to detect any signs of bone marrow suppression. Approximately 3 to 5% of patients experience pancreatitis, and both conditions completely rule out the possibility of relapsing. Blood tests can be used to screen for hepatotoxicity, which is less common, every six to twelve months. These medications have been linked to an increased risk of skin cancers other than melanoma and lymphoma.

Thiopurine methyltransferase (TPMT), an enzyme that changes azathioprine and 6-mercaptopurine into their active metabolites 6-thioguanine (6-TG) and 6-methylmercaptopurine (6-MMP), should be tested on patients before beginning these medications. Genotype testing for known low-activity variants of this enzyme should also be performed on patients. To help ensure safe and effective drug dosages, it is helpful to measure levels of 6-TG and 6-MMP after starting these medications. 6-TG levels between 230 and 450 picomoles per 8×10^8 red blood cells (RBCs) are correlated with therapeutic efficacy. 6-TG levels above 450 have the potential to cause myelotoxicity. When 6-MMP levels are greater than 5700 picomoles per 8×10^8 RBCs, hepatotoxicity may result. In nonresponding patients, the metabolite concentrations can also be used to differentiate between resistance and nonadherence.

5.5.3.2. Methotrexate

Many patients with corticosteroid-dependent or corticosteroid-refractory Crohn's disease benefit from methotrexate, even those who have not responded to azathioprine or 6-mercaptopurine.

Nausea, vomiting, and abnormal liver tests are among the side effects. One daily dose of 1 mg of folate may lessen some of the negative effects. When taking methotrexate, both men and women should make sure the female partner uses an oral contraceptive, intrauterine device, or contraceptive implant. It is best to discourage the use of less effective forms of contraception like cervical caps, diaphragms, spermicides, condoms, and intermittent abstinence. Men and women alike should discontinue methotrexate at least three months before attempting to conceive. For the first three months of therapy, complete blood counts and liver tests with albumin should be performed monthly. After that, they should be performed every eight to twelve weeks. Hepatotoxicity risk factors include alcohol consumption, hepatitis B and C, obesity, diabetes, and possibly psoriasis. Methotrexate treatment for these patients should ideally be avoided. Liver biopsies performed before treatment are not advised; instead, they should be performed if the results of six out of twelve tests conducted within a year indicate elevated aspartate aminotransferase (AST) levels. Methotrexate therapy may also result in nephrotoxicity, pulmonary toxicity, and myelosuppression.

5.5.3.3. Cyclosporine and Tacrolimus

Patients with severe ulcerative colitis who are not responsive to corticosteroids and biologic agents and who might otherwise need a colectomy may benefit from cyclosporine, which inhibits lymphocyte activation. The only Crohn's disease patients for whom it has a documented use are those who have pyoderma or refractory fistulas. Multiple adverse effects (e.g., renal toxicity, seizures, opportunistic infections, hypertension, neuropathy) make long-term use (> 6 months) contraindicated. Unless there is a compelling reason to forego the less risky curative option of colectomy, patients with severe ulcerative colitis who are not responsive to corticosteroids and biologics are typically not offered cyclosporine. When using the medication, trough blood levels should be maintained between 200 and 400 ng/mL (166 and 333 nmol/L), and prophylactic treatment for Pneumocystis jirovecii should be taken into consideration while concurrently taking antimetabolite, cyclosporine, and corticosteroid medication.

In patients with severe or refractory ulcerative colitis who do not require hospitalization, tacrolimus, an immunosuppressant also used in transplant patients, appears to be as effective as cyclosporine. It is recommended to maintain the trough blood levels between 10 and 15 ng/mL (12 and 25 nmol/L). For the short term, perianal and cutaneous fistulas associated with Crohn's disease can be treated with tacrolimus.

5.5.4. Biologic Agents

5.5.4.1. Anti-TNF Medications

Tumor necrosis factor antibodies include infliximab, certolizumab, adalimumab, and golimumab (TNF). When treating Crohn's disease, infliximab, certolizumab, and adalimumab are helpful, especially when it comes to preventing or delaying postoperative recurrence. Golimumab, adalimumab, and infliximab are helpful in treating refractory or corticosteroid-dependent ulcerative colitis.

For Crohn's disease and ulcerative colitis, infliximab is administered as a single intravenous infusion at a dose of 5 mg/kg spread over two hours. Repeat infusions occur at weeks two and six after it. It is then administered every eight weeks. Within a year or so, the dose must be increased or the interval must be shortened to maintain remission in many, if not most, of the patients. More than 5 mcg/mL is the approved therapeutic serum level.

Adalimumab is beneficial for ulcerative colitis and Crohn's disease. It is administered subcutaneously with a loading dose of 160 mg at week one and 80 mg at week two. Following that, 40 mg is administered subcutaneously every two weeks. > 7.5% mcg/mL is the approved therapeutic serum level. Adalimumab therapy may be helpful for patients who are intolerant of infliximab or who have lost their initial response to it.

For Crohn's disease, certolizumab is helpful. It is administered subcutaneously as 400 mg for three doses every two weeks, and then once every four weeks for maintenance. Certolizumab may be helpful for patients who are intolerant of infliximab or who have lost their initial response to it. More than 20 mcg/mL is the approved therapeutic serum level.

Patients suffering from ulcerative colitis benefit from golimumab. It is administered subcutaneously with a 200 mg loading dose at week one and 100 mg at week two. Following that, 100 mg is administered every four weeks. Golimumab therapy may be helpful for patients who are intolerant to infliximab or who have not responded to it at first.

Anti-TNF agent monotherapy is unquestionably effective for both remission induction and maintenance; however, some studies indicate that anti-TNF agents work better when started in combination with methotrexate or a thiopurine, such as azathioprine. However, recommendations for treatment should be tailored to the patient because combination therapy may increase side effects. After two weeks, corticosteroid tapering may start. Adverse reactions that occur during infusion include fever, chills, headaches, nausea, and instant hypersensitivity reactions (such as rash, itching, and occasionally anaphylactoid reactions). Hypersensitivity reactions that are delayed have also happened. Anti-TNF medications administered subcutaneously, such as adalimumab, can result in localized erythema, pain, and itching (injection site reaction), but they do not cause infusion reactions.

Anti-TNF medications should not be used in cases of uncontrolled bacterial infection because they have been linked to multiple sepsis-related deaths in patients. Anti-TNF medications have also been linked to reactivation of hepatitis B and tuberculosis (TB). For this reason, screening for latent TB (using interferon-gamma release assay and/or tuberculin skin tests) and hepatitis B is necessary before therapy. It is advisable to document varicella immunity. Additionally, serologic testing for cytomegalovirus and Epstein-Barr virus may be advised.

Other potential concerns with anti-TNF drug treatment include lymphoma and possibly other cancers (e.g., nonmelanoma skin cancer), demyelinating disease (e.g., multiple sclerosis, optic neuritis), heart failure, and liver and hematologic toxicity.

5.5.4.2. Other Biologic Agents

Numerous immunosuppressive interleukins and anti-interleukin antibodies are being investigated for Crohn's disease, and they may also lessen the inflammatory response.

Leukocyte adhesion molecules are the target of the antibodies natalizumab and vedolizumab. Vedolizumab is a treatment for Crohn's disease and moderate-to-severe ulcerative colitis. IV vedolizumab dosage recommendations are 300 mg at 0, 2, and 6 weeks, and then every 8 weeks thereafter. It is safer than natalizumab, which is only prescribed as a second-line treatment under a restricted prescription program for the most refractory Crohn's disease cases, because its effect is thought to be restricted to the gut. Vedolizumab's recognized therapeutic serum level is greater than 20 mcg/mL. These drugs raise the possibility of infections and can result in hypersensitivity reactions. At present, natalizumab can only be obtained through a limited-use program due to its potential to cause progressive multifocal leukoencephalopathy (PML). Since vedolizumab and natalizumab belong to the same class of medications, there is a potential risk of PML.

Ustekinumab, an anti-IL-12/23 antibody, is available for patients with moderate to severe Crohn disease or ulcerative colitis. The initial loading dose is a single IV dose based on weight:

- < 55 kg: 260 mg
- 55 to 85 kg: 390 mg
- 85 kg: 520 mg

After the loading dose, patients are given a maintenance dose of 90 mg subcutaneously every 8 weeks.

Other anticytokine, anti-integrin, small-molecule agents, and growth factors are being studied, along with the depletion of activated immune cells through leukapheresis therapy. An anti-IL-23 antibody called Risankizumab is available for people with moderate to severe Crohn's disease. 600 mg IV is the induction dose given at weeks 0, 4, and 8. After week 12, the maintenance dose is 180–360 mg administered subcutaneously every 8 weeks. It is advised to use the lowest dose necessary to maintain endoscopic remission. Liver tests ought to be performed both at baseline and throughout the induction phase. Biologic drugs that closely resemble a reference biologic product are known as biosimilars. Commercialization of biosimilars for anti-TNF medications has occurred.

5.5.4.3. Small-Molecule Agents

Drugs that are small enough to enter cells, usually around 900 daltons, and affect cellular processes known as small-molecule agents. A few of these are being developed or are currently being used to manage IBD. They are administered orally and don't elicit the same immune response as monoclonal antibodies.

A small-molecule medication called tofacitinib is available for adult patients with moderate to severe ulcerative colitis. It inhibits Janus kinase 1–3. For at least eight weeks, the immediate-release form's starting dosage is 10 mg taken twice daily. After that, the dosage can be either 5 or 10 mg taken twice daily. For at least eight weeks, the extended-release form's starting dosage is 22 mg taken once daily; after that, it is 11 mg taken once daily. Raised cholesterol, rash, headaches, diarrhea, herpes zoster, nasopharyngitis, increased blood creatine phosphokinase, and upper respiratory tract infections are possible side effects. Opportunistic infections and cancer are two other rare side effects. Furthermore, the U. S. The Food and Drug Administration issued a warning to patients using tofacitinib for rheumatoid arthritis regarding an increased risk of fatal pulmonary embolism and death.

A small molecule called upadacitinib selectively inhibits Janus kinase 1. Compared to other small molecule agents like tofacitinib, this has less of an impact on the depletion of natural killer cells because it inhibits signaling related to IL-6 and IFN-gamma. For both ulcerative colitis and Crohn's disease, the maintenance dose is 15 mg once daily; in patients with refractory, severe, or extensive disease, the dose can be titrated to 30 mg once daily. The induction dose is 45 mg once daily for eight weeks and 45 mg once daily for twelve weeks. If the 30-mg dose does not result in remission, the medication should be stopped. Acne vulgaris, folliculitis, upper respiratory tract infection, hypersensitivity, nausea, and abdominal pain are the most frequent side effects. The majority of the time, the adverse effects resemble those of other Janus kinase (JAK) inhibitors, such as tofacitinib.

Ozanimod is a medication used to treat adults with moderate to severe active ulcerative colitis. It is a sphingosine 1-phosphate (S1P) receptor modulator. The starting dosage is 0.23mg mg once daily for days 1 through 4, and 0.46mg once daily for days 5 through 7. Beginning on day 8, the maintenance dose is 0.92mg taken once daily by mouth. In the event that a dose is skipped within the first 14 days of treatment, the oral titration regimen containing 0.23mg once daily should be resumed. After 14 days of treatment, if a dose is missed, the course of action should be followed. Those who have had a myocardial infarction within the previous six months, as well as those who have unstable angina or heart failure, should not take ozanimod. Additionally, unless they have a working pacemaker, patients with Mobitz type II 2nd-degree block, 3rd-degree atrioventricular block, sick sinus syndrome, or sinoatrial block should not take this medication. Those who have experienced a stroke or transient ischemic attack within the previous six months ought to refrain from using ozanimod. Additionally, those taking monoamine oxidase inhibitors and those with severe untreated sleep apnea should refrain from using ozanimod. Ozanimod has been linked to liver damage, bradyarrhythmia, decreased lymphocyte counts, and an increased risk of infections. Before beginning ozanimod treatment, a varicella zoster virus antibody test and an ECG should be performed.

5.5.5. Antibiotics and Probiotics

1. Antibiotics

In cases of"toxic colitis, antibiotics are not very useful in ulcerative colitis but may be in Crohn's disease. For four to eight weeks, 500–750 mg of metronidazole taken orally three times a day may help heal fistulas and manage mild Crohn's disease. Unfortunately, side effects—especially neurotoxicity—often make it impossible to finish treatment. Oral ciprofloxacin 500–750 mg twice a day might be less harmful. Combining metronidazole and ciprofloxacin is advised by many experts. For the treatment of active Crohn's disease, nonabsorbable antibiotic rifaximin at a dose of 200 mg orally three times a day or 800 mg orally twice a day may also be helpful.

2. Probiotics

Consistent daily administration of nonpathogenic microorganisms (e.g., commensal Escherichia coli, Lactobacillus species, Saccharomyces) functions as a probiotic and may be useful in preventing pouchitis; however, their other therapeutic functions remain unclear. Trichuris suis infection has been used therapeutically to try to increase T2-helper cell immunity and potentially reduce ulcerative colitis disease activity. (Baker, 2006; Malfertheiner et al, 2006; DeCamp et al, 2008; Liu et al, 2011)

A Closer Look

Diagnosis of Constipation in Elderly

The diagnosis process starts with a thorough medical history and examination. History can be used to diagnose drug-induced constipation, prolonged inactivity-induced constipation, and changes in diet and fluid intake. When constipation appears suddenly or gets worse, has blood in the stools, causes unexplained weight loss, fever, nausea, vomiting, appetite loss, or has a family history of inflammatory bowel disease or colon cancer in older adults over 50, it is important to thoroughly rule out other conditions that could be the cause of the constipation, including rectal and colon cancer.

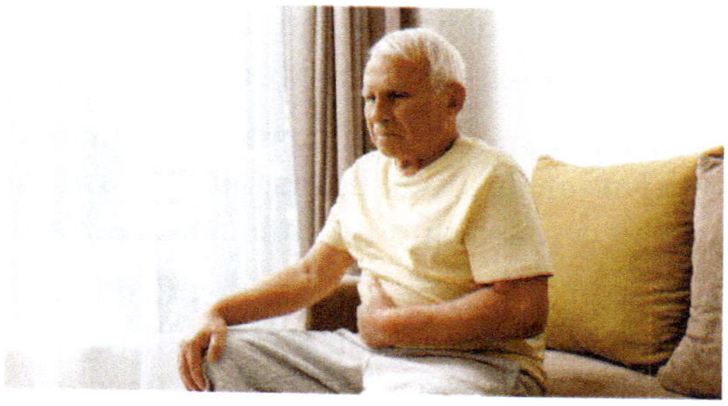

Source: https://dailycaring.com/constipation-in-seniors-6-effective-home-remedies/

A general examination is next undertaken to evaluate the presence of other causes of constipation. Other causes that may affect other body systems and manifest as constipation include:

- heart diseases like heart failure
- Diabetes mellitus
- hypothyroidism (underactive thyroid)
- hypercalcemia (increased blood calcium)
- hypokalemia (low blood potassium)
- hypermagnesemia (increased blood magnesium)
- hyperparathyroidism (overactive parathyroid glands) etc.

Constipation can be brought on by many muscle and nerve conditions, such as dermatomyositis, autonomic neuropathy, systemic sclerosis, Parkinson's disease, spinal cord lesion (tumors or injury), dementia, and depression. Constipation can also result from certain gastrointestinal disorders. These include rectal prolapse, diverticular disease, strictures, anal fissures, volvulus, megacolon, and irritable bowel syndrome.

The Bristol stool chart is used to record and categorize the type and consistency of the stool. This aids in figuring out the colonic transit duration. In the case of the stool, Type 1 takes roughly 100 hours to transit (slow transit), whereas Type 7 transits quickly in about 10 hours.

Summary

- Gastrointestinal diseases refer to diseases involving the gastrointestinal tract, namely the esophagus, stomach, small intestine, large intestine and rectum, and the accessory organs of digestion, the liver, gallbladder, and pancreas.
- The drugs for the gastrointestinal system are designed for care and treatment of the digestive system organs (including the liver, biliary tract and pancreas) and diseases that may affect those organs.
- Acid peptic diseases result from distinctive but overlapping pathogenic mechanisms that typically involve acid effects on diminished mucosal defense.
- A peptic ulcer is histologically defined as a mucosal defect that extends to or beyond the muscularis mucosa, with mucosal damage due to pepsin and gastric acid secretion.
- Acid-related disorders influence the quality of life and productivity of afflicted patients and are common and important causes of morbidity and mortality.
- Laxatives are a category of medications frequently used to address constipation and various other gastrointestinal medical conditions.
- Hemorrhoids is a very common anorectal disease defined as the symptomatic enlargement and/or distal displacement of anal cushions, which are prominences of anal mucosa formed by loose connective tissue, smooth muscle, arterial and venous vessels.
- Inflammatory bowel disease (IBD), which includes Crohn's disease and ulcerative colitis, is a relapsing and remitting condition characterized by chronic inflammation at various sites in the gastrointestinal tract, which results in diarrhea and abdominal pain

References

1. Aigner, F., Gruber, H., Conrad, F., Eder, J., Wedel, T., Zelger, B., Engelhardt, V., Lametschwandtner, A., Wienert, V., Böhler, U., et al. (2009). Revised morphology and hemodynamics of the anorectal vascular plexus: Impact on the course of hemorrhoidal disease. *International Journal of Colorectal Disease, 24*(1), 105–113. https://doi.org/10.1007/s00384-008-0593-4.
2. Athmann, C., Zeng, N., Scott, D. R., & Sachs, G. (2000). Regulation of parietal cell calcium signaling in gastric glands. *American Journal of Physiology–Gastrointestinal and Liver Physiology, 279*(6), G1048–G1058. https://doi.org/10.1152/ajpgi.2000.279.6.G1048.
3. Baker, H. (2006). Hemorrhoids. In J. L. Longe (Ed.), *Gale Encyclopedia of Medicine* (3rd ed., pp. 1766–1769). Thomson Gale.
4. Brand, S. J., & Stone, D. (1988). Reciprocal regulation of antral gastrin and somatostatin gene expression by omeprazole-induced achlorhydria. *Journal of Clinical Investigation, 82*(3), 1059–1066. https://doi.org/10.1172/JCI113558.
5. Camilleri, M., & Bharucha, A. E. (2010). Behavioral and new pharmacological treatments for constipation: Getting the balance right. *Gut, 59*(9), 1288–1296. https://doi.org/10.1136/gut.2010.219505.
6. Chang, L., Chey, W. D., Imdad, A., Almario, C. V., Bharucha, A. E., Diem, S., Greer, K. B., Hanson, B., Harris, L. A., Ko, C., Murad, M. H., Patel, A., Shah, E. D., Lembo, A. J., & Sultan, S. (2023). American gastroenterological association-American college of gastroenterology clinical practice

guideline: Pharmacological management of chronic idiopathic constipation. *Gastroenterology, 164*(7), 1086–1106. https://doi.org/10.1053/j.gastro.2023.01.027.

7. Cui, G., & Waldum, H. L. (2007). Physiological and clinical significance of enterochromaffin-like cell activation in the regulation of gastric acid secretion. *World Journal of Gastroenterology, 28*(10), 493–496. https://doi.org/10.3748/wjg.v28.i10.493.

8. DeCamp, L. R., Byerley, J. S., Doshi, N., & Steiner, M. J. (2008). Use of antiemetic agents in acute gastroenteritis: A systematic review and meta-analysis. *Archives of Pediatrics & Adolescent Medicine, 162*(9), 858–865. https://doi.org/10.1001/archpedi.162.9.858.

9. Fallon, R., Boulger, S., Fraser, C., & Moriarty, K. (2010). Recommended drug options for nausea and vomiting. *Prescriber, 21*, 18–33.

10. Krogh, K., Chiarioni, G., & Whitehead, W. (2017). Management of chronic constipation in adults. *United European Gastroenterology Journal, 5*(4), 465–472. https://doi.org/10.1177/2050640617709274.

11. Kulaksiz, H., Arnold, R., Goke, B., et al. (2000). Expression and cell-specific localization of the cholecystokinin B/gastrin receptor in the human stomach. *Cell and Tissue Research, 299*(2), 289–298. https://doi.org/10.1007/s004410051293.

12. Leung, L., Riutta, T., Kotecha, J., & Rosser, W. (2011). Chronic constipation: An evidence-based review. *Journal of the American Board of Family Medicine, 24*(4), 436–451. https://doi.org/10.3122/jabfm.2011.04.100239.

13. Liu, L. W. (2011). Chronic constipation: Current treatment options. *Canadian Journal of Gastroenterology, 25*(Suppl B), 22B–28B. https://doi.org/10.1155/2011/691239.

14. Mahajan, R. (2019). Prucalopride: A recently approved drug by the Food and Drug Administration for chronic idiopathic constipation. *International Journal of Applied and Basic Medical Research, 9*(1), 1–2. https://doi.org/10.4103/ijabmr.IJABMR_4_19.

15. Malfertheiner, P., Fass, R., Quigley, E. M., et al. (2006). Review article: From gastrin to gastro-oesophageal reflux disease–A century of acid suppression. *Alimentary Pharmacology & Therapeutics, 15*(5), 683–690. https://doi.org/10.1111/j.1365-2036.2006.02958.x.

16. Manela, F. D., Ren, J., Gao, J., McGuigan, J. E., & Harty, R. F. (1995). Calcitonin gene-related peptide modulates acid-mediated regulation of somatostatin and gastrin release from rat antrum. *Gastroenterology, 109*(2), 701–706. https://doi.org/10.1016/0016-5085(95)90677-2.

17. Masri, Y., Abubaker, J., & Ahmed, R. (2010). Prophylactic use of laxative for constipation in critically ill patients. *Annals of Thoracic Medicine, 5*(4), 228–231. https://doi.org/10.4103/1817-1737.72395.

18. O'Brien, S. H., Fan, L., & Kelleher, K. J. (2010). Inpatient use of laxatives during opioid administration in children with sickle cell disease. *Pediatric Blood & Cancer, 54*(4), 559–562. https://doi.org/10.1002/pbc.22579.

19. Orlando, L. A., Lenard, L., & Orlando, R. C. (2007). Chronic hypergastrinemia: Causes and consequences. *Digestive Diseases and Sciences, 52*(9), 2482–2489. https://doi.org/10.1007/s10620-006-9661-3.

20. Peghini, P. L., Annibale, B., Azzoni, C., et al. (2002). Effect of chronic hypergastrinemia on human enterochromaffin-like cells: Insights from patients with sporadic gastronomes. *Gastroenterology, 123*(1), 68–85. https://doi.org/10.1053/gast.2002.34034.

21. Riss, S., Weiser, F. A., Schwameis, K., Riss, T., Mittlböck, M., Steiner, G., & Stift, A. (2012). The prevalence of hemorrhoids in adults. *International Journal of Colorectal Disease, 27*(2), 215–220. https://doi.org/10.1007/s00384-011-1370-5.

22. Rohde, H., & Christ, H. (2004). Haemorrhoids are too often assumed and treated: Survey of 548 patients with anal discomfort. *Deutsche Medizinische Wochenschrift, 129*(38), 1965–1969. https://doi.org/10.1055/s-2004-828457.

23. Roila, F., Herrstedt, J., Aapro, M., Gralla, R. J., Einhorn, L. H., Ballatori, E., et al. (2010). ESMO/MASCC Guidelines Working Group. Guideline update for MASCC and ESMO in the prevention of chemotherapy- and radiotherapy-induced nausea and vomiting: Results of the Perugia consensus conference. *Annals of Oncology, 21*(Suppl 5), v232–v243. https://doi.org/10.1093/annonc/mdq278.

24. Sachs, G., Shin, J. M., Vagin, O., Lambrecht, N., Yakubov, I., & Munson, K. (2007). The gastric H, K-ATPase as a drug target: Past, present, and future. *Journal of Clinical Gastroenterology, 41*(Suppl 2), S226–S242. https://doi.org/10.1097/01.mcg.0000242150.64773.4d.

25. Sandler, R. S., Everhart, J. E., Donowitz, M., et al. (2002). The burden of selected digestive diseases in the United States. *Gastroenterology, 122*(5), 1500–1511. https://doi.org/10.1053/gast.2002.32982.

26. Schmitz, F., Goke, M. N., Otte, J. M., et al. (2001). Cellular expression of CCK-A and CCK-B/gastrin receptors in human gastric mucosa. *Regulatory Peptides, 102*(2), 101–110. https://doi.org/10.1016/S0167-0115(01)00253-5.

27. Schubert, M. L., Hightower, J., & Makhlouf, G. M. (1989). Linkage between somatostatin and acid secretion: Evidence from use of pertussis toxin. *American Journal of Physiology, 256*(3), G418–G422. https://doi.org/10.1152/ajpgi.1989.256.3.G418.

28. Schubert, M. L., Jong, M. J., & Makhlouf, G. M. (1991). Bombesin/GRP-stimulated somatostatin secretion is mediated by gastrin in the antrum and intrinsic neurons in the fundus. *American Journal of Physiology, 261*(5), G885–G889. https://doi.org/10.1152/ajpgi.1991.261.5.G885.

29. Tari, A., Kamiyasu, T., Yonei, Y., et al. (1997). Role of gastrin/CCK-B receptor in the regulation of gastric acid secretion in rat. *Digestive Diseases and Sciences, 42*(9), 1901–1907. https://doi.org/10.1023/A:1018888529468.

30. Tonini, M., Cipollina, L., Poluzzi, E., Crema, F., Corazza, G. R., & De Ponti, F. (2004). Review article: Clinical implications of enteric and central D2 receptor blockade by antidopaminergic gastrointestinal prokinetics. *Alimentary Pharmacology & Therapeutics, 19*(4), 379–390. https://doi.org/10.1111/j.1365-2036.2004.01838.x.

31. Tucker, H., George, E., Barnett, D., & Longson, C. (2008). NICE Technology Appraisal on Stapled Haemorrhoidopexy for the Treatment of Haemorrhoids. *Annals of the Royal College of Surgeons of England, 90*(1), 82–84. https://doi.org/10.1308/003588408X271375.

32. Yeung, T. M., & D'Souza, N. D. (2013). Quality analysis of patient information on surgical treatment of hemorrhoids on the internet. *Annals of the Royal College of Surgeons of England, 95*(5), 341–344. https://doi.org/10.1308/003588413X13629981489258.

33. Zanner, R., Hapfelmeier, G., Gratzl, M., & Prinz, C. (2002). Intracellular signal transduction during gastrin-induced histamine secretion in rat gastric ECL cells. *American Journal of Physiology-Cell Physiology, 282*(2), C374–C382. https://doi.org/10.1152/ajpcell.00130.2

Chapter

DRUGS ACTING ON THE CENTRAL NERVOUS SYSTEM

6

Contents

Introduction

The brain and spinal cord make up the central nervous system. It is the center of the autonomic nervous system, awareness, and behavior involving motor coordination, thoughts, and memory. It has been demonstrated that numerous neurotransmitters play a role in the regulation of these functions in various brain regions. To coordinate and regulate the various processes, neurotransmitter pairs are found in most locations, acting in opposition to one another. Any abnormality in the way that neurotransmitters function can result in the emergence of mental or neurological conditions.

Orientation and Directional Terms

Term	Definition	Illustration
Hypnotic	Hypnotic, or soporific drugs, commonly known as sleeping pills, are a class of (and umbrella term for) psychoactive drugs whose primary function is to induce sleep (or surgical anesthesia) and to treat insomnia (sleeplessness).	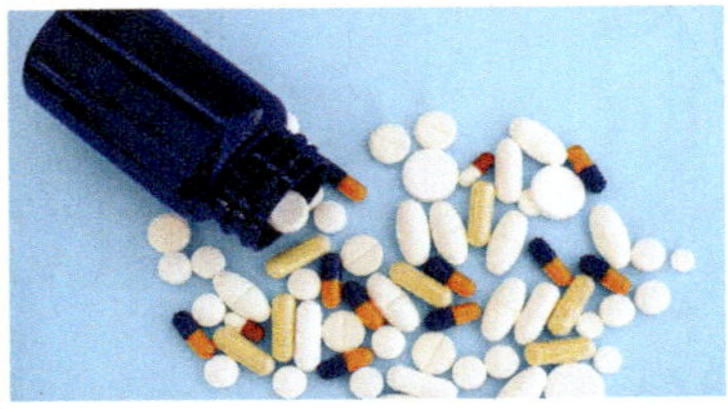
Agranulocytosis	Agranulocytosis is a life-threatening condition that involves having severely low levels of white blood cells called neutrophils. White blood cells are part of your immune system. They protect your body from infection by fighting off germs that make you sick.	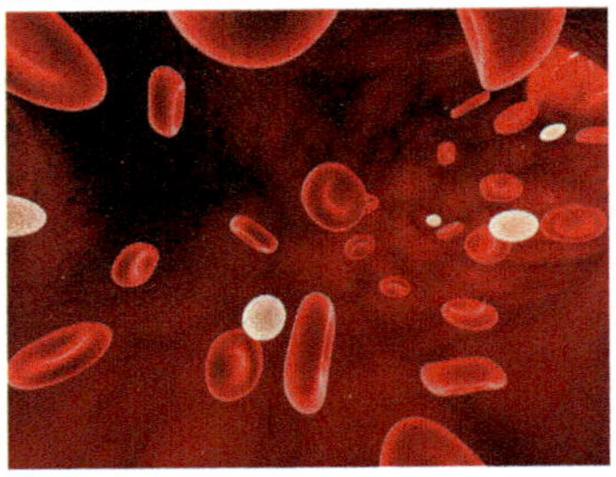
Psychological therapies	Psychological therapies, also known as psychotherapy or talk therapy, are evidence-based treatments that can help improve mental and physical health. They can help people identify and change troubling thoughts, emotions, and behaviors.	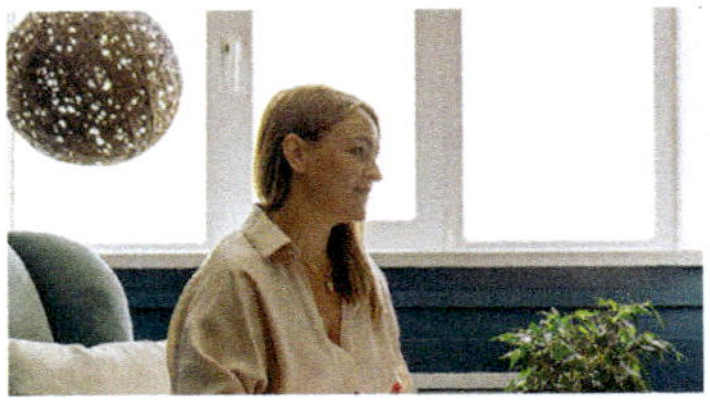
Opioid-inclusive anesthesia (OIA)	Opioid-inclusive anesthesia (OIA) is a type of anesthesia that uses opioids to supplement sedation and provide analgesia. Opioids are often used in breast cancer surgery, and are administered intravenously as repeat injections or a continuous infusion.	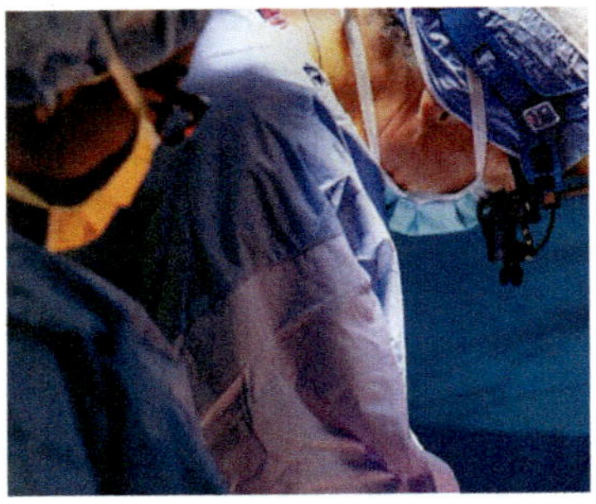
Piroxicam	Piroxicam is a nonsteroidal anti-inflammatory drug of the oxicam class used to relieve the symptoms of painful inflammatory conditions like arthritis.	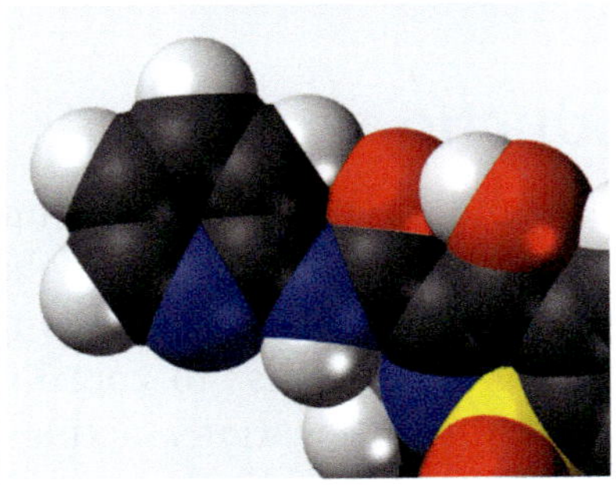

6.1. Sedatives and Hypnotics

Agents that calm people down and lessen anxiety while having little to no impact on cognitive or motor abilities are known as sedatives, also known as anxiolytics. Drugs known as hypnotics induce drowsiness and promote the initiation and maintenance of sleep.

For centuries, the only substances with sedative-hypnotic properties were opium and alcohol. A liquid solution of bromide salts was the first drug introduced expressly for use as a sedative and hypnotist in the 1800s. As a synthetic sedative-hypnotic, chloral hydrate, a derivative of ethyl alcohol, was first introduced in 1869 and was infamously used as "knock-out" drops. In the 1880s, paraldehyde was first used in clinical medicine. In 1903, barbital was synthesized. After phenobarbital became accessible in 1912, a lengthy list of additional barbiturates was introduced over the course of the following 20 years. New classes of sedative-hypnotic medications were created in the middle of the 20th century, with benzodiazepines being the most common.

6.1.1. Barbiturates

Barbituric acid is the chemical source of a class of depressant medications known as barbiturates. In addition to having the potential for overdose and physical and psychological addiction, they are useful when used medicinally as hypnotics, anticonvulsants, and anxiolytics. Because of the risks involved in their recreational use, they are controlled in the majority of countries despite their historical use for their sedative and anti-anxiety effects.

Because benzodiazepines and nonbenzodiazepines("Z-drugs") have a much lower risk of overdose and the lack of antidote for barbiturates, they have largely replaced barbiturates in routine medical practice, especially when treating anxiety disorders and insomnia. Barbiturates are still used today for many conditions, including general anesthesia, epilepsy, treating acute tension headaches, acute migraines or cluster headaches, euthanasia, the death penalty, and assisted suicide.

Barbituric acid is the source of barbiturates. They are CNS depressants in general. The specific barbiturates used and their dosage can result in sedation, hypnosis, and general anesthesia. Barbiturates cause dose-dependent central nervous system depression. Barbiturates are typically used as a sedative and to reduce anxiety when taken in small doses. At hypnotic dosages, they induce sleep that is comparable to regular physiological sleep. Long-acting barbiturates are especially known to cause hangovers. They have the potential to be abused and produce physical dependence.

The important therapeutic uses of this class of compounds are:

- To produce sedation and hypnosis.
- Anticonvulsant action: Phenobarbital is drug of choice.
- For general anesthesia: Ultra short acting barbiturates are used.
- As preanesthetic medication.
- As obstetrical analgesic.

6.1.1.1. Side Effects

Pregnant women and older adults should take particular precautions. The body's capacity to eliminate barbiturates decreases with age. Because of this, individuals over 65 are more likely to suffer from the negative effects of barbiturates, such as drug dependence and accidental overdose. Barbiturates crosses the placenta and enters the fetus when taken during pregnancy. The baby may have breathing difficulties and withdrawal symptoms after birth. Furthermore, barbiturates may pass from nursing mothers to their infants through breast milk. Stevens-Johnson syndrome is an uncommon adverse reaction to barbiturates that mainly affects the mucous membranes.

Common side effects

- Nausea
- Hypotension
- Headache
- Drowsiness
- Skin rash

Serious side effects

- Confusion
- Coma
- Hallucination
- Fainting
- Slow breathing

Rare side effects

- Agranulocytosis
- Stevens–Johnson syndrome
- Liver injury
- Megaloblastic anemia

6.1.1.2. Tolerance and dependence

Tolerance to barbiturates' effects grows with continued use. According to research, tolerance can form after just one barbiturate administration. Barbiturate withdrawal is similar to benzodiazepine withdrawal and delirium tremens, but it is more severe due to its more direct mechanism of GABA agonism. This is because, like all GABAergic drugs, barbiturate withdrawal can result in potentially fatal effects like seizures. It's regarded as one of the riskiest withdrawal symptoms from any known addictive substance. Longer-acting barbiturates cause a less severe withdrawal syndrome than short-acting and ultra-short-acting barbiturates, much like benzodiazepines do. Higher users experience more severe withdrawal symptoms than those on lower dosages. Withdrawal symptoms are dose-dependent.

The long-term pharmacological management of barbiturate withdrawal frequently entails switching the patient to a long-acting benzodiazepine (i.e., Valium), then weaning off the benzodiazepine gradually. Addiction specialists strongly recommend counseling and support groups for individuals experiencing mental cravings for barbiturates, which may persist for months or even years. Due to the high lethality and relatively quick onset of the withdrawal, patients should never attempt to stop using barbiturates on their own without first speaking with a doctor. Attempting to quit "cold turkey" may result in neurological damage due to excitotoxicity, severe physical injuries received during convulsions, and even death resulting from arrhythmias during Grand-Mal seizures, delirium tremens.

6.1.1.3. Overdose

Sluggishness, incoordination, trouble thinking, slurred speech, poor judgment, drowsiness, shallow breathing, stagger, and, in extreme situations, coma or death are some of the symptoms of an overdose. Barbiturates have a wide range of lethal dosages depending on tolerance and individual differences. The class of barbiturates varies greatly in terms of the lethal dose; super potent barbiturates, like pentobarbital, have the potential to be fatal at much lower doses than low-potency barbiturates, like butalbital. The development of tolerance is still an issue in inpatient settings because stopping a drug after dependence has set in can cause unpleasant and dangerous withdrawal symptoms. Barbiturates are generally inappropriate for long-term psychiatric use because tolerance to their anxiolytic and sedative effects tends to develop more quickly than tolerance to their effects on smooth muscle, respiration, and heart rate. Nonetheless, anticonvulsants remain a good option for long-term epilepsy treatment because tolerance to their effects tends to correlate more with tolerance to physiological effects.

Combining barbiturates excessively with other CNS (central nervous system) depressants (e.g. Because of their combined effects on the central nervous system and respiratory system, alcohol, opiates, and benzodiazepines are even more harmful. Barbiturates enhance the binding affinity of the benzodiazepine binding site, which causes the effects of benzodiazepines to be amplified in addition to their additive effects. The combined effects of the drugs increase the overall function of the channels by 900%, not 600% if a benzodiazepine increases the frequency of channel opening by 300% and a barbiturate increases the duration of their opening by 300%.

The longest-acting barbiturates cause the drug to bioaccumulate in the body because they have half-lives of a day or longer. Even when taken at the therapeutic or recommended dose, long-acting barbiturates' effects wear off much more quickly than they can be eliminated, which means that even though the user experiences little to no effects from the drug's plasma-bound concentrations, the drug can still accumulate to toxic levels in the blood after repeated administration. After the effects of the drug have worn off but before it has cleared the system, users who drink alcohol or take other sedatives may experience a greatly amplified effect from the other sedatives, which can be fatal or severely incapacitating.

Barbiturates stimulate several hepatic CYP enzymes, including CYP2C9, CYP2C19, and CYP3A4. As a result, many prodrugs have their effects amplified, and drugs that are converted to inactive metabolites by these enzymes have their effects diminished. This can lead to lethal overdoses from medications like codeine, tramadol, and carisoprodol, which increase in potency significantly upon CYP enzyme metabolism. While all known members of the class are capable of inducing relevant enzymes, there is a wide range in both the overall degree of induction and the impact on individual enzymes; the most potent inducers of enzymes in the class are phenobarbital and secobarbital, while some of the weakest inducers of enzymes are butalbital and talbutal.

6.1.1.4. Mechanism of Action

Barbiturates function as positive allosteric modulators and, at higher levels, as agonists of GABAA receptors, which are affected by the principal inhibitory neurotransmitter in the mammalian central nervous system (CNS), GABA. Barbiturates attach to the GABAA receptor at multiple homologous transmembrane pockets located at subunit interfaces, separate from GABA and benzodiazepine binding sites. Similar to benzodiazepines, barbiturates enhance the impact of GABA at this receptor. Additionally, barbiturates block AMPA and kainate receptors, types of ionotropic glutamate receptors, which are influenced by the principal excitatory neurotransmitter in the mammalian CNS, glutamate. The combination of barbiturates' enhancement of inhibitory GABAA receptors and inhibition of excitatory AMPA receptors can clarify why these agents have stronger CNS-depressant effects compared to other GABA potentiating agents. At higher concentrations, barbiturates impede the Ca2+-dependent release of neurotransmitters like glutamate by affecting P/Q-type voltage-dependent calcium channels. The pharmacological effects of barbiturates involve prolonging the opening of chloride ion channels at the GABAA receptor, enhancing the efficacy of GABA, while benzodiazepines increase the frequency of chloride ion channel opening, enhancing GABA potency. The direct opening of chloride ion channels is the reason behind the heightened toxicity of barbiturates in overdose compared to benzodiazepines.

Furthermore, barbiturates are relatively non-selective substances that bind to multiple members of the GABAA receptor channel superfamily of ligand-gated ion channels. The neuronal nACh receptor channel, the 5-HT_3 receptor channel, and the glycine receptor channel are members of the Cys-loop receptor superfamily of ion channels. Barbiturates and other general anesthetics increase GABAA receptor currents, but they also block ligand-gated ion channels, which are primarily permeable to cationic ions. For instance, clinically relevant anesthetic concentrations of both thiopental and pentobarbital block neuronal nAChR channels. These results link certain barbiturates' (side) effects to (non-GABA-ergic) ligand-gated ion channels, such as the neuronal nAChR channel. When barbiturates are used in anesthetic concentration, this mechanism accounts for their (mild to moderate) anesthetic effect at high doses.

6.1.1.5. Interactions

Drug interactions with barbiturates are:

- alcohol
- opioids
- benzodiazepines
- anticoagulants
- antihistamines
- atazanavir
- birth-control pills
- boceprevir

6.1.1.6. Caution

Caution is needed in people using:

- Medications such as opioids or benzodiazepines
- Alcohol

Caution is also required in patients with:

- Asthma
- Kidney- or liver-problems
- Heart-disease
- Substance use disorder
- Depression
- History of suicidal thoughts

6.1.2. Benzodiazepines

A benzene ring and a diazepine ring combine to form the basic chemical structure of benzodiazepines, a class of depressant medications. They are prescribed to treat ailments like seizures, insomnia, and anxiety disorders. Leo Sternbach made the accidental discovery of the first benzodiazepine, chlordiazepoxide (Librium), in 1955. Hoffmann-La Roche then commercialized the drug in 1960, and in 1963, diazepam (Valium) was released. When selective serotonin reuptake inhibitors (SSRIs) were introduced, among other factors, prescription rates for benzodiazepines decreased, but they are still widely used globally. By 1977, benzodiazepines were the most prescribed drugs worldwide.

Benzodiazepines are depressants that exert a sedative, hypnotic (sleep-inducing), anxiolytic (anti-anxiety), muscle relaxant, and anticonvulsant effect by amplifying the action of the neurotransmitter gamma-aminobutyric acid (GABA) at the GABAA receptor. Anterograde amnesia and dissociation can also be brought on by high dosages of several shorter-acting benzodiazepines. Withdrawal from alcohol, agitation, seizures, insomnia, anxiety, panic disorder, muscle spasms, and premedication for dental or medical procedures are among the conditions for which benzodiazepines are beneficial. There are three types of benzodiazepines: short-, intermediate-, and long-acting. For the treatment of insomnia, short- and intermediate-acting benzodiazepines are preferred; longer-acting benzodiazepines are advised for the treatment of anxiety.

For brief periods of time—two to four weeks—benzodiazepines are thought to be safe and effective, though they can have paradoxical side effects like aggression or behavioral disinhibition as well as cognitive impairment. Long-term use may result in "impaired thinking or memory loss," according to the Department of Health (Victoria). Depression and anxiety. agitation, hostility, paranoia, etc. A small percentage of people experience paradoxical side effects from benzodiazepines, like increased anxiety or agitation. Because of their negative withdrawal effects, impulsivity, and aggression, benzodiazepines are linked to an increased risk of suicide. Because of worries about physical dependence, benzodiazepine withdrawal syndrome, declining effectiveness, and an elevated risk of dementia and cancer, long-term use of these drugs is controversial. Because older adults are more likely to experience negative side effects in the short and long term, benzodiazepines are all included in the Beers List of drugs that are not appropriate for older adults. The safety of benzodiazepines during pregnancy is a topic of debate. They are known to cause withdrawal symptoms in the newborn, but it is unclear whether they cause neurobehavioral effects due to prenatal exposure or if they cause cleft palate in a small number of babies. Regardless, they are not major teratogens.

Although benzodiazepines are less toxic than their predecessors, the barbiturates, when taken in excess, they can still result in dangerous deep unconsciousness, and fatalities are rare when benzodiazepines are used alone. When combined with other depressants of the central nervous system (CNS), like alcohol and opioids, there is a greater chance of toxicity and lethal overdose. Benzodiazepines are regulated in the majority of nations and are frequently used recreationally. They are also frequently taken in conjunction with other addictive substances.

6.1.2.1. Medical Uses

The psycholeptic, sedative, hypnotic, anxiolytic, anticonvulsant, muscle relaxant, and amnesic properties of benzodiazepines are helpful for many conditions, including alcoholism, seizures, anxiety disorders, panic attacks, restlessness, and insomnia. The majority are taken orally, but they can also be injected into the muscle, or taken rectally. Benzodiazepines are generally well tolerated and, for a variety of conditions, safe and effective short-term medications. In addition to the possibility of dependence and the development of tolerance to their effects, there's also a chance of withdrawal symptoms upon cessation. Their long-term applicability is limited by these factors as well as other potential side effects such as psychomotor, cognitive, or memory impairments following prolonged use. Long-term use or misuse has the potential to cause or exacerbate depression, anxiety, and cognitive deficits. The British Columbia College of Physicians and Surgeons advises against giving benzodiazepines to people taking opioids or who have used them for an extended period of time. These results support clinical and regulatory efforts to reduce benzodiazepine usage, particularly when combined with non-benzodiazepine receptor agonists, as benzodiazepines can have serious adverse health effects.

1. Panic disorder

Benzodiazepines are widely used to treat anxiety related to panic disorder due to their efficacy, tolerability, and quick onset of anxiolytic action. Expert groups disagree, nevertheless, about the long-term benefits of benzodiazepines for panic disorder. There are differing opinions regarding the effectiveness of benzodiazepines over the long term. Some believe they should only be used for patients who are not responding to treatment, while others believe they are just as effective as selective serotonin reuptake inhibitors (SSRIs).

According to the American Psychiatric Association (APA) guidelines, benzodiazepines are generally well tolerated and have been shown in multiple controlled trials to be an effective initial treatment for panic disorder. According to the American Psychological Association, there is not enough data to favor one of the approved treatments for panic disorder over another. Treatment options include tricyclic antidepressants, benzodiazepines, selective serotonin reuptake inhibitors (SNRIs), benzodiazepines, and psychotherapy; the selection should be based on the patient's history, preferences, and other unique characteristics. Although many patients with panic disorder may benefit most from selective serotonin reuptake inhibitors (SSRIs), benzodiazepines are still frequently prescribed and may even be used more frequently than SSRIs, according to certain studies. Benzodiazepines have the advantage of relieving anxiety symptoms considerably more quickly than antidepressants, which makes them a possible choice for patients whose quick symptom relief is essential. Nevertheless, the risk of becoming dependent on benzodiazepines outweighs this benefit. Benzodiazepines are not advised by the American Psychological Association for people who have depressive symptoms or a recent history of substance abuse disorders. According to the American Psychological Association guidelines, treatment with benzodiazepines for panic disorder should be continued for at least a year, as clinical experience suggests, to prevent recurrence. Despite significant worries about benzodiazepine tolerance and withdrawal, long-term benzodiazepine users do not appear to have experienced a significant dose escalation. Stable dosages of benzodiazepines continue to be effective for many of these patients for several years.

The National Institute for Health and Clinical Excellence (NICE), a UK-based organization that issues guidelines, used a different methodology to conduct a systematic review and reached a different conclusion. They questioned the validity of non-placebo-controlled studies. Furthermore, they advise against using benzodiazepines for longer than two to four weeks due to the rapid development of tolerance and physical dependence, which results in withdrawal symptoms like rebound anxiety after six weeks or longer of use, according to the results of placebo-controlled studies. Although specific antidepressants and psychological therapies are advised as first-line treatments for anxiety disorders, benzodiazepines are still prescribed for long-term use. Pregabalin, an anticonvulsant medication, is indicated as a second- or third-line treatment and is suitable for long-term use. According to NICE, clinical guidelines do not recommend the long-term use of benzodiazepines for panic disorder, with or without agoraphobia, as it is an unlicensed indication lacking long-term efficacy. For panic disorder, psychological therapies like cognitive behavioral therapy are advised as a first line of treatment; the use of benzodiazepines has been found to impede the therapeutic benefits of these therapies.

Although lorazepam or diazepam are rarely given intravenously to treat panic attacks, benzodiazepines are typically taken orally.

2. Generalized anxiety disorder

While benzodiazepines have demonstrated strong short-term efficacy in treating generalized anxiety disorder (GAD), they have not been demonstrated to be effective in promoting overall long-term improvement. The National Institute for Health and Clinical Excellence (NICE) states that benzodiazepines may be used, if necessary, to treat GAD right away. They shouldn't, however, typically be administered for more than two to four weeks. Antidepressants are the only drugs that NICE suggests for the long-term treatment of GAD.

Alprazolam, bromazepam, lorazepam, and diazepam are among the benzodiazepines that the Canadian Psychiatric Association (CPA) only suggests as a second-line option in the event that treatment with two separate antidepressants proves to be ineffective. Benzodiazepines are second-line medications, but they can be used briefly to treat severe anxiety and agitation. According to CPA guidelines, benzodiazepines are less effective than antidepressants at reducing ruminative worry, the primary symptom of generalized anxiety disorder (GAD), and their effects may eventually reach the level of a placebo after 4–6 weeks. Nonetheless, there are situations where benzodiazepines can be used in addition to antidepressants for a longer period of time.

3. Anxiety

Benzodiazepines may be prescribed to alleviate acute anxiety because they provide quick and significant relief of symptoms for most people. However, it is advisable not to use them for more than 2–4 weeks as they can lead to tolerance, dependence, and do not show long-term effectiveness. As for insomnia, they may also be used on an irregular/"as-needed" basis, such as in cases where said anxiety is at its worst.

When benzodiazepines are stopped, there is a twice as high chance of the underlying condition returning than with other pharmaceutical treatments. For the long-term treatment of generalized anxiety disorder, pharmacological therapies as well as psychological therapies are advised. In general, antidepressants are safe and effective both in the short and long term, and they have higher rates of remission.

4. Insomnia

For the short term, benzodiazepines can be helpful in treating insomnia. Due to the possibility of dependence, using them for longer than two to four weeks is not advised. In cases where long-term benzodiazepine use for insomnia is indicated, the Committee on Safety of Medicines report suggested treating insomnia with intermittent therapy whenever feasible. Benzodiazepines should ideally be taken at the lowest feasible dosage and sporadically. By extending sleep duration, decreasing wakefulness overall, and cutting down on the amount of time spent in bed before falling asleep, they help with sleep-related issues. But because they promote lighter sleep while decreasing deep sleep, they degrade the quality of our sleep. Additional side effects of hypnotics, such as benzodiazepines, include decreased slow-wave sleep, rebound insomnia, potential tolerance to their effects, and a withdrawal period marked by protracted anxiety and agitation.

The approved list of benzodiazepines for treating insomnia is consistent across most countries, but the designation of first-line hypnotics for insomnia treatment varies by country. Benzodiazepines with longer-acting effects, like nitrazepam and diazepam, are not generally recommended due to their residual effects that can linger into the next day.

Since the introduction of nonbenzodiazepines, or "z-drugs," in 1992 in response to safety concerns, people with insomnia and other sleep disorders have received more prescriptions for nonbenzodiazepines (23% in 1993 to 13% in 2010) and benzodiazepines (23.5% in 1993 to 10.8% in 2010) less frequently. Whether the new non-benzodiazepine hypnotics (Z-drugs) are superior to the short-acting benzodiazepines is unclear. These two classes of drugs have comparable levels of efficacy. Indirect comparison suggests that side effects from benzodiazepines may occur roughly twice as frequently as those from nonbenzodiazepines, according to the US Agency for Healthcare Research and Quality. Certain experts recommend nonbenzodiazepines as the first-choice, long-term treatment for insomnia. The UK's National Institute for Health and Clinical Excellence, however, was unable to locate any solid proof in support of Z-drugs. The NICE review noted that in clinical trials, long-acting benzodiazepines and short-acting Z-drugs were not appropriately compared. Trials comparing appropriate dosages of short-acting benzodiazepines with Z-drugs that act quickly have not been conducted. NICE advised selecting the hypnotic based on the patient's preference and cost as a result.

Benzodiazepines shouldn't be used by older adults to treat insomnia unless all other options have been exhausted. Patients who use benzodiazepines should talk to their doctor, their caregivers, and themselves about the increased risks of side effects. Research indicates that patients who drive have twice the risk of traffic accidents, and older patients are more likely to fall and break their hip.

5. Seizures

Fast-acting benzodiazepines are strong anticonvulsants that are typically effective in treating prolonged convulsive epileptic seizures, which are considered a medical emergency. The first-choice medications in a hospital setting are intravenous clonazepam, lorazepam, and diazepam. Since intravenous administration is impractical in the community, buccal midazolam or rectal diazepam are used instead; buccal is preferred because it is easier to administer and more socially acceptable.

Benzodiazepines were widely used to treat all types of epilepsy when they were first introduced. But with prolonged use, drowsiness and tolerance develop into issues, and none of the options are now regarded as first-line for long-term epilepsy therapy. Worldwide, specialized epilepsy clinics use clobazam extensively, and clonazepam is well-liked in the Netherlands, Belgium, and France. In the US, clobazam's use was authorized in 2011. Clobazam and clonazepam are second-line options for treating various types of epilepsy in the United Kingdom. Clobazam is also helpful in the treatment of catamenial epilepsy and very short-term seizure prevention. Given the potential for rebound seizures, it is especially important to exercise extra caution when stopping long-term epilepsy medication. As a result, the dosage is gradually reduced over a minimum of six months.

6. Alcohol withdrawal

Although diazepam can be used as an alternative, chlordiazepoxide is the most frequently used benzodiazepine for alcohol detoxification. Both are short-term prescriptions meant to minimize the possibility of tolerance and dependence on the benzodiazepine medication itself. They are utilized in the detoxification of people who are motivated to stop drinking. Longer half-lived benzodiazepines facilitate detoxification and reduce the risk of hazardous (and possibly fatal) alcohol withdrawal symptoms. However, it is not advised to use short-acting benzodiazepines for detoxification in an outpatient setting as they may cause breakthrough seizures. Since oxycodone and lorazepam are metabolized differently from other benzodiazepines through conjugation, they are frequently prescribed to patients who are at risk of drug accumulation, including the elderly and those with cirrhosis.

When it comes to treating alcohol withdrawal syndrome, benzodiazepines are the recommended option because they can prevent and treat dangerous seizure complications and calm extremely severe delirium. The most successful benzodiazepine for both preventing and treating acute seizures is lorazepam, which is the only one with consistent intramuscular absorption.

7. Contraindications

In those who are vulnerable, benzodiazepines may induce respiratory depression due to their muscle relaxant effect. As such, they should not be used in patients with COPD, bronchitis, sleep apnea, or myasthenia gravis. Because benzodiazepines frequently cause paradoxical reactions, care must be taken when administering them to individuals with personality disorders or intellectual disabilities. They are occasionally used for suicidal overdoses and can trigger suicidal thoughts in people suffering from major depression. Benzodiazepines should not be taken by anyone with a history of excessive alcohol consumption or non-medical use of opioids or barbiturates because these medications carry a risk of potentially fatal interactions.

8. Pregnancy

The Food and Drug Administration in the US has classified benzodiazepines as either category D or X, indicating that there is proof of a potential risk to the fetus.

While some studies find no correlation between benzodiazepines and cleft palate, exposure to these drugs during pregnancy has been linked to a slightly increased (from 0.06 to 0.07%) risk of cleft palate in newborns. When used by expectant mothers in the final stages of pregnancy, they may cause the syndrome known as floppy infants. This condition typically affects newborns and causes hypotonia, hypothermia, lethargy, and difficulties with feeding and breathing. Babies who were repeatedly exposed to benzodiazepines while still in utero have been reported to have cases of neonatal withdrawal syndrome. Since this syndrome can appear several days after delivery—it can appear as late as 21 days in the case of chlordiazepoxide—it may be challenging to diagnose. For as long as three to six months, the symptoms—which include tremors, hypertonia, hyperreflexia, hyperactivity, and vomiting—may persist. Reducing the dosage while pregnant might make it less severe. Benzodiazepines with a longer and better safety record—like diazepam or chlordiazepoxide—are advised against potentially more dangerous ones—like temazepam or triazolam—when used during pregnancy. The risks to the fetus are reduced when the lowest effective dose is used for the shortest amount of time.

9. Elderly

In the elderly, benzodiazepines have the least advantages and the highest risks. The American Geriatrics Society lists them as a potentially inappropriate medication for older adults. The long-term effects of benzodiazepines and benzodiazepine dependence in the elderly can resemble dementia, depression, or anxiety syndromes, and they worsen over time. The elderly are more susceptible to dependence and to its side effects, which include memory loss, daytime sedation, impaired motor coordination, an increased risk of motor vehicle accidents and falls, and an increased risk of hip fractures. It is possible to confuse adverse effects on cognition for the effects of aging. Withdrawal has several advantages, such as enhanced mobility, alertness, and cognition; it also lowers the risk of incontinence and fractures and falls. Benzodiazepines can be tapered down gradually with equal success in older adults as in younger adults. Elderly patients should only receive low-dose, short-term prescriptions for benzodiazepines, and with extreme caution. For elderly patients, short- to intermediate-acting benzodiazepines like temazepam and oxazepam are recommended. The elderly should not take long-acting benzodiazepines or the strong benzodiazepines triazolam and alprazolam due to increased side effects. Low dosages of sedating antidepressants and nonbenzodiazepines like zolpidem and zaleplon are occasionally used as benzodiazepine substitutes.

Reducing prescription levels is likely to lower the risk of dementia because long-term benzodiazepine use is linked to an increased risk of cognitive impairment and dementia. Uncertainty surrounds the relationship between benzodiazepine use in the past and cognitive decline; some studies report a lower risk of cognitive decline in former users, while others find no association and still others indicate an increased risk.

Benzodiazepines are sometimes used treat dementia's behavioral symptoms. Though antipsychotics have demonstrated some benefit, they, like antidepressants, have little evidence of efficacy. Dementia can be made worse by the benzodiazepine's cognitively impairing effects, which are common in the elderly.

6.1.2.2. Adverse Effect

The sedative and muscle-relaxing effects of benzodiazepines are the most frequent side effects. They consist of fatigue, lightheadedness, and a decline in focus and alertness. Injuries and falls can occur from poor coordination, especially in the elderly. Impaired driving abilities and a higher risk of traffic accidents are further outcomes. A common side effect is decreased libido and difficulties getting an erection. Disinhibition and depression could surface. Intravenous use may result in hypotension and suppressed breathing, or hypoventilation. A less frequent range of adverse effects includes vomiting, altered appetite, depersonalization, euphoria, confusion, and nightmares. Although they are extremely rare, cases of liver toxicity have been reported. Long-term benzodiazepine use can lead to affective and behavioral issues, as well as cognitive impairment. There may also be feelings of chaos, trouble thinking clearly, loss of sex drive, agoraphobia, social anxiety, rising anxiety and depression, loss of interest in hobbies and leisure activities, and an inability to feel or communicate emotions. However, not everyone has issues after prolonged use. Moreover, there may be changes in one's perception of oneself, one's surroundings, and one's relationships. According to a 2020 study, long-term prescription benzodiazepine use is linked to a higher all-cause death rate in people under 65, but not in people over 65. The study also discovered that, only in patients 65 years of age or younger, the all-cause death rate was higher in situations where benzodiazepines and opioids were prescribed together as opposed to separately.

Hospital visits involving benzodiazepines had a 66% higher risk of a serious adverse health outcome when compared to other sedative-hypnotics. The odds of a serious health outcome were nearly four times higher for visits involving benzodiazepines and non-benzodiapine receptor agonists. This included hospitalization, patient transfer, or death.

September of 2020 saw the U.S. Food and Drug Administration (FDA) mandated that the risks of abuse, misuse, addiction, physical dependence, and withdrawal reactions be consistently described in the boxed warning for all benzodiazepine medications.

1. Cognitive effects

The most significant of these negative effects of short-term benzodiazepine use on cognition is its interference with the formation and consolidation of new material memories, which can lead to complete anterograde amnesia. Regarding the consequences of continuous administration, researchers disagree. According to one perspective, many of the short-term effects persist and sometimes even get worse over time when benzodiazepines are stopped. According to a different perspective, chronic benzodiazepine users experience cognitive deficits only briefly after taking the medication, and these deficits are thought to be caused by the anxiety disorder.

A 2004 meta-analysis of 13 small studies supported the former view, even though the conclusive studies are still lacking. According to this meta-analysis, extended use of benzodiazepines was linked to moderate to severe negative effects on all areas of cognition, with the most frequent impairment found to be in visuospatial memory. Reduced IQ, visiomotor coordination, information processing, verbal learning, and concentration were among the other impairments mentioned. The subjects were primarily recruited from withdrawal clinics; the coexisting drug use, alcohol use, and psychiatric disorders were not defined; and several of the included studies carried out the cognitive assessments during the withdrawal period. These factors, according to the authors of the meta-analysis and a subsequent reviewer, limit the applicability of this meta-analysis.

2. Paradoxical effects

Sometimes there are paradoxical reactions, including increased seizures in epileptics, violence, impulsivity, aggression, irritability, and suicidal thoughts and actions. These responses have been described as the result of losing control over socially unacceptable behavior due to disinhibition. In the general population, paradoxical reactions are uncommon, occurring at a rate of less than 1% and being comparable to placebo. However, those who abuse drugs recreationally, those who suffer from borderline personality disorder, kids, and patients on high dosage regimens experience them more frequently. In these populations, learning disabilities and neurological disorders are also major risk factors for disinhibition; however, impulse control issues may be the most important risk factor. High dosages of strong benzodiazepines are involved in the majority of reports of disinhibition. Adverse effects can also arise from long-term benzodiazepine use.

3. Long-term worsening of psychiatric symptoms

While some patients may benefit from benzodiazepines in the short term for their anxiety, agitation, and sleep, prolonged use (i.e., more than two to four weeks) can exacerbate the very symptoms that these drugs are intended to treat. Possible explanations include compounding the cognitive issues associated with anxiety disorders, generating or exacerbating depression and suicidality, interfering with deep stage sleep and disrupting sleep architecture, causing withdrawal symptoms or rebound symptoms between doses that resemble or exacerbate underlying anxiety or sleep disorders, impeding the benefits of psychotherapy by impeding memory consolidation and lowering fear extinction, and lowering stress/trauma coping and making one more susceptible to stress in the future. Benzodiazepines may be harmful or ineffective in treating PTSD and phobias, according to the latter two theories. Although withdrawal symptoms such as anxiety, insomnia, and irritability may worsen for a while, psychiatric symptoms after stopping benzodiazepines are typically less severe than they were when using them. After stopping, functioning considerably improves after a year.

6.1.2.3. Benzodiazepine Overdose

The term "benzodiazepine overdose" refers to the ingestion of a benzodiazepine drug in amounts that exceed what is generally advised or used. The most typical signs of an overdose are ataxia, slurred speech, depression of the central nervous system (CNS), and impaired balance. Respiratory depression and coma are examples of severe symptoms. The cornerstone of treatment for benzodiazepine overdose is supportive care. Flumazenil is an antidote; however its application is debatable.

Overdose deaths resulting from benzodiazepine overdoses are rare, especially after hospital admission. Nevertheless, it is especially risky to combine large doses of benzodiazepines with alcohol, barbiturates, opioids, or tricyclic antidepressants as this can result in serious side effects like coma or even death. Benzodiazepines were implicated in 31% of the estimated 22,767 prescription drug overdose deaths that occurred in the US in 2013. Subsequently, the US Food and Drug Administration (FDA) released a black box warning about using opioids and benzodiazepines at the same time. One of the most frequently prescribed drug classes is benzodiazepines, which are also frequently used to self-poison. In the UK, benzodiazepines, with or without alcohol, have been linked to 1512 fatal poisonings over a ten-year period. It has been demonstrated that temazepam is more toxic than most benzodiazepines. According to an Australian study, when benzodiazepines are overdosed, temazepam is more toxic and sedative than oxazepam.

6.1.3. Zopiclone

Among other names for it, zopiclone is a nonbenzodiazepine that is prescribed to treat insomnia. Zopiclone belongs to the cyclopyrrolone class of medications and differs molecularly from benzodiazepine medications. However, by modulating GABAA receptors in a manner akin to that of benzodiazepine drugs, zopiclone increases the normal transmission of the neurotransmitter gamma-aminobutyric acid (GABA) in the central nervous system similar to the effects of benzodiazepines. It is a sedative, zopiclone. It functions by tranquilizing or depressing the central nervous system. The effects of zopiclone can become accustomed to the body after extended use. Withdrawal symptoms could happen if the medication is suddenly stopped or the dose is lowered. These may include a variety of symptoms resembling the withdrawal symptoms from benzodiazepines. While the symptoms of withdrawal from zopiclone and its isomers at therapeutic dosages (i.e., eszopiclone) do not usually cause convulsions and are therefore not thought to be life-threatening, but patients may become so agitated or anxious that they go to the emergency room. While eszopiclone, the active stereoisomer of zopiclone, is commercially available in the US, zopiclone is not. In the US, Japan, Brazil, New Zealand, and several European nations, zopiclone is a controlled substance; it may be against the law to possess without a prescription.

Zopiclone is known colloquially as a "Z-drug." Other Z-drugs include zaleplon and zolpidem and were initially thought to be less addictive than benzodiazepines. However, this appraisal has shifted somewhat in the last few years as cases of addiction and habituation have been presented. Zopiclone is recommended to be taken at the lowest effective dose, with a duration of 2–3 weeks for short-term insomnia. Daily or continuous use of the drug is not usually advised, and caution must be taken when the compound is used in conjunction with benzodiazepines, sedatives or other drugs affecting the central nervous system.

6.1.3.1. Medical Uses

For the short term treatment of insomnia when the inability to fall asleep or stay asleep is a major symptom, zolpicol is used. Given the potential for tolerance, dependence, and addiction, prolonged use is not advised. More research in this area has been recommended. A low-quality study revealed that zopiclone is ineffective in increasing sleep duration or improving sleep quality in shift workers.

When treating insomnia, cognitive behavioral therapy has been shown to be more effective than zopiclone and to have long-lasting effects on sleep quality that last for at least a year after therapy.

6.1.3.2. Specific Populations

1. Elderly

Like other benzodiazepines and nonbenzodiazepine hypnotic medications, zolpicol impairs a person's ability to maintain balance and stand steadily when they wake up in the middle of the night or early the following day. Hip fractures and falls are commonplace. These impairments are made worse by the combination with alcohol consumption. Tolerance to these impairments develops, albeit incompletely. Along with increased cognitive side effects, zopiclone causes postural sway and an increase in falls among the elderly. An important cause of death for the elderly is falls.

There is strong evidence of the efficacy and long-term advantages of non-pharmacological treatments for insomnia, according to a thorough evaluation of the medical literature on the topic of managing insomnia in the elderly. Nonbenzodiazepine sedative-hypnotics, like zopiclone, have little to no advantage over benzodiazepines in terms of efficacy or tolerability in older adults. Elderly patients with chronic insomnia may respond better to newer, more effective treatments, such as melatonin receptor agonists. There is no evidence to support the long-term use of sedative-hypnotics for insomnia, and it is not advised due to possible side effects like motor incoordination, sedation during the day, cognitive impairment (anterograde amnesia), and an increased risk of falls and auto accidents. Furthermore, it is still unknown how safe and effective it is to use nonbenzodiazepine hypnotic medications over the long term.

2. Liver disease

In addition to eliminating zopiclone far more slowly than healthy patients with liver disease also experience amplified pharmacological effects from the medication.

6.1.3.3. Adverse Reactions

There is a higher risk of death linked to sleeping pills, such as zopiclone. The British National Formulary states adverse reactions as follows: "taste disturbance (some report a metallic taste); less commonly nausea, vomiting, dizziness, drowsiness, dry mouth, headache; rarely amnesia, confusion, depression, hallucinations, nightmares; very rarely light headedness, incoordination, paradoxical effects and sleep-walking also reported."

6.1.3.4. Contraindications

Driving abilities are similarly affected by zolpidem like they are by benzodiazepines. Long-term hypnotic drug users for sleep disorders only partially adapt to the negative effects on driving; even one year after starting treatment, hypnotic drug users still have a higher rate of motor vehicle accidents. Patients who operate motor vehicles shouldn't take zopiclone because doing so greatly increases their risk of having an accident. A psychomotor impairment is brought on by zolpicolone. After taking zopiclone, one should avoid operating machinery or driving since side effects, such as poor hand-eye coordination, can persist into the following day.

According to a double-blind study, melatonin (which has no effect), zaleplon, temazepam, and zopiclone were the drugs listed in increasing order of performance impact duration. This information is relevant to military personnel who may need to be awakened to perform their duties. Measures were taken of the effects on multitask (MT), serial subtraction (SST), logical reasoning (LRT), and serial reaction time (SRT). The times to return to normal performance for

SRT were 3.25, 6.25, and 5.25 hours for zaleplon (10 mg), 7.5 mg for zopiclone, and 15 mg for temazepam. Similarly, for LRT, the times were 3.25, >6.25, and 4.25 hours; for SST, they were 2.25, >6.25, and 4.25 hours; and for MT, they were 2.25, 4.25, and 3.25 hours. The drugs' ability to promote sleep was not taken into account in the study.

6.1.3.5. Overdose

Sometimes people use zopiclone as a means of suicide. With the exception of temazepam, which is extremely toxic in overdose, it has a fatality index comparable to benzodiazepine medications. Overdosing on zopiclone alone or in combination with other drugs has resulted in fatalities. A zopiclone overdose may cause excessive drowsiness and decreased breathing, which could lead to a coma and even death. Combining zopiclone with opiates, alcohol, or other drugs that depress the central nervous system may increase the risk of lethal overdoses. Flumazenil, a GABAA receptor benzodiazepine site antagonist, can be used to treat zopiclone overdose by displacing the drug from its binding site and quickly undoing its effects. When combined with piperazine, a zopiclone overdose can also have serious cardiac effects.

The number of deaths linked to zopiclone is increasing, according to death certificates. It usually has no fatal effects when taken by itself, but the risk of a serious and deadly overdose rises when combined with alcohol, other drugs, like opioids, or in patients who have liver or respiratory conditions.

6.1.3.6. Interactions

Zopiclone also interacts with trimipramine and caffeine.

When alcohol is mixed with zopiclone, it has an additive effect that greatly increases the side effects, including the potential for overdose. When using zopiclone, alcohol should be avoided due to these risks and the increased risk of dependence.

Erythromycin seems to speed up zopiclone's absorption and extend its half-life of elimination, raising plasma levels and intensifying its effects. The pharmacokinetics of zopiclone are similarly affected by itraconazole and erythromycin. The drug interaction between erythromycin and itraconazole when used with zopiclone may be more severe in the elderly. It might be necessary to temporarily lower the dosage during combined therapy, particularly in the elderly. Zopiclone's half-life and peak plasma levels are significantly shortened by rifampicin, which significantly lessens the drug's hypnotic effect. Carbamazepine and phenytoin may also cause comparable interactions. Both sulfaphenazole and ketoconazole affect zopiclone metabolism. Nefazodone inhibits the metabolism of zopiclone, which raises levels of the drug and causes noticeable sedation the following day.

6.1.4. Zolpidem

One of the main uses of zolpidem, which is marketed under several brands including Ambien, is the temporary management of sleep disorders. According to guidelines, it should only be used after behavioral modifications like improving sleep hygiene and cognitive behavioral therapy for insomnia have been tried. In larger doses, it helps people stay asleep longer and reduces the time it takes for sleep to start by about fifteen minutes. It is taken orally and comes in tablet, sublingual tablet, and oral spray form.

Headache, nausea, diarrhea, and daytime sleepiness are typical side effects. More serious adverse effects include confusion and delusions. While the effects of zolpidem can be reversed by the GABAA-receptor antagonist flumazenil, supportive care is typically the only course of action advised in cases of overdose.

Z-drug, also known as nonbenzodiazepine, zolpidem is a sedative and hypnotic. Zolpidem belongs to the imidazopyridine class of GABAA receptor agonists. By attaching to GABAA receptors in the same spot as benzodiazepines, it increases the effects of GABA in the central nervous system. Its half-life is typically two to three hours. However, individuals with liver issues experience an increase in this.

In 1992, zolpidem received FDA approval for use in medicine. In 2007, it was made accessible as a generic drug. According to the Controlled Substances Act of 1970 (CSA), zolpidem is classified as a Schedule IV controlled substance. It's one of the most widely prescribed treatments for sleep disorders, with over 10 million prescriptions filled annually in the US. With over 10 million prescriptions, it was the 63rd most frequently prescribed drug in the US in 2021.

6.1.4.1. Medical Uses

The lowest dose of zolpidem is recommended for the short-term (typically two to six week) treatment of insomnia. It can be applied to enhance falling asleep, staying asleep, and sleep onset latency.

According to guidelines from the American College of Physicians, NICE, and the European Sleep Research Society, medication for insomnia (possibly zolpidem) should only be used as a second line of treatment after non-pharmacological options (such as cognitive behavioral therapy) have been exhausted. This is partially based on a 2012 review that concluded psychological effects account for almost half of zolpidem's effectiveness rather than the drug itself.

6.1.4.2. Contraindications

Those who suffer from respiratory depression, myasthenia gravis, severe liver disease, obstructive sleep apnea, children, or psychotic illnesses shouldn't take zolpidem. Those who are or have been addicted to other substances shouldn't take it.

The use of zolpidem may impede one's ability to drive, increasing the chance of an accident. This side effect happens with other hypnotic medications as well, not just zolpidem. Motor vehicle drivers ought to drive cautiously. Due to reduced function the day after taking the medication, the FDA recommended in 2013 that prescribers consider lowering dosages for men and women.

Elderly people should not be prescribed zolpidem because they are more susceptible to the side effects of hypnotics like zolpidem and are more likely to fall or experience other negative cognitive effects like delirium and neurocognitive disorder.

The FDA has not classified zolpidem as being in a pregnancy category. At doses greater than seven times the maximum recommended human dose or higher, animal studies have shown evidence of incomplete ossification and increased intrauterine fetal death; however, teratogenicity was not observed at any dose level. In human pregnancy, no controlled data exist. In one case report, cord blood from the newborn contained zolpidem. Use of zolpidem during pregnancy is advised only in situations where advantages outweigh risks.

6.1.4.3. Adverse Effects

The most common adverse effects of short-term use include headache (reported by 7% of people in clinical trials), drowsiness (2%), dizziness (1%), and diarrhea (1%); the most common side effects of long-term use included drowsiness (8%), dizziness (5%), allergy (4%), sinusitis (4%), back pain (3%), diarrhea (3%), drugged feeling (3%), dry mouth (3%), lethargy (3%), sore throat (3%), abdominal pain (2%), constipation (2%), heart palpitations (2%), lightheadedness (2%), rash (2%), abnormal dreams (1%), amnesia (1%), chest pain (1%), depression (1%), flu-like symptoms (1%), and sleep disorder (1%).

Zolpidem has been linked to an increased risk of death as well as an increased risk of depression, falls, fractures, impaired driving, and suppressed breathing. Additionally common are upper and lower respiratory infections, affecting 1–10% of the population.

After being administered at night, residual "hangover" effects, such as drowsiness and diminished psychomotor and cognitive function, may last throughout the day. These side effects could make it more difficult for users to drive safely and raise the possibility of hip fractures and falls. Approximately 3% of zolpidem users may break a bone in a fall as a result of the medication's decreased coordination.

While taking zolpidem, some users have experienced unexplained sleepwalking, sleep driving, night eating syndrome, and the inability to perform other daily tasks while asleep. According to research conducted by the National Prescribing Service in Australia, these side effects typically manifest themselves a few days or after the first dose is taken. The Australian Therapeutic Goods Administration included a boxed warning about this side effect in February 2008.

1. Tolerance, dependence and withdrawal

Zolpidem is only prescribed for severe insomnia and for brief periods of time at the lowest effective dose because it is linked to drug tolerance and substance dependence. Some people can become tolerant to zolpidem's effects in a matter of weeks. When used for extended periods of time and at high doses, abrupt withdrawal can have negative effects such as delirium, seizures, or other health problems. Treatment usually involves a gradual dose reduction over several months to minimize withdrawal symptoms, which can mimic those experienced during benzodiazepine withdrawal, when drug tolerance and physical dependence to zolpidem develop. If that doesn't work, some people might need to try an alternate approach, like switching to a longer-acting benzodiazepine medication that has a benzodiazepine equivalent dose, like diazepam or chlordiazepoxide, and then gradually lowering the dose of the long-acting benzodiazepine. Flumazenil can be administered intravenously to patients who are hard to treat. This allows for the fast and competitive binding of flumazenil as an antagonist to the GABAA-receptor, effectively blocking the ability of zolpidem to bind as an agonist. As a result, drug dependence or addiction to zolpidem will gradually go away.

Abuse or physical dependence on zolpidem may be more likely in alcoholics or those in recovery from alcoholism. Those with a history of alcoholism, recreational drug use, physical dependence, or psychological dependence on sedative-hypnotic drugs are not usually prescribed it. According to a 2014 review, there was evidence of drug-seeking behavior, with zolpidem prescriptions accounting for 20% of forged or falsified prescriptions.

Studies on the ability of zolpidem to induce tolerance in rodents have revealed that it is less capable of doing so than benzodiazepines;

however, in primates, zolpidem's capacity to induce tolerance was equivalent to that of benzodiazepines.

2. Overdose

Overdosing may result in death or a coma. There are frequently additional drugs in the victim's system when overdosing occurs. The GABAA receptor antagonist flumazenil can be used to treat zolpidem overdose by displacing zolpidem from its binding site on the GABAA receptor and quickly undoing the drug's effects.

3. Detection in body fluids

Zolpidem can be measured in blood or plasma to support a hospitalized patient's diagnosis of poisoning, to offer proof in an arrest for driving while intoxicated, or to support a medicolegal death investigation. Zolpidem concentrations in blood or plasma typically range from 30–300 μg/L in patients receiving the medication therapeutically, 100–700 μg/L in drivers arrested for driving while intoxicated, and 1000–7000 μg/L in acute overdose victims. Generally speaking, analytical techniques use liquid or gas chromatography.

6.1.4.4. Pharmacology

1. Mechanism of action

In the central nervous system, zolpidem is a ligand of high-affinity positive modulator sites of GABAA receptors that strengthens GABAergic inhibition of neurotransmission. It attaches itself specifically to the pentameric ion channel's α_1 subunits. As such, it possesses potent hypnotic qualities along with weaker myorelaxant, anticonvulsant, and anxiolytic effects. Zolpidem can bind to binary αβ GABA receptors in contrast to diazepam; here, it has been demonstrated to bind to the α_1–α_1 subunit interface. When compared to α_1, zolpidem's affinity for the α_2- and α_3-subunits is about 10 times lower, and it has almost no affinity for receptors that contain the α_5 subunit. The GABAA receptors classified as ω_1 type are mainly located in the brain, while the receptors classified as ω_2 type are mainly found in the spine and contain the α_2-, α_3-, α_4-, α_5-, or $\alpha_6$subunits. Because of this, zolpidem prefers to bind to GABAA receptors in the brain as opposed to the spine. Like most benzodiazepine-like drugs, zolpidem also lacks affinity for receptors containing α_4 and α_6, and it has no affinity for receptors containing the γ_1 and γ_3 subunits. Without influencing desensitization or peak currents, zolpidem modulates the receptor most likely by causing a conformational change in the receptor that permits an increased binding strength of the orthosteric agonist GABA towards its cognate receptor.

Similar to zaleplon, zolpidem has no effect on stage 2 sleep but may increase slow wave sleep. Few consistent differences were found between zolpidem and benzodiazepines in terms of sleep onset latency, total sleep duration, number of awakenings, quality of sleep, adverse events, tolerance, rebound insomnia, and daytime alertness, according to a meta-analysis comparing benzodiazepines against nonbenzodiazepines.

2. Pharmacokinetics

According to microsome studies, CYP3A4 (61%), CYP2C9 (22%), CYP1A2 (14%), CYP2D6 (<3%), and CYP2C19 (<3%) are the enzymes that metabolize zolpidem. Urine contains less than 1% of the substance unaltered. Three metabolites are primarily produced by it, but none of them are thought to have pharmacological activity. About 70% of zolpidem is bioavailable in its entirety. In healthy adults, the medication has a half-life of two to three hours and reaches peak concentration in about two hours. Children have a shorter half-life of zolpidem than do the elderly and those with liver problems. Men may metabolize zolpidem more quickly than women, according to certain studies, but this may be because of testosterone. According to a review, women's clearance was only 33% lower than men's, which may indicate that the FDA's 50% dosage reduction for women was excessive.

6.1.4.5. Interactions

When taking zolpidem, people shouldn't drink alcohol. They also shouldn't be prescribed opioid medications or use illegal opioids for recreational purposes. Additionally, opioids may raise the possibility of developing a zolpidem psychological dependence. The risk of respiratory depression and death rises when opioids and zolpidem are used together. Patients taking benzodiazepines or other drugs that depress the central nervous system (CNS) should not be denied access to the opioid addiction medications buprenorphine and methadone, according to advice from the US Food and Drug Administration (FDA). If someone takes zolpidem along with antipsychotics, other sedatives, anxiolytics, antidepressants, antiepileptic medications, and antihistamines, the sedation the next day may get worse. When taking zolpidem along with antidepressants, some patients experienced visual hallucinations.

A given dosage of zolpidem will have greater effects when combined with cytochrome P450 inhibitors, especially CYP3A4 and CYP1A2 inhibitors like fluvoxamine, ciprofloxacin, and clarithromycin. Activators of cytochrome P450, such as St. John's Wort may lessen zolpidem's action. According to one study, caffeine raises the concentration of zolpidem over time by roughly 20%. It also doesn't fully make up for the cognitive impairment that zolpidem causes. According to other research, caffeine has no effect on the metabolism of zolpidem. (Katzung et al, 2009; Aubrun et al, 2019; Crockett et al, 2019)

6.2. Narcotic Analgesics

Analgesics are medications (natural or synthetic) that block the central nervous system (CNS) or peripheral pain pathways to reduce pain without knocking out. Analgesics fall into two primary categories:

a. Opioid/narcotic/morphine like analgesics.

b. Non-opioid/non-narcotic/aspirin-like analgesics.

Narcotic analgesics, often known as opioids, are pharmaceuticals derived from morphine. The Papaver somniferum opium poppy is the source of opium. It contains two kinds of alkaloids, such as derivatives of phenanthrene (morphine, codeine, and thebaine) and derivatives of benzylisoquinoline (papaverine and noscapine).

6.2.1. Opioids

A class of medications known as opioids is derived from or imitates natural substances present in the opium poppy plant. Opioids have many effects on the brain, one of which is the reduction of pain. They are a class of drugs that have morphine-like effects by binding to opioid receptors. Although the terms "opioid" and "opiate" are occasionally used synonymously, there are important distinctions between them because of how these drugs are made.

In medicine, their main application is in the treatment of pain, including anesthesia. Additional medical applications include treating opioid use disorder with replacement therapy, treating diarrhea, stopping an opioid overdose, and suppressing cough. Strong opioids like carfentanil are only permitted for use in veterinary medicine. In addition, opiates are commonly used recreationally for the euphoric effects or to avoid withdrawal symptoms. In the US, opioids have been used in executions and have the potential to be fatal.

Opioid side effects can include euphoria, constipation, nausea, sedation, itching, and respiratory depression. Long-term drug use can result in physical dependence, which means that abruptly stopping the drug causes unpleasant withdrawal symptoms, and tolerance, which means that higher doses are needed to get the same effect. The high encourages recreational use, and regular, increasing recreational use of opioids leads to addiction most of the time. Respiratory depression is a common cause of death from drugs that depressants like benzodiazepines, whether taken in excess or in combination with them.

Opioid receptors, which are primarily located in the central and peripheral nervous systems as well as the gastrointestinal tract, are the site of action for opioids. These receptors mediate opioids' somatic and psychoactive effects. Opioid medications include partial agonists, such as loperamide, which prevents diarrhea, and antagonists, such as naloxegol, which treats constipation brought on by opioids. While they do not cross the blood-brain barrier, they can prevent other opioids from binding to the same receptors in the myenteric plexus.

The majority of opioids are controlled substances due to their potential for addiction and deadly overdose. Approximately 28 to 38 million individuals used opioids illegally in 2013 (or 0.6 to 0.8% of the world's population between the ages of 15 and 65). An estimated 4 million Americans either depended on opioids or used them recreationally in 2011. As of 2015, cheap illicit heroin and overprescription of opioid drugs were to blame for rising rates of addiction and recreational use.

On the other hand, concerns about opioid addiction, overprescribing, and inflated side effects are also held responsible for the undertreatment of pain.

6.2.1.1. Medical Uses

1. Pain

For the treatment of mild pain, the weak opioid codeine is frequently found in prescription medications and over-the-counter in combination with one or more other drugs in low doses. Usually, moderate to severe pain relief is the only use for other opioids.

2. Acute pain

When it comes to treating acute pain, such as pain after surgery, opioids work well. Opioids are often the first choice for treating moderate to severe acute pain because of their quick onset, high efficacy, and low dependence risk. A recent study, however, demonstrated a definite risk of long-term opioid use when opioid analgesics are started for the acute treatment of pain following surgery or trauma. They've also been shown to be crucial in palliative care, helping with the severe, persistent, incapacitating pain that can accompany degenerative diseases like rheumatoid arthritis and some terminal illnesses like cancer. Opioids are frequently a successful long-term care option for cancer patients experiencing chronic pain.

In the United States, just over half of the states have passed legislation limiting the prescription or dispensing of opioids for acute pain.

3. Chronic non-cancer pain

Guidelines have indicated that when opioids are used to treat the majority of chronic non-cancer conditions, such as back pain, headaches, and fibromyalgia, their risks are probably greater than their benefits. As such, their use in chronic non-cancer pain should be done so with caution.

The advantages and disadvantages should be reevaluated if utilized, ideally every three months. Opioids are a treatment option for chronic pain that should be explored only after less dangerous options such as NSAIDs like ibuprofen or naproxen or paracetamol/acetaminophen have been exhausted. Certain types of chronic pain, such as pain from migraines or fibromyalgia, are better treated with medications other than opioids. It's unclear if taking opioids will help reduce chronic neuropathic pain.

As a first-line treatment for headaches, opioids are not recommended due to their tendency to impair alertness, cause dependence, and raise the possibility that episodic headaches will become chronic. Additionally, opioids may increase sensitivity to headache pain. If the patient can be closely watched to prevent the development of chronic headache, opioids may be appropriate for treating headache when other treatments are ineffective or unavailable.

More often than not, opioids are used to treat chronic non-malignant pain. Due to this practice, there is currently a new and expanding issue with opioid addiction and misuse. Opioids should not be used for long-term chronic pain management due to many adverse effects unless all other less dangerous painkillers have been proven to be ineffective. Pain that is not always severe, like that caused by fibromyalgia, migraines, or nerve pain, is often better managed with non-opioid medications. Safer substitutes include nonsteroidal anti-inflammatory medications like ibuprofen and naproxen as well as paracetamol/tylenol/acetaminophen. They are commonly used in combination with opioids, such as ibuprofen and hydrocodone (Vicoprofen) or paracetamol and oxycodone (Percocet), to increase pain relief while also discouraging recreational use.

6.2.1.2. Adverse Effects

Over 15 million people suffer from opioid addiction, and 69,000 people globally pass away from opioid overdoses every year.

In older adults, opioid use is associated with increased adverse effects such as "sedation, nausea, vomiting, constipation, urinary retention, and falls." As a result, older adults taking opioids are at greater risk for injury. Opioids do not cause any specific organ toxicity, unlike many other drugs, such as aspirin and paracetamol. They are not associated with upper gastrointestinal bleeding and kidney toxicity.

Opioid prescriptions for osteoarthritis treatment and acute low back pain appear to have long-term negative consequences.

The USCDC reports that between 1999 and 2010, methadone was implicated in 31% of opioid-related deaths in the US and 40% of cases where methadone was the only drug involved, a significantly higher percentage than other opioids. Research on long-term opioid use has shown that many people stop using them and that mild side effects are typical. Addiction was present in roughly 0.3% of cases. One in seven Americans died from an opioid overdose in the United States in 2016.

1. Nausea and vomiting

It takes 7–10 days to reach tolerance to nausea, during which time antiemetics, e.g. Haloperidol at a low dose (once at night) works wonders. Haloperidol is no longer often used because of serious side effects like tardive dyskinesia. Prochlorperazine, a comparable medication, is used more frequently despite having comparable risks. Even though they are more expensive, stronger antiemetics like tropisetron or ondansetron are occasionally used when nausea is severe or persistent and bothersome. Dopamine antagonists like metoclopramide and domperidone are less costly options. Domperidone inhibits the opioid emetic action in the chemoreceptor trigger zone but does not cross the blood–brain barrier or have negative central antidopaminergic effects. This medication cannot be purchased in the U.S.

Certain antihistamines possessing anticholinergic qualities (e.g., Diphenhydramine and orphenadrine) might also work well. Hydroxyzine, a first-generation antihistamine, is widely used and has the added benefits of not causing movement disorders and having analgesic-sparing properties. In addition to producing analgesia that may permit lower doses of opioids with less nausea and vomiting, Δ9-tetrahydrocannabinol relieves nausea and vomiting.

- 5-HT3 antagonists (e.g. ondansetron)
- Dopamine antagonists (e.g. domperidone)
- Anti-cholinergic antihistamines (e.g. diphenhydramine)
- Δ9-tetrahydrocannabinol (e.g. dronabinol)

Aside from direct action on the chemoreceptor trigger zone of the area postrema, the brain's vomiting center, esophageal reflux, epigastric fullness, large-volume vomiting, and briefly relieved nausea all contribute to vomiting-induced edema. Prokinetic medications, such as metoclopramide or domperidone, can therefore stop vomiting. These medications must be given by a non-oral method (e.g., subcutaneous for metoclopramide, rectally for domperidone) if vomiting has already begun.

- Prokinetic agents (e.g. domperidone)
- Anti-cholinergic agents (e.g. orphenadrine)

Research indicates that postoperative nausea and vomiting are linked to opioid-inclusive anesthesia. Opioids for chronic pain resulted in modest improvements in pain and physical functioning but also increased risk of vomiting in these patients.

2. Drowsiness

Usually, a tolerance to drowsiness takes 5–7 days to develop, but if it becomes problematic, switching to a different opioid usually helps. Some opioids, like oxycodone, tilidine, and meperidine (pethidine), tend to produce relatively less sedation than other opioids, like morphine, fentanyl, and diamorphine (heroin). However, patient responses can vary greatly, so some trial and error may be required to determine which opioid is best for a given patient. Other than that, CNS stimulant therapy is usually successful.

3. Itching

When opioids are used for pain relief, itching usually doesn't pose a serious issue; however, antihistamines can help when it does. Non-sedating antihistamines, like fexofenadine, are frequently recommended because they prevent the drowsiness caused by opioids from getting worse. On the other hand, a few sedative antihistamines, like orphenadrine, can work in concert to relieve pain, allowing for the use of lower dosages of opioids. As a result, many opioid/antihistamine combination products, including Diconal (dipipanone/cyclizine) and Meprozine (meperidine/promethazine), have been put on the market. These products may also lessen the nausea that opioids cause.

The most severe adverse effect linked to opioid use is respiratory depression, which typically occurs when an opioid-naïve patient takes an intravenous dose. Tolerance to respiratory depression develops quickly in patients who regularly take opioids for pain relief, so it is not a clinical concern. Many medications have been created that can partially block respiratory depression, but doxapram, the only respiratory stimulant that is currently approved for this use, is only moderately effective in this regard. More recent medications like CX-546 and BIMU-8 might be far more successful.

4. Increased pain sensitivity

Some people have reported experiencing opioid-induced hyperalgesia, a condition in which those taking opioids for pain relief paradoxically feel more pain as a result of the drug. Even though it's rare, some palliative care patients experience this phenomenon; it usually occurs when the dosage is increased quickly. Rotating between multiple opioid painkillers may help prevent the development of exacerbation if it occurs. While chronic use or short-term high doses are the most common causes of opioid-induced hyperalgesia, very low doses may also cause it, according to some research.

Long-term use of opioid analgesics may cause side effects like hyperalgesia and allodynia, which are occasionally accompanied by a worsening of neuropathic pain. This is particularly likely to occur when increasing tolerance leads to a loss of efficacy and a progressive dose escalation over time. This appears to be primarily caused by the way opioid drugs act on targets other than the three classic opioid receptors, such as the sigma, nociceptin, and Toll-like receptor 4. Antagonists at these targets, such as J-113,397, BD-1047, or (+)-naloxone, can reverse this in animal models. As of right now, no medication is licensed expressly to treat opioid-induced hyperalgesia in humans. In extreme circumstances, stopping the use of opioid analgesics and switching to non-opioid analgesic medications may be the only viable course of action. However, many patients can avoid this side effect by simply reducing the dose of the opioid drug (usually accompanied by the addition of a supplemental non-opioid analgesic), rotating between different opioid drugs, or switching to a milder opioid with a mixed mode of action that also counteracts neuropathic pain, particularly tramadol or tapentadol. Individual sensitivity to the development of this side effect is highly dose-dependent and may vary depending on which opioid analgesic is used.

6.2.2. Agonist-Antagonist

The term "agonist-antagonist" or "mixed agonist/antagonist" in pharmacology describes a drug that, depending on the situation, acts as an antagonist (a material that binds to a receptor but does not activate and can block the activity of other agonists) or as an agonist (a substance that fully activates the receptor that it binds to). Receptor ligands that function as an agonist for some receptor types and an antagonist for others, or that function as an agonist in some tissues and an antagonist in others, are examples of mixed agonist/antagonists (also known as selective receptor modulators).

6.2.2.1. Synaptic Receptors

An agonist for synaptic receptors is a substance that either binds to the receptor directly or lengthens the duration that neurotransmitters are present in the synaptic cleft. A substance that has the opposite effect of an agonist is called an antagonist. By binding and preventing neurotransmitters from binding, or by shortening the duration of neurotransmitter presence in the synaptic cleft, it reduces the activation of a synaptic receptor. There are several ways to accomplish these goals. Reuptake inhibition is a common mechanism of action for agonists, in which the agonist prevents neurotransmitters from reentering the pre-synaptic axon terminal. As a result, the neurotransmitter has more time to interact with the synaptic receptors in the synaptic cleft. On the other hand, antagonists frequently attach themselves directly to synaptic cleft receptors, preventing neurotransmitters from binding.

At the alpha adrenoceptors, (*R*)-3-nitrobiphenyline is an α_{2C} selective agonist as well as a weak antagonist at the α_{2A} and α_{2B} subtypes.

6.2.2.2. Agonist-Antagonist Opioids

The best-known agonist-antagonists are opioids. Examples of such opioids are:

- pentazocine, agonist at the kappa (κ) and sigma (σ) and has a weak antagonist action at the mu opioid receptor (μ)
- butorphanol, partial agonist at μ- and a pure agonist at κ-opioid receptor and antagonist activity at the delta opioid receptor (δ)
- nalbuphine, κ-agonist/μ-antagonist analgesic

Opioids that are antagonist-antagonists typically have a ceiling effect, meaning that they don't become more potent over a certain dosage. As a result, agonist-antagonist opioids are more likely to cause psychotomimetic effects and have a lower potential for addiction while also having a lower analgesic efficacy.

Opioid antagonist-antagonist drugs provide analgesia without causing tolerance by blocking delta opioid receptors and activating mu-opioid receptors. (Katzung et al, 2009; Aubrun et al, 2019; Crockett et al, 2019)

6.3. Non-Narcotic Analgesics (NSAIDs)

Non-opioid or non-narcotic analgesics are other names for non-steroidal anti-inflammatory drugs (NSAIDs). They have antipyretic properties as well as the ability to reduce pain without interfering with opioid receptors, depress the central nervous system, or cause drug dependence or abuse. They mainly increase the pain threshold by acting on peripheral pain mechanisms and the central nervous system.

NSAIDs have effects that are related to analgesia, antipyretics, and anti-inflammatory. Arachidonic acid is released from the phospholipid portion of the cell membrane during pain, fever, and inflammation. It is subsequently transformed into prostaglandins (PGs) by the cyclooxygenase pathway.

6.3.1. Individual Agents

These can be put into the following categories

1. Salicylates

Salicylates work both centrally and peripherally to reduce pain. The hypothalamus appears to be the location of central analgesia's action. They are helpful in treating headaches, dysmenorrhea, throbbing pain in the muscles and joints, dull itching, and toothaches, among other conditions. Salicylates bring down the body's elevated temperature. Salicylates' antipyretic effect is most likely brought on by their inhibition of PG synthesis. Salicylates increase oxygen consumption, mostly by the skeletal muscles, which promotes respiration. By preventing prostaglandin synthesis, salicylates reduce the clinical manifestations of rheumatoid arthritis and other associated inflammatory diseases.

The main therapeutic uses of salicylates as given below:

i. As analgesic-antipyretic. Salicylates are effective in the treatment of mild to moderate types of pain. They are used in the treatment of headache, toothache, body ache, arthralgias, neuralgias and dysmenorrhea. They are also effective in fever of any origin.

ii. As an anti-inflammatory, anti-rheumatic, anti-gout and as an anti-platelet agent.

2. **Phenylbutazone:** It has strong anti-inflammatory properties. Its antipyretic and analgesic properties are lacking. The way it works is comparable to that of other NSAIDs. It is recommended in cases of acute gout, rheumatoid arthritis, osteoarthritis, rheumatic fever, fractures, blunt trauma, tooth extraction, and vasectomy.

3. **Indomethacin:** This medication has strong anti-inflammatory properties as well as good analgesic and antipyretic effects. It is used to treat gout, osteoarthritis, rheumatoid arthritis, and ankylosing spondylitis.

4. **Propionic Acid Derivatives:** Medications such as naproxen, ibuprofen, ketoprofen, and flurbiprofen, etc. have anti-inflammatory properties comparable to those of aspirin, but less toxicity and fewer severe side effects. They are recommended for mild to moderate pain, including dysmenorrhea, soft tissue injuries, fractures, rheumatoid and osteoarthritis, ankylosing spondylitis, and postoperative analgesia.

5. **Anthranilic Acid Derivatives:** Mefenamic acid and enfenamic acid are examples of cyclooxygenase inhibitors that have antipyretic, analgesic, and anti-inflammatory qualities. They are recommended as an antipyretic, for dental pain, postoperative or postpartum pain, rheumatoid and osteoarthritis, dysmenorrhea, and muscle, joint, and soft tissue pain.

6. **Piroxicam:** The novel NSAID piroxicam has analgesic, antipyretic, and anti-inflammatory properties. It offers efficient and durable pain and stiffness relief. In addition to other rheumatic disorders like osteoarthritis, ankylosing spondylitis, cervical spondylosis, acute gouty arthritis, and acute musculoskeletal disorders, it is indicated for use in both acute and chronic cases of rheumatoid arthritis.

7. **Diclofenac:** An NSAID with strong antirheumatic, anti-inflammatory, analgesic, and antipyretic qualities is diclofenac. Additionally, it has a strong analgesic effect on moderate to severe pain that is not related to rheumatism. It is utilized to treat rheumatoid arthritis, ankylosing spondylitis, osteoarthritis, spondylarthritis, painful spinal column syndromes, nonarticular rheumatism, and acute gout attacks. It is also used to treat inflammatory and degenerative forms of rheumatism.

8. **Paracetamol:** It acts on the CNS to produce analgesia and antipyretic effects. It has negligible anti-inflammatory action peripherally in therapeutic uses. It is a poor inhibitor of PG synthesis in peripheral tissues. It also raises the pain threshold. Paracetamol is used for the rapid relief of fever, pains and aches such as headache, earache, toothache, fibrositis, myalgia, neuralgia, arthralgia, osteoarthritis and postoperative pain.

9. **Ketorolac:** This medication acts as an analgesic, an antipyretic, and an inflammatory. It is recommended for

the short-term treatment of acute pain and pain following surgery.

10. **Celecoxib:** One NSAID with COX-2 selectivity is celecoxib. Its anti-inflammatory, analgesic, and antipyretic properties are thought to result from COX-2 inhibition. In humans, celecoxib does not inhibit the COX-1 enzyme at therapeutic doses. It is used to treat rheumatoid arthritis, osteoarthritis, neuralgia, gout, ankylosing spondylitis, and other ailments.

6.3.2. Drugs Used in Rheumatoid Arthritis

An inflammatory joint disease that is chronic and autoimmune is rheumatoid arthritis (RA). It's a progressive, symmetrical, deforming, and destructive polyarthritis that primarily affects the proximal small and large joints of the hand. NSAIDs and low-dose corticosteroids make up the initial course of treatment. Disease-modifying medications (DMDs) are added as a second line of treatment if the symptoms are not under control. DMDs are started early and continued indefinitely with regular monitoring because joint damage occurs early, spontaneous remissions are uncommon, and the disease progresses.

The disease-modifying drugs (DMDs/DMARDs) used are gold, D-penicillamine, hydroxychloroquine, sulfasalazine and immunosuppressants like methotrexate, azathioprine, cyclosporin, etc.

6.3.3. Drugs for Gout

Hyperuricemia, or elevated serum uric acid levels, is the cause of gout. A normal range for serum uric acid is 1–5 mg/dl. Purine metabolism results in the formation of uric acid. High blood uric acid levels cause precipitation in the kidney, subcutaneous tissues, joints, and cartilage, resulting in a variety of symptoms.

Drugs used for gout can be divided into two groups:

a. Drugs for acute attack of gout: NSAIDs, colchicine, corticosteroids.

b. Drugs for chronic gout/hyperuricemia: Can be uric acid synthesis inhibitors (allopurinol) and uricosurics (allopurinol) and uricosurics (increase renal excretion of uric acids) e.g. probenecid and sulfinpyrazone.

1. **Colchicine**: It works well to treat gout attacks that are acute. Colchicine helps treat gout by inhibiting the release of glycoproteins from granulocytes in inflamed joints, which stops uric acid crystals from forming and lysosomal enzymes from being released.

2. **Allopurinol**

   In cases of primary hyperuricemia from gout, secondary hyperuricemia from myeloid metaplasia, radiation, chemotherapy for cancer, and thiazide diuretics, allopurinol is indicated.

3. Probenecid

   It prevents uric acid from being reabsorbed from kidney tubules, which leads to an increase in uric acid excretion.

4. Sulfinpyrazone

   Pyrazolone derivative related to phenylbutazone. It has uricosuric action. It also inhibits platelet aggregation. (Katzung et al, 2009; Aubrun et al, 2019; Crockett et al, 2019)

6.4. General Anesthetics

The class of medications known as general anesthetics causes a temporary loss of consciousness and pain perception. There are many different drugs that can be used alone or in combination to achieve the appropriate depth of anesthesia for performing surgical procedures. Each drug has a distinct function. While there are several ways to administer general anesthetics, the most reliable methods are inhalation or intravenous because these methods provide more consistent results in terms of both the effective dose and the time course of action.

Inhalational and intravenous anesthetics are the two primary categories of general anesthetics.

6.4.1. Inhalational Anesthetics

i. **Nitrous Oxide (N_2O):** Anesthesia is induced and maintained with nitrous oxide. In general anesthesia, it is frequently utilized as a carrier gas for additional volatile agents. When administered in combination with air, nitrous oxide causes delirium, excitement, and amnesia. Thus, the moniker "laughing gas." Because of its analgesic properties at subanesthetic concentrations, nitrous oxide is used for painful procedures like dressing burns and minor surgeries like tooth extractions. It is inexpensive and widely utilized.

ii. Volatile Liquids:

a. **Ether (Diethyl Ether):** It was among the first substances used to induce general anesthesia. Ether is rarely used these days due to its slow induction and recovery, irritant property, and other drawbacks. In children, however, it may occasionally be added as a supplement to nitrous oxide-oxygen mixture.

b. **Halothane:** Because of its quick and easy induction, halothane is the most commonly used volatile anesthetic. Laryngeal and pharyngeal reflexes are inhibited by it. Recuperation proceeds easily and fairly quickly. This anesthetic is currently one of the most widely used because of its pleasant, quick-acting, non-irritating, and non-inflammable properties.

6.4.2. Intravenous Anesthetics

The primary purpose of intravenous anesthetics is to quickly induce anesthesia, which is subsequently sustained by an inhalational agent. Additionally, they help to lessen the need for maintenance anesthetics.

i. Barbiturates:

a. **Thiopentone Sodium:** Thiopentone Sodium is a thiobarbiturate with extremely rapid onset of action. Induction typically occurs smoothly and takes 10 to 15 seconds. Painful procedures shouldn't be performed while under the influence of this drug unless nitrous oxide or an opioid has been administered due to its poor analgesic property. Sometimes, thiopentone is used to quickly stop convulsions. Because it heals quickly, methylhexitone sodium is recommended for outpatient procedures and brief surgeries over thiopentone sodium. It acts faster and for a shorter duration than thiopentone sodium, making it about three times more potent.

ii. Non-Barbiturate Intravenous Anesthetics:

a. **Propanidid:** Compared to thiopentone, propanidid is a less potent oily liquid. It is a cosmetic intravenous that acts quickly and is specifically used for quick outpatient surgeries and dental procedures. Ketamine is a novel non-barbiturate anesthetic that shares pharmacological similarities with the hallucinogen phencyclidine. Within 30 seconds, intravenous ketamine causes analgesia and unconsciousness.

b. **Diazepam:** It may be used to produce light sedation and amnesia for unpleasant procedures by intravenous injection. It has also been used for induction and to supplement nitrous oxide anesthesia.

6.4.3. Preanesthetic Medication

Preanesthetic medication is the term for the use of medications to make an anesthetic agent administration more comfortable and safe for the patient. Depending on the situation, a combination of two or three medications is used to accomplish all the goals. Opioids, sedative-hypnotics, antianxiety medications, anticholinergics, neuroleptics, and antiemetics are among the medications that are frequently used.

1. Opioids

   These drugs are the most often used ones. Due to their sedative and analgesic effects, morphine and pethidine are commonly used medications. They produce analgesia both before and after surgery, lessen fear and anxiety, and facilitate a smooth induction.

2. Sedative-Hypnotics

   Barbiturates such as butobarbitone, secobarbitone, and pentobarbitone have been used to induce sedation and reduce anxiety before surgery. Since it rarely causes respiratory depression, promethazine, an antihistaminic with sedative, antiemetic, and anticholinergic qualities, is typically used in children.

3. Antianxiety Drugs

   Nowadays, preanesthetic medications are more often prescribed as tranquillizers, such as benzodiazepines, due to their ability to induce calm, improve muscle relaxation, and smoothen induction. Phenothiazines are additional tranquilizer compounds that have sedative, antiemetic, and antihistaminic effects. They can be administered parenterally or orally.

4. Anticholinergics

   To decrease salivary and bronchial secretions, morphine is typically administered in conjunction with tropine or scopolamine to block the vagal action. Hyoscine has both an antiemetic and amnesic effects.

5. Neuroleptics

   Preanesthetic drugs include triflupromazine, haloperidol, and chlorpromazine. They facilitate a smooth induction and lessen emesis and anxiety. These substances do, however, exacerbate respiratory depression.

6. Antiemetics

   Roperidol and hydroxyzine are occasionally utilized due to their antiemetic properties. Additionally, hydroxyzine possesses anticholinergic, antihistaminic, and antianxiety qualities.

6.5. Antiepileptic Drugs

Epilepsy is a neurological condition with episodes of motor, sensory, or psychological dysfunction due to abnormal electrical activity in the brain. It is caused by sudden and excessive discharge in the brain's grey matter. Anti-epileptic drugs help control this abnormal activity with minimal effect on the central nervous system.

1. **Phenobarbitone**

   Grandmal epilepsy can be effectively treated with phenobarbitone because it eliminates the tonic phase and increases the threshold for seizures. When treating grandmal, focal, temporal lobe, and occasionally petitmal epilepsy, phenobarbitone is helpful. Additionally, it helps with the management of febrile convulsions.

2. **Primidone**

   The drug primidone has twice the potency of phenobarbitone. It works well against all forms of seizures, including myoclonic, focal, psychomotor, and grandmal epilepsy. In cases of petitmal epilepsy, it is ineffective.

3. Diphenylhydantoin (Phenytoin)

   Because phenytoin stabilizes the neuronal membrane, it inhibits the repetitive detonation of these healthy brain cells. It is used as a preventative measure for all types of partial epilepsy, regardless of whether a seizure develops secondary generalization. Additionally, it is used to treat status epilepticus and as a preventive measure for generalized convulsive seizures.

4. Carbamazepine

   It is effective in grand mal and psychomotor epilepsy.

5. Ethosuximide

   Ethosuximide was the most commonly used antiepileptic agent in the treatment of petit mal epilepsy.

6. Methsuximide

   It is similar to ethosuximide and used along with the other drugs in the treatment of temporal lobe epilepsy.

7. Sodium Valproate (Valproic Acid)

   Valproate is a broad-range antiepileptic drug. It is commonly employed in the treatment of absence seizures.

8. Clonazepam

   Clonazepam is used in the treatment of petitmal epilepsy not responding to ethosuximide and sodium valproate.

9. Topiramate

   It is used as an adjunctive treatment for seizures including refractory seizures, and simple and complex partial seizures.

10. Gabapentin

    It is a new anticonvulsant drug used as adjunctive therapy in the treatment of partial seizures with or without secondary generalization in adults.

11. Vigabatrin

    It is used in partial seizure with or without generalization. Lamotrigine It is phenyltriazine compound, chemically unrelated to existing antiepileptic drugs. It is mainly used as adjunctive therapy in patients for simple partial seizures, complex partial seizures, secondary generalised tonic and clonic seizures.

6.6. Psychopharmacological Agents

Three major categories can be used to categorize psychopharmacological agents, which are used in different stages of psychological disorders.

1. Antipsychotic drugs used in all types of psychosis mainly schizophrenia.
2. Antianxiety drugs used in anxiety.
3. Antidepressants for minor and major depressive disorders and mood stabilizers (antimanic drugs) for mania.

6.6.1. Antipsychotic Drugs

They are mainly divided into two main groups and certain newer compounds.

i. **Phenothiazines:** These drugs cause sedation that doesn't turn into anesthesia. Without influencing wakefulness, they lessen the psychotic patient's agitation, anxiety, and aggression. They alleviate thought disorders, blunted affect, withdrawal, and self-centered behavior in patients with schizophrenia. They also enhance delusions and hallucinations. Chlorpromazine functions as a potent antiemetic by depressing the chemoreceptor trigger zone (CTZ).

It is used in the following conditions:

1. Treatment of psychosis (schizophrenia): Schizophrenia is a split mind or splitting of perception from reality. The patient of schizophrenia is dissociated from the world around him and lives in their own world which is characterized by aggression, anxiety, restlessness, hallucinations and delusions. Phenothiazines reduce the hallucinations, aggression, anxiety and make them acceptable and cooperative.
2. In treatment of manic-depressive psychosis (mania).
3. In alcoholic hallucinosis and Huntington's disease.
4. As an antiemetic in drug and disease induced vomiting. Also useful in morning sickness but are ineffective in motion sickness.
5. In the treatment of intractable hiccough.
6. In the treatment of behavioral disorders in children.
7. As preanesthetic medication.
8. To produce hypothermia.

ii. **Butyrophenones Haloperidol:** It is a strong antipsychotic. It doesn't result in gaining weight. Its effects on pharmacology are comparable to those of phenothiazines. Antiemetic neuroleptanalgesia, Huntington's disease, anxiety disorders, acute mania, and behavioral disorders in children are among the conditions for which it is indicated.

iii. Other Newer Compounds:

- **Loxapine:** It is the antipsychotic agent resembling chlorpromazine in pharmacological actions. It is used in manifestation of psychotic disorders, acute and chronic paranoid schizophrenia.
- **Clozapine:** Clozapine is an unusual medication for neuroleptics. Few extrapyramidal symptoms are produced by it. It is recommended for all forms of schizophrenia, including persistent schizophrenia and resistant cases that do not improve with traditional antipsychotics.

6.6.2. Antianxiety Drugs

Anxiety is a fearful emotional state accompanied by unease and discomfort. Anti-anxiety medications are used to manage anxiety symptoms without interfering with other bodily or mental processes. They can be broadly classified into two categories.

i. **Benzodiazepines:** They have selective action on the limbic system and have little effect on other body systems. They help in improving the anxiety and stress-related symptoms. They are widely used because of lower dependence producing liability and a wide margin of safety.

ii. **Azapirones:** Buspirone is a member of the azapirones, a different class of compounds both pharmacologically and chemically. It partially agonistically interacts with dopamine and serotonin receptors. It is used to treat anxiety disorders temporarily and relieve anxiety symptoms, whether or not depression is present.

iii. **Others:** With antiemetic, sedative, anticholinergic, and local and esthetic properties, hydroxyzine is an antihistaminic agent. It is used as an adjunct therapy for both acute and chronic alcoholism and anxiety. By reducing the symptoms of sympathetic overactivity, such as palpitations, tremors, elevated blood pressure, etc., beta-blockers help patients with their symptoms. They function as benzodiazepine adjuvants.

6.6.3. Antidepressants

Agents used to treat depression are called antidepressants. There are two primary categories for these agents.

i. **MAO Inhibitors:** By indirectly acting as sympathomimetic amines, MAO inhibitors raise the catecholamine content of different organs, causing more catecholamine to be released.

ii. **Tricyclic and Related Compounds:** The most widely prescribed medications for the treatment of depression are tricyclic antidepressants, or TCAs. Imipramine is a medication that effectively reduces depression. Patients with depression experience an improvement in mood after taking the medication for roughly three weeks. It is recommended for all forms of depression, sleep apnea syndrome, narcolepsy, intractable chronic pain, nocturnal enuresis, and mood disorders. Amitryptaline is recommended for the treatment of depression, anxiety-related illnesses, agitation, restlessness, and sleep disturbances; masked depression; dysphoria and depression in alcoholism; and bedwetting in children. It is also helpful in the prevention of migraines.

Sertaline is a type of medication known as a selective serotonin reuptake inhibitor (SSRI), which is widely used in the treatment of depression. It works by blocking the reabsorption of serotonin in the brain, helping to alleviate symptoms of depression and anxiety. Sertaline is also effective in preventing the return of depressive episodes and managing symptoms of obsessive-compulsive disorder.

6.6.4. MOOD Stabilizers (Antimanic Drugs)

The preferred medication for treating bipolar disorders is lithium carbonate. Its narrow therapeutic index necessitates a facility for therapeutic serum lithium level monitoring during treatment. It is recommended in cases of agranulocytosis, schizoaffective psychosis, acute hypomania, mania, recurrent mania, mental depression, cluster headaches, and leukopenia brought on by chemotherapy.

6.7. CNS Stimulants

These medications belong to the class that stimulates the central nervous system. Some of them are also referred to as analeptics, but because of their non-selectivity of action, they are not very helpful in clinical settings.

- **Analeptics**

These medications, despite their small margin of safety, are sometimes used to induce breathing in coma patients or those who are fainting. The use of Nikethamide has ended. Doxapram increases blood pressure and speeds up breathing.

- **Psychostimulants**

Amphetamines, such as methamphetamine, dexamphetamine, and others. serve as primary sympathomimetics. These are addictive substances, and continued use of them can lead to persistent behavioral abnormalities and even the onset of psychosis.

- **Convulsants**

  Because of its convulsive qualities, strychnine, an alkaloid derived from Strychnos nux vomica seeds, was utilized in the past. Fish berries contain picrotoxin, a strong convulsant. It is no longer in use. Synthetic convulsant bicuculline acts similarly to a picrotoxin. A CNS stimulant, pentylenetetrazol works by directly depolarizing central neurons.

  But none of these compounds are used therapeutically and their use is restricted to laboratories as research tools.

- **Cerebroactive Drugs**

  Certain substances in this category are used to treat dementia and other brain disorders that are related to it. In ischemic areas, pyritinol promotes cerebral microcirculation and cholinergic transmission. It shields the neurons from hypoxia and disruptions in the metabolism of glucose. It is recommended in cases of encephalitis, perinatal distress, senility, organic brain syndrome, alcohol withdrawal, and cerebrovascular accidents. Piracetam enhances both normal and abnormal brain functioning related to cognitive functions, such as memory, cognition, and learning. It is indicated in cases of cerebral insufficiency, senile dementia, learning disabilities and mental retardation in children, dementia and confusion in the elderly, and behavioral issues in the former.

- **Drugs Used in Alzheimer's Disease**

  The majority of those affected by Alzheimer's disease (AD), a progressive neurodegenerative disorder, are elderly. It is the most frequent cause of dementia, characterized by a decline in personality, intellect, and memory without a noticeable impairment in motor function. (Katzung et al, 2009; Aubrun et al, 2019; Crockett et al, 2019)

6.8. Pharmacological Treatment of Parkinson's Disease

One of the most prevalent long-term degenerative disorders of the nervous system is Parkinson's disease (PD). Although there isn't a cure for Parkinson's disease (PD), several medications can help manage its motor symptoms. Even though these medications can significantly improve motor function, they may also have unfavorable side effects, especially as the disease worsens.

Parkinson's disease (PD) is a neurological disorder that worsens over time. PD currently has no disease-modifying treatments available, and the mainstay of medical care is medication-assisted motor symptom control. Due to the protracted nature of the illness, patients may need to adhere to complex drug regimens intended to manage their motor symptoms, which may have unfavorable side effects. The primary cause of Parkinson's disease (PD) is the selective loss of neurons in the substantia nigra pars compacta, which leads to dopamine depletion in the striatum. Currently, the cornerstone of PD treatment is the use of dopaminergic medications, which are intended to mimic the effects of dopamine in the depleted striatum.

Drugs that block the breakdown of endogenous dopamine, activate the dopamine receptor, or are metabolized to dopamine can all accomplish this. There is no one-size-fits-all approach to treatment; instead, drug regimens are customized for each patient according to the intensity and timing of their symptoms as well as any adverse effects they may be experiencing. This chapter will address pharmacological treatment strategies in this context, focusing primarily on dopamine replacement therapies.

6.8.1. Current Treatments

Although there aren't any disease-modifying medications available for Parkinson's disease (PD), there are treatments that can significantly reduce motor symptoms. In terms of the non-motor symptoms of Parkinson's disease, they don't really help patients clinically. To lessen the severity of side effects, treatment is typically started after the patient's symptoms become bothersome.

6.8.1.1. Levodopa

Levodopa-based preparations are the cornerstone of today's Parkinson's disease (PD) treatment regimen, acting as a dopamine substitute in the striatum. It is not possible to treat Parkinson's disease (PD) with dopamine alone because it cannot cross the blood-brain barrier. Levodopa, on the other hand, is a dopamine precursor that can be given as a medication and crosses the blood-brain barrier. DOPA decarboxylase transforms it into the neurotransmitter dopamine after it has been absorbed and passed through the blood-brain barrier. Levodopa is typically started on a low dose for patients, and the dose is gradually increased based on how well the patient responds to treatment and how well the side effects are managed. The majority of patients need multiple daily doses within the range of 150–1000 mg. Levodopa typically has a rapid clinical effect that can last for several hours, especially in the early stages of the disease. However, the drug's effects usually wear off after shorter periods of time as the disease progresses, necessitating more frequent dosing.

Despite its effectiveness, levodopa has many serious side effects that play a major role in the patient's illness, especially when the disease is advanced. Some of its related side effects are caused by DOPA decarboxylase's peripheral conversion of levodopa to dopamine, which occurs outside of the central nervous system. As will be covered below, administering levodopa in conjunction with peripheral DOPA decarboxylase inhibitors reduces these effects. Extended usage may lead to severe on-off motor fluctuations and major motor complications, such as dyskinesias.

Involuntary twisting hyperkinetic movements, or dyskinesias, typically happen when a drug is at its highest dosage, though they can also happen when the drug is wearing off or even during off-periods. Levodopa dosage reduction may be used to treat problematic dyskinesias. This means that a challenging balance must be struck between maximizing motor symptom control and minimizing side effects. Deep brain stimulation may be taken into consideration for patients who have previously responded well to levodopa but have developed problematic dyskinesias. This may allow for the control of motor symptoms on a lower dosage of levodopa. The term "on-off phenomenon" describes the sudden changes in motor function that patients with advanced Parkinson's disease may encounter. While in the "on" state, levodopa's effects wear off quickly, leaving the patient in the "off" state with severe Parkinsonian motor features. During this time, the patient's motor symptoms are largely under control. These variations can seriously impair function and be especially troublesome. Variable drug absorption and transit across the blood-brain barrier, along with the ensuing oscillations in pre-synaptic and post-synaptic dopamine levels in the nigrostriatal pathway, are likely the root causes of these motor symptoms. Orthostatic hypotension and gastrointestinal disorders like nausea and vomiting are significant additional side effects. Dopamine's "off-target" effects in extranigral brain regions may give rise to neuropsychiatric features such as anxiety and hallucinations.

6.8.1.2. Dopamine Agonists

In 1978, dopamine receptor agonists were introduced to the market to treat Parkinson's disease. Based on receptor specificity, the widely used agonists can be divided into ergot and non-ergot derived groups. All agonists have an ethanolamine moiety. Unlike levodopa, these medications do not require conversion into dopamine to activate the dopamine system. Instead, they bind to dopaminergic receptors. For PD patients, especially those who are younger, dopamine agonists are frequently prescribed as an initial treatment.

Some of these medications come in tablet, patch, and injection form in controlled or extended release formulations. For example, rotigotine patches come in handy for patients who are nil-by-mouth during surgery or who are unable to take oral medications. To make sure a patient is receiving enough medication when switching to rotigotine patches in this situation, the levodopa-equivalent dose of their current treatment plan must be calculated. Dopamine agonists can be helpful in patients with mild symptoms, in those who cannot tolerate levodopa, or as an adjunct to levodopa therapy, even though they may be less effective than levodopa in controlling the motor symptoms of Parkinson's disease (PD), with the majority of patients eventually requiring levodopa therapy.

Patients and the kind of agonist prescribed will determine how long a drug will take to take effect and how long its half-life is. When starting dopamine agonists, the dosage is typically increased gradually in accordance with the patient's response and any side effects that may occur. Among the frequently prescribed dopamine agonists, the typical dosage is as follows: up to 4.5mg of pramipexole, divided into three doses; 0.75-3 (Maximum 3 mg per day} of ropinirole divided into three to four doses; andReplace with : 1-8mg of Rotigotine patch applied once daily.. Although it is not as commonly used, apomorphine can be helpful when administered as a subcutaneous injection to treat severe "off" episodes or as a subcutaneous infuse-on to patients who still experience severe motor fluctuations even after other medications have been optimized. Dopamine agonists may have antioxidant qualities and slow the loss of dopaminergic neurons, according to certain preclinical and imaging research, but there isn't enough proof to support the idea that these medications can alter the course of the disease.

Compared to levodopa, treatment with dopamine agonists has been demonstrated to reduce the incidence and severity of dystonia, motor fluctuations, and dyskinesia. They might, however, have additional serious negative effects. Frequent adverse effects include dry mouth, insomnia, peripheral edema, constipation, fainting, hallucinations, nausea, vomiting (caused by stimulation of the area postrema, which is located in the medulla at a site in which the BBB is disrupted), and sleepiness.

Impulse control disorder (ICD), a behavioral disorder characterized by compulsive and impulsive behaviors, is arguably the most significant side effect of dopamine agonists. Hypersexuality, gambling, compulsive shopping, binge eating, punding, and hobbyism are some possible symptoms. After starting dopamine agonists, it is critical for clinicians to be on the lookout for these issues because they can cause serious financial and social problems for the patient. Interpersonal relationships, caregiver well-being, and overall quality of life can all suffer from ICD. ICD is more common in people with a history of addiction (such as alcohol or gambling), and certain behaviors may be more common in men or women (such as compulsive shopping or hypersexuality). Fifteen to twenty percent of Parkinson's disease patients who take dopamine agonists experience ICD; levodopa also increases the risk of ICD, but it is significantly lower than that of dopamine agonists. Dopamine agonists' effects on the opiate and serotonin systems, the orbitofrontal cortex, and the mesolimbic dopaminergic pathway have all been suggested as possible mechanisms.

The possibility of developing dopamine agonist withdrawal syndrome (DAWS), which can happen when someone with compulsive or impulsive behavior either quits using dopamine agonists altogether or lowers their dosage, is another crucial factor to take into account. Anxiety, panic attacks, sleeplessness, restlessness, dysphoria, agitation, exhaustion, orthostatic hypotension, diaphoresis, and cravings for drugs are some of the symptoms of withdrawal syndrome. As a result, stopping dopamine agonists gradually and keeping a close eye out for these issues is necessary. Similar to ICD, DAWS can have serious psychosocial repercussions.

6.8.1.3. Monoamine Oxidase B (MAO-B) Inhibitors

Inhibiting the enzymes responsible for dopamine metabolism, as employed by other Parkinson's disease medications, maintains endogenous dopamine levels. MAO-B inhibitors are one member of this class. Reduced activity of MAO-B leads to increased dopaminergic activity within the striatum, which is mediated by endogenous dopamine. As was previously discussed, MAO-B is one of the primary enzymes involved in the breakdown of dopamine. Their use reduces motor symptoms in patients with Parkinson's disease (PD), and similar to dopamine agonists, they can be used as a first line of treatment to postpone the need for levodopa therapy and lower the risk of motor complications from levodopa. While in the early stages of the disease they may be adequate for symptom control, levodopa-based treatment is ultimately necessary for the majority of patients. To lower the levodopa dosage, MAO-B inhibitors can also be used in conjunction with preparations based on levodopa.

Rasagiline (Azilect) and selegiline (Deprenyl, Eldepryl, Zelapar) are two commonly used MAO-B inhibitors. Safinamide, also known as Xadago, was recently approved for use in the treatment of Parkinson's disease (PD). The drug appears to have several modes of action, one of which is thought to be the inhibition of MAO-B. For selegiline, the recommended dosage is 5–10 mg daily; for rasagiline, it is 0–5–1 mg once daily. The most frequent side effect of MAO-B inhibitors is gastrointestinal distress, which is otherwise well tolerated. Aching joints, melancholy, exhaustion, dry mouth, sleeplessness, lightheadedness, disorientation, hallucinations, flu-like symptoms, indigestion, and headache are some additional side effects.

6.8.1.4. Catechol-O-Methyl Transferase Inhibitors

As was previously mentioned, COMT is an additional enzyme that contributes to the breakdown of dopamine. Because they lessen the breakdown of endogenous dopamine, inhibitors of COMT also provide a therapeutic way to maintain endogenous dopamine levels. They are primarily used in conjunction with levodopa to extend the latter's duration of action by boosting the latter's half-life and cerebral delivery. Compared to standard levodopa/DOPA decarboxylase inhibitor combinations, this reduces off time and allows for control of motor symptoms in some patients. When levodopa therapy alone is not enough to address end-of-dose "wearing-off," these are frequently prescribed to the patients.

COMT inhibitors are available as tablets and are not typically prescribed as monotherapy because of their limited ability to treat Parkinson's disease symptoms on their own. Entacapone (Comtan), tolcapone (Tasmar), and opicapone (Ongentys) are a few examples of COMT inhibitors. In combination preparations with carbidopa and levodopa, entacapone is frequently used (Stalevo, Sastravi). The two most widely used COMT inhibitors are tolcapone (100 mg three times a day) and entacapone (200 mg four to eight times a day) with each levodopa dosage. It should be highlighted that COMT inhibitors may require a decrease in the levodopa dosage because they can exacerbate levodopa-induced side effects, such as dyskinesias. Since tolcapone carries a rare but potentially dangerous risk of hepatotoxicity, entacapone is typically recommended. Therefore, it is necessary to monitor liver function tests while on tolcapone treatment. Sleepiness, nausea, appetite loss, diarrhea, dizziness, orange urine discoloration, hallucinations, headaches, confusion, dry mouth, and chest pain are other infrequent side effects.

6.8.1.5. Anticholinergics

All of the drugs that have been covered thus far are intended to raise dopaminergic activity in the striatum. Not all medications used to treat Parkinson's disease (PD) work via dopaminergic pathways. The anticholinergic drug class is one example of this. Through their antagonistic effects on cholinergic receptors, these decrease the activity of the neurotransmitter acetylcholine. They may help reduce rigidity and tremor in Parkinson's disease (PD), despite their limited use and infrequency of prescription. The normal balance between dopamine and acetylcholine in the brain is disrupted when dopaminergic neurons are lost, but anticholinergic medications may help to restore and maintain this normal balance.

These medications are primarily used to treat mild movement symptoms, especially tremors and muscle stiffness, in young patients who are still in the early stages of the illness. In the early stages of tremor-predominant Parkinson's disease (PD), anticholinergic medications may be used as monotherapy. Anticholinergics, however, are typically taken in conjunction with levodopa and the other drugs mentioned above when they are used. The class of drugs in question may cause confusion in older or cognitively impaired patients, so it is generally advised to avoid them in these populations. There are preparations for tablets and oral suspensions. Trihexyphenidyl, procyclidine, orphenadrine, and benztropine are a few anticholinergics. Blurred vision, dry mouth, constipation, drowsiness, difficulty urinating, urine retention, confusion, cognitive impairment, hallucinations, dizziness, difficulty swallowing, dyskinetic movements, and memory issues are among the common side effects. Although anticholinergics are known to cause dry mouth, in patients for whom drooling is a particular problem, the reduced salivation caused by these drugs is a desirable effect, and they can even be used to treat the symptom.

6.8.1.6. Amantadine

Amantadine, also known as Symmetrel, was first created as an antiviral medication to treat the flu, but it has since been used to treat Parkinson's disease (PD). It may provide a transient improvement in symptoms and be used to treat rigidity, rest tremor, and occasionally fatigue. Additionally, it might make it possible to use less levodopa, which would lower the risk of dyskinesia. That being said, its most advantageous characteristic is presumably its ability to reduce the severity of dyskinesias brought on by levodopa. Be aware that there is little evidence to support the use of amantadine in treating Parkinson's disease symptoms.

It is the chemical derivative of adamantine, also known as 1-aminoadamantane or 1-adamantylamine. Although amantadine acts as a weak glutamate antagonist at the N-methyl-D-aspartate receptor (NMDAR), its potential anti-Parkinsonian effect is unclear. Similar to the majority of other anti-Parkinson medications that have been discussed, this one is titrated up from a low initial dose. It is available as liquid syrup and tablet form. Although amantadine is usually well tolerated, there are many potential adverse effects that can arise from using it, such as hallucinations, livedo reticularis, leg swelling, blurred vision, nausea, vomiting, appetite loss, insomnia, nightmares, sweating, agitation, and headache.

6.8.2. Emerging Treatments

The medications that have been discussed help manage the symptoms of Parkinson's disease (PD), but none of them change how the illness progresses. Even though there aren't any disease-modifying therapies for Parkinson's disease (PD) at the moment, several intriguing new strategies are being researched. In addition to novel experimental compounds, drug repurposing—the application of pharmaceuticals with a recognized clinical indication in an unproven setting—also attracts a lot of interest. Because these medications have already been used, safety information about them is already available, which could speed up the clinical trial process. Apart from novel medications, several regenerative methods are either in the process of entering or have already entered clinical trials. The use of stem cells and gene therapies, such as ProSavin, a lentivirus vector containing the genes encoding TH, GTPCH1, and DOPA decarboxylase, are among them. These regenerative therapies aim to restore dopaminergic activity in the striatum in a more physiological way than what is currently possible with dopaminergic medications, potentially with a lower risk of levodopa's side effects. Instead of providing a disease-modifying effect.

There is a plethora of evidence suggesting that alpha-synuclein (α-synuclein) aggregation plays a central role in the pathogenesis of PD. Thus, there is much interest in how this process may be targeted by potential therapies. Therapeutic approaches have been developed aiming to:

- reduce α-synuclein production
- inhibit α-synuclein aggregation
- increase intracellular and extracellular degradation of α-synuclein aggregates
- reduce uptake of extracellular α-synuclein by neighboring cells

Clinical trials for immunotherapies that target α-synuclein are currently underway. Affiris recently concluded a Phase 1 clinical trial using the synthetic vaccine AFFITOPE PD03A, which contains a peptide mimicking α-synuclein. In 36 patients with early-stage Parkinson's disease (PD), this formulation was tested and found to be very well tolerated with only mild side effects when administered subcutaneously. Phase 1a and Phase 1b clinical trials have also evaluated PRX002, (Prothena), a passive immunotherapeutic agent that targets α-synuclein. This humanized monoclonal antibody was found to reduce free serum levels of α-synuclein by 96.5%. With no significant adverse effects or toxicity, the medication has advanced to Phase 2 clinical trials. BIIB-054 (Biogen), an additional α-synuclein-based passive immunotherapy, was discovered to have a good pharmacokinetic profile and be well tolerated. Numerous additional experimental immunotherapeutic agents are being studied as well. Furthermore, medications that seek to enhance the extracellular degradation of α-synuclein—such as the serine protease Kallikrein 6—are being explored as possible PD treatments.

Apart from augmenting α-synuclein clearance, a plausible approach would be to diminish α-synuclein production, which could be accomplished via RNA interference (RNAi) technology. *In vitro* and animal studies have produced some intriguing results, even though this has not yet reached the stage of human trials. For instance, lentiviral delivery of short hairpin RNA (shRNA) targeting α-synuclein to rats resulted in the silencing of ectopic human α-synuclein expression in the striatum. After a two-week infusion, small interfering RNA (siRNA) administered into the mouse hippocampus likewise reduced the expression of endogenous α-synuclein without causing any harm. Subsequent application of siRNA in non-human primates revealed a 40–50% decrease in α-synuclein levels. Unfortunately, a lack of funding prevented this strategy from moving forward with clinical trials. Additionally, rats given shRNA showed a 35% decrease in α-synuclein levels. Naturally, the issue with severely reducing α-synuclein levels is that the protein's typical functionality is compromised. A considerable decrease in α-synuclein levels was linked in certain investigations to increased neurotoxicity, and a few even revealed nigrostriatal system degeneration. Therefore, to proceed with clinical trials involving these techniques, extensive preclinical safety data will be required.

Reducing α-synuclein's transcriptional expression is an additional strategy for lowering its synthesis. It has been suggested that beta-2-adrenoreceptor (beta-2AR) agonists, like clenbuterol, can accomplish this. They have been shown to reduce α-synuclein expression in rat cortical neurons and a neuroblastoma cell line by more than 35%. It has been suggested that they function by acetylating α-synuclein promoters and enhancers on histone 3 lysine 27. Two large-scale epidemiological studies conducted in Norway provide supportive data for the potential benefit of these medications. These studies indicate that beta-2AR agonists are worthy of additional research and may eventually be used to treat Parkinson's disease (PD).

Two of the other medications currently under consideration for repurposing—nilotinib, a chemotherapy agent, and exenatide, a glucagon-like peptide-1 receptor agonist—have advanced to clinical trials. A c-Abl tyrosine kinase inhibitor called nilotinib is used to treat chronic myelogenous leukemia (CML). In the brain tissue of Parkinson's disease patients, there has been an increase in c-abl activity. This could result in increased α-synuclein phosphorylation and aggregation, as well as decreased activity of the Parkin protein, which is involved in mitochondrial biogenesis. In A53T transgenic mice, nilotinib reduced α-synuclein levels while also offering a certain level of neuroprotection. Nilotinib has entered a Phase 2a trial in 2017, and there is great hope regarding its treatment potential because it has been observed to be well tolerated by patients with Parkinson's disease (PD), albeit at a much lower dosage than what is typically prescribed for the treatment of CML. The poor transit across the BBB of c-abl inhibitors, however, may be a drawback to their use in Parkinson's disease (PD), necessitating the development of novel agents to overcome this.

In a similar vein, exenatide, a well-known treatment for type 2 diabetes, is showing promise as a PD treatment. Preclinical disease models have demonstrated neuroprotective potential, and a preliminary clinical trial found long-lasting clinical improvements. Subsequently, it was advanced to a single-center, randomized, double-blind, placebo-controlled Phase 2 clinical trial where patients received a weekly subcutaneous dose of 2 mg. Similar gains in motor scores were noted, and these continued after the course of treatment was stopped. (Katzung et al, 2009; Aubrun et al, 2019; Crockett et al, 2019)

A Closer Look

Drug-related Changes in the Central Nervous System

The discussion focuses on the clinical and imaging characteristics of central nervous system complications linked to prescription drugs and drugs of abuse.

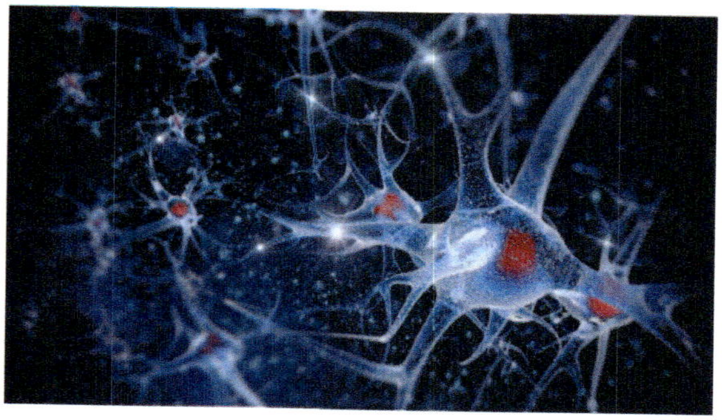

Source: https://www.rehabclinic.org.uk/long-term-effects-drugs-body-mind/

Drug misuse is a serious issue in today's society and is linked to high rates of morbidity and death. Many drugs have been linked to major brain-related side effects. To promptly provide medical management, it is crucial to identify the imaging findings of these side effects. Addiction-related substances and certain prescription drugs target the central nervous system (CNS). The Central Nervous System (CNS) is affected by the abuse of cocaine, heroin, alcohol, amphetamines, toluene, and cannabis. Antiepileptics, nitrous oxide, immunosuppressants, and total parenteral nutrition are examples of prescribed drugs or medical treatments that can have an impact on the central nervous system. These medications can cause neurovascular problems, encephalopathy, atrophy, infection, alterations in the corpus callosum, and other nonspecific changes in the central nervous system. Imaging abnormalities suggestive of these complications can be recognized on computed tomography (CT) and magnetic resonance imaging (MR) scans. It is essential for radiologists to identify iatrogenic side effects from different medications as well as complications linked to drug abuse. Consequently, the identification and prompt treatment of medication-related consequences in the central nervous system can be greatly aided by diagnostic imaging modalities like CT and MR imaging.

Summary

- The central nervous system consists of the brain and the spinal cord. It is the seat of the autonomic nervous system, consciousness, motor coordination behavior, thoughts and memory processes.
- Sedatives (anxiolytic) are the agents that reduce anxiety and exert a calming effect with little or no effect on motor or mental functions.
- Barbiturates are a class of depressant drugs that are chemically derived from barbituric acid. They are effective when used medically as anxiolytics, hypnotics, and anticonvulsants, but have physical and psychological addiction potential as well as overdose potential among other possible adverse effects.
- Analgesics are drugs (natural or synthetic origin) that relieve pain by acting on CNS or peripheral pain mechanisms without causing loss of consciousness.
- Opioids are a class of drugs that derive from, or mimic, natural substances found in the opium poppy plant. Opioids work in the brain to produce a variety of effects, including pain relief.
- For synaptic receptors, an agonist is a compound that increases the activation of the receptor by binding directly to it or by increasing the amount of time neurotransmitters are in the synaptic cleft.
- Non-steroidal anti-inflammatory drugs (NSAIDs) are also known as non-opioid or non-narcotic analgesics. They relieve pain without interacting with opioid receptors and do not depress CNS and have no drug dependence or drug abuse property and possess antipyretic activity also.
- Salicylates relieve pain by both central and peripheral action. The site of action of central analgesia seems to be the hypothalamus.
- General anesthetics are the group of drugs that bring about a reversible loss of pain sensation and consciousness.
- Epilepsy is a neurological disorder characterized by short, recurrent and periodic attacks of motor, sensory or psychological malfunction.

References

1. Adaikpoh, M. A., Orhue, N. E. J., & Igbe, I. (2007). The protective role of *Scoparia dulcis* on tissue antioxidant defense system of rats exposed to cadmium. *African Journal of Biotechnology, 6*(10), 1192–1196.
2. Aiyer, R., Mehta, N., Gungor, S., & Gulati, A. (2018). A systematic review of NMDA receptor antagonists for treatment of neuropathic pain in clinical practice. *Clinical Journal of Pain, 34*(5), 450–467. https://doi.org/10.1097/AJP.0000000000000610.
3. AlDakheel, A., Kalia, L. V., & Lang, A. E. (2014). Pathogenesis-targeted, disease-modifying therapies in Parkinson disease. *Neurotherapeutics, 11*(1), 6–23. https://doi.org/10.1007/s13311-013-0211-1.
4. Aubrun, F., Nouette-Gaulain, K., Fletcher, D., Belbachir, A., Beloeil, H., Carles, M., Cuvillon, P., Dadure, C., Lebuffe, G., Marret, E., Martinez, V., Olivier, M., Sabourdin, N., & Zetlaoui, P. (2019).

Revision of expert panel's guidelines on postoperative pain management. *Anesthesia, Critical Care & Pain Medicine, 38*(4), 405–411. https://doi.org/10.1016/j.accpm.2018.12.003.

5. Barkin, R. L. (2015). Topical nonsteroidal anti-inflammatory drugs: The importance of drug, delivery, and therapeutic outcome. *American Journal of Therapeutics, 22*(5), 388–407. https://doi.org/10.1097/MJT.0000000000000127.
6. Connolly, B. S., & Lang, A. E. (2014). Pharmacological treatment of Parkinson disease: A review. *JAMA, 311*(16), 1670–1683. https://doi.org/10.1001/jama.2014.3654.
7. Crockett, S. D., Greer, K. B., Heidelbaugh, J. J., Falck-Ytter, Y., Hanson, B. J., & Sultan, S. (2019). American Gastroenterological Association Institute guideline on the medical management of opioid-induced constipation. *Gastroenterology, 156*(1), 218–226. https://doi.org/10.1053/j.gastro.2018.09.063.
8. Dawood, M. Y. (2006). Primary dysmenorrhea: Advances in pathogenesis and management. *Obstetrics & Gynecology, 108*(2), 428–441. https://doi.org/10.1097/01.AOG.0000230213.35273.1f.
9. Dhawan, K., Dhawan, S., & Chhabra, S. (2003). Attenuation of benzodiazepine dependence in mice by a tri-substituted benzoflavone moiety of *Passiflora incarnata Linneaus*: A non-habit-forming anxiolytic. *Journal of Pharmacy & Pharmaceutical Sciences, 6*(2), 215–222.
10. Dowell, D., Haegerich, T. M., & Chou, R. (2016). CDC guideline for prescribing opioids for chronic pain—United States, 2016. *JAMA, 315*(15), 1624–1645. https://doi.org/10.1001/jama.2016.1464.
11. Eisenhofer, G., Kopin, I. J., & Goldstein, D. S. (2004). Catecholamine metabolism: A contemporary view with implications for physiology and medicine. *Pharmacological Reviews, 56*(3), 331–349. https://doi.org/10.1124/pr.56.3.1.
12. Freire, S. M. F., Emim, J. A. S., Lapa, A. J., Souccar, C., & Torres, L. M. B. (1993). Analgesic and anti-inflammatory properties of *Scoparia dulcis* L. extracts and gulitol in rodents. *Phytotherapy Research, 7*(6), 408–414. https://doi.org/10.1002/ptr.2650070605.
13. Hayashi, T., Kawasaki, M., Miwa, Y., Taga, T., & Morita, N. (1990). Antiviral agents of plant origin. III. Scopadulin, a novel tetracyclic diterpene from *Scoparia dulcis* L. *Chemical and Pharmaceutical Bulletin, 38*(4), 945–947. https://doi.org/10.1248/cpb.38.945.
14. Jankovic, J. (2008). Parkinson's disease: Clinical features and diagnosis. *Journal of Neurology, Neurosurgery, and Psychiatry, 79*(4), 368–376. https://doi.org/10.1136/jnnp.2007.131045.
15. Katzung, B. G., Masters, S. B., & Trevor, A. J. (2009). *Basic and Clinical Pharmacology* (11th ed.). McGraw-Hill.
16. Latha, M., Pari, L., Sitasawad, S., & Bhonde, R. (2004). Insulin-secretagogue activity and cytoprotective role of the traditional antidiabetic plant *Scoparia dulcis* (Sweet broomweed). *Life Sciences, 75*(16), 2003–2014. https://doi.org/10.1016/j.lfs.2004.05.012.
17. Latha, M., Ramkumar, K. M., Pari, L., Damodaran, P. N., Rajeshkannan, V., & Suresh, T. (2006). Phytochemical and antimicrobial study of an antidiabetic plant: *Scoparia dulcis* L. *Journal of Medicinal Food, 9*(3), 391–394. https://doi.org/10.1089/jmf.2006.9.391.
18. May, J. J., Lovell, G., & Hopkins, W. G. (2007). Effectiveness of 1% diclofenac gel in the treatment of wrist extensor tenosynovitis in long-distance kayakers. *Journal of Science and Medicine in Sport, 10*(1), 59–65. https://doi.org/10.1016/j.jsams.2006.06.010.

19. Musacchio, J. M. (2013). Enzymes involved in the biosynthesis and degradation of catecholamines. In L. Iverson (Ed.), *Biochemistry of Biogenic Amines* (pp. 1–35). Springer. ISBN 978-1-4684-3171-1.

20. National Collaborating Centre for Chronic Conditions. (2006). *Parkinson's Disease*. London: Royal College of Physicians. ISBN 1-86016-283-5.

21. Orhue, N. E. J., & Nwanze, E. A. C. (2009). Anti-anemic properties of *Scoparia dulcis* in *Trypanosoma brucei* infected rabbits. *African Journal of Biochemistry Research, 3*(5), 245–249.

22. Oyler, D. R., Parli, S. E., Bernard, A. C., Chang, P. K., Procter, L. D., & Harned, M. E. (2015). Nonopioid management of acute pain associated with trauma: Focus on pharmacologic options. *Journal of Trauma and Acute Care Surgery, 79*(3), 475–483. https://doi.org/10.1097/TA.0000000000000721.

23. Palfi, S., Gurruchaga, J. M., Lepetit, H., Howard, K., Ralph, G. S., Mason, S., & Salgado, N. (2018). Long-term follow-up of a phase I/II study of ProSavin, a lentiviral vector gene therapy for Parkinson's disease. *Human Gene Therapy Clinical Development, 29*(3), 148–155. https://doi.org/10.1089/humc.2018.001.

24. Pari, L., & Latha, M. (2004). Protective role of *Scoparia dulcis* plant extract on brain antioxidant status and lipid peroxidation in STZ diabetic male Wistar rats. *BMC Complementary and Alternative Medicine, 4*, 16. https://doi.org/10.1186/1472-6882-4-16.

25. Phillips, W. J., & Currier, B. L. (2004). Analgesic pharmacology: II. Specific analgesics. *Journal of the American Academy of Orthopedic Surgeons, 12*(4), 221–233. https://doi.org/10.5435/00124635-200407000-00004.

26. Samii, A., Nutt, J. G., & Ransom, B. R. (2004). Parkinson's disease. *Lancet, 363*(9423), 1783–1793. https://doi.org/10.1016/S0140-6736(04)16245-7.

27. Seeman, P. (2009). Historical overview: Introduction to the dopamine receptors. In K. Neve (Ed.), *The Dopamine Receptors* (pp. 1–22). Springer. ISBN 978-1-60327-333-6.

28. Shekelle, P. G., Newberry, S. J., FitzGerald, J. D., Motala, A., O'Hanlon, C. E., Tariq, A., Okunogbe, A., Han, D., & Shanman, R. (2017). Management of gout: A systematic review in support of an American College of Physicians clinical practice guideline. *Annals of Internal Medicine, 166*(1), 37–51. https://doi.org/10.7326/M16-0570.

29. Smischney, N. J., Pollard, E. M., Nookala, A. U., & Olatoye, O. O. (2018). Serotonin syndrome in the perioperative setting. *American Journal of Case Reports, 19*, 833–835. https://doi.org/10.12659/AJCR.911763.

30. Sveinbjornsdottir, S. (2016). The clinical symptoms of Parkinson's disease. *Journal of Neurochemistry, 139*(Suppl 1), 318–324. https://doi.org/10.1111/jnc.13691.

31. van den Bekerom, M. P. J., Sjer, A., Somford, M. P., Bulstra, G. H., Struijs, P. A. A., & Kerkhoffs, G. M. M. J. (2015). Non-steroidal anti-inflammatory drugs (NSAIDs) for treating acute ankle sprains in adults: Benefits outweigh adverse events. *Knee Surgery, Sports Traumatology, Arthroscopy, 23*(8), 2390–2399. https://doi.org/10.1007/s00167-015-3522-3.

32. Zacher, J., Altman, R., Bellamy, N., Brühlmann, P., Da Silva, J., Huskisson, E., & Taylor, R. S. (2008). Topical diclofenac and its role in pain and inflammation: An evidence-based review. *Current Medical Research and Opinion, 24*(4), 925–950. https://doi.org/10.1185/030079908X282098.

Chapter

CHEMOTHERAPEUTIC DRUGS

7

Contents

Introduction

Uncontrolled cell proliferation, invasion, and checkpoint evasion of abnormal, mostly nonfunctional cells are characteristics of cancer. To put it mildly, smoking, genetic mutations, and inadequate diets can all lead to cancer. The incidence of cancer is rising as a result of sedentary lifestyles, crowded, dirty megacities, and people's rising preference for processed foods with additives and preservatives. It would be difficult, if not impossible, to treat cancers that are discovered in their late stages because they may not show symptoms when they first appear. Tumors are primarily made up of two components: the stroma, which is made up of connective tissue and blood vessels, and the proliferating cells. Chemotherapy has proven to be one of our most effective treatments for cancer.

Chemotherapy is the process of killing cancer cells by administering a variety of medications and chemicals, either separately or in combination. Chemotherapeutic medications target and eradicate cancer cells throughout the patient's body, whereas radiation and surgery target specific areas of the body. Chemotherapies aim to achieve three goals: relief, control, and cure. When chemotherapy drugs are used to kill cancer cells, the situation is defined as "Control," meaning that achieving a full remission seems unlikely. As a result, the goal of treatment would be to reduce the size of the tumor or to slow down its growth and angiogenesis. Palliation is the process of reducing the discomfort, side effects, and illnesses brought on by cancer. Most often, it is done when cancer has progressed to the point where it cannot be completely cured; in this case, our goal would be to enhance the quality of life.

The methods for prescribing chemotherapy depend on many factors, such as the type and stage of the cancer, the patient's age, general health, other coexisting medical conditions, and previous chemotherapy experiences. The other essential factor in obtaining the best outcome is following the recommended dosage because chemotherapeutic medications are unable to discriminate between cancerous and healthy cells. The patient's weight, body surface area, age, nutritional status, history of radiation therapy, and blood cell count all affect how much is administered. Additionally, a good drug administration schedule may help achieve the least amount of side effects and the most effective anti-cancer activity.

Different phases of the cell cycle are the focus of chemotherapeutic agents. Based on how they interfere with cell reproduction in different stages of the cell cycle and damage DNA by alkylating substrates, they are categorized into distinct groups. These factors have an effect on somatic cells as well as bone marrow stem cells, which makes them a better choice for solid tumors and leukemia. Conversely, antimetabolite agents—also referred to as RNA and DNA blockers—replace the conventional structures of RNA and DNA. The so-called process prevents chromosomes from multiplying, which is why these medications are effective against ovarian, breast, and leukemia cancers. However, anti-tumor antibiotics inhibit the activity of enzymes linked to DNA duplication, in contrast to conventional antibiotics. These are called anthracyclines, and many cancers have been treated with them. However, non-Anthracyclines have been developed to lessen these side effects because permanent heart failure is one of their serious side effects. Additionally, topoisomerase I and II inhibitors block topoisomerase activity, which prevents DNA replication. However, topoisomerase II inhibitors increase the likelihood of developing secondary cancers, including acute myeloid leukemia (AML). Furthermore, compounds derived from plants known as mitotic inhibitors disrupt distinct stages of the cell cycle, obstructing cell proliferation. However, one drawback of these compounds is that they may cause unintentional harm to the nervous system. Lastly, the chemotherapy drug's side effects, like nausea, vomiting, and allergic reactions, have been treated with corticosteroids (Table 7.1).

Table 7.1. *The Category of Chemotherapy Drugs*

Category	Drugs	Mechanisms of action
Alkylating agents	Altretamine	Damage the DNA
Busulfan		
Carboplatin		
Carmustine		
Chlorambucil		
Cisplatin		
Cyclophosphamide		
Dacarbazine		
Lomustine		
Melphalan		
Oxaliplatin		
Temozolomide		
Thiotepa		
Antimetabolite	5-fluorouracil (5-FU)	Substitute the RNA and DNA blocks
6-mercaptopurine (6-MP)		
Capecitabine (Xeloda)		
Cytarabine (Ara-C)		
Floxuridine		
Fludarabine		
Gemcitabine (Gemzar)		
Hydroxyurea		
Methotrexate		
Pemetrexed (Alimta)		

Anti-tumor Antibiotics	Anthracyclines	Epirubicin	Interfere with the activity of DNA replication enzymes
		Idarubicin	
		Daunorubicin	
		Doxorubicin (Adriamycin)	
	non-Anthracyclines	Actinomycin-D	
		Bleomycin	
		Mitomycin-C	
		Mitoxantrone	
Topoisomerase inhibitors	Topoisomerase inhibitor I	Topotecan	Interfere with the topoisomerase enzymes and incorporate the unwinding DNA in replication and transcription
		Irinotecan (CPT-11)	
	Topoisomerase inhibitor II	Etoposide (VP-16)	
		Teniposide	
		Mitoxantrone	
Mitotic inhibitors		Docetaxel	Hinder the cell proliferation and division
Estramustine			
Ixabepilone			
Paclitaxel			
Vinblastine			
Vincristine			
Vinorelbine			
Corticosteroids		Prednisone	Palliate the chemotherapy side effects
Methylprednisone (Solumedrol)			
Dexamethasone (Decadron)			
EGFR inhibitors		Tarceva (Erlotinib)	Blocks the epidermal growth factor receptors on tumor cells
Erbitux (Cetuximab)			
Iressa (Gefitinib)			

Source: https://www.ncbi.nlm.nih.gov/pmc/articles/PMC7938256/table/tbl0001/?report=objectonly.

That being said, chemoresistance and tumor recurrence are two important and serious side effects of chemotherapy. Resistance can be intrinsic or extrinsic (acquired); multi-drug resistance is one way that cancer cells develop resistance to various chemotherapeutic drugs through shared resistance mechanisms. Other mechanisms by which cancer cells become resistant to drugs include improved DNA repair mechanisms, increased drug efflux, reduced apoptosis, improved detoxification, and changed expression of the drug target.

We have chosen members of each chemotherapeutic drug family to talk about their cellular and molecular pathways that lead to cell resistance and death in this regard. Additionally, we have provided an overview of the current uses for combination chemotherapy, which includes a wide range of encapsulated and combined chemotherapy drugs. We also talked about how next-generation sequencing (NGS), whole-exome sequencing (WES), machine learning, and precision medicine could be used to advance cancer immunotherapies. To provide a realistic view of the future of therapies in cancer cases, some of the most recent clinical trials of the application of immunotherapies and combination chemotherapies were also included.

Orientation and Directional Terms

Term	Definition	Illustration
Chemotherapy	Chemotherapy is the type of cancer treatment that uses one or more anti-cancer drugs in a standard regimen. Chemotherapy may be given with a curative intent, or it may aim only to prolong life or to reduce symptoms.	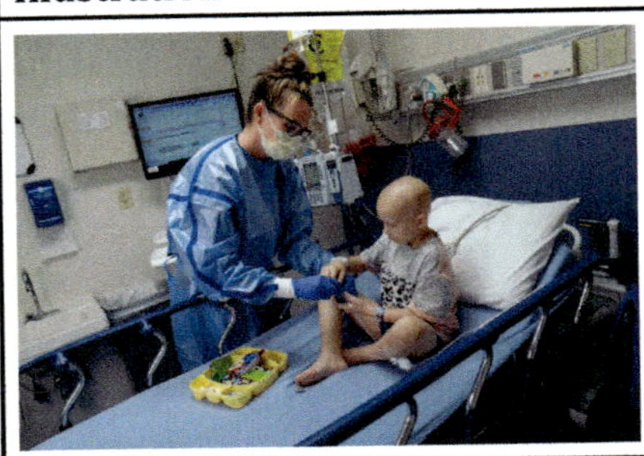
Leukemia	Leukemia is a type of blood cancer that causes the bone marrow to produce an abnormal amount of white blood cells. These abnormal white blood cells, also known as blasts or leukemia cells, are unable to fight infection and prevent the bone marrow from producing healthy red blood cells and platelets.	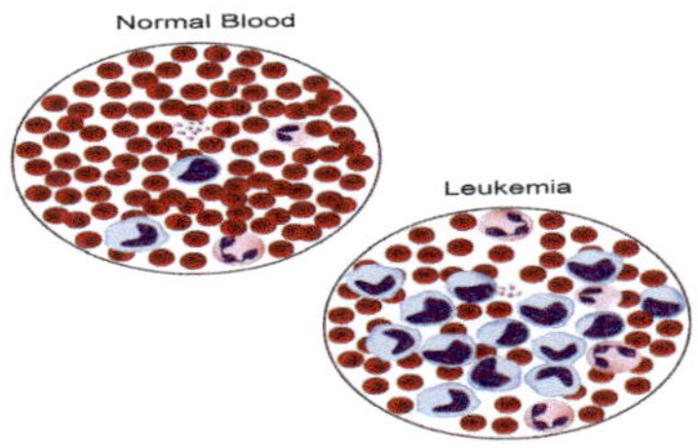
Nucleotide excision repair (NER)	Nucleotide excision repair (NER) is a DNA repair mechanism that removes damaged DNA strands. It's a multistep process that can remove a wide variety of DNA lesions, including: Cyclobutane pyrimidine dimers (CPD), 6-4 photoproducts (6-4PP), Base adducts, and Reactive oxygen species (ROS)-induced base modifications	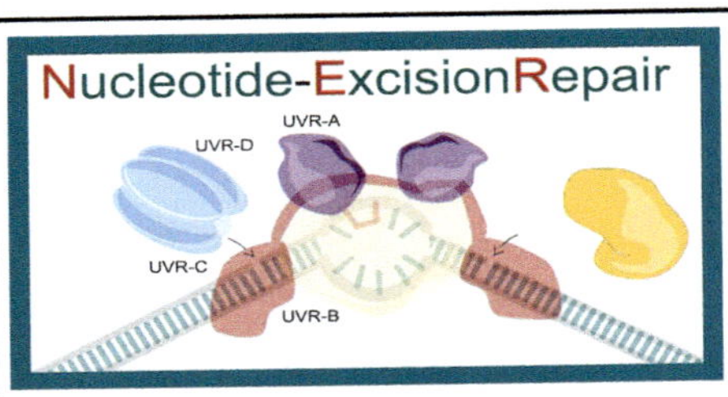
Phagocytosis	Phagocytosis is the process by which a cell uses its plasma membrane to engulf a large particle (≥ 0.5 **µm**), giving rise to an internal compartment called the phagosome. It is one type of endocytosis. A cell that performs phagocytosis is called a phagocyte.	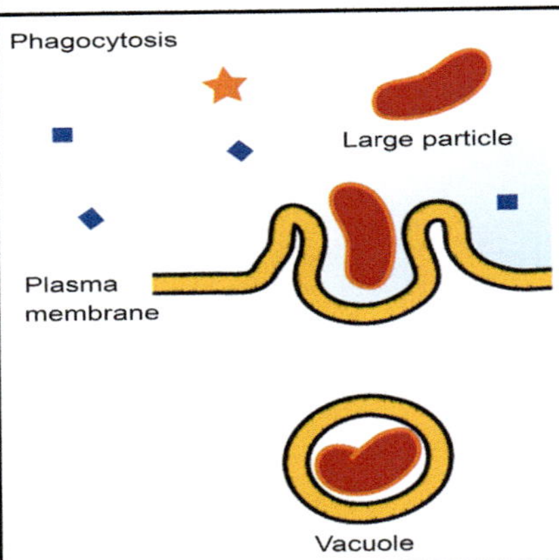
Cell proliferation	Cell proliferation is the process by which cells grow and divide to produce more cells. It's a vital mechanism for tissue growth, wound healing, and the growth of multicellular organisms.	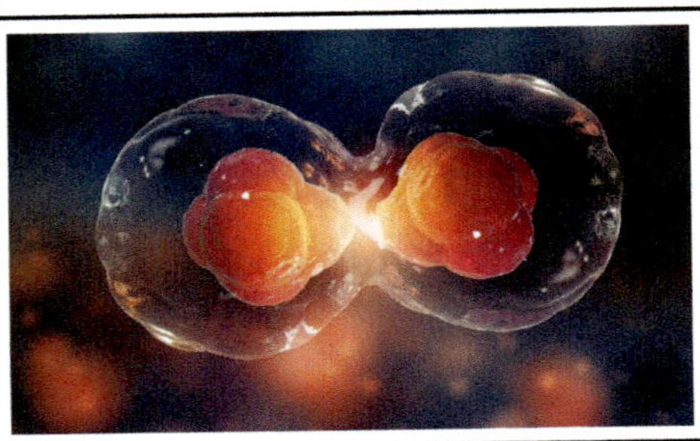

7.1. Current Chemotherapeutic Drugs and Their Mechanisms of Action

7.1.1. Cisplatin

7.1.1.1. Cisplatin Mechanism of Action

One of the most useful chemotherapeutic medications is cisplatin, or isoamminedichloroplatinum, which is prescribed for half of all malignancies. When cisplatin is injected intravenously, it binds to albumin and other plasma proteins to travel through the bloodstream and eventually enter target cells through copper transporters. It's interesting to note that only 1% of the drug that is administered affects DNA. The platinum-based combinations found in cisplatin create intra- and interstrand adducts between guanine and adenine in the opposing strands of DNA, which cause cell cycle arrest and trigger apoptosis. Cisplatin creates these adducts in two stages to demonstrate this. It first bonds with N7 guanine and then forms a second link with either guanine or adenine in the same strand or in the opposite strand. A general distortion in the DNA framework results from cisplatin's formation of multiple adducts and cross-links within the DNA structure, which is made possible by the readily accessible N7 atoms in guanine and adenine.

Mechanisms of cisplatin in signaling cascades-mediated cell cisplatin binds to DNA, the structure of the DNA is bent. This bend is recognized by a variety of proteins, including the high mobility group (HMG), a type of non-histone- and chromosome-structural protein that binds to cisplatin adducts in DNA with preference. Because HMG proteins prevent nucleotide excision repair (NER) and mismatch repair (MMR) from identifying the damaged DNA, p53, the genome security guard, is activated. This raises the activity of waf1, p21, and MDM2, which results in cell cycle arrest. To elaborate, cisplatin causes oxidative stress in cells. Reactive oxygen species (ROS) damage cell lipids, proteins, and DNA. BCL2 inhibition and caspase activation initiate the intrinsic pathway of apoptosis, assuming the damage is significant or irreversible. The integrity of the mitochondrial membrane is also impacted by BCL2 inhibition. Furthermore, cisplatin lowers glutathione levels in the mitochondria, which produces hydroxyl radicals and oxidative stress, both of which compromise the integrity of the mitochondrial membrane. As a result, cytochrome C is released and continues to interact with Apaf-1. Poly ADP-ribose polymerase (PARP) is cleaved and activated as a result of this interaction activating pro-caspase 9, which in turn activates caspases 3 and 7, also referred to as the executioner caspases. Due to DNA fragmentation, loss of function, and the breakdown of several essential proteins, PARP initiates cell death.

Furthermore, cisplatin is thought to target DNA in the mitochondria. Since there are many guanine-rich stretches in mitochondrial DNA (mtDNA), cisplatin forms more adducts within the mtDNA structure than it does in cellular DNA. It follows that mitochondrial functions would also probably be compromised.

Furthermore, research has clearly demonstrated that cisplatin affects the MAPK family. Serine/threonine kinases like JNK, p38, and ERK are included in MAPK and are essential for cell survival and proliferation. To exemplify this, consider the following: cisplatin stimulates ERK, which in turn permits p53's phosphorylation and activation, instigating BAX transcription, p21 overexpression, and cell cycle arrest. Additionally, cisplatin-induced DNA damage from platinum-based combinations activates JNK, which in turn stabilizes and activates pro-apoptotic protein p73. P73 cooperates with JNK to facilitate apoptosis induced by cisplatin. Moreover, P18 interacts with p53 in a way that stabilizes and strengthens the correlation between p53 and the pro-apoptotic gene NOXA. For this reason, cisplatin may also activate the pathways leading to cell death via p18-p38. It's interesting to note that p38 also contributes to the cisplatin-induced cell death process by activating EGFRs and causing them to internalize.

Furthermore, it has been documented that cisplatin phosphorylates Chk1 and Chk2, which stops the cell cycle at the G2 phase. Moreover, it promotes Cdc25C activation and trafficking to the cytoplasm, obstructing the cell cycle's transition to the M phase.

The mechanisms underlying cisplatin resistance via signaling cascades and strategies for addressing them Chemoresistance is an undesirable trait in cancer cells. It has restricted the use of different medications to treat different types of cancer. More specifically, there are two main subcategories of chemoresistance: 1) innate resistance, where the drug that is administered has no effect at all, and 2) acquired resistance, where the drug that is administered initially as a chemotherapeutic loses its beneficial effects over time. Changes in the cellular drug absorption pattern, drug influx and efflux patterns, conjugation to glutathione or metallothionein, increased drug detoxification, activation of DNA repair mechanisms, and inhibition of apoptosis pathways are the causes of the so-called condition.

Arguments concerning cisplatin resistance in patients with ovarian, lung, and colorectal cancer have been made.

Numerous mechanisms have been demonstrated in the context of cisplatin resistance; including:

1. Tumor cells increase drug efflux, therefore decreasing the intracellular accumulation of cisplatin;
2. Escalated intracellular levels of glutathione and metallothioneins, that are intracellular scavengers, increase drug detoxification;
3. Stimulation of DNA repair machinery such as nucleotide excision repair (NER), inter-strand bound repair and mismatch repair (MMR) which attenuates the impact of cisplatin; and finally
4. Adjustment in the approaches of apoptosis-based cell death.

The previously mentioned processes result in cisplatin inactivation and stop cisplatin-DNA adduct formation. In the transportation of cisplatin, three copper transporters (CTRs) have different functions. Although studies on human ovarian carcinoma have shown a decrease in CTR1 expression level, CTR1 improves cisplatin uptake. Consequently, it has been observed that loss of CTR1 reduces the intracellular build-up of cisplatin, resulting in cisplatin resistance. Furthermore, it has been demonstrated that elevated levels of ATP7A and ATP7B, which support copper efflux, improve cisplatin resistance.

Furthermore, a variety of substances, including RNA, thiol peptides, and cell microfilaments, attach to cisplatin after it accumulates intracellularly, causing cisplatin to become blocked. Thiol peptides and RNA strands form adducts with cisplatin inside the cell to demonstrate this. The enzyme glutathione S transferase (GST) controls the conjugation of glutathione and cisplatin. It possesses a regulatory sensor made of cysteine residues. Consequently, this also leads to the inhibition of cisplatin-DNA adducts. Studies show a correlation between cisplatin resistance and high glutathione and GST levels. Moreover, metallothionein binds to cisplatin, reducing the dosage that is given and promoting drug resistance and inactivation.

Numerous proteins, including replication protein A (RPA), xeroderma pigmentosum A (XPA), and XPG, are implicated in NER. Research has shown that deficiencies in NER heighten the susceptibility to platinum-based chemotherapeutic agents. Consequently, it is thought that NER protein overexpression is associated with cisplatin resistance.

Moreover, a higher tumor mass is associated with abnormal activation of signaling pathways related to cell survival, such as PI3K, AKT, and mTOR. It has been demonstrated that RSK proteins, such as Ras-ERK mediators, which are important for cell survival, activate BCL-2 and NHE1 to inhibit apoptotic pathways (Figure 7.1).

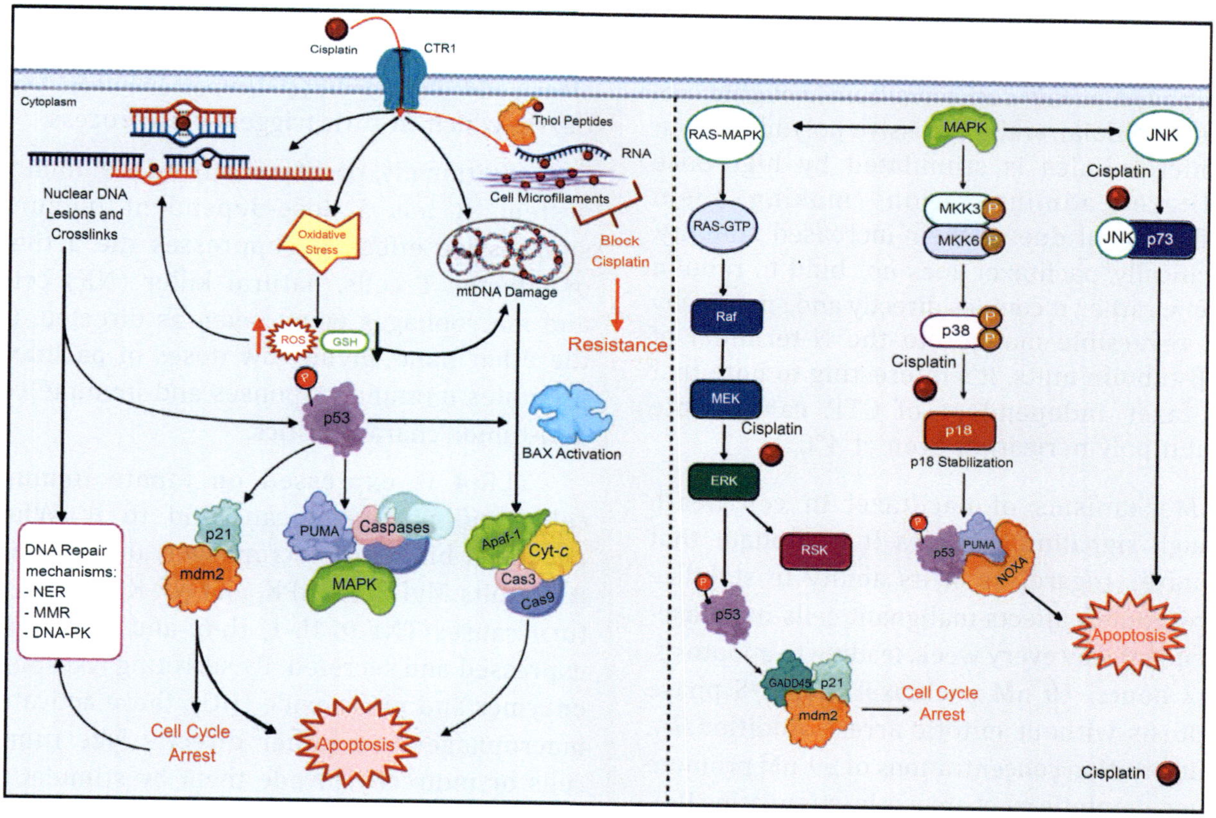

Figure 7.1. *Platinum-based combinations in cisplatin constructs inter- and intrastrand adducts, namely lesions, within the nuclear and mitochondrial DNA.*

Source: ncbi.nlm.nih.gov/pmc/articles/PMC7938256/.

7.1.2. Paclitaxel

7.1.2.1. Paclitaxel Mechanism of Action

Paclitaxel is a member of the taxane family of chemotherapeutic drugs, which stimulates tubulin polymerization. Except vinblastine, which stacks tubulin and depolymerizes the microtubules, all taxanes stabilize microtubules. The building blocks of microtubule structure are called tubulins. In metaphase and anaphase, taxanes can obstruct cell division by hindering the polymerization of microtubules. It goes without saying that microtubules are essential for many cellular processes, such as phagocytosis, mitosis, transport, cell shape maintenance, and secretion. Targeting these microtubules, paclitaxel causes severe damage to spindles in the G2 and M phases, particularly during prophase. Horwitz states that paclitaxel stops cell division and replication by making β-tubulin microtubules more polymerized and inhibiting their depolymerization. As a result, poisoned cells will be stopped in the G2/M phases and will undergo apoptosis. Recent data has revealed that microtubule depolymerization is inhibited at low concentrations, roughly less than nanomolar, while excessive polymerization of microtubules is stimulated by high-dose paclitaxel administration, making them nonfunctional due to their increased stability. Specifically, paclitaxel does not bind to tubulin dimers; rather, it couples directly and specifically in a reversible manner to the N-terminal of the β-tubulin units. It's interesting to note that paclitaxel, independent of GTP, canpromote tubulin polymerization even at 4°C.

Mechanisms of paclitaxel in cell death through signaling cascades It is thought that paclitaxel, regardless of its ability to stabilize microtubules, affects malignant cells in a dose-dependent way every week, leading to apoptosis. In 12 hours, 10 nM paclitaxel causes S phase apoptosis without mitotic arrest. Additionally, administration concentrations of ≥9 nM promote further apoptotic mechanisms by stimulating Raf-1 activation, while administration concentrations of ≤9 nM induce p53 and p21, further apoptosis independent of Raf-1 activation.

Furthermore, paclitaxel cantrigger additional pro-apoptotic pathways. Paclitaxel's ability to cause cell death is linked to the JNK, MAPK, NF-KB, JAK, and STAT pathways, which are all related to the toll-like receptor-4 (TLR-4) pathway. The apoptosis cascade is eventually triggered by the phosphorylation of Bcl2 and the dephosphorylation of Bad and Bax, which are caused by the activation of MAPK.

Paclitaxel administered once a week has also demonstrated anti-angiogenic effects. Put differently, data points to the inhibition of vascular endothelial growth factor (VEGF) expression following low-dose paclitaxel administration.

The induction of ROS generation is how paclitaxel achieves its other mode of action. Nicotinamide adenine dinucleotide phosphate (NADPH) oxidase induction causes oxidative stress and the ensuing pathways leading to cell death, which in turn triggers this process.

Additionally, paclitaxel affects the immune system. It has a dose-dependent immune-suppressive effect. It suppresses the activity of effector T cells, natural killer (NK) cells, and macrophages when taken as directed. On the other hand, giving low doses of paclitaxel promotes immune responses and immune cell anti-tumor characteristics.

TLR-4 is expressed on innate immune cells, and paclitaxel can bind to it. When paclitaxel binds to macrophages, for example, it recruits MyD88, MAPK, and NF-KB, which in turn causes TNF-α, IL-1, IL-6, and IL-8 to be expressed and secreted. By secreting lysosomal enzymes and nitric oxide (NO), these activated macrophages can either directly lyze tumor cells or indirectly invade them by stimulating dendritic cells (DCs), NK cells, and cytotoxic T lymphocytes (CTLs). Furthermore, paclitaxel can also directly stimulate DCs via TLR-4. Upregulating the expression of genes linked to antigen presentation, costimulatory molecules, and IL-12P70 causes DC maturation. As a result, it enhances DCs' ability to activate T cells and trigger anti-tumor responses.

It is now widely understood that tumor cells can reduce MHC class I and specific tumor antigens to elude cytotoxic T lymphocytes. On the other hand, NK cells appear to help eradicate tumors in this way. It has been demonstrated that paclitaxel stimulates NK cell capacity to kill tumor cells by inducing mRNA transcription and protein expression of perforin. But it's important to remember that paclitaxel also has a dose-dependent effect on NK cells.

There are additional effects of paclitaxel on immune-related processes. To demonstrate this, consider the fact that paclitaxel increases mannose-6-phosphate, which raises granzyme B cellular permeability and enhances T lymphocyte cytotoxicity. Moreover, it stimulates the release of type I cytokines, such as IFN-γ from CD^{8+} T cells and IL-2 from $CD4^{+}$ T cells. Upon further differentiation, activated CD^{8+} T cells can become MHC I-CTL type 1 (Tc1) secreting IFN-γ, which is accountable for the lysis of tumor cells. It is well known that $CD^{4+}CD^{25+}$ Tregs support tumor cells by thwarting immunological responses and accelerating the development of cancer. Studies on mice have shown that paclitaxel increases the anti-tumor capabilities of immune cells by reducing Treg size and number. Additionally, paclitaxel increased the pro-apoptotic factor Bax in Tregs while decreasing the expression level of the anti-apoptotic agent Bcl-2, making Tregs more prone to apoptosis.

Moreover, an ultra-low dose of paclitaxel dampens myeloid-derived suppressor cells (MDSCs), which tumor cells are using to proliferate and inhibit immune responses in a study conducted on C57Bl/6 mice. More specifically, paclitaxel at ultra-low doses promotes MDSC differentiation into DCs without the need for TLR-4. Because of the previously mentioned information, paclitaxel can stimulate immune responses against tumor cells and trigger the apoptotic pathways within these cells in addition to suppressing Tregs.

Many genes are correlated with paclitaxel resistance, but not all of them have been thoroughly elucidated. Mechanisms of paclitaxel resistance through signaling cascades and how to be addressed Multifactor approaches. It has been suggested that paclitaxel-resistant cells primarily have altered levels of mRNA and protein synthesis, including multiple transcriptional factors and ribosomal genes. They also show changes in the glutathione metabolism pathways, glycolysis (ADH1A, HK1, and ENO3), and genes linked to oxidative stress (UGT1A6, MAOA, and CYBA). This theory has been supported by research results wherein tumor cells were treated with paclitaxel and other chemotherapeutic medications. Put differently, out of 845 genes, 337 had altered levels of expression. Changes in their gene expression profiles disrupt the effects of drugs, the cellular structure, the tumor microenvironment, and changes in metabolism that can cause resistance in tumor cells.

Additionally, because cancers proliferate aggressively, new, malformed vessels are created to meet their oxygen needs; however, the rate at which they grow causes hypoxia and oxygen depletion. In response to this microenvironment, tumor cells change and adapt. As a result, they continue to exist and have the capacity to multiply, spread, invade, progress, and lose sensitivity to chemotherapy.

This process does not stop here; hypoxia causes resistance to chemotherapy by altering both genomic and proteomic profiles. Essentially, the lack of oxygen triggers the activation of P53, inhibits cell death, and promotes blood vessel formation by increasing VEGF and angiogenin levels. It also boosts the production and release of growth factors like PDGF, TGF-β, and IGF, and encourages glycolysis, all of which support cell survival. Tumor cells evade cell death, thanks to the hypoxic environment and HIF-1, which halts cell growth at a certain stage and makes them less susceptible to drugs like paclitaxel. In addition, other factors like NF-KB and STAT3, which stimulate inflammation, cell survival, blood vessel formation, cell growth, and cancer spread, are activated at low oxygen levels. Furthermore, paclitaxel enhances the activity of BCL-2, an anti-cell death protein, through NF-KB under hypoxic circumstances, which helps to resist cell death and withstand chemotherapy. Studies have found that inhibiting STAT3 can decrease resistance to paclitaxel. The activation of certain genes, enzymes, and inflammatory substances also contributes to resistance against paclitaxel in hypoxic conditions.

One common mechanism of chemoresistance in tumor cells treated with different chemotherapeutic drugs is drug efflux. P-glycoprotein (P-gp) and other ATP-binding cassette (ABC) transporters facilitate drug efflux. MDR-1 encodes P-gp, which has been demonstrated to increase paclitaxel chemosensitivity. According to reports, tumor cells resistant to paclitaxel overexpress P-gp.

Furthermore, it has been suggested that tubulin-related pathways contribute to paclitaxel resistance. They are insufficient for paclitaxel to act because of a decrease in their intracellular concentration. Conversely, paclitaxel resistance is a result of point mutations in tubulin genes and variations in the expression level of different tubulin isotypes, including class-III β-tubulin (Figure 7.2).

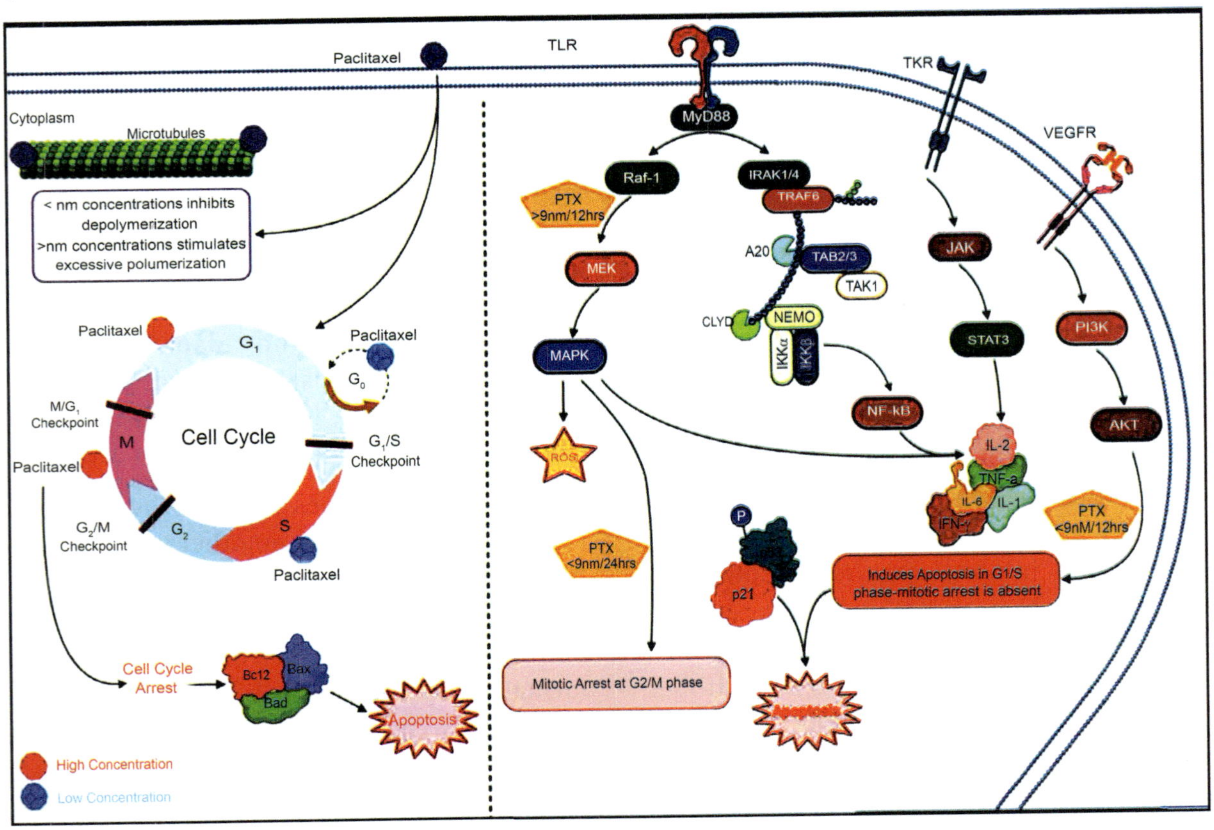

Figure 7.2. *Paclitaxel targets microtubules and wreck havoc on spindles in G2, prophase, and M phases.*

Source: https://www.ncbi.nlm.nih.gov/pmc/articles/PMC7938256/.

7.1.3. Gefitinib and Erlotinib

7.1.3.1. Gefitinib and Erlotinib Mechanism of Action

Tyrosine kinase inhibitors (TKIs) are structurally identical to adenosine triphosphate (ATP) and are non-peptide combinations that are prescribed orally. They fight for the ATP-binding domains in kinases, which halts the signaling transduction that follows and eventually results in cell proliferation inhibition and apoptosis. TKIs are represented by erlotinib, gefitinib, and lapatinib. Because cancer cells express more tyrosine kinase receptors of epidermal growth factors, drugs like gefitinib are used to block these receptors. EGFRI-gefitinib inhibits growth signaling via EGFRs, preventing cell division and survival. Although gefitinib has shown promise in treating non-small cell lung cancer and shrinking thyroid tumors, chemoresistance is unavoidable. Similar mechanisms of action are used by erlotinib; however, its use is restricted by chemoresistance and high cost. Erlotinib has a half-life of approximately 36 hours and exhibits a strong affinity for plasma proteins, including albumin and α-1 acid glycoprotein. Cytochrome P450 (CYP) 3A4 is the primary metabolizer of erlotinib; however, CYP1A2 may also slightly metabolize it. Erlotinib's plasma level has reportedly increased when it is administered in combination with ketoconazole, a CYP3A4 inhibitor.

Reasons for gefitinib and erlotinib's involvement in signaling cascade-mediated cell death EGFRs are overexpressed in many cancers, such as non-small cell lung cancer (40–80%), colorectal cancer (72–28%), head and neck cancer (95–20%), breast cancer (14–51%), and renal cell cancer (50–90%). Furthermore, many studies suggested that the VEGF and EGFR pathways interact.

As previously indicated, gefitinib and erlotinib inhibit the tyrosine kinase domain of EGFRs by acting as an ATP antagonist and competing with it for intracellular binding sites. This lowers the tyrosine kinase activity of EGFRs. ErbB-2/Neu/HER2, ErbB-3/HER3, and ErbB-4/HER4 are the other members of the ErbB family, which includes the 170-kDa transmembrane glycoprotein known as EGFR. These cell surface receptors support cell survival, differentiation, and growth regulation. EGFR dimerizes in a hetero- or homo-modal manner depending on which way its extracellular domain attaches to its ligand. The intracellular domains' tyrosine kinase activity is made possible by this dimerization, and as a result, their cytoplasmic tyrosine residues undergo autophosphorylation. The tyrosine residues additionally offer a docking platform on which a range of intracellular signaling proteins attach and become active, ultimately affecting the degree of gene expression.

Different central downstream signaling cascades are linked to the activation of EGFR. These cascades include Ras/Raf mitogen-activated protein, phospholipase C (PLCγ), extracellular signal-regulated kinase (ERK1,2), PI3/Akt, Jak2/STAT3, and modulation of calcium channels. While they prevent apoptosis, these cascades also encourage angiogenesis, invasion, metastasis, and cell proliferation. Thus, blocking EGFRs and the downstream signaling cascades they trigger reduces angiogenesis, invasion, metastasis, and cell proliferation. It also induces apoptosis and supports concurrent radiation treatments.

Finding somatic mutations in the ATP-binding domain of EGFR genes recently has provided insight into how to get the desired effects from EGFR-TKIs like erlotinib and gefitinib. Specifically, the most intriguing mutations were missense mutations at codon 858, which result in the substitution of arginine for leucine in exon 21 with a frequency of 35–45%, and frame deletion mutations in exon 19, codons 746–750, which have a frequency of 45–50% among all

EGFR mutations. Following the administration of EGFR-TKIs, a subset of non-small cell lung cancer patients with the previously mentioned somatic mutations showed improved outcomes. At least one of these EFGR gene mutations is present in erlotinib/gefitinib responders, according to recent studies.

Apart from the comparable roles that various TKIs play, gefitinib also has additional effects. Put differently, during sub-G1/G1 phases of the cell cycle, gefitinib administration results in a reduction of cyclin D1 and Cdk4 and an increase in P27. Furthermore, gefitinib reduces the phosphorylation of GSK-3β, a target of AKT kinase, glycogen synthase kinase. A large body of research suggests that gefitinib causes apoptosis in part by raising P38 MAPK levels, dephosphorylating FOXOs, which increases P27 levels later on, and upregulating caspase 3 and BIM expression. Furthermore, it has been documented that the administration of gefitinib results in the down-regulation of mTOR signaling. Mechanisms of erlotinib and gefitinib resistance through signaling cascades and strategies for addressing them: Most patients become resistant to TKIs in less than a year. Many mechanisms remain elusive, despite the fact that some have been found thus far.

It has been shown that dysregulated microRNAs play a role in TKI-chemoresistance. More specifically, in erlotinib-resistant non-small cell lung cancer, miR-21 is markedly overexpressed. This leads to the downregulation of PTEN and PDCD4, which in turn increases the proliferation and progression of the cancer by activating AKT. However, it has been demonstrated that tumor-suppressive miR-34 is downregulated in cancers that are resistant to TKIs, including those that have received erlotinib treatment. Overexpression of MiR-34 has been used to resensitize tumors and encourage cell cycle arrest, either in conjunction with erlotinib therapy or independently. It's interesting to note that miR-147b has been shown to modify the TCA cycle to promote resistance against osimertinib, the third generation of EGFR TKIs. Additionally, miR-17–5p and miR-641 contribute to resistance to erlotinib. In non-small cell lung cancer, it has been demonstrated that overexpression of miR-17–5p resensitizes tumor cells to erlotinib through EZH1; however, overexpression of miR-641 promotes erlotinib resistance by downregulating NF1. A. Pal, S., and others. have unequivocally shown that the regulation of erlotinib resistance and drug efflux is mediated by miR-5693, miR-3618, and miR-432–5p. Additionally, the effects of miR-3618, miR-5693, and miR-432–5p were assessed in conjunction with gefitinib and afatinib, two additional EGFR TKIs. It's interesting to note that in the presence of these TKIs, they have considerably accelerated cancer progression and cell proliferation.

According to recent research, EGFR TKI resistance is increased when the epithelial-mesenchymal transition (EMT) is stimulated. It is widely known that the transforming growth factor-beta (TGF-β) pathway, which induces migration in a variety of cancers, including lung malignancies, appears to be one of the primary drivers of tumor invasiveness and metastasis. TGF-β ligands bind to the TGF-β receptor complex, which is made up of TGF-βRI and TGF-βRII, to demonstrate this. Subsequently, Smad2 and Smad3 are phosphorylated and activated by the receptor. These transcriptional factors, along with Smad4, form a transcriptional complex that can induce the expression of genes linked to tumor progression. Consequently, TGF-β overexpression promotes the growth, division, and metastasis of tumors. It has been hypothesized that EGFR TKIs can reduce cell migration brought on by TGF-β. That being said,

Serizawa et al. have demonstrated that EGFR TKIs like erlotinib and gefitinib, when combined with TGF-β inhibitors like LY364947, slow down the growth and invasion of cancer cells resistant to EGFR TKIs.

Furthermore, integrins have been linked to malignancies that are resistant to erlotinib. Kanda and associates. have demonstrated that the levels of β_1, α_2, and α_5 integrins were elevated in all resistant cells. Moreover, they demonstrated how integrin β1 could be knocked down using siRNA to resensitize cancerous cells to erlotinib, which resulted in a complete dampening of Akt phosphorylation. This idea indicates that integrin β_1 silencing reduces erlotinib-chemoresistance. However, in these cancers, Akt phosphorylation was moderately inhibited by silencing α_2 and α_5 integrins. Furthermore, it was observed that integrin α_5 expression was downregulated upon integrin β_1 silencing, indicating a potential correlation between the two integrins. These results collectively indicate the function of integrins in erlotinib-chemoresistance.

Additionally, in non-small cell lung cancer, EGFR TKI resistance is mediated by ras-associated binding protein-25 (Rab25). Regarding this, Wang et al. have revealed that erlotinib resistance was triggered by Rab25 overexpression. Specifically, Rab25 binds to integrin β_1, promoting its passage toward the membrane and triggering Akt phosphorylation there. It additionally initiates the Wnt/β-catenin signaling cascade, facilitating cell division and the advancement of cancer. Additionally, they demonstrated how Akt-related signaling cascades, Wnt/β-catenin, and Rab25 silencing could dampen them and make cancer cells more susceptible to erlotinib.

Gefitinib resistance is also correlated with the activation of EGFR downstream cascades. Within breast cancer models, intrinsic and acquired resistance is partly attributed to the hyperactivation of the MAPK pathway, particularly P42-MAPK. Thus, by inhibiting MAPK-related pathways, it was possible to witness the induction of apoptosis and the inhibition of cell proliferation. Interestingly, some research has suggested that gefitinib has a transcriptional function. This is achieved by boosting the importation and nuclear accumulation of neuregulin, a HER ligand, as well as the expression of HER-specific ligands. Additionally, some results showed that another factor contributing to gefitinib resistance is the upregulation of PI3K, which is caused by a non-functioning PTEN. Put differently, studies conducted on subtypes of breast cancer that overexpress EGFR but lack PTEN activity showed that gefitinib prevented EGFR and MAPK from becoming phosphorylated while maintaining AKT. However, in the case of the PTEN-restored cell populations treated with gefitinib, there was a reduction in the phosphorylation of AKT, GSK-3β, and the translation repressor protein 4EBP1. Additionally, they developed a resensitization to gefitinib and were halted at the G1 phase.

Gefitinib chemoresistance is also correlated with other pathways pertaining to the interaction between EGFRs and the hepatocyte growth factor receptor (MET). Gefitinib resistance and the advancement of breast cancer are linked to MET, a tyrosine kinase receptor that raises EGFR phosphorylation by activating c-Src kinase. It has been demonstrated that MET inhibition in EGFR-overexpressed and HER-2 positive breast cancers reduced cell proliferation and made cells more sensitive to gefitinib (Figure 7.3).

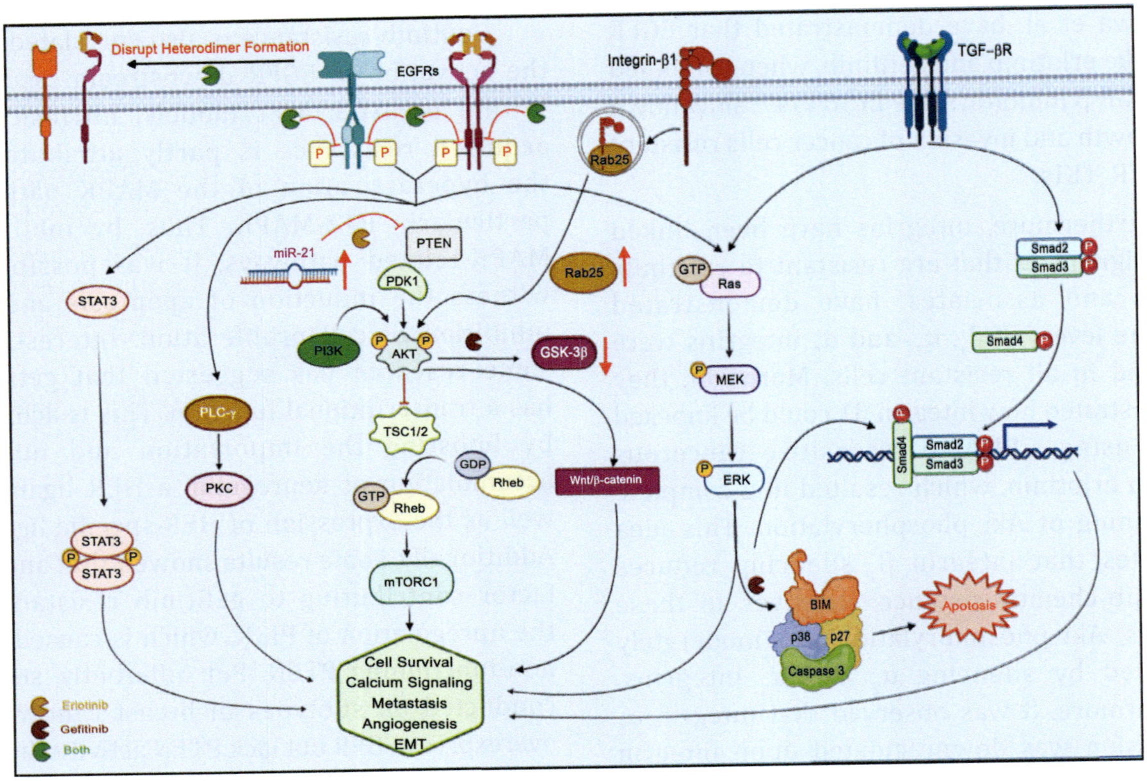

Figure 7.3. *Tyrosine kinase inhibitors (TKIs) are similar to ATP; hence they compete for ATP-binding domains in kinases of EGFRs.*

Source: https://www.ncbi.nlm.nih.gov/pmc/articles/PMC7938256/.

Because tyrosine kinase inhibitors (TKIs) and ATP are similar, they compete with one another for ATP-binding domains in EGFR kinases. If the aforementioned pathways are absent, they can activate the machinery of apoptosis because they inhibit PI3K/Akt, JAK/STAT, PLCγ, and Ras/Raf. Moreover, gefitinib raises p27 levels and activates p38-MAPK, both of which lead to apoptosis. TGF-β signaling is one important way that cells become resistant to EGFR TKIs. Cell survival and EMT are stimulated by recruiting Smads 2, 3, and 4. Additionally, Rab25, which closely interacts with integrin β1, is correlated with resistance to TKIs. More specifically, it phosphorylates Akt, which in turn helps signaling cascades related to proliferation and survival.

7.1.4. Gemcitabine

7.1.4.1. Gemcitabine Mechanism of Action

Under a process known as "masked chain termination," 2□,2□-difluoro-2□-deoxycytidine (dFdCTP), also referred to as gemcitabine, functions as the analog of deoxycytidine. By using dFdCTP, it is possible to replace it with a regular nucleoside, which halts DNA duplication and DNA polymerase activity. However, gemcitabine is not able to separate from the DNA strands by DNA repair mechanisms.

Gemcitabine functions through two mechanisms. The first involves enhancing its ability to inhibit key enzymes involved in the metabolism of deoxynucleotides. dFdCTP and dFdCDP, respectively, directly and indirectly, inhibit the enzyme deoxycytidylate deaminase (dCTD). More specifically, dFdCDP binds covalently to the active sites of ribonucleotide reductase (RR), preventing ribonucleotides from being converted to deoxynucleotides and causing a shortage in the dNTP pool. As a result of this shortfall, dCTD activity is subsequently reduced. Furthermore, because dCTP modulates deoxycytidine kinase (dCK), a reduced-dNTP pool induces dFdC phosphorylation by activating dCK, which raises the amount of dFdCTP and causes interference with the DNA structure.

Furthermore, gemcitabine's third known mechanism of action that causes cell apoptosis is caspase signaling cascades.

One of the most potent chemotherapeutic medications, gemcitabine is prescribed for a variety of cancers, including breast, pancreatic, bladder, and non-small cell lung cancer. The results for gemcitabine's approval as a treatment for ovarian cancer are encouraging. Gemcitabine is a better choice for chemotherapies because, among other things, it is less toxic and has fewer side effects than other chemotherapeutic agents. However, the results are not always satisfactory, which creates a need for new regimens or even new approaches to its application, such as combination chemotherapy.

Mechanisms of gemcitabine in signaling cascade-mediated cell death It's interesting to note that gemcitabine activates p38 mitogen-activated protein kinase (MAPK), which causes cancer cells to undergo apoptosis while sparing healthy cells. Additionally, heat-shock protein-27 (HSP-27) is phosphorylated when gemcitabine activates MAPK-activated protein kinase (MK2). This inhibits the growth of tumor cells.

Evidence suggests that gemcitabine treatment can activate and slow down the S-phase checkpoint, leading to breaks and lesions in DNA replication. When replication is halted, ATM and Chk2 are activated to manage cell cycle arrest, apoptosis, and DNA repair. Additionally, DNA lesions can activate ATR, Chk1, and the 9–1-1 complex to inhibit cell cycle progression, stabilize the replication fork, and induce DNA repair mechanisms. This indicates that gemcitabine treatment initially causes cell cycle arrest, but ATM can still facilitate cell cycle progression independent of p53. Research by Larry et al. further supports the idea that the depletion of ATM can make tumors more sensitive to gemcitabine treatment.

Gemcitabine resistance mechanisms through signaling cascades and strategies for intervention As with other chemotherapeutic drugs, tumor cells develop acquired or intrinsic resistance to gemcitabine. The first-line therapy for pancreatic cancer has been gemcitabine. However, the extensive desmoplastic reaction, which forms about 90% of the tumor mass, is a significant barrier to treating pancreatic cancer. Poor drug delivery and innate-gemcitabine chemoresistance in pancreatic cancer cases are explained by the desmoplastic reaction. Furthermore, a unique role for Hedgehog (Hh) signaling has been demonstrated in gemcitabine chemoresistance. Hormone H signaling is associated with changes in the extracellular matrix's construction, morphogenesis, tumorigenesis, and desmoplastic response. To this end, genetic analyzes were performed to identify common mutations found in pancreatic tumors. The cancer's most genetically altered signaling is hh. Remarkably, Olive et al. have demonstrated that they can boost intratumor drug delivery by up to 60% in mice by blocking Hh signaling.

Furthermore, following gemcitabine administration, MK2 activation is crucial for inducing apoptosis. An investigation conducted by Cöpper et al. has demonstrated that the inhibition of MK2 activation by polymerase activity has ultimately improved osteosarcoma survival.

Assuring the intended chemotherapy responses begins with effective drug delivery, so any hiccups or dysfunctions in this process could encourage chemoresistance. According to research, pancreatic cancer patients who have low levels of hENT1, the main transporter of gemcitabine, are more likely to develop gemcitabine resistance and have a poor prognosis.

Gemcitabine is a prodrug that requires dCK processing, which is well understood. There is proof that gemcitabine resistance is linked to the loss of dCK mRNA in pancreatic and ovarian cancer cell lines.

Furthermore, it has been demonstrated that the holoenzyme ribonucleotide reductase (RR), which is composed of RRM1 and RRM2, lowers the activity of gemcitabine. A higher concentration of these subunits has been linked to gemcitabine resistance, according to fragments of evidence.

Gemcitabine resistance is also caused by transcription factors. Among them is high mobility group A1 (HMGA1), a class of transcription factors related to the framework that modulate different genes and are elevated in different types of tumors. Furthermore, the other transcription factor linked to gemcitabine resistance is NF-KB. Arlt and associates. showed that resistant cell lines, such as BxPc-3, Capan-1, and PancTu-1, had an overexpressed level of NF-KB among five distinct pancreatic cancer cell lines. Gemcitabine-resistant cells with overexpressed NF-KB may be related to the effect of redox factor-1 and pururinic/apyrimidinic endonuclease on transcription factor activation, including NF-KB. Furthermore, it has been demonstrated that NF-KB promotes gemcitabine resistance in pancreatic cancer cell lines by suppressing the expression of the nucleoside transporter hCNT1. Gemcitabine resistance is facilitated by hypoxia-inducible factor 1-α (HIF-1α), which is targeted by an excessive build-up of NF-KB in cells. First, there is HIF-1, a transcription factor involved in angiogenesis, metastasis, invasiveness, and chemoresistance in tumors; second, there is evidence to suggest that HIF-1α down-regulates hENT1 and hENT2. Additionally, NF-KB and HIF-1α may operate through additional pathways that lead to gemcitabine resistance. As an example, consider how the CXCL12/CXCR4 downstream pathway activates factors involved in cell survival and proliferation, like NF-KB. According to credible witnesses, the interaction between CXCL12 and CXCR4 stimulates PI3K/Akt, ERK, and FAK in pancreatic cancer cells, which in turn leads to gemcitabine resistance. Furthermore, gemcitabine increases the invasiveness of pancreatic cancer cells by inducing the expression of CXCR4 through NF-KB and HIF-1α. This is consistent with other studies showing that pancreatic and non-small cell lung cancers express more NF-KB when exposed to low doses of gemcitabine. Furthermore, studies indicate that the NF-KB-mediated CXCL12/CXCR4 downstream pathway stimulates Hh signaling. all combine to produce a cycle that may be the main factor in gemcitabine resistance and promotes cancer cell survival through NF-KB signaling. Additionally, Nagano, et al. have demonstrated that in pancreatic cell lines, miRNA-29a causes gemcitabine resistance via Wnt/β-catenin. The Wnt/β-catenin signaling pathway plays a role in cell proliferation, differentiation, the initiation of many types of cancer, and chemoresistance. Research findings indicate that approximately 65% of patients with pancreatic cancer exhibit activated Wnt/β-catenin signaling, a factor that contributes to the development of chemoresistant cancer stem cells. Furthermore, Kapinas et al. have demonstrated that miRNA-29a activates Wnt/β-catenin via Dikkopf-1 (Dkk1), Kremen2, and secreted frizzled-related protein 2 (sFRP2).

Gemcitabine is the best option for treating pancreatic cancer, as was previously mentioned. Nevertheless, the hypoxic central tumor state prevents satisfactory responses to chemotherapy. Hypoxia is linked to poor prognosis, inhibition of apoptosis, metastasis, and resistance to chemotherapy and radiation. Under hypoxic conditions, PI3K, Akt, and MAPK—essential downstream signaling pathways linked to cell proliferation, migration (including metastasis), inhibition of apoptosis, and responding to growth factors—become phosphorylated and activated. Yokoi and associates. have demonstrated an increase in NF-KB's DNA-binding activity as well as the activation of PI3K/Akt and MAPK under hypoxia, which causes L3.6pl cells to become gemcitabine resistant. Nevertheless, they were able to cause apoptosis in this cell population by blocking PI3K with PKI166.

Annexin II is another factor linked to gemcitabine resistance. While there is evidence linking pancreatic cancer patients receiving gemcitabine to tumor relapses associated with overexpression of Annexin II, gemcitabine's toxicity has increased when Annexin II is inhibited. Additionally, Kagawa et al. have shown that to put it mildly, Annexin-II-related gemcitabine resistance is mediated by Akt/mTOR signaling.

By the time gemcitabine is given, it has already activated p38-MAPK, which starts apoptosis by phosphorylating HSP-27 and triggering MK2. Additionally, the DNA damage brought on by gemcitabine activates the S phase checkpoint, recruits ATM/Chk2 and ATR/Chk1, and together they phosphorylate and activate p53 in conjunction with the 9–1-1 complex. In terms of resistance, Hh signaling appears to be involved in the desmoplastic reaction, which explains the inadequate drug delivery. It has also been demonstrated that RR reduces gemcitabine's activity. Moreover, CXCL12/CXCR4 increases NF-KB, ERK, and PI3K/Akt, which together with Wnt/β catenin reduces the effectiveness of gemcitabine therapy.

7.1.5. Doxorubicin

7.1.5.1. Doxorubicin Mechanism of Action

Doxorubicin is a class I anthracycline chemotherapeutic agent that is non-selective and contains sugar and aglyconic components. After being administered, it attaches itself to the carriers of plasma proteins and passively diffuses into the target cell, where it further accumulates intracellularly. Subsequently, it primarily enters the nucleus and increases its cytosolic concentration. It is mostly prescribed for soft tissue sarcoma, thyroid cancer, lung, stomach, ovaries, and breast cancer.

It is thought to function as an anti-cancer agent through two primary mechanisms, despite having a complex mechanism of action. a) Doxorubicin interferes with DNA and, through a process called intercalation, slows down the production of many macromolecules and stops topoisomerase II from progressing. To put it another way, doxorubicin prevents the release of the DNA double helix, which further forbids DNA replication, by stabilizing the DNA after the breaks caused by topoisomerase II. b)

Doxorubicin increases free radical production, which in turn causes damage to membranes, proteins, and DNA.

Mechanisms of doxorubicin-induced cell death via signaling cascades: Doxorubicin undergoes oxidation to form semiquinone, an unstable metabolite that produces reactive oxygen species (ROS). To put it mildly, proteins, DNA, and organelle membranes are harmed by ROS. In addition, it triggers apoptotic pathways, raises lipid peroxidation and alkylation, and produces oxidative stress. For example, when cells are unable to repair damaged DNA, the apoptotic pathway is activated, resulting in cell cycle arrest during the G1 and G2 phases.

Moreover, in reaction to DNA damage, doxorubicin triggers autophagy. It is well known that the nuclear enzyme poly (ADP-ribose) polymerase-1 (PARP-1) must be activated for cells to undergo autophagy or not. Stresses involving DNA can trigger PARP-1 hyperactivation, which exacerbates the deficiency of ATP and NAD+. As a result, cells would exhaust their energy reserves, which, if it is irreversible, drives them to undergo apoptosis. These results confirm that the cellular energy collapse that follows PARP-1 hyperactivation drives cells toward autophagy and necrosis when doxorubicin is administered at a normal dose, but not at a high dose.

Furthermore, doxorubicin promotes AMP-activated protein kinase (AMPK) activation. By triggering ROS-dependent liver kinase B1 (LKB1), which provides AMPK with the required upstream signals, this activation is achieved. Serine 15 in P53 is activated and phosphorylated by activated AMPK, which in turn causes B16 melanoma cells to undergo apoptosis. Thus, in insulin-secretor β-Langerhans cells and the liver, AMPK activates JNK kinase, thereby initiating cell death pathways.

Furthermore, research on MCF-7 cells has demonstrated that doxorubicin increases the quantity of Bax, an agent that inhibits Bcl-2, while decreasing the concentration of Bcl-2, an anti-apoptotic agent. First, it was hypothesized that doxorubicin reduces Bcl-2 mRNA levels in a way that is independent of P53. However, because caspases require a change in the Bcl-2/Bax ratio to be activated, it has been proposed that doxorubicin affects the expression level of Bcl-2 through P53, as per MCF-7 studies.

Furthermore, some claimed that doxorubicin functions in part by enlisting certain elements of the Fas/Fas-ligand apoptotic pathway; however, other findings were inconsistent.

How to address the mechanisms of doxorubicin resistance through signaling cascades Autophagy can either promote or inhibit chemoresistance, depending on the type of tumor, the drug, the length of the treatment, and how the drug affects metabolic stress. Highly mobile group box 1 protein (HMGB1) is an essential modulator of autophagy, both non-selective and selective. It is also essential for DNA repair and replication processes. Research has shown that tumor cells become doxorubicin-sensitive by the time autophagy and HMGB1 are inhibited, indicating that HMGB1 plays a role in doxorubicin resistance as tumors grow. Stated differently, doxorubicin administration results in increased HMGB1 mRNA and protein levels. Additionally, HMGB1 and Bcl-2 compete with one another for binding to BECN1, which leads to the formation of the BECN1-PtdIns3KC3 complex, which in turn initiates autophagy and autophagosome formation. Moreover, the interaction between HMGB1 and BECN1 depends on the upstream signal, specifically ULK1-mATG12-FIP200.

Ceramides have sparked curiosity regarding their potential role in doxorubicin resistance as well. Ceramide is a cellular lipid messenger that regulates the death of cells caused by doxorubicin in a unique way. The findings show that doxorubicin increases ceramide levels in cells, which causes glucosylceramide synthase (GCS) to be upregulated. Cellular drug resistance is the consequence of increased ceramide glycosylation and cellular stress brought on by doxorubicin administration. The exact mechanism by which doxorubicin raises ceramide levels is still somewhat of a mystery, but some speculate that it is either activated ceramide synthesis-related enzymes or stimulates sphingomyelinase.

Additionally, it has been reported that ABCB8 significantly modulates doxorubicin resistance in melanoma cells, which may contribute to the preservation of the mitochondrial genome, though the precise mechanisms underlying this are still unknown. While ATP-binding cassette (ABC) proteins are implicated in many chemoresistant tumors, it is important to note that ABCB8 is specifically linked to doxorubicin resistance, but not in resistance to other chemotherapy agents. It has been suggested that doxorubicin resistance may be reduced by ABCB8 knockdown with particular shRNA. In addition, it has been demonstrated that doxorubicin resistance is partially correlated with ABCB1 (MDR1, Pgp), ABCC1 (MRP1), ABCC2, ABCC3, ABCG2, and RAPBP1.

In addition, another established mechanism for doxorubicin resistance is the replication of the TOP2A gene. There have been reports that the doxorubicin response is impacted by this gene's amplification. It's interesting to note that HER-2, a marker for the advancement of breast cancer and the effectiveness of chemotherapy, interacts with TOP2A nearby. It is now evident that the doxorubicin response is impacted by HER-2 amplification as well.

Intercalation is the process by which doxorubicin combines with DNA and Topoisomerase to form adducts. When DOX enters the target cell, it oxidizes to semiquinone, producing ROS along the way. Furthermore, ROS damages protein, DNA, and organelle membranes in addition to causing lipid peroxidation. When DNA damage occurs, PARP-1 is triggered, which directs the cell to either G1/S arrest and apoptosis or autophagy (assuming low ATP and NAD+ resources). Additionally, protein damage results in G2/M arrest, which triggers apoptosis. Additionally, DOX can phosphorylate and activate p53 via p38-MAPK, JNK, and AMPK. On the other hand, a rise in HMGB1 protein or mRNA levels promotes cell survival and resistance by inhibiting apoptosis. (Galanski et al, 2005; Yen et al, 2005; Anand et al, 2008; Houles & Roux, 2018)

7.1.6. Etoposide

Etoposide mechanism of action: Generally speaking, etoposide is an anti-topoisomerase II and a semi-synthetic podophyllotoxin derivative agent that inhibits DNA replication as well as other processes like chromatin remodeling, DNA transcription, and DNA repair that depend on topoisomerase II. To produce a temporary break in the double helix strain, topoisomerase needs to undergo two crucial transesterification reactions. During the first step, the tyrosine motif at the enzyme's active site forms a covalent bond with one phosphate residue in the DNA backbone, causing a brief disruption in the integrity of the DNA strain. By releasing the DNA break, a second reaction occurs to re-ligate the double helix. The first reaction's cleaved double-helix DNA is transient, but it can be stabilized with toxic substances.

One of the suggested medications is etoposide, which poisons the complex known as topoisomerase-II cleavage (TopoIIcc) and stops the second transesterification reaction, or re-ligation. More specifically, by stabilizing the short-term topoisomerase-cleaved DNA, etoposide exhibits a high affinity toward the Topo-II-DNA complex while demonstrating a low affinity toward naked DNA. There are two isotypes of Topoisomerase II: Topo-IIα and Topo-IIβ. Topo-IIα supports cell cycle processes like chromosome segregation, DNA replication, and DNA repair; on the other hand, Topo-IIβ is primarily involved in transcription and the development of new cells. Etoposide functions as a topo-inhibitor by interfering with particular amino acid residues in the structures of the two isotypes of topoisomerase.

In addition, etoposide has been shown to have a strong affinity for chromatin and histones, which raises the possibility of additional mechanisms of action.

It has also been noted that etoposide affects the replication machinery in other ways. Stated differently, etoposide has a progressive effect on the distribution of replication proteins during the S phase. Replication sites are dispersed throughout the DNA strain as a result, resulting in massive nuclear foci that contain the single-strand DNA binding protein RPA.

Eptoside also acts through a different mechanism that involves inhibiting the transcription of particular genes. Takami along with others. have shown that the heterodimeric E2F-4/DP complexes in the nucleus are responsible for the downregulation and inhibition of the transcription of certain genes as a result of the transcription factor E2F-4's binding to etoposide.

Mechanisms of etoposide in signaling cascade-mediated cell death A 5′-phosphodiesterase has been found to be able to break down Topo-II-DNA bonds and fix DNA damage caused by topoisomerase. This can be demonstrated by the fact that TRAF and TNF receptor-associated protein (TTRAP), which was renamed TDP2 (tyrosine phosphodiesterase 2) recently, is an Mg^{2+}/Mn^{2+}-dependent member of the phosphodiesterase group that allows the cleaved double helix strain to religate its 5′-phosphate residues. TDP2 depletion has been shown to enhance cellular susceptibility to double-strand breaks induced by etoposide, indicating a potential role for TTRAP/TDP2 in the etoposide chemotherapeutic response.

Additionally, Adachi et al. have shown that cells repair the DNA damage caused by etoposide primarily through the low-fidelity non-homologous end-joining (NHEJ) pathway. Put another way, depending on which stage of the cell cycle the damage occurred in, cells repair DNA damage in different ways. For example, homologous recombination (HR) is used to repair G1 damages while NHEJ is used to repair those in the S and G2 phases. It has been demonstrated that DT40 cells are extremely sensitive to etoposide when the NHEJ pathway is dampened by knocking out the DNA ligase IV and Ku70 subunit (LIG4−/−, Ku70−/−). Nevertheless, etoposide significantly lessens the sensitivity of RAD54−/− knocked-out cells, which are HR-defective. Rad54 is a DNA repair and recombination protein. Malik and colleagues have provided evidence in favor of this theory by highlighting the significance of Ku70 and Ku80 existence for NHEJ and cell survival following etoposide treatment. Chen et al. have also confirmed that defective Ku70 reduces the ability of cells exposed to etoposide early on to repair DNA. Furthermore, the effect of Ku70 acetylation in histone deacetylase (HDAC) inhibitors has been mentioned. More specifically, it has been demonstrated that mutations in Ku70 resemble the acetylation of specific lysine residues. This results in Ku70's inability to bind DNA, which in turn increases the sensitivity of prostate cancer cells to etoposide.

Furthermore, ataxia-telangiectasia mutated (ATM) and its downstream kinase, checkpoint kinase 2 (Chk2), are activated in response to etoposide. As a result of ATM kinase activation, the Mre11/Rad50/NSB1 (MRN) complex and ionizing radiation-induced foci (IRIF) are created, both of which are indicative of significant DNA damage. Hypersensitivity to etoposide is caused by ATM mutations. Furthermore, even though etoposide administration has resulted in DNA breaks and chromosomal abnormalities, AT cells' loss of the G2/M checkpoint permits mitosis to occur.

Moreover, bridging integrator-1 (BIN1) promoter and transcription factor E2F1 interact more when etoposide is administered. It has been demonstrated that the cell-death rate mediated by the interaction of E2F1 and etoposide is reduced when BIN1 is dampened using an antisense RNA.

Moreover, etoposide also has an effect on the alternative splicing mechanism. The administration of etoposides induces the dephosphorylation of serine/arginine-rich splicing factor-1 (SRSF1), a splicing element that oversees and modulates the alternative splicing of pro- or anti-apoptotic genes, including the tumor suppressor BIN1 and the Ron oncogene. Furthermore, the alternative splicing pattern of caspase 9 is modified by changes in the phosphorylation of SRSF1 following DNA damage. This indicates that etoposide actively affects alternative splicing pathways and that it is correlated with target cell apoptosis modulation.

High etoposide concentrations have been shown to activate cytochrome C-caspase-9-mediated pathways, according to many studies. By activating Apaf1, it creates an apoptosome complex that can cleave pro-caspase 9 into active caspase 9, which in turn causes the cleavage and activation of caspase 3 and 7, which ultimately causes cellular apoptosis.

Furthermore, fresh data indicate the role of Fas/FasL in etoposide-induced apoptosis. This is demonstrated by the fact that the administration of etoposide causes the interaction between FasL and its receptor, FasR, which in turn creates a death-inducing signaling complex (DISK), in which FADD activates pro-caspase 8 into functional caspase 8, which in turn activates caspase 7.

Additionally, etoposide causes resting cells such as T lymphocytes and tumor cells to initiate DNA damage responses (DDRs). In this sense, ATM phosphorylation leads to the phosphorylation of p53 and H2AX. In the end, this results in the activation of p53-upregulated modulator of apoptosis (PUMA), a pro-apoptotic protein. It has been observed that blocking ATM activities in quiescent cells with Ku55933 reduces DDR and apoptosis by lowering PUMA expression and caspase activation; however, carrying out the same process in malignant cells amplifies the cytotoxic effect of etoposide.

It should be mentioned that p53 is involved in etoposide-induced cell death in a different way. More specifically, Nemo-like serine/threonine kinase (NLK) is required for p53 activation after etoposide-induced DDR. The precise mechanism is still unknown, but DDR causes an upregulation of NLK. By blocking the ubiquitin-proteasome system and Double Minute 2 (MDM2)-mediated protein degradation, NLK stabilizes p53. Additionally, it has been proposed that NLK increases cellular etoposide sensitivity by inhibiting certain transcription factors, like NF-KB.

Additionally, research has demonstrated that the administration of etoposide triggers several stress pathways, such as JNK and MAPK. These pathways are thought to play opposing roles in both pro- and anti-apoptotic pathways. WWOX is a tumor suppressor and oxidoreductase that works by stabilizing p53, which causes cell death. WWOX has reportedly been shown to rise after etoposide-induced DDR.

Chemoresistance is a side effect of etoposide treatment, and similar to other chemotherapeutic regimens, there are mechanisms of etoposide resistance through signaling cascades and how to address them. The MDM2 gene plays a role in etoposide resistance by encoding ubiquitin ligase, an enzyme involved in protein degradation. Stated differently, the upregulation of MDM2 is caused by a single-nucleotide polymorphism called SNP 309 T/G that is found within its promoter. This leads to a decreased response to various drugs that damage DNA, including etoposide. Homogyote-SNP309 cell lines have been reported to be resistant to etoposide. In these cell lines, MDM2 indicated a greater propensity to bind and degrade Topo-II. Moreover, Topo-II had stabilized and etoposide resistance had reduced by the time RNAi knocked down MDM2.

Moreover, Zhang and colleagues. have revealed that etoposide resistance is caused by a proteasome-mediated degradation process. They have demonstrated that MG132 dampening proteasome attenuates etoposide-mediated DNA damages using knock-out and knock-down Topo-IIβ mice.

Numerous pieces of evidence have demonstrated the connection between MAGE family proteins and the control of cell survival. According to reports, HDACs are recruited by MageA2 to the P53 transcription sites, where they promote histone hypoacetylation and thereby inhibit the activity of the transcription factor in melanoma cells. As a result, melanoma cells that express MAGE-A genes are immune to the apoptotic effects of etoposide.

A growing body of research indicates that etoposide plays a role in autophagy as well. Katayama and associates. have demonstrated the viability of ATP production in glioma cells that is dependent on autophagy. It is surprising that it not only doesn't kill them but also helps them survive; as a result, it may help develop resistance to etoposide. It has been suggested that even in cases where cells go without glucose, this crisis is irreversible. However, preincubation with the autophagy inhibitor 3-methyladenine (3-MA), the mitochondrial inhibitor oligomycin, and the siRNA-mediated downregulation of beclin 1 can all inhibit it. These measures lower the autophagy-induced ATP level and cause non-apoptotic cell death in the cells.

In addition, Alpsoy and colleagues. have shown that the primary contributions to etoposide efflux and chemoresistance are made by MRP1 (ABCC1 transporter). Furthermore, it has been reported that MCF7-etoposide-resistant cells involve mismatch repair mechanisms. Put differently, the argument put forth was that etoposide-resistant cells exhibit a significant downregulation of MLH1 and MSH2, two proteins involved in DNA damage repair. Additionally, they have looked into the rates of expression for E3 ubiquitin-protein ligase EDD and topoisomerase IIβ-binding protein 1 (TOPBP1). TOPBP1 is involved in signaling pathways for DNA damage response, proliferation, and replication. It initiates the apoptotic pathway and results in cell cycle arrest. One of the tumor suppressor protein EDD's interaction partners is DNA damage signaling and checkpoint responses. Alpsoy et al. discovered a reduction in TOPBP1 and EDD expression. It tackles resistance in etoposide-treated cells as a whole.

The anti-topoisomerase II substance etoposide poisons the TopoIIcc and stops DNA strands from religating. After etoposide causes persistent DNA damage, ATM/Chk2 are recruited and, with the help of Mre11/Rad50/NSB1, cause the S phase arrest that results in apoptosis. Additionally, ATM is phosphorylated by alternative signaling, specifically NLK, which in turn phosphorylates and activates p53, resulting in p53. However, SNP mutations such as SNP 309 T/G create a distinct subtype of MDM2, which inactivates p53 and sometimes explains etoposide resistance. Other potential mechanisms implicated in etoposide-cell death mechanisms described include Cyto C/Apaf-1/Cas-9 and Fas/FasL/Cas-8, 10. (Galanski et al, 2005; Yen et al, 2005; Anand et al, 2008; Houles & Roux, 2018)

7.2. The Role of mTOR /Akt/ Pi3k Signaling Pathways in Human Cancer

Under both normal and pathological circumstances, such as cell survival, proliferation, apoptosis, and invasion, the phosphatidylinositol-3-kinase/Akt signaling cascades and the mammalian target of rapamycin (mTOR) signaling pathway serve as an essential double-edged sword. To put it mildly, these pathways are intricately linked to a variety of cell signaling pathways, including NF-KB and HIF.

The PI3K/Akt signaling cascade is thought to be the key regulator that promotes cell survival in stressful conditions. To demonstrate this, consider the lipid kinase family known as PI3K, which is capable of phosphorylating the inositol rings 3?-OH found in inositol phospholipids. Catalytic subunits (CAT), specifically p110, and the adaptor-regulatory domain, p85, combine to form class-I PI3K. Accordingly, tyrosine kinases in growth factor receptors are stimulated and phosphorylated to start the signaling cascade. Subsequently, the adaptor subunit's SH2 domains attract PI3K to the cell membrane, where it binds to receptor tyrosine residues. This results in the activation of the CAT residue, which in turn triggers the production of the second messenger, phosphatidylinositol-3,4,5-triphosphate (PI3,4,5-P3). Next, other signaling proteins such as Akt/protein kinase B (PKB) and protein serine/threonine kinase-3?-phosphoinositide-dependent kinase 1 (PDK1) are recruited by PI3,4,5-P3, and they go on to control cell survival and cell cycle progression.

In terms of cell survival, Akt/PKB inhibits the expression of apoptotic elements like Fas/FasL and inactivates pro-caspase and Bad. It also attenuates associated transcription factors. Moreover, TNF-related apoptosis-induced ligand (TRAIL)/APO-2L has been modulated by Akt/PKB to function as a resistance-inducing agent. Additionally, it triggers IKB kinase (IKK), the survival signaling element in NF-KB signaling.

Many processes related to protein synthesis, glycogen metabolism, and cell cycle regulation interact closely with downstream signaling pathways of Akt, such as mTOR, glycogen synthase kinase-3 (GSK-3), insulin receptor substrate-1 (IRS-1), p21, p27, and Raf-1, in relation to the progression of the cell cycle.

Conversely, AMP/GMP kinases and protein kinase C (PKC) are correlated with Akt kinases, which are members of the AGC family. Specifically, the three primary domains that make up Akt kinases are the regulatory hydrophobic residue (C-terminal), the CAT domain (central domain), and the PH domain (N-terminal). The CAT domain is closely linked to PKC, PKA, and SGK and is highly conserved throughout the entire Akt family.

Because it influences several facets of cell fate, MTOR is regarded as the most important component in the field of cell signaling. Put differently, mTOR functions via its two primary complexes. The components of the mTOR complex-1 (mTORC1) are mTOR, Raptor, mLST8, and PRAS40. It generally stimulates S6K and dampens 4E-BP1, which results in protein translation and cell growth. It is highly sensitive to rapamycin. mTOR, Rictor, Sin 1, and mLST8 combine to form mTORC2, which is less susceptible to rapamycin. It is recognized that Akt is stimulated by mTORC2, and this enhances cell survival and proliferation. The canonical pathway of mTOR signaling is thought to function via Ras/MEK/ERK and PI3K/Akt.

In healthy cells, several upstream signaling pathways control mTOR. Positive and negative modulators are two subcategories of these regulators. Positive regulators, such as vascular endothelial growth factor receptors (VEGFRs) and their ligands, human epidermal growth factor receptors (HER family) and their ligands, and insulin growth factor-1 (IGF-1) and its receptor, channel signals through PI3K/Akt. However, the energy-sensing element LKB1, phosphatase and tensin homolog (PTEN), tuberous sclerosis complex-1 (TSC-1), and -2 (TSC-2) are among the negative regulators. To put it another way, TCS-2 releases its inhibitory effects on mTOR by the time it is phosphorylated by Akt, and PTEN performs its detrimental effects through PI3K/Akt.

The regulator of the PI3K/Akt/mTOR signaling cascades is PTEN. Further, PTEN affects proteins as well as lipids. It is a tumor-suppressor drug that promotes apoptosis in target cells and aids in preventing cell division. But PTEN is mutated in many cancers; for example, it is mutated in Cowden's syndrome, which puts the patient at a high risk of receiving multiple cancer diagnoses at the same time. While PTEN does function as a negative regulator of PI3K/Akt signaling, when PTEN activity is lost, PI3K/Akt signaling is continuously and uncontrollably activated in cells, resulting in excessive and needless cell survival and proliferation.

The intracellular buildup of DNA damage, amino acids, glucose, ATP, and oxygen, as well as external and internal stimuli such as growth factors, nutrients, and hormones, all activate mTORC1 signaling. For example, following damage to DNA, p53 dampens mTORC1, which triggers TSC-2 activation. Additionally, after a period of energy exhaustion, AMPK is stimulated, resulting in the formation of the TSC1/2 complex, which phosphorylates Raptor and inhibits mTORC1.

But as was previously mentioned, by the time mTORC1 is activated, it has already sent signals to S6K and 4E-BP1. Eukaryotic initiation factor (eIF)-4E and eukaryotic initiation factor-3 (eIF-3) are recruited subsequent to the involvement of S6K and 4E-BP1, thereby promoting ribosomal biogenesis. As an example, consider how low mTORC1 activity phosphorylates and activates 4E-BP1, starting protein translation. Additionally, S6K phosphorylates S6 ribosomal protein (S6RP) and elF-4B, enabling the translation process to proceed and initiate the elongation phase. After that, elF-4E forms the elF-4F complex, which promotes protein translation—a crucial step if the G1/S transition is involved. Thus, it is hypothesized that mTORC1 activation promotes oncogenic protein translation, which results in cell invasion, metastasis, and proliferation. Furthermore, the activation of mTORC1 also affects other elements, such as HIF-α, STAT3, and Protein phosphatase 2A (PP2A), which helps malignant cells make vital lipids, proteins, and nucleotides that aid in their survival, growth, and invasion.

However, the mechanisms by which mTORC2 carries out its regulatory effects are still somewhat unclear, most likely as a result of the intricate distinction between mTORC1 and mTORC2. Both mTORC1 and PI3K/Akt signaling influence mTORC2. In this sense, in both healthy and pathological conditions, PI3K stimulates mTORC2 to bind to ribosomes. Studies have supported Akt's increased expression level in various malignancies, where it gathers signals from PI3K/mTORC2 and PI3K/PDK1, which promotes cell survival and proliferation. Akt and mTORC2 have a strong correlation. Furthermore, Akt affects mTORC1 through additional complex mechanisms.

The fact that mTORC1 negatively regulates mTORC2 is widely known. More precisely, mTORC2 and PI3K/Akt signaling are inhibited when S6K1 promotes the degradation of insulin receptor substrate-1 (IRS-1). Moreover, mTORC1 recruits Grb-10, which inhibits mTORC2.

In mTORC2-related signaling cascades, glucocorticoid kinase (SGK) and protein kinase C (PKC) are important phosphorylation substrates that promote cell survival in conditions such as hypoxia, malnutrition, and PI3K blockage. Research has shown that mTORC2 influences cytoskeletal reorganization and cell movement, crucial for cell invasion and tumorigenesis, through activation of different PKC members.

In summary, mTOR is closely linked to the pathophysiology of various tumors because it controls the synthesis of many essential proteins and is involved in a variety of signaling processes, including cell survival, proliferation, glucose metabolism, cell cycle, and protein and lipid synthesis. Additionally, mTOR contributes to chemoresistance. Put another way, certain components, such as cyclin D1 and HIF, are among the crucial proteins that interact with the signaling pathways mentioned above and cause the cell cycle to advance, thereby promoting the expression of angiogenic factors like VEGF, and ultimately leading to the survival and growth of tumors. More significantly, it has been reported that mTOR and its downstream and upstream signaling pathways both directly and indirectly contribute to the onset of various malignancies.

MTOR serves multiple cellular functions in both physiological and pathological conditions, making it the crossroads and essential signaling cascade in the field of intracellular signaling. It primarily functions via the mTORC1 and mTORC2 complexes. These complexes interact closely with Ras/ERK, AMPK, and PI3K/Akt, three upstream signaling cascades. The upstream signaling phosphorylates Akt, which lessens the inhibitory effect of TCS 2 and permits mTORC1 to function. Moreover, the mTORC1 controls $E-BP1, S6K1, SREBP, STAT3, HIF-α, and PP2A to promote angiogenesis, cell cycle progression, and the synthesis of lipids, proteins, and nucleotides. Conversely, mTORC2 is influenced by mTORC1 via Grb-10 (in a feedback loop) and IRS-1, ultimately supporting cytoskeletal reorganization, cell migration, and proliferation. (Galanski et al, 2005; Yen et al, 2005; Anand et al, 2008; Houles & Roux, 2018)

7.3. Recent Outcomes in the Application of Combination Chemotherapy

The majority of the time, tumor relapse and chemoresistance have restricted the use of single-chemotherapy. Each chemotherapeutic drug targets distinct cell cycle phases and intracellular signaling cascades. As a result, administering combination chemotherapy appears to increase responses to chemotherapy; however, this application has been restricted by antagonistic effects, differences in pharmacokinetics, and disparate drug distribution patterns.

For example, cisplatin and gemcitabine were combined and applied to multiple solid tumors. Studies conducted *in vitro* in this area have shown that gemcitabine and cisplatin have synergistic effects, which appear to be caused by an increase in platinum-DNA adducts. The combination of gemcitabine and etoposide therapy for lung and ovarian cancer was also shown to exhibit synergism. Additionally, the effects of gemcitabine-nab-paclitaxel, gemcitabine-capecitabine, and nanoliposomal irinotecan-5-fluorouracil-leucovorin were examined in elderly patients with pancreatic cancer. Beneficiary outcomes for these combination therapies were demonstrated by the results.

Additionally, 113 patients with advanced gastric cancer who received combination chemotherapy consisting of paclitaxel, 5-fluorouracil, and leucovorin (TFL) as their first-line treatment protocol were included in a retrospective study. The results showed a moderate toxicity rate of 43.4% overall response. That being said, Wan-Cai et al. asserted that TFL is a safe and proactive treatment for these patients. Still, Choi et al. have noted that there is considerable disagreement regarding the effectiveness of combination chemotherapy in treating patients with primary or recurrent gastric cancer. They went on to say that while combination chemotherapy is advised for these patients, in some circumstances—particularly with older patients—single chemotherapy administration may make sense.

In a different retrospective study, patients with advanced gastric cancer received first-line treatment every 14 days consisting of paclitaxel and oxaliplatin. With an approximately 80% disease control, this combination therapy is a novel, safe, and effective regimen for these patients. Furthermore, improved chemotherapy approaches are necessary because peritoneal metastasis is a common cause of death for patients with advanced or recurrent gastric cancer; unfortunately, the current treatments remain inadequate. Ohnuma and companions. have recommended that patients be prescribed S-1, cisplatin, and docetaxel as a workable and efficient combination chemotherapy.

Gemcitabine has long been used in the treatment of pancreatic cancer. However, the use of this regimen has been severely restricted due to chemoresistance. Li along with others. have used valproic acid (VPA) and gemcitabine together and documented the dose-dependent synergistic effects of both drugs. According to reports, this combination therapy with high-dose VPA may effectively raise the gemcitabine sensitivity of pancreatic cancer cells. However, they also showed that by raising ROS levels and activating Akt, STAT3, and Bmi1, low-dose VPA in combination with gemcitabine enhanced the migration and invasion potency in pancreatic cancer cells. On the other hand, high-dose VPA-gemcitabine administration increased excessive ROS retention, which prompted p38 activation and the inactivation of Bmi1 and STAT3.

Additionally, in a study, patients with advanced non-small cell lung cancer received bevacizumab in addition to chemotherapy that included gemcitabine and cisplatin (GC). By splitting the cases into two groups, GC was given to one as the control group and GC-bevacizumab was given to the other as the observation group. The outcomes showed some promise. Duan and associates. revealed that in the control group, the efficiency rate and disease control were roughly 41% and 71%, respectively, while in the observation group, they were 71% and 90%, respectively. Additionally, there was a significant decrease in the concentration of serum vascular endothelial growth factor (VEGF) and tumor markers, specifically CYFRA21-1 and CEA.

Additionally, combination chemotherapy has shown promise in treating cancers that are resistant to multiple drugs. To demonstrate this, doxorubicin and cisplatin were encapsulated in polymeric nanogels. The fact that they were able to kill more cancer cells and introduce a higher concentration of the drug into MCF7/ADR cells supports the synergistic effects of the drug. Moreover, magnetic nano-carriers were used for multidrug delivery. Rahimi and companions. have created magnetic nanoparticles coated in mPEG and grafted with dendritic chitosan to deliver methotrexate and doxorubicin to MCF7 cells. They showed that these nano-carriers could bind to many peripheral bloodstream proteins, enhancing the delivery of drugs. Furthermore, they verified that the combined drug's anticancer activity was substantially higher than that of the individual drugs.

In a different study, recombinant high-density lipoprotein nanoparticles (rHDL) were used to co-encapsulate paclitaxel and doxorubicin. The outcomes demonstrated improved cytotoxicity characteristics as well as increased drug intracellular accumulation. Zhu et al. have encapsulated paclitaxel and doxorubicin using bilayered folate (FA) receptor-targeted polymersomes. Compared to a free drug cocktail, the results showed more sustainability in drug release and more adequate damping of cell growth. Additionally, this method has been tested on brain-metastasizing breast cancers. Because of inadequate drug delivery to the brain, current chemotherapies are not effective in curing this subtype. Thus, Bao has encapsulated paclitaxel (PTX) and oleanolic acid (OA), a potent anti-tumor agent that penetrates the brain, in nanoparticle form. They described how the combination chemotherapy of PTX, OA, and NPs effectively slowed the progression of breast and metastatic brain cancer.

Polymers appear to be intriguing for drug delivery methods involving encapsulation as well. We used an armed amphiphilic star copolymer to encapsulate avasimibe and doxorubicin. According to the cytotoxicity tests, synergistic anticancer activity was taken into account. Additionally, co-administration of avasimibe may lessen the dosage of doxorubicin needed, thereby lowering its side effects and pointing to a potentially effective combination therapy against HeLa and K562 cells.

Before beginning any combination chemotherapy protocol, there are important risk factors that must be considered. For example, even though patients with urothelial cancer (UC) now typically receive combined gemcitabine-cisplatin (GC) chemotherapy, one significant drawback in this regard is still the hematological toxicity that follows. A retrospective study's findings showed that 21% of all cases had grade 3 thrombocytopenia and 48% of patients had grade 4 neutropenia. They also talked about neutrophil count, platelet count, and K level as significant risk factors among UC patients receiving GC combined therapy-induced hematological toxicity, even though some people thought that age was the main risk factor. Furthermore, Toffalorio's study examined the relationship between the expression level of cN-II and the outcome of gemcitabine-platinum combination chemotherapy in patients with non-small-cell lung cancer.

In addition, as was previously mentioned, MDR, or multiple drug resistance, is a difficult side effect of chemotherapy. Consequently, it is critical to address this crisis by boosting the intracellular build-up of chemotherapy medications. To address this problem, celastrol (CST) and doxorubicin (DOX) were combined to form CST/DOX NPs, which are carrier-free nanoparticles that help overcome DOX resistance. With any luck, this formulation has reduced the necessary DX dosage and increased water solubility. As a result, it may greatly raise the concentration of the drug within the target cells, activate heat-shock factor-1 (HSF-1), dampen NF-KB to inhibit P-gp expression, and ultimately cause autophagy and apoptosis in DOX-resistant cells by way of the ROS/JNK signaling cascade.

Although paclitaxel has been prescribed for many types of cancer, its use has been restricted due to chemoresistance and adverse effects like neuro-, hepato-, and cardiotoxicity. Shafiqadeh and associates. have found that paclitaxel and curcumin, which functions as an anti-tumor and anti-inflammatory agent, when combined, effectively increase the anti-tumor potency and reduce the main side effects of paclitaxel administration alone.

Applications of combination chemotherapy yield results in patients not only with good prognoses. In an interesting case report study, a 79-year-old man with hilar cholangiocarcinoma that had spread to his lymph nodes was given a neoadjuvant combination of gemcitabine, cisplatin, and S-1. Despite the liver's severe impairments making it unsalvageable, the results of the biopsy and cytology revealed no localized cancer cells following resection. In contrast, dabrafenib and trametinib combined to cause a potentially fatal arrhythmia in a 61-year-old man with stage IV papillary and anaplastic thyroid cancer in another case study. Because of the patient's extreme condition, the chemotherapeutic drugs were removed through plasmapheresis.

The regimens listed above are not the only combinations of chemotherapy that can be used. These findings support the possibility that this strategy could be used to combat a variety of malignancies. Beneficiary responses also exist, even though in certain cases the results may be disappointing. However, more research is needed to pinpoint the precise mechanisms of action that underpin the combined effects of drugs to create combinations that produce fewer side effects and better results. (Galanski et al, 2005; Yen et al, 2005; Anand et al, 2008; Houles & Roux, 2018)

7.4. The Contribution of Precision Medicine in Chemotherapy

Even though cancers may be pathologically identical, different cancer subtypes may react differently to a given chemotherapy drug. The majority of the time, the cellular and genetic mechanisms that underlie chemoresistance are used to guide chemotherapy selections; however, tumor- and patient-specific factors also play a role in chemotherapy response. To achieve the best possible response, therefore, particular measurements are needed in addition to an optimized drug to choose chemotherapeutic drugs and their administration schedule based on the unique pharmacokinetics and pharmacodynamics of each patient.

While novel chemotherapeutic agents are being created and combination chemotherapies are increasingly popular, certain cases do not yield completely satisfactory results. This is because different patients have different underlying causes for the start of their cancer cases. Instead of using stochastic chemotherapy, current advancements in genomics and next-generation sequencing (NGS) can help identify genetic variations in different patients, allowing drug development to focus on precise, single-patient approaches for each patient's unique biological, molecular, and cellular variations. Additionally, for roughly 50 years, the variety of natural compounds has aided in the creation of novel chemotherapeutic agents. By combining high-throughput technology with chemistry, it will be possible to anticipate the behavior of individual molecules, create customized chemotherapy regimens, and overcome chemoresistance according to the needs of each individual situation.

In this sense, omics technologies and mathematical models are crucial. For example, McKenna, et al. have produced a plethora of evidence. that in the field of precision medicine, mathematical models can be used to predict, specify, and enhance chemotherapy treatments for breast cancer.

Furthermore, oral squamous cell carcinoma is a complicated cancer that can exhibit tumor heterogeneity and plasticity in various circumstances. These variations are being addressed by omics technologies. Omics are high throughput technologies that can perform both qualitative and quantitative screening of various target molecules. To put it another way, personalized biomarkers can be discovered in tumor biopsies, circulating tumor cells, or bodily fluids like saliva by using genomics, transcriptomics, proteomics, and metabolomics. Unlike traditional chemotherapies, which only target one signaling cascade, one can target cells and molecules more precisely and obtain a comprehensive and objective view through targeted genomics and proteomics when utilizing omics.

Remarkably, Cammarota et al. have also talked about the use of machine learning, big data mining, and gut microbiota in the context of precision medicine. The gut microbiome is as unique to each person as their fingerprints and has complicated cancer treatments by promoting tumor growth, influencing tumor tolerability, and influencing the immune system's reaction to cancer. Beneficiary data can be gathered through omics, and more precise approaches can be designed through data mining. Furthermore, machine learning is evolving swiftly and is turning into a key component of precision medicine. This technology is not limited to proteomics and genomics; it gathers all available data and can help with precision medicine through the development of various algorithms. As an example, Lee et al. have shown promise as a method for determining molecular traits to create more individualized targeted treatments for acute myeloid leukemia (AML). Using multi-omic computational algorithms, in-vitro testing of 160 drug sensitivity of chemotherapeutic drugs, and the collection of genome-wide gene expression data, they were able to identify SMARCA4 as a marker and driver of sensitivity to topoisomerase II inhibitors, mitoxantrone, and etoposide in AML.

The development of targeted and predictive biomarkers has also affected the chemotherapy regimens for patients with ovarian cancer. Even within a particular histological subtype of ovarian cancer, there exist distinct molecular characteristics. As a result, the one-size-fits-all approach to treating ovarian cancer has given way to a precise treatment plan that includes targeted therapy, chemotherapy, and surgery. Furthermore, advances in NGS aim to identify multiple unique biomarkers and genetic variations, which collectively support the creation of novel therapeutic strategies for individual ovarian cancer patients.

Another strategy that has been proven to help cancer patients is immunotherapy; however, a significant drawback is that stimulating the immune system can lead to autoimmune disorders and unneeded inflammatory reactions. Nevertheless, because of their higher survival rate in advanced cancers, their uses and clinical trials are growing. Tumor mutational burden (TMB) is a reliable method in personalized medicine for identifying particular biomarkers. Precision medicine has been applied to non-small-cell lung cancer, wherein multiple FDA-approved targeted therapies, including immune-checkpoint inhibitors, have been developed based on identified biomarkers, including EGFR, ALK, ROS1, and BRAF. Both whole-exome sequencing (WES) and NGS can be used to evaluate TMB, however NGS is more widely available and less expensive. A growing body of research has validated the use of TMB in the process of identifying potential personalized immune-checkpoint inhibitor therapies.

Furthermore, because there are numerous mutations in head and neck squamous cell carcinoma (HNSCC) without any clear guidelines, treating this cancer requires a complex process. While radiation and surgery are the standard treatments for HNSCC, checkpoint inhibitors, precision medicine, and targeted immunotherapy—such as anti-PD-L1 and anti-CTLA-4—can help discover new and more effective ways to treat HNSCC. (Galanski et al, 2005; Yen et al, 2005; Anand et al, 2008; Houles & Roux, 2018)

A Closer Look

Adjuvant Therapy

To enhance the efficacy of the primary or initial therapy, adjuvant therapy is administered in addition to it. The phrase is now primarily used to refer to adjuvant cancer treatments because of the surgeries and intricate treatment plans involved in cancer therapy. The additional treatment typically administered following surgery in cases where all detectable diseases have been removed but where there is still a statistical risk of relapse because of the presence of undetected disease is an example of adjuvant therapy. Further treatment is not technically adjuvant if the surgery leaves known disease behind.

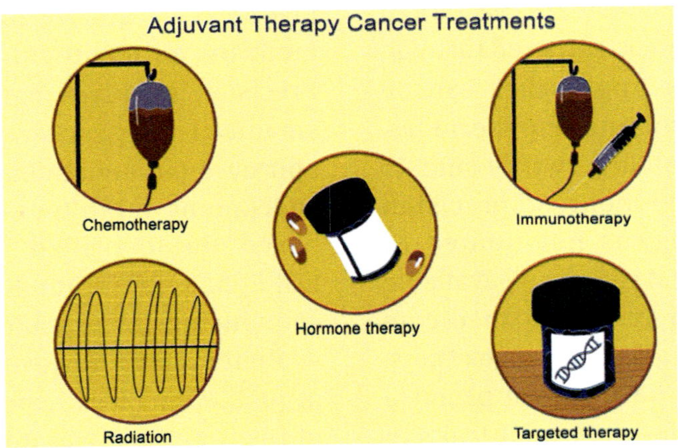

Source: https://www.verywellhealth.com/adjuvant-therapy-5198903

When an adjuvant is used alone, it particularly refers to a substance that enhances a vaccine's effectiveness. Add-on medications are those that supplement primary medications.

- ***Neoadjuvant therapy***

Unlike adjuvant therapy, neoadjuvant therapy is administered before the primary treatment. Neoadjuvant chemotherapy, for instance, is systemic treatment for breast cancer administered before breast excision. Neoadjuvant cancer therapy is most frequently used to shrink the tumor to enable more successful surgery.

Administering neoadjuvant chemotherapy before surgery can enhance patient survival in the case of breast cancer. If no active cancer cells are present in a tissue extracted from the tumor site after neoadjuvant therapy, physicians classify a case as "pathologic complete response" or "pCR." While the response to therapy has been demonstrated to be a strong predictor of outcome, the medical community has still not reached a consensus in regard to the definition of pCR across various breast cancer subtypes. It remains unclear whether pCR can be used as a surrogate endpoint in breast cancer cases.

Ø *Adjuvant cancer therapy*

For instance, systemic therapy or radiotherapy is frequently administered as an adjuvant after breast cancer surgery. Chemotherapy, immunotherapy, biological response modifiers, or hormone therapy comprise systemic therapy. Before selecting an adjuvant therapy, oncologists use statistical data to estimate the chance of disease relapse. Improving both overall survival and disease-specific symptoms is the goal of adjuvant therapy. Given that adjuvant therapy treats a risk rather than a proven illness, it is acknowledged that some patients will have already recovered from their initial surgery before beginning adjuvant therapy.

For many cancers, including pancreatic, colon, lung, breast, prostate, and certain gynecological cancers, adjuvant systemic therapy and radiation therapy are frequently administered after surgery. However, adjuvant therapy is ineffective for certain types of cancer. Renal cell carcinoma and some types of brain cancer are examples of these cancers.

Another type of adjuvant therapy that is occasionally used in conjunction with chemotherapy or radiation therapy to enhance the efficacy of these traditional treatments for advanced cancers is heat therapy, also known as hyperthermia therapy. By heating the tumor, the surrounding tissue becomes more sensitive to the other therapies being used. It is safe, affordable, and appears to have a bright future in the treatment of cancer.

Summary

- Cancer is characterized by the uncontrolled cell proliferation, invasion, and check-point evasion of abnormal cells that are mostly non-functional.
- Chemotherapy is defined as the administration of numerous drugs and chemicals either alone or in combination to kill the cancer cells.
- Cis-diamminedichloroplatinum, known as cisplatin, is one of the most beneficial chemotherapeutic drugs which is prescribed for half of the malignancies.
- Paclitaxel is a member of the chemotherapeutic drug family known as taxane, which agitates the polymerization of tubulins.
- Tyrosine kinase inhibitors (TKIs) are non-peptide combinations prescribed orally and are structurally identical to adenosine triphosphate (ATP). They compete for the ATP-binding domains in kinases, therefore stopping the subsequent signaling transduction, which ultimately leads to apoptosis and the prevention of cell proliferation.
- Doxorubicin is a non-selective class-I anthracycline chemotherapeutic agent that contains aglyconic and sugar components. It binds to the plasma protein carriers and enters its target cell through passive diffusion after its administration, where it further accumulates intracellularly.
- The mammalian target of rapamycin (mTOR) and phosphatidylinositol-3-kinase/Akt signaling cascades act as a crucial double-edged sword within intracellular signaling pathways under both physiological and pathological conditions, including cell survival, cell proliferation, apoptosis, and invasion.
- Although current chemotherapy selections are mostly based on the cellular and genetic mechanisms underlying chemoresistance, various tumor-specific and patient-specific criteria contribute to chemotherapy response.

References

1. Alexandre, J., Hu, Y., Lu, W., Pelicano, H., & Huang, P. (2007). Novel action of paclitaxel against cancer cells: Bystander effect mediated by reactive oxygen species. *Cancer Research, 67*(8), 3512–3517. https://doi.org/10.1158/0008-5472.CAN-06-3560.
2. Anand, P., Kunnumakara, A. B., Sundaram, C., Harikumar, K. B., Tharakan, S. T., Lai, O. S., Sung, B., & Aggarwal, B. B. (2008). Cancer is a preventable disease that requires major lifestyle changes. *Pharmaceutical Research, 25*, 2097–2116. https://doi.org/10.1007/s11095-008-9661-9.
3. Basu, A., & Tu, H. (2005). Activation of ERK during DNA damage-induced apoptosis involves protein kinase Cδ. *Biochemical and Biophysical Research Communications, 334*, 1068–1073. https://doi.org/10.1016/j.bbrc.2005.06.188.
4. Belotti, D., Vergani, V., Drudis, T., Borsotti, P., Pitelli, M. R., Viale, G., Giavazzi, R., & Taraboletti, G. (1996). The microtubule-affecting drug paclitaxel has antiangiogenic activity. *Clinical Cancer Research, 2*(11), 1843–1849.
5. Bogoyevitch, M. A., & Court, N. W. (2004). Counting on mitogen-activated protein kinases—ERKs 3, 4, 5, 6, 7 and 8. *Cellular Signaling, 16*, 1345–1354. https://doi.org/10.1016/j.cellsig.2004.04.002.

6. Bracci, L., Schiavoni, G., Sistigu, A., & Belardelli, F. (2014). Immune-based mechanisms of cytotoxic chemotherapy: Implications for the design of novel and rationale-based combined treatments against cancer. *Cell Death and Differentiation, 21*(1), 15–25. https://doi.org/10.1038/cdd.2013.67.

7. Byrd-Leifer, C. A., Block, E. F., Takeda, K., Akira, S., & Ding, A. (2001). The role of MyD88 and TLR4 in the LPS-mimetic activity of Taxol. *European Journal of Immunology, 31*(8), 2448–2457. https://doi.org/10.1002/1521-4141(200108)31:8<2448::AID-IMMU2448>3.0.CO;2-P.

8. Chang, L., & Karin, M. (2001). Mammalian MAP kinase signaling cascades. *Nature, 410*, 37–40. https://doi.org/10.1038/35065000.

9. Cohen, S. M., & Lippard, S. J. (2001). Cisplatin: From DNA damage to cancer chemotherapy. *Inorganic Chemistry, 40*, 1–20.

10. De Luca, A., Parker, L. J., Ang, W. H., Rodolfo, C., Gabbarini, V., Hancock, N. C., Palone, F., Mazzetti, A. P., Menin, L., & Morton, C. J. (2019). A structure-based mechanism of cisplatin resistance mediated by glutathione transferase P1-1. *Proceedings of the National Academy of Sciences, 116*, 13943–13951. https://doi.org/10.1073/pnas.1902718116.

11. DeHaan, R. D., Yazlovitskaya, E. M., & Persons, D. L. (2001). Regulation of p53 target gene expression by cisplatin-induced extracellular signal-regulated kinase. *Cancer Chemotherapy and Pharmacology, 48*, 383–388. https://doi.org/10.1007/s002800100365.

12. Dempke, W., Voigt, W., Grothey, A., Hill, B. T., & Schmoll, H. J. (2000). Cisplatin resistance and oncogenes-A review. *Anti-Cancer Drugs, 11*, 225–236. https://doi.org/10.1097/00001813-200003000-00001.

13. Eckardt, J. R. (1997). Antitumor activity of docetaxel. *American Journal of Health-System Pharmacy, 54*, S2–S6. https://doi.org/10.1093/ajhp/54.suppl_5.S2.

14. Elmore, S. (2007). Apoptosis: A review of programmed cell death. *Toxicologic Pathology, 35*, 495–516. https://doi.org/10.1080/01926230701320337.

15. Florea, A. M., & Büsselberg, D. (2011). Cisplatin as an anti-tumor drug: Cellular mechanisms of activity, drug resistance and induced side effects. *Cancers, 3*, 1351–1371. https://doi.org/10.3390/cancers3011351.

16. Fuertes, M. A., Alonso, C., & Pérez, J. M. (2003). Biochemical modulation of cisplatin mechanisms of action: Enhancement of antitumor activity and circumvention of drug resistance. *Chemical Reviews, 103*, 645–662. https://doi.org/10.1021/cr0204579.

17. Galanski, M., Jakupec, M. A., & Keppler, B. K. (2005). Update of the preclinical situation of anticancer platinum complexes: Novel design strategies and innovative analytical approaches. *Current Medicinal Chemistry, 12*, 2075–2094. https://doi.org/10.2174/0929867054637626.

18. Garcia, J. A., & Danielpour, D. (2008). Mammalian target of rapamycin inhibition as a therapeutic strategy in the management of urologic malignancies. *Molecular Cancer Therapeutics, 7*, 1347–1354. https://doi.org/10.1158/1535-7163.MCT-08-0061.

19. Gillet, J. P., & Gottesman, M. M. (2010). Mechanisms of multidrug resistance in cancer. In *Multi-drug Resistance in Cancer* (pp. 47–76). Springer.

20. Gligorov, J., & Lotz, J. P. (2004). Preclinical pharmacology of the taxanes: Implications of the differences. *The Oncologist, 9*, 3–8. https://doi.org/10.1634/theoncologist.9-3-3.

21. Gumulec, J., Balvan, J., Sztalmachova, M., Raudenska, M., Dvorakova, V., Knopfova, L., Polanska, H., Hudcova, K., Ruttkay-Nedecky, B., & Babula, P. (2014). Cisplatin-resistant prostate cancer model: Differences in antioxidant system, apoptosis and cell cycle. *International Journal of Oncology, 44*, 923–933. https://doi.org/10.3892/ijo.2014.2242.

22. Hadzic, T., Aykin-Burns, N., Zhu, Y., Coleman, M. C., Leick, K., Jacobson, G. M., & Spitz, D. R. (2010). Paclitaxel combined with inhibitors of glucose and hydroperoxide metabolism enhances breast cancer cell killing via H_2O_2-mediated oxidative stress. *Free Radical Biology and Medicine, 48*(8), 1024–1033. https://doi.org/10.1016/j.freeradbiomed.2010.01.035.

23. Haldar, S., Basu, A., & Croce, C. M. (1997). Bcl2 is the guardian of microtubule integrity. *Cancer Research, 57*, 229–233.

24. Hennequin, C., Giocanti, N., & Favaudon, V. (1995). S-phase specificity of cell killing by docetaxel (Taxotere) in synchronized HeLa cells. *British Journal of Cancer, 71*, 1194–1198. https://doi.org/10.1038/bjc.1995.230.

25. Holzer, A. K., & Howell, S. B. (2006). The internalization and degradation of human copper transporter 1 following cisplatin exposure. *Cancer Research, 66*, 10944–10952. https://doi.org/10.1158/0008-5472.CAN-06-1865.

26. Holzer, A. K., Katano, K., Klomp, L. W., & Howell, S. B. (2004). Cisplatin rapidly down-regulates its own influx transporter hCTR1 in cultured human ovarian carcinoma cells. *Clinical Cancer Research, 10*, 6744–6749. https://doi.org/10.1158/1078-0432.CCR-04-0677.

27. Holzer, A. K., Manorek, G. H., & Howell, S. B. (2006). Contribution of the major copper influx transporter CTR1 to the cellular accumulation of cisplatin, carboplatin, and oxaliplatin. *Molecular Pharmacology, 70*, 1390–1394. https://doi.org/10.1124/mol.106.027011.

28. Houles, T., & Roux, P. P. (2018). Defining the role of the RSK isoforms in cancer. In *Seminars in Cancer Biology* (pp. 53–61). Elsevier. https://doi.org/10.1016/j.semcancer.2018.01.006.

29. Huang, C. Y., Ju, D. T., Chang, C. F., Reddy, P. M., & Velmurugan, B. K. (2017). A review on the effects of current chemotherapy drugs and natural agents in treating non–small cell lung cancer. *Biomedicine, 7*, 10. https://doi.org/10.4103/2221-1691.207198.

30. Imamura, T., Izumi, H., Nagatani, G., Ise, T., Nomoto, M., Iwamoto, Y., & Kohno, K. (2001). Interaction with p53 enhances binding of cisplatin-modified DNA by high mobility group 1 protein. *Journal of Biological Chemistry, 276*, 7534–7540. https://doi.org/10.1074/jbc.M009252200.

31. Ishida, S., Lee, J., Thiele, D. J., & Herskowitz, I. (2002). Uptake of the anticancer drug cisplatin mediated by the copper transporter Ctr1 in yeast and mammals. *Proceedings of the National Academy of Sciences, 99*, 14298–14302. https://doi.org/10.1073/pnas.212502399.

32. Jamieson, E. R., & Lippard, S. J. (1999). Structure, recognition, and processing of cisplatin–DNA adducts. *Chemical Reviews, 99*, 2467–2498. https://doi.org/10.1021/cr980421n.

33. Jansen, B. A., Brouwer, J., & Reedijk, J. (2002). Glutathione induces cellular resistance against cationic dinuclear platinum anticancer drugs. *Journal of Inorganic Biochemistry, 89*, 197–202. https://doi.org/10.1016/S0162-0134(01)00382-1.

34. Javeed, A., Ashraf, M., Riaz, A., Ghafoor, A., Afzal, S., & Mukhtar, M. M. (2009). Paclitaxel and immune system. *European Journal of Pharmaceutical Sciences, 38*(4), 283–290. https://doi.org/10.1016/j.ejps.2009.08.004.

35. Jiang, X. (2014). Harnessing the immune system for the treatment of breast cancer. *Journal of Zhejiang University-Science B, 15*(1), 1–15. https://doi.org/10.1631/jzus.B1300195.

36. Johnson, G. L., & Lapadat, R. (2002). Mitogen-activated protein kinase pathways mediated by ERK, JNK, and p38 protein kinases. *Science, 298*, 1911–1912. https://doi.org/10.1126/science.1072682.

37. Jones, E. V., Dickman, M. J., & Whitmarsh, A. J. (2007). Regulation of p73-mediated apoptosis by c-Jun N-terminal kinase. *Biochemical Journal, 405*, 617–623. https://doi.org/10.1042/BJ20061538.

38. Kampan, N. C., Madondo, M. T., McNally, O. M., Quinn, M., & Plebanski, M. (2015). Paclitaxel and its evolving role in the management of ovarian cancer. *BioMed Research International, 2015*, 1–21. https://doi.org/10.1155/2015/413076.

39. Kaneno, R., Shurin, G. V., Tourkova, I. L., & Shurin, M. R. (2009). Chemomodulation of human dendritic cell function by antineoplastic agents in low noncytotoxic concentrations. *Journal of Translational Medicine, 7*(1), 58. https://doi.org/10.1186/1479-5876-7-58.

40. Kartalou, M., & Essigmann, J. M. (2001). Mechanisms of resistance to cisplatin. *Mutation Research/Fundamental and Molecular Mechanisms of Mutagenesis, 478*, 23–43. https://doi.org/10.1016/S0027-5107(01)00184-5.

41. Kelland, L. (2007). The resurgence of platinum-based cancer chemotherapy. *Nature Reviews Cancer, 7*, 573–584. https://doi.org/10.1038/nrc2167.

42. Kim, H. S., Kim, S. J., Bae, J., Wang, Y., Park, S. Y., Min, Y. S., Je, H. D., & Sohn, U. D. (2016). The p90rsk-mediated signaling of ethanol-induced cell proliferation in HepG2 cell line. *Korean Journal of Physiology and Pharmacology, 20*, 595–603. https://doi.org/10.4196/kjpp.2016.20.6.595.

43. Klauber, N., Parangi, S., Flynn, E., Hamel, E., & D'Amato, R. J. (1997). Inhibition of angiogenesis and breast cancer in mice by the microtubule inhibitors 2-methoxyestradiol and taxol. *Cancer Research, 57*(1), 81–86.

44. Kohno, K., Wang, K. Y., Takahashi, M., Kurita, T., Yoshida, Y., Hirakawa, M., Harada, Y., Kuma, A., Izumi, H., & Matsumoto, S. (2015). Mitochondrial transcription factor A and mitochondrial genome as molecular targets for cisplatin-based cancer chemotherapy. *International Journal of Molecular Sciences, 16*, 19836–19850. https://doi.org/10.3390/ijms160919836.

45. Kreis, T., & Vale, R. (1993). *Guidebook to the Cytoskeletal and Motor Proteins*. Oxford University Press.

46. Kubo, M., Morisaki, T., Matsumoto, K., Tasaki, A., Yamanaka, N., Nakashima, H., Kuroki, H., Nakamura, K., Nakamura, M., & Katano, M. (2005). Paclitaxel probably enhances cytotoxicity of natural killer cells against breast carcinoma cells by increasing perforin production. *Cancer Immunology, Immunotherapy, 54*(5), 468–476. https://doi.org/10.1007/s00262-004-0627-y.

47. Kushi, L. H., Doyle, C., McCullough, M., Rock, C. L., Demark-Wahnefried, W., Bandera, E. V., Gapstur, S., Patel, A. V., Andrews, K., & Gansler, T. (2012). American Cancer Society guidelines on nutrition and physical activity for cancer prevention: Reducing the risk of cancer with healthy food choices and physical activity. *CA: A Cancer Journal for Clinicians, 62*, 30–67. https://doi.org/10.3322/caac.20140.

48. Lafarga, V., Cuadrado, A., & Nebreda, A. R. (2007). p18Hamlet mediates different p53-dependent responses to DNA damage inducing agents. *Cell Cycle, 6*, 2319–2322. https://doi.org/10.4161/cc.6.18.4681.

49. Lau, D. H., Xue, L., Young, L. J., Burke, P. A., & Cheung, A. T. (1999). Paclitaxel (Taxol): An inhibitor of angiogenesis in a highly vascularized transgenic breast cancer. *Cancer Biotherapy & Radiopharmaceuticals, 14*(1), 31–36. https://doi.org/10.1089/cbr.1999.14.31.

50. Mansouri, A., Ridgway, L. D., Korapati, A. L., Zhang, Q., Tian, L., Wang, Y., Siddik, Z. H., Mills, G. B., & Claret, F. X. (2003). Sustained activation of JNK/p38 MAPK pathways in response to cisplatin leads to Fas ligand induction and cell death in ovarian carcinoma cells. *Journal of Biological Chemistry, 278*, 19245–19256. https://doi.org/10.1074/jbc.M301630200.

51. Markasz, L., Stuber, G., Vanherberghen, B., Flaberg, E., Olah, E., Carbone, E., Eksborg, S., Klein, E., Skribek, H., & Szekely, L. (2007). Effect of frequently used chemotherapeutic drugs on the cytotoxic activity of human natural killer cells. *Molecular Cancer Therapeutics, 6*(2), 644–654. https://doi.org/10.1158/1535-7163.MCT-06-0541.

52. McKenna, M. T., Weis, J. A., Brock, A., Quaranta, V., & Yankeelov, T. E. (2018). Precision medicine with imprecise therapy: Computational modeling for chemotherapy in breast cancer. *Translational Oncology, 11*, 732–742. https://doi.org/10.1016/j.tranon.2018.03.006.

53. Meijer, C., Timmer, A., De Vries, E. G., Groten, J. P., Knol, A., Zwart, N., Dam, W. A., Sleijfer, D. T., & Mulder, N. H. (2000). Role of metallothionein in cisplatin sensitivity of germ-cell tumours. *International Journal of Cancer, 85*, 777–781. https://doi.org/10.1002/(SICI)1097-0215(20000315)85:6<777::AID-IJC12>3.0.CO;2-P.

54. Mentella, M. C., Scaldaferri, F., Ricci, C., Gasbarrini, A., & Miggiano, G. A. D. (2019). Cancer and the Mediterranean diet: A review. *Nutrients, 11*, 2059. https://doi.org/10.3390/nu11092059.

55. Metzger, R., Bollschweiler, E., Hölscher, A. H., & Warnecke-Eberz, U. (2010). ERCC1: Impact in multimodality treatment of upper gastrointestinal cancer. *Future Oncology, 6*, 1735–1749. https://doi.org/10.2217/fon.10.127.

56. Midha, S., Chawla, S., & Garg, P. K. (2016). Modifiable and non-modifiable risk factors for pancreatic cancer: A review. *Cancer Letters, 381*, 269–277. https://doi.org/10.1016/j.canlet.2016.08.004.

57. Moggs, J. G., Szymkowski, D. E., Yamada, M., Karran, P., & Wood, R. D. (1997). Differential human nucleotide excision repair of paired and mispaired cisplatin-DNA adducts. *Nucleic Acids Research, 25*, 480–490. https://doi.org/10.1093/nar/25.3.480.

58. Nagai, N., Okuda, R., Kinoshita, M., & Ogata, H. (1996). Decomposition kinetics of cisplatin in human biological fluids. *Journal of Pharmacy and Pharmacology, 48*, 918–924. https://doi.org/10.1111/j.2042-7158.1996.tb07043.x.

59. Nakayama, K., Miyazaki, K., Kanzaki, A., Fukumoto, M., & Takebayashi, Y. (2001). Expression and cisplatin sensitivity of copper-transporting P-type adenosine triphosphatase (ATP7B) in human solid carcinoma cell lines. *Oncology Reports, 8*, 1285–1287. https://doi.org/10.3892/or.8.6.1285.

60. Neuss, N., Mallett, G., Brannon, D., Mabe, J., Horton, H., & Huckstep, L. (1974). Vinca alkaloids XXXIII. Microbiological conversions of vincaleukoblastine (VLB, vinblastine), an antitumor alkaloid from Vinca rosea. *Helvetica Chimica Acta, 57*, 1886–1890. https://doi.org/10.1002/hlca.19740570709.

61. Niedner, H., Christen, R., Lin, X., Kondo, A., & Howell, S. B. (2001). Identification of genes that mediate sensitivity to cisplatin. *Molecular Pharmacology, 60*, 1153–1160. https://doi.org/10.1124/mol.60.6.1153.

62. Nuñez, G., Benedict, M. A., Hu, Y., & Inohara, N. (1998). Caspases: The proteases of the apoptotic pathway. *Oncogene, 17*, 3237–3245. https://doi.org/10.1038/sj.onc.1202581.

63. Payet, D., Gaucheron, F., Sip, M., & Leng, M. (1993). Instability of the monofunctional adducts in cis-[Pt (NH3)2(N7-N-methyl-2-diazapyrenium)Cl]2+-modified DNA: Rates of cross-linking reactions in cis-platinum modified DNA. *Nucleic Acids Research, 21*, 5846–5851. https://doi.org/10.1093/nar/21.24.5846.

64. Perez, R. P. (1998). Cellular and molecular determinants of cisplatin resistance. *European Journal of Cancer, 34*, 1535–1542. https://doi.org/10.1016/S0959-8049(98)00235-7.

65. Petrović, M., & Todorović, D. (2016). Biochemical and molecular mechanisms of action of cisplatin in cancer cells. *Facta Universitatis, Series: Medicine and Biology, 18(1), 12–18.*

66. Pfannenstiel, L. W., Lam, S. S., Emens, L. A., Jaffee, E. M., & Armstrong, T. D. (2010). Paclitaxel enhances early dendritic cell maturation and function through TLR4 signaling in mice. *Cellular Immunology, 263*(1), 79–87. https://doi.org/10.1016/j.cellimm.2010.03.007.

67. Pinto-Leite, R., Botelho, P., Ribeiro, E., Oliveira, P. A., & Santos, L. (2009). Effect of sirolimus on urinary bladder cancer T_{24} cell line. *Journal of Experimental & Clinical Cancer Research, 28*, 3. https://doi.org/10.1186/1756-9966-28-3.

68. Rabik, C. A., & Dolan, M. E. (2007). Molecular mechanisms of resistance and toxicity associated with platinating agents. *Cancer Treatment Reviews, 33*, 9–23. https://doi.org/10.1016/j.ctrv.2006.09.006.

69. Raimondi, S., Maisonneuve, P., & Lowenfels, A. B. (2009). Epidemiology of pancreatic cancer: An overview. *Nature Reviews Gastroenterology & Hepatology, 6*, 699. https://doi.org/10.1038/nrgastro.2009.177.

70. Rao, S., Orr, G. A., Chaudhary, A. G., Kingston, D. G. I., & Horwitz, S. B. (1995). Characterization of the Taxol binding site on the microtubule 2-(m-azidobenzoyl) taxol photolabels a peptide (amino acids 217-231) of β-tubulin. *Journal of Biological Chemistry, 270*, 20235–20238. https://doi.org/10.1074/jbc.270.34.20235.

71. Reardon, J. T., Vaisman, A., Chaney, S. G., & Sancar, A. (1999). Efficient nucleotide excision repair of cisplatin, oxaliplatin, and bis-aceto-ammine-dichloro-cyclohexylamine-platinum (IV) (JM216) platinum intrastrand DNA diadducts. *Cancer Research, 59*, 3968–3971. https://doi.org/10.1016/S0006-291X(03)01018-5.

72. Romeo, Y., Moreau, J., Zindy, P. J., Saba-El-Leil, M., Lavoie, G., Dandachi, F., Baptissart, M., Borden, K. L., Meloche, S., & Roux, P. P. (2013). RSK regulates activated BRAF signaling to mTORC1 and promotes melanoma growth. *Oncogene, 32*, 2917–2926. https://doi.org/10.1038/onc.2012.319.

73. Romeo, Y., Zhang, X., & Roux, P. P. (2012). Regulation and function of the RSK family of protein kinases. *Biochemical Journal, 441*, 553–569. https://doi.org/10.1042/BJ20111306.

74. Rowinsky, E. K., Onetto, N., Canetta, R., & Arbuck, S. (1992). Taxol: The first of the taxanes, an important new class of antitumor agents. *Seminars in Oncology, 19*, 646–662.

75. Saad, S. Y., Najjar, T. A., & Alashari, M. (2004). Role of non-selective adenosine receptor blockade and phosphodiesterase inhibition in cisplatin-induced nephrogonadal toxicity in rats. *Clinical and Experimental Pharmacology and Physiology, 31*, 862–867. https://doi.org/10.1111/j.1440-1681.2004.04088.x.

76. Sako, T., Burioka, N., Yasuda, K., Tomita, K., Miyata, M., Kurai, J., Chikumi, H., Watanabe, M., Suyama, H., & Fukuoka, Y. (2004). Cellular immune profile in patients with non-small cell lung cancer after weekly paclitaxel therapy. *Acta Oncologica, 43*(1), 15–19. https://doi.org/10.1080/02841860310020618.

77. Salvesen, G. S., & Abrams, J. M. (2004). Caspase activation–stepping on the gas or releasing the brakes? Lessons from humans and flies. *Oncogene, 23*, 2774–2784. https://doi.org/10.1038/sj.onc.1207510.

78. Schiff, P. B., & Horwitz, S. B. (1980). Taxol stabilizes microtubules in mouse fibroblast cells. *Proceedings of the National Academy of Sciences, 77*, 1561–1565. https://doi.org/10.1073/pnas.77.3.1561.

79. Schiff, P. B., Fant, J., & Horwitz, S. B. (1979). Promotion of microtubule assembly in vitro by taxol. *Nature, 277*, 665–667. https://doi.org/10.1038/277665a0.

80. Selvakumaran, M., Pisarcik, D. A., Bao, R., Yeung, A. T., & Hamilton, T. C. (2003). Enhanced cisplatin cytotoxicity by disturbing the nucleotide excision repair pathway in ovarian cancer cell lines. *Cancer Research, 63*, 1311–1316.

81. Sève, P., & Dumontet, C. (2005). Chemoresistance in non-small cell lung cancer. *Current Medicinal Chemistry–Anti-Cancer Agents, 5*, 73–88. https://doi.org/10.2174/1568011053352908.

82. Sevko, A., Kremer, V., Falk, C., Umansky, L., Shurin, M. R., Shurin, G. V., & Umansky, V. (2012). Application of paclitaxel in low non-cytotoxic doses supports vaccination with melanoma antigens in normal mice. *Journal of Immunotoxicology, 9*(3), 275–281. https://doi.org/10.3109/1547691X.2011.639795.

83. Siddik, Z. H. (2003). Cisplatin: Mode of cytotoxic action and molecular basis of resistance. *Oncogene, 22*, 7265–7279. https://doi.org/10.1038/sj.onc.1206911.

84. Siegsmund, M. J., Marx, C., Seemann, O., Schummer, B., Steidler, A., Toktomambetova, L., Köhrmann, K. U., Rassweiler, J., & Alken, P. (1999). Cisplatin-resistant bladder carcinoma cells: Enhanced expression of metallothioneins. *Urological Research, 27*, 157–163. https://doi.org/10.1007/s002400050116.

85. Szakács, G., Paterson, J. K., Ludwig, J. A., Booth-Genthe, C., & Gottesman, M. M. (2006). Targeting multidrug resistance in cancer. *Nature Reviews Drug Discovery, 5*(3), 219–234. https://doi.org/10.1038/nrd1984.

86. Tacar, O., Sriamornsak, P., & Dass, C. R. (2013). Doxorubicin: An update on anticancer molecular action, toxicity and novel drug delivery systems. *Journal of Pharmacy and Pharmacology, 65*, 157–170. https://doi.org/10.1111/j.2042-7158.2012.01567.x.

87. ter Haar, E., Kowalski, R. J., Hamel, E., Lin, C. M., Longley, R. E., Gunasekera, S. P., Rosenkranz, H. S., & Day, B. W. (1996). Discodermolide, a cytotoxic marine agent that stabilizes microtubules more potently than taxol. *Biochemistry, 35*, 243–250. https://doi.org/10.1021/bi952152a.

88. Vaisman, A., Varchenko, M., Umar, A., Kunkel, T. A., Risinger, J. I., Barrett, J. C., Hamilton, T. C., & Chaney, S. G. (1998). The role of hMLH1, hMSH3, and hMSH6 defects in cisplatin and

oxaliplatin resistance: Correlation with replicative bypass of platinum-DNA adducts. *Cancer Research, 58*, 3579–3585.

89. Wang, A. C., Ma, Y. B., Wu, F. X., Ma, Z. F., Liu, N. F., Gao, R., Gao, Y. S., & Sheng, X. G. (2014). TLR4 induces tumor growth and inhibits paclitaxel activity in MyD88-positive human ovarian carcinoma in vitro. *Oncology Letters, 7*(3), 871–877. https://doi.org/10.3892/ol.2013.1806.

90. Wang, T., Chan, Y., Chen, C., Kung, W., Lee, Y., Wang, S., Chang, T., & Wang, H. (2006). Paclitaxel (Taxol) upregulates expression of functional interleukin-6 in human ovarian cancer cells through multiple signaling pathways. *Oncogene, 25*(29), 4857–4866. https://doi.org/10.1038/sj.onc.1209462.

91. Welsh, C., Day, R., McGurk, C., Masters, J. R., Wood, R. D., & Köberle, B. (2004). Reduced levels of XPA, ERCC1 and XPF DNA repair proteins in testis tumor cell lines. *International Journal of Cancer, 110*, 352–361. https://doi.org/10.1002/ijc.20121.

92. Winograd-Katz, S., & Levitzki, A. (2006). Cisplatin induces PKB/Akt activation and p38 MAPK phosphorylation of the EGF receptor. *Oncogene, 25*, 7381–7390. https://doi.org/10.1038/sj.onc.1209715.

93. Woźniak, K., & Błasiak, J. (2002). Recognition and repair of DNA-cisplatin adducts. *Acta Biochimica Polonica, 49*, 583–596.

94. Wu, X., Obata, T., Khan, Q., Highshaw, R., White, R. D. V., & Sweeney, C. (2004). The phosphatidylinositol-3 kinase pathway regulates bladder cancer cell invasion. *BJU International, 93*, 143–150. https://doi.org/10.1111/j.1464-410x.2004.04590.x.

95. Yakirevich, E., Sabo, E., Naroditsky, I., Sova, Y., Lavie, O., & Resnick, M. B. (2006). Multidrug resistance-related phenotype and apoptosis-related protein expression in ovarian serous carcinomas. *Gynecologic Oncology, 100*(1), 152–159. https://doi.org/10.1016/j.ygyno.2005.07.103.

96. Yen, H. C., Tang, Y. C., Chen, F. Y., Chen, S. W., & Majima, H. J. (2005). Enhancement of cisplatin-induced apoptosis and caspase 3 activation by depletion of mitochondrial DNA in a human osteosarcoma cell line. *Annals of the New York Academy of Sciences, 1042*, 516–522. https://doi.org/10.1196/annals.1338.051.

97. Yoon, S., & Seger, R. (2006). The extracellular signal-regulated kinase: Multiple substrates regulate diverse cellular functions. *Growth Factors, 24*, 21–44. https://doi.org/10.1080/08977190600564865.

98. Zamble, D. B., Mikata, Y., Eng, C. H., Sandman, K. E., & Lippard, S. J. (2002). Testis-specific HMG-domain protein alters the responses of cells to cisplatin. *Journal of Inorganic Biochemistry, 91*, 451–462. https://doi.org/10.1016/S0162-0134(02)00046-1.

99. Zhang, D., Yang, R., Wang, S., & Dong, Z. (2014). Paclitaxel: New uses for an old drug. *Drug Design, Development and Therapy, 8*, 279–284. https://doi.org/10.2147/DDDT.S56874.

100. Zhu, Y., Liu, N., Xiong, S., Zheng, Y., & Chu, Y. (2011). CD4+ Foxp3+ regulatory T-cell impairment by paclitaxel is independent of toll-like receptor 4. *Scandinavian Journal of Immunology, 73*(4), 301–308. https://doi.org/10.1111/j.1365-3083.2010.02494.x.

Chapter

ENDOCRINE PHARMACOLOGY

8

Contents

Introduction

Hormones are endogenous chemicals that the endocrine system uses to help maintain internal homeostasis. Generally speaking, a hormone is thought of as a chemical messenger that is released into the bloodstream and affects target cells that are located a certain distance from the site of hormonal release. Hormones that aid in controlling physiological functions like energy metabolism, growth and development, reproduction, fluid and electrolyte balance, and reaction to stress and injury are produced and released by a variety of endocrine glands.

Pharmacology plays a significant role in the regulation and control of endocrine function through drug use. Hormones are drugs in the sense that the body produces them for the patient. This provides a clear window of opportunity to mimic or reduce the effects of particular hormones during endocrine dysfunction using exogenous chemicals.

In cases of hormonal insufficiency, patients may be prescribed medication as replacement therapy (e.g., insulin for diabetes mellitus). Similarly, exogenous hormone analogs, such as glucocorticoids to help treat inflammation, can enhance the effects of their endogenous counterparts. Drugs, on the other hand, can be used to treat endocrine hyperactivity; one such example is the treatment of hyperthyroidism with antithyroid drugs. Lastly, medications have the ability to control normal endocrine function to produce a desired result. One example of this is the way that oral contraceptives inhibit ovulation. (Falkenstein et al, 2000; Schacke et al, 2002; Nelson, 2002; Nelson et al, 2002)

Orientation and Directional Terms

Term	Definition	Illustration
Glaucoma	Glaucoma is a group of eye diseases that damage the optic nerve, which can lead to vision loss or blindness. It's often called the "silent thief of sight" because vision loss usually occurs gradually over time.	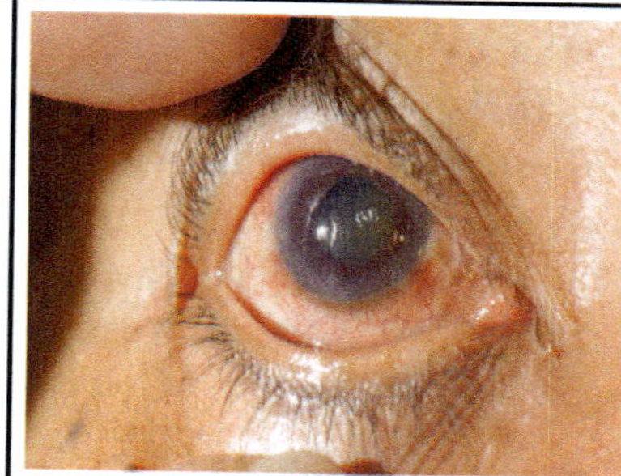
Bone resorption	Bone resorption is the process by which osteoclasts break down bone tissue, releasing minerals and calcium into the blood. It's a natural process that's important for normal bone development and remodeling. However, excessive resorption can lead to bone loss and increase the risk of fractures.	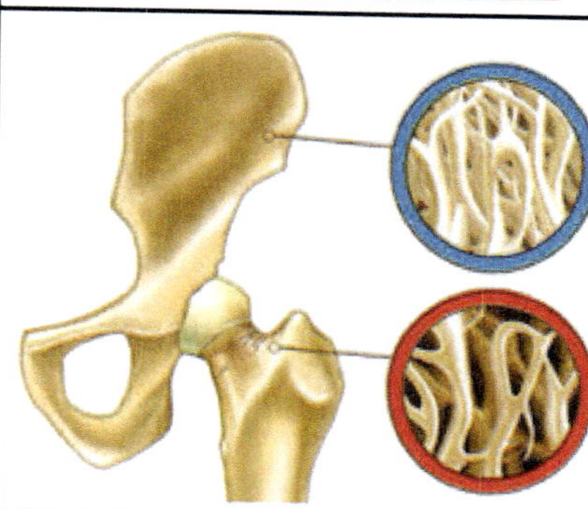
Thromboembolism	Thromboembolism is a condition in which a blood clot (thrombus) breaks off from its original site and travels through the bloodstream (as an embolus) to obstruct a blood vessel, causing tissue ischemia and organ damage. Thromboembolism can affect both the venous and arterial systems, with different clinical manifestations and management strategies.	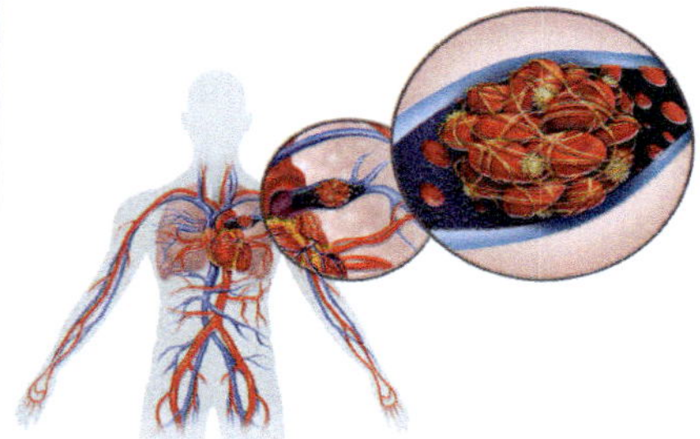
Somatomedins	Somatomedins are a group of proteins produced predominantly not by the liver when growth hormones act on target tissue. Somatomedins inhibit the release of growth hormones by acting directly on anterior pituitary and by stimulating the secretion of somatostatin from the hypothalamus.	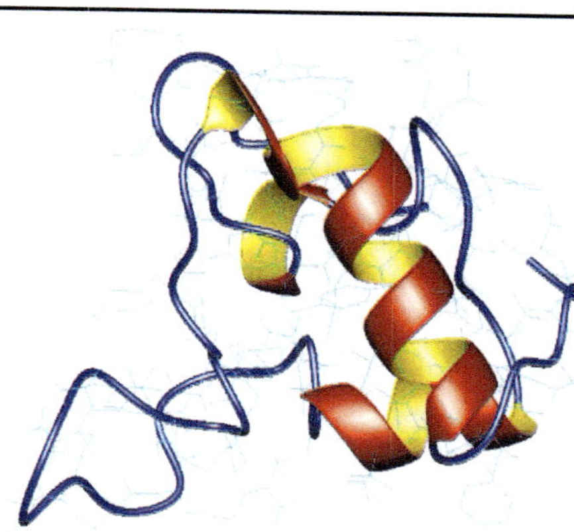

8.1. Diabetes Mellitus

Before the discovery of insulin, type 1 diabetes was always fatal due to insulin deficiency's potential to cause ketoacidosis. The goal of treatment for diabetic ketoacidosis has shifted to preventing long-term vascular complications since the discovery of insulin. In addition to causing symptoms directly related to hyperglycemia (polyuria, polydipsia, and blurred vision; see below), type 2 diabetes—where insulin resistance and a relative lack of insulin lead to hyperglycemia—is also a significant risk factor for atheromatous disease. Both diabetes mellitus and glucose intolerance are becoming more common in developed and developing nations, and they pose a serious threat to public health. It is important to address risk factors other than blood glucose, such as hypertension; this is addressed elsewhere.

8.1.1. Pathophysiology

The β-cells, also referred to as B-cells, located in the islets of Langerhans secrete insulin. In addition to lowering blood sugar, it also modifies how fats, amino acids, and carbohydrates are metabolized. It is secreted along with inactive C-peptide, which serves as a helpful indicator of insulin secretion: in patients with type 1 diabetes, its plasma concentration is either nonexistent or very low, whereas in patients with insulinomas, an uncommon tumor that secretes insulin to cause hypoglycemia, it is highly concentrated. This is not the same as "C-reactive peptide" (CRP), an acute phase protein produced by the liver that is utilized as a general indicator of inflammation. Patients with insulin injection-induced hypoglycemia do not have elevated C-peptide concentrations.

An absolute or relative lack of insulin is the cause of diabetes mellitus, which is defined as a fasting blood glucose concentration of ≥ 7 mmol/L. Insulin deficiency is the only condition associated with type 1 diabetes. These patients typically present as young, non-obese individuals. An inherited propensity exists. However, concordance in identical twins is reportedly less than 50%, suggesting that environmental factors must also be encountered by genetically predisposed individuals. One such element is viruses, such as the Coxsackie and Echo viruses, which can start an autoimmune reaction that eventually results in the islet cells being destroyed.

Type 2 diabetes is characterized by a notable resistance to the action of insulin and a relative lack of insulin secretion. More discriminating assays show that there is an increase in proinsulin and a decrease in true insulin concentration, while standard assays, which do not distinguish well between insulin and pro-insulin, may show a normal or even increased circulating concentration of immunoreactive insulin. These patients are typically obese and middle-aged or older when they first present. In nearly all identical twins, this type of diabetes is congruent. Diabetic ketoacidosis is a rare side effect of type 2 diabetes; however, it can also cause complications such as non-ketotic hyperosmolar coma or, in rare cases (when combined with biguanide medication, like metformin; refer below), lactic acidosis.

An increased concentration of glucose in the circulating blood gives rise to osmotic effects:

1. diuresis (polyuria) with consequent circulating volume reduction, causing thirst and polydipsia;
2. the refractive index of a high glucose concentration solution in the eye differs from healthy aqueous humor, causing blurred vision

Furthermore, glycosuria increases the risk of Candida infection, particularly in females. The inability to store energy as fat or glycogen or to bind protein in muscle is accompanied by calorie loss in the urine, and uncontrolled diabetics frequently experience weight loss accompanied by a loss of muscle and fat (a condition known as "amyotrophy").

Vascular complications complicate both forms of diabetes mellitus. Retinopathy, which comprises hard exudates and blot hemorrhages that do not in and of themselves endanger vision, and proliferative retinopathy, which can result in retinal hemorrhage and blindness, are examples of microvascular complications. Often, cataracts occur. Diabetic neuropathy results in painful paresthesia and loss of sensation in the gloves and stockings. Renal failure is the result of diabetic nephropathy, which affects about one-third of patients with diabetes. An early sign of overt diabetic nephropathy is microalbuminuria. Accelerated atheroma leads to macrovascular disease, which increases the risk of myocardial infarction, peripheral vascular disease, and stroke. Reaven in 1988 at the American Diabetes Association annual meeting highlighted the strong correlation between diabetes and obesity, hypertension and dyslipidemia (particularly hypertriglyceridemia), and the strong link between type 2 diabetes and endothelial dysfunction, an early event in atherogenesis.

8.1.2. Principles of Management

Setting high but attainable goals for every patient is crucial. There is strong evidence that better diabetic control lowers microvascular complications in young type 1 patients. To prevent the development of such complications, it is highly worthwhile to make a concerted effort to minimize the metabolic disruption associated with diabetes mellitus. To encourage the patient to learn how to modify their insulin dosage for the best possible glycemic control, education and support are crucial. This can only be accomplished if the patient learns to monitor their blood sugar levels at home and modify their insulin dosage accordingly. A customized treatment plan is required. To provide a low, stable background level of insulin during the night, a common approach is to combine injections of a short-acting insulin before each meal with a once-daily injection of a long-acting insulin. Follow-up care needs to be structured and involve regular screening for signs of microvascular disease as well as an assessment of chronic glycemic control using the HbA1c test. Given that prophylactic laser therapy can prevent blindness in cases of proliferative retinopathy and maculopathy, this is particularly crucial.

In contrast, it is only appropriate in certain situations to aim for strict blood sugar control in type 2 patients. Although strict control lowers macrovascular problems, it also increases the risk of hypoglycemic episodes, and a significant number of patients must receive this kind of care to avoid a single cardiovascular event. On the other hand, patients with hypertension can benefit greatly from aggressive treatment, and their goal blood pressure should be lower than that of people without diabetes. The goal of hypoglycemic therapy for older type 2 patients is to reduce hyperosmolar coma risk and symptoms of polyuria, polydipsia, and recurrent Candida infections.

8.1.3. Diet in Diabetes Mellitus

Maintaining ideal body weight on a diet that does not promote atherosclerosis is crucial. Insulin injections should be carefully matched with caloric intake. Patients using injected insulin should time their meals accordingly. To avoid postprandial hyperglycemia, it is advised to limit intake of simple sugars and replace them with foods that have a low glycemic index. Artificial sweeteners can be a useful alternative for those who have a sweet tooth. A diet high in fiber can help regulate glucose levels and reduce insulin needs. Beans and lentils can help stabilize blood sugar levels. Limiting saturated fat and cholesterol intake and opting for lean sources of protein is recommended. There is no need for expensive "special diabetic foods" that are often high in fat and calories, instead focus on complex carbohydrates.

8.1.4. Drugs Used to Treat Diabetes Mellitus

8.1.4.1. Insulins

Insulin, a polypeptide, has largely been replaced by recombinant human insulin and similar analogs in animals due to their consistent quality and reduced allergic effects. Different formulations of insulin with protamine and/or zinc have varying pharmacokinetic properties, affecting absorption rates and duration of action. "Designer" insulins are synthetic polypeptides resembling insulin but with slight amino acid composition changes, altering their properties. For instance, insulin lispro absorbs rapidly and has a quick onset, while insulin glargine acts slowly to maintain a low level of insulin activity over a 24-hour period.

1. Use

Insulin is recommended for approximately one-third of patients with type 2 diabetes and for all patients with type 1 diabetes mellitus, though it is not strictly required during the early "honeymoon" period before islet cell destruction is finished. Typically, insulin is injected subcutaneously, but type 2 diabetics now have access to an inhaled formulation as well. (Note: Due to its lack of commercial success, this has been removed from sale in the UK). Because blocking antibodies are not produced, the effective dose of human insulin is typically lower than that of animal insulins. As a result, when converting from animal to human insulin, the dosage is decreased.

Soluble insulin is the preferred choice for intravenous administration, particularly in diabetic emergencies. It is also commonly given subcutaneously before meals for long-term management. There are various formulations of human insulins available, with different ratios of short-acting and longer-lasting forms. Some of these formulations come in pre-filled injection devices, known as pens, which are convenient for patients. Soluble insulin helps control hyperglycemia immediately after administration, but it can also lead to hypoglycemia, especially in the early morning hours. When starting a patient on a twice-daily insulin regimen, it is recommended to divide the daily dose, with two-thirds given before breakfast and one-third before the evening meal. Adjustments may need to be made for individuals engaging in strenuous physical activity to prevent exercise-induced hypoglycemia.

Insulin is necessary for type 2 diabetics who are symptomatic and do not respond well to diet or oral hypoglycemic drugs. However, insulin can make weight loss more challenging as it increases appetite, but it can be beneficial for patients with diabetic amyotrophy. In addition, insulin is essential for acute diabetic emergencies like ketoacidosis, during pregnancy, before and after surgery, and in cases of severe illness such as infections, heart attacks, and burns.

Intercurrent infections can cause an increase in insulin requirements of up to one-third, so patients should be advised to intensify home blood glucose monitoring (even if they are not eating as much as usual) and increase their insulin dosage as needed when they have a cold or other infection. After the infection has cleared, the dosage will need to be lowered. Patients who vomit frequently mistakenly quit injecting insulin because they are afraid of hypoglycemia, which can lead to ketoacidosis.

Before any elective surgery, patients should switch to soluble insulin. It is possible to infuse soluble insulin during surgery. v. with glucose to generate a 6–8 mmol/L blood glucose concentration. This is maintained until oral feeding and sporadic subcutaneous insulin injections can be resumed following surgery. For emergency operations, a similar regimen is appropriate, but more frequent blood glucose testing is necessary. Insulin may not always be necessary for the management of type 2 diabetes patients; however, frequent blood glucose monitoring is necessary during the post-operative phase.

2. Ketoacidosis

Since glucose is not available intracellularly in diabetic ketoacidosis (DKA) despite elevated plasma glucose concentrations, the metabolic alterations are similar to those of starvation ("starving amidst plenty"). Electrolyte loss and osmotic diuresis are the results of hyperglycemia. When faced with acidosis and osmotic diuresis, conservation of potassium is even less effective than that of nain; large intravenous potassium replacements are frequently required to make up for the significant loss of total body potassium. Nonetheless, a shift from the intracellular to the extracellular compartment in DKA can cause an increase in plasma potassium concentration; therefore, large doses of potassium chloride should be avoided until high urine output and plasma electrolyte concentrations are established. Adipose tissue mobilization releases free fatty acids, which are then converted to acetyl coenzyme A (CoA) through β-oxidation. Acetyl CoA is converted to acetoacetate, acetone, and β-hydroxybutyrate (ketones) in the absence of glucose breakdown.

These are buffered by plasma bicarbonate, leading to a fall in bicarbonate concentration (metabolic acidosis – with an increased 'anion gap' since anionic ketone bodies are not measured routinely) and compensatory hyperventilation ('Küssmaul' breathing). There are therefore many metabolic abnormalities:

- **Deficit in sodium and potassium:** To replenish extracellular fluid volume, an intravenous dose of physiological saline (0.09% sodium chloride) must be administered in large quantities. Urine output needs to be watched. In cases where blood glucose levels are less than 17 mmol/L, normal saline solution is substituted with 5% glucose. It is necessary to replenish potassium, and if the urine production is adequate and the plasma potassium concentration is 3.5 mEq/L, up to 20 mmol/hour of potassium chloride can be administered. The rate of replacement is determined by regular measurements of the plasma potassium concentration and electrocardiogram monitoring.
- **Hyperglycemia:** Using a syringe pump, intravenous insulin is injected up to 0.1 units/kg/hour until ketosis is resolved (as determined by blood pH, serum bicarbonate, and blood or urine ketones).
- **Metabolic acidosis:** This condition usually goes away with proper insulin and physiological sodium chloride therapy. It is debatable whether treating extracellular metabolic acidosis with bicarbonate will improve intracellular and cerebrospinal fluid acidosis. When a patient's arterial pH is less than 7 points, they should be managed in an

intensive care unit and may require inotropic support. Bicarbonate is often given to them in this situation.

- Treatment of the coma's precipitating cause (e.g., gastric stasis) and aspiration of the stomach are additional measures, as aspiration can be severe and even fatal. g. antibiotics for infections caused by bacteria.

3. Hyperosmolar non-ketotic coma

   Because the blood pH is normal and insulin sensitivity is maintained, less insulin is needed in this scenario. Physiological saline (0.5%, or half-strength, saline) is used to replace lost fluid; large doses of intravenous potassium are frequently needed. As long as renal function is normal, magnesium deficiency should be treated because it is common and makes it more difficult to correct the potassium deficit. Due to the increased blood viscosity in this hyperosmolar state, prophylaxis against venous thrombosis should be explored with a heparin preparation.

4. Mechanism of action

   Insulin acts by binding to transmembrane glycoprotein receptors. Receptor occupancy results in:

1. Activation of insulin-dependent glucose transport processes (in adipose tissue and muscle) via a transporter known as 'Glut-4';
2. Inhibition of adenylyl cyclase-dependent metabolism (lipolysis, proteolysis, glycogenolysis);
3. Intracellular accumulation of potassium and phosphate, which is linked to glucose transport in some tissues.

Increased oxidative phosphorylation, increased DNA and RNA synthesis, and increased cellular amino acid uptake are examples of secondary effects.

5. Adverse reactions

i. The most significant and serious side effect of insulin therapy is hypoglycemia. For patients who are unconscious, the treatment is an intravenous injection of glucose; for those with less severe symptoms, sugar is administered as a sweet drink. If the patient is unconscious and intravenous access cannot be obtained, 1 mg of glucagon administered intramuscularly may be repeated after a few minutes if needed (e.g., to an ambulance staff member or a close relative).

ii. The Somogyi effect, or insulin-induced post-hypoglycemic hyperglycemia, happens when hypoglycemia (e.g., causes an excess of hormones (adrenaline, growth hormone, glucocorticosteroids, and glucagon) in the early morning hours, which raises blood sugar (higher blood sugar upon awakening). It is possible to misinterpret the situation and think that more insulin is needed, which would lead to more hypoglycemia.

iii. Local or systemic allergic reactions to insulin, with itching, redness and swelling at the injection site.

iv. The loss of subcutaneous fat at or close to injection sites is known as lipodystrophy. Rotating injection locations reduces atrophy. If the same location is injected repeatedly, fatty tumors may develop.

v. Insulin resistance is unusual because it is caused by antibodies and is arbitrarily defined as a daily requirement of more than 200 units. Switching to a highly pure insulin preparation and starting with a low dose helps prevent hypoglycemia.

6. Pharmacokinetics

Insulin is administered by injection and is metabolized by the kidney, liver, and stomach. Three to five minutes is the $_{t1/2}$. Insulin glutathione transhydrogenase, a liver and renal enzyme, is primarily responsible for its metabolism into inactive α and β peptide chains. Presystemic metabolism is the process by which up to 60% of the insulin produced by the pancreas is broken down in the liver before it is released into the bloodstream. Insulin is primarily released into the portal circulation. Additionally crucial to insulin metabolism is the kidney, and individuals with progressive renal impairment frequently require less insulin overall. There is no proof that increased hepatic insulin destruction causes diabetes, but cirrhosis increases the risk of hypoglycemia because the liver is unable to inactivate insulin.

8.1.4.2. Oral Hypoglycemic Drugs and Type 2 Diabetes

Oral hypoglycemic drugs are useful in type 2 diabetes as adjuncts to continued dietary restraint. They fall into four groups:

1. Biguanides (Metformin);
2. Sulphonylureas and related drugs;
3. Thiazolidinediones (Glitazones); and
4. α-glucosidase inhibitors (acarbose).

Many patients with type 2 diabetes can achieve proper control through diet and medication. In cases where drugs are not effective (primary failure), insulin may be necessary. Secondary failure, occurring in about one-third of patients after initially effective treatment, also requires insulin. Inhaled insulin is a costly but effective option, though its efficacy can be impacted by smoking and respiratory infections. Patients with asthma or COPD should use inhaled insulin with caution.

1. Biguanides: Metformin

- **Uses**

In the UK, biguanide is only available as metformin. It is used in patients with type 2 diabetes whose diet control is insufficient. If there are no contraindications, it is the first choice medication for obese type 2 patients because of its anorectic effect, which helps with weight loss.

It must not be used in patients at risk of lactic acidosis and is contraindicated in:

- renal failure (it is eliminated in the urine, see below);
- alcoholics;
- cirrhosis;
- chronic lung disease (because of hypoxia);
- cardiac failure (because of poor tissue perfusion);
- congenital mitochondrial myopathy (which is often accompanied by diabetes);
- acute myocardial infarction and other serious intercurrent illness (insulin should be substituted).

Before a major elective surgery, metformin should be stopped and insulin should be used instead. Testing for liver function and plasma creatinine should be done both before and after using it.

- **Mechanism of action**

This remains uncertain. Biguanides do not produce hypoglycemia and are effective in pancreatectomized animals. Effects of metformin include:

- reduced glucose absorption from the gut;
- facilitation of glucose entry into muscle by a non-insulin-responsive mechanism;
- inhibition of gluconeogenesis in the liver;
- suppression of oxidative glucose metabolism and enhanced anaerobic glycolysis.

- **Adverse effects**

Anorexia, vomiting, diarrhea, nausea, and a metallic taste are all side effects of metformin. When treatment first starts, the symptoms are at their worst, and some patients are unable to take even tiny dosages. With a reported mortality rate exceeding 60%, lactic acidosis is rare as long as the aforementioned contraindications are adhered to. Treatment options include peritoneal or hemodialysate to reduce sodium overload and circulatory collapse, as well as drug withdrawal. Metformin was not as frequently linked to this issue as phenformin, which was withdrawn in the USA and the UK. Metformin decreases vitamin B_{12} absorption, however this is rarely clinically significant.

- **Pharmacokinetics**

Metformin is absorbed 50–60% through the mouth; it is excreted unchanged by the kidneys, where its active secretion into the tubular fluid causes a higher clearance rate than the glomerular filtration rate. Metformin builds up in individuals with impaired renal function. Although the plasma $t_{1/2}$ spans from 1:45 to 4:45 hours, its half-life is significantly longer, allowing for twice-daily administration.

- **Drug interactions**

Metformin and other oral hypoglycemic medications interact. Ethanol increases the risk of lactic acidosis caused by metformin.

2. Sulphonylureas and Related Drugs

- **Use**

Sulphonylureas, such as tolbutamide, glibenclamide, and gliclazide, are prescribed to type 2 diabetics whose diets alone or diet plus metformin have not produced the desired results. They alleviate polyuric and polydipsic symptoms, but they also increase appetite—as opposed to metformin. The longest-acting medication in this class, chlorpropamide, should be avoided because it has a higher frequency of side effects than other medications (particularly hypoglycemia). It is rarely used because of its prolonged effect and decreased renal clearance in elderly and renal dysfunction patients. Gliclazide and tolbutamide are preferred in the elderly because they have a lower risk of hypoglycemia due to their shorter half-lives compared to glibenclamide. Although they act at the same receptor, related medications (such as nateglinide and repaglinide) differ chemically. Even though they are more costly, they have a shorter half-life than tolbutamide. They're taken before meals.

- **Mechanism of action**

The hypoglycemic impact of these medications is contingent upon the existence of functional B cells. Similar to glucose, sulphonylureas cause B cells to depolarize and release insulin. They achieve this by attaching themselves to sulphonyl urea receptors (SUR) and obstructing ATP-dependent potassium channels (KATP); the depolarization that follows opens voltage-sensitive Ca^{2+} channels, which allows Ca^{2+} ions to enter and insulin to be secreted.

- **Adverse effects**

Hypoglycemia can occur from sulphonylureas. The longest-acting medication, chlorpropamide, was the cause of numerous cases. When ethanol is consumed by susceptible individuals, it can also result in dilutional hyponatremia and flushing. Sulphonyl urea-induced allergic reactions can manifest as rashes, drug fever, gastrointestinal disturbances, temporary jaundice (typically cholestatic), and alterations in hematopoietic function, such as pancytopenia, thrombocytopenia, and neutropenia. It is rare to have serious consequences other than hypoglycemia.

- **Pharmacokinetics**

The main distinctions between sulphonylureas, which are readily absorbed from the gastrointestinal tract, are their respective potencies and rates of clearance. The liver almost entirely breaks down glibenclamide into weakly active metabolites, which are then eliminated in the urine and bile. These metabolites' activity is only clinically significant in patients with renal failure, where it can build up and result in hypoglycemia. The liver transforms tolbutamide into inactive metabolites, which are then eliminated through the urine. Although there is significant inter-individual variability, the $t_{1/2}$ is typically four to eight hours. Although gliclazide is extensively metabolized, up to 20% of it is eliminated unaltered in the urine. There is a 6–14 hour range for the plasma $t_{1/2}$. Both repaglinide and nateglinide have quick onset and offset kinetics, quick absorption (maximum plasma concentration reached in about 55 minutes following oral administration), and quick elimination (approximately three-hour half-life). These characteristics result in a brief onset of action and a minimal risk of hypoglycemia. In patients with type 2 diabetes, they are given just before a meal to lessen the rise in blood sugar that occurs after a meal.

- **Drug interactions**

Through an unidentified mechanism, monoamine oxidase inhibitors increase the potency of sulphonylureas. Many medications, such as growth hormone and glucocorticosteroids, counteract the hypoglycemic effects of sulphonylureas by affecting insulin sensitivity or release. (Falkenstein et al, 2000; Schacke et al, 2002; Nelson, 2002; Nelson et al, 2002)

3. Thiazolidinediones (Glitazones)

The development of glitazones (such as pioglitazone and rosiglitazone) resulted from the accidental discovery that a fibrate medication raised insulin sensitivity.

- **Use**

Glitazones are used to treat type 2 diabetes mellitus in patients whose blood glucose and hemoglobin A1c (HbA1c) cannot be adequately controlled with diet alone or in combination with other oral hypoglycemic medications. Although their impact on mortality or diabetic complications is still unknown, their use has expanded quickly.

- **Mechanism of action**

Glitazones bind to the nuclear receptor known as peroxisome-proliferating activator receptor γ (PPARγ), which is primarily present in adipocytes but is also present in hepatocytes and myocytes. It acts gradually, perhaps through effects of circulating fatty acids on glucose metabolism, to increase sensitivity to insulin.

- **Adverse effects**

Due to their severe hepatotoxicity, the first two glitazones are no longer in use. Although rosiglitazone and pioglitazone are contraindicated in patients with hepatic impairment and liver function should be monitored during their use, hepatotoxicity has not been demonstrated to be an issue with these medications. The most frequent side effects are fluid retention brought on by PPARγ receptors' impact on renal tubular sodium ion absorption and weight gain, which may be directly related to their effect on adipocytes. They should not be used in heart failure because they can worsen cardiac dysfunction. Osteoporosis and an increase in bone fractures have been linked recently. They should not be used while pregnant. Although there has been some debate over the data, rosiglitazone may increase the risk of myocardial infarction.

- **Pharmacokinetics**

Pharmacokinetics: Pioglitazone and rosiglitazone are both highly protein bound, well absorbed drugs that are metabolized by the liver.

- **Drug interactions**

Glitazones can be taken in addition to other oral hypoglycemic medications. They potentiate insulin, but while this combination is commonly used in the USA, it is contraindicated in Europe due to concerns that it may raise the risk of heart failure. Due to pioglitazone-caused CYP3A induction, concurrent administration of drugs that are CYP3A substrates (such as reproductive steroids) may result in treatment failure.

4. Acarbose

When a patient's type 2 diabetes is not well controlled with diet alone or with diet plus other oral hypoglycemic medications, patients may be prescribed acarbose. Acarbose inhibits intestinal α-glucoside hydrolases in a reversible competitive manner, delaying the absorption of starch and sucrose while leaving intact the absorption of glucose that has been consumed. Following a meal containing complex carbohydrates, the postprandial glycemic rise is lowered and its peak is postponed. Increased gas production from the fermentation of unabsorbed carbohydrates in the gut causes flatulence, distension of the abdomen, and sporadically diarrhea. Blood glucose needs to be closely watched in diabetic patients as with any changes to their medication, food, or activities. (Falkenstein et al, 2000; Schacke et al, 2002; Nelson, 2002; Nelson et al, 2002)

8.2. Thyroid

In vertebrates, the thyroid, or thyroid gland, is an endocrine gland. It is located in the neck of humans and is made up of two connected lobes. The isthmus, a narrow band of tissue, connects the lower two thirds of the lobes. The thyroid is a butterfly-shaped gland that sits beneath the Adam's apple in the neck. The spherical thyroid follicle, which is surrounded by a lumen-containing colloid and lined with follicular cells (thyrocytes) occasionally, is the functional unit of the thyroid gland under the microscope. The two thyroid hormones, thyroxine (T_4) and triiodothyronine (T_3), as well as the peptide hormone calcitonin, are secreted by the thyroid gland. Thyroid hormones affect children's growth and development, protein synthesis, and metabolic rate. A component of calcium homeostasis is calcitonin. The anterior pituitary gland secretes thyroid-stimulating hormone (TSH), which controls the secretion of the two thyroid hormones. Thyrotropin-releasing hormone (TRH), which is generated by the hypothalamus, controls TSH.

The thyroid gland's under- or overactivity can be effectively treated with medication. As the serum TSH level accurately reflects thyroid state, sensitive and accurate TSH assays have greatly aided in the diagnosis of abnormal thyroid function and therapy monitoring. In contrast, the interpretation of serum concentrations of T_3 and T_4 is complicated by extensive and somewhat variable protein binding. Serum TSH is raised when the thyroid gland is primary failing, and it is lowered when the gland is overactive thanks to the negative feedback of biologically active thyroid hormones. Relatively rare hypothyroidism brought on by hypopituitarism is linked to decreased sex hormone and cortical function in the adrenal glands. It is exceedingly uncommon for hyperthyroidism to result from elevated TSH.

8.2.1. Pathophysiology and Principles of Treatment

Thyroid disease can present as goiter or as either an overactive or underactive gland. It is more common in women than in men. In particular, hypothyroidism is prevalent in the elderly. If left untreated, it typically results in the clinical manifestation of myxoedema and is brought on by autoimmune destruction of the gland. The course of treatment involves thyroxine replacement for life.

Hyperthyroidism is also common and again autoimmune processes are implicated. Treatment options comprise:

- Antithyroid drugs;
- Radioactive iodine;
- Surgery.

Antithyroid medications help keep the thyroid levels balanced until the disease resolves or further treatment with radioactive iodine or surgery is pursued. Radioactive iodine treatment is safe and does not have the risks associated with surgery, such as damage to the laryngeal nerve. Surgery is typically recommended for cases where there are mechanical issues like tracheal compression.

Multinodular toxic goiter is the most common cause of hyperthyroidism in elderly patients. Graves' disease, in which an immunoglobulin binds to and stimulates the TSH receptor, is typically the cause in young women. It promotes the synthesis and release of T_3 and T_4, which are then independent of TSH. Mucopolysaccharide is frequently deposited in addition to a smooth vascular goiter; this is especially noticeable in the extrinsic eye muscles, which thicken and result in proptosis. Graves' illness progresses in a remitting/relapsing manner and frequently results in hypothyroidism in the end. Acute postpartum hyperthyroidism, iatrogenic iodine excess, and acute viral or autoimmune thyroiditis are other causes of hyperthyroidism that typically go away on their own.

8.2.2. Iodine

Iodine is concentrated in the thyroid gland. The average daily intake of dietary iodide is between 100 and 200 mg, which is absorbed actively from the stomach and small intestine. Iodide is oxidized to iodine in the thyroid gland after systemic absorption and uptake. Iodine is the precursor to several iodinated tyrosine compounds, such as T3 and T_4. Iodine deficiency is treated with iodine to treat simple non-toxic goiter. Potassium iodide (3 mg daily p.o.) stops the gland from growing further, but it rarely truly shrinks. In regions where the diet is iodine deficient, iodized salt is used to prevent this kind of endemic goiter, per a World Health Organization (WHO) policy.

To lessen the gland's vascularity and stop the release of thyroid hormones, preoperative treatment with Lugol's iodine solution—an aqueous solution of iodine and potassium iodide—in conjunction with carbimazole or propylthiouracil is employed. If the cause of the hyperthyroidism is not addressed, the effect of iodine in suppressing thyroid hormone release is only maintained for a duration of one to two weeks, following which there is a noticeable increase in thyroid hormone release.

8.2.3. Thyroxine and Tri-Iodothyronine

- **Use**

Simple hypothyroidism is treated with L-thyroxine, with a dose customized based on serum TSH levels. Every four weeks, the dose is increased or decreased until the patient has shown a clinical response and the TSH level has returned to a normal range. Overdosing can cause heart problems, especially in those with ischemic heart disease, for whom a lower initial dosage is recommended. In the event that angina pectoris restricts the thyroxine dosage, adding a beta-blocker (e.g. atenolol) will permit additional increases in the dosage of thyroxine. Chronic overdosage is undesirable because it increases the risk of osteoporosis and cardiac dysrhythmias.

Similar measures are taken for congenital hypothyroidism, and thyroxine needs to be administered as soon as possible. The Guthrie test's introduction in the UK has substantially aided in the early identification of newborn hypothyroidism.

T3's quick action is helpful in the treatment of myxoedema coma. It is administered intramuscularly as a precursor to thyroxine maintenance therapy. In certain cases, hypothyroidism coexists with Addison's disease, which has an autoimmune etiology. Patients suffering from myxoedema coma are empirically treated with hydrocortisone.

Hypopituitarism may lead to hypothyroidism. Oral thyroxine is also used to treat this, at the regular dosages. If glucose corticosteroid replacement is not initiated initially, acute adrenal insufficiency may develop.

- **Mechanism of action**

Thyroxine is a prohormone. After entering cells it is converted to T_3, which binds to the thyroid hormone nuclear receptor and the ligand–receptor complex increases the transcription of genes involved in the following cellular functions:

- stimulation of metabolism – raised basal metabolic rate;
- promotion of normal growth and maturation, particularly of the central nervous system and skeleton;
- sensitization to the effects of catecholamines.

- **Adverse effects**

Angina, myocardial infarction, congestive heart failure, and cardiac dysrhythmia are among the physiologically related side effects of thyroid hormones. These hormones have toxic effects that vary in dose and can cause tremor, restlessness, heat intolerance, diarrhea, and other symptoms of hyperthyroidism. An indirect cause of osteoporosis is a long-term excess of thyroxine.

- **Pharmacokinetics**

The stomach is where thyroid hormones are absorbed. When taking T_4 on a regular basis, the effects usually take up to 24 hours to become apparent, and it takes several days to reach maximum activity. T_3 starts to take effect in six hours and reaches its peak activity in twenty-four. In euthyroid individuals, the half-life ($_{t1/2}$) of T_4 is six to seven days, but in hypothyroidism, it can be much longer. The half-life ($t_{1/2}$) of T_3 is two days or less. Giving thyroid hormones more often than once a day is not necessary. Thyroid hormones are conjugated in the liver and then recirculated enterohepatically.

8.2.4. Antithyroid Drugs

8.2.4.1. Carbimazole

- **Use**

Carbimazole is a medication used to treat hyperthyroidism. Typically, patients achieve a normal thyroid function within four to six weeks of treatment, after which the dosage is decreased. Treatment usually lasts one to two years, and then the medication is slowly discontinued. In case of a relapse, the dosage is increased until symptoms improve. If regulating the dosage is challenging, a combination of thyroxine replacement and carbimazole blocking doses may help achieve better control.

- **Mechanism of action**

Through its active metabolite methimazole, which is a substrate-inhibitor of peroxidase and is iodinated and degraded within the thyroid, carbimazole acts by preventing thyroglobulin from being synthesized from oxidized iodine and by reducing the production of thyroid hormones. Thyroid follicular cells, neutrophils, macrophage/monocytes, and salivary glands are among the peroxidase-containing cells that concentrate methimazole. It suppresses the immune system in the thyroid. and prevents macrophages from producing oxygen radicals, which disrupts lymphocytes' ability to present antigens. Methimazole has no direct effect on hormone secretion. As a result, following a latent period during which the thyroid depletes its hormone reserves, hormone release declines.

- **Adverse effects**

While it is fairly common to experience rashes and pruritus, carbimazole is generally well tolerated. Most of the time, these react when propylthiouracil is used instead. One uncommon but potentially deadly side effect is neutropenia. Patients should be advised to report any sore throat or other infection-related symptoms right away, to get a white blood cell count as soon as possible, and to stop taking the medication immediately if they exhibit neutropenia. Rare but known side effects include arthralgia, leukopenia, drug fever, nausea, and hair loss. Pregnancy-related carbimazole use has sporadically been linked to neonatal aplia cutis.

- **Pharmacokinetics**

After oral administration, carbimazole is quickly absorbed and hydrolyzes to methimazole, which is concentrated in the thyroid within minutes. The apparent volume of distribution of methimazole is comparable to that of body water, and the $t_{1/2}$ varies with thyroid status, being roughly seven, nine, and fourteen hours in patients with hyperthyroidism, euthyroidism, and hypothyroidism, respectively. The thyroid and liver are where it is metabolized.

8.2.4.2. Propylthiouracil

- **Use**

Apart from its similar actions, uses, and toxic effects to carbimazole, propylthiouracil also prevents T_4 from being converted to active T3 in the peripheral tissues. Similar to carbimazole, dangerous leukopenia is extremely uncommon but can occur. Similar to carbimazole, the strategy involves starting with a high dose and gradually lowering it to achieve a euthyroid state. The intestine quickly absorbs propylthiouracil. Propylthiouracil can be taken once daily, just like carbimazole, but its duration of action within the thyroid is prolonged, despite its short plasma $t_{1/2}$. It is used (by experts) during pregnancy (see below) and is superior to carbimazole in certain situations.

8.2.4.3. -Adrenoceptor Antagonists

Beta-blockers improve symptoms of hyperthyroidism, including anxiety, tachycardia and tremor. They inhibit the conversion of T_4 to T_3 in the tissues. They are useful:

- while awaiting laboratory confirmation, if the diagnosis is in doubt;
- during initiation of therapy with antithyroid drugs;
- before treatment with radio-iodine, because they do not interfere with the uptake of iodine by the gland;

- in thyroid crisis;
- with iodine, as a rapid preparation for surgery on a hyperactive thyroid goiter;
- in neonatal hyperthyroidism due to thyroid-stimulating immunoglobulin from the mother – this remit within about six weeks as maternal-derived immunoglobulin is cleared by the infant

Even though they seem clinically euthyroid, beta-blocker-treated hyperthyroid patients are not biochemically euthyroid, and if treatment is stopped, thyroid crisis, or "storm," may develop.

8.2.4.4. Radioactive Iodine

When treating thyrotoxicosis brought on by toxic nodular goiter or Graves' disease, radioactive iodine is a useful oral medication. It is safe, doesn't hurt the patient, and has mostly taken the place of surgery, except situations in which there are local mechanical issues, like tracheal compression. It should not be used while pregnant. There has been debate regarding dosage. To prevent late-onset undiagnosed hypothyroidism, many units now routinely administer an ablative dose followed by replacement therapy with thyroxine. With a half-life of eight days, ^{131}I is the isotope that is typically used. After four to six weeks, replacement therapy with thyroxine is initiated and maintained for life. When ^{131}I is used therapeutically, there is no increased risk of leukemia, thyroid, or any other cancer; however, the use of ^{131}I in young women or children raises concerns. There is no proof that therapeutic doses of radioactive iodine harm germ cells or lower fertility, though the radiation dose to the gonads is lower than that of many radiological procedures. Because it harms the fetus and results in congenital hypothyroidism and mental retardation, it is not recommended during pregnancy. After a negative pregnancy test and for the first 10 days of the menstrual cycle, patients are typically treated as outpatients. After treatment, a woman should refrain from getting pregnant for at least four months and stop nursing her baby for at least two months. Patients with well-differentiated thyroid carcinoma are treated with high-dose ^{131}I to ablate any remaining tumor following surgery. To encourage the gland to absorb the isotope, TSH levels must rise, which can only be achieved by stopping thyroid medication at least one month before treatment. To safeguard possible contacts, patients are initially kept apart in the hospital for a few days following dosage.

8.2.5. Special Situations

8.2.5.1. Graves' Ophthalmopathy

Regardless of the thyroid's condition, eye symptoms typically appear within 18 months of the start of Graves' disease and usually go away over the course of a year or two. There is a strong clinical impression that iatrogenic hypothyroidism can exacerbate eye disease, so overly aggressive treatment of hyperthyroidism in patients with eye signs should be avoided. Elevating the head of the bed while you sleep can help minimize peri-orbital oedema. Basic hydrating eye drops (e.g., hypromellose) could be advantageous. In severe cases, tarsoroplasty is recommended to prevent corneal abrasion. When Graves' ophthalmopathy is moderate and does not pose a threat to vision, radiation therapy may be utilized. Exophthalmos that is severe and upsetting calls for a prednisolone trial. If medical treatment fails and optic nerve compression results in deteriorating visual acuity, immediate surgical decompression of the orbit is necessary.

8.2.5.2. Thyroid Crisis

A severe, sudden flare-up of hyperthyroidism accompanied by hyperpyrexia, tachycardia, vomiting, dehydration, and shock is known as a thyroid crisis. It may develop after surgery, after receiving radioiodine therapy, or in conjunction with an ongoing infection. Rarely, it appears on its own in a patient who has never had a diagnosis or treatment. Death rates are high.

Urgent treatment comprises:

- β-adrenoceptor antagonists;
- intravenous saline;
- cooling;
- propylthiouracil;
- Lugol's iodine;
- glucocorticoids;
- fast atrial fibrillation can be especially difficult to treat: DC cardioversion may be needed.

Salicylate displaces bound T_4 and T_3, and it also uncouples oxidative phosphorylation, exacerbating the metabolic state. For these reasons, aspirin should be avoided.

8.2.5.3. Pregnancy and Breast-Feeding

Pregnancy is a complete contraindication for radioactive iodine, and surgery should be avoided whenever feasible. Because T_4 and T_3 do not sufficiently cross the placenta, hypothyroid fetuses have congenital hypothyroidism, which is characterized by maldevelopment of the central nervous system and mental retardation. Carbimazole and propylthiouracil are antithyroid medications that cross the placenta and end up in breast milk. Pregnancy-related hyperthyroidism management calls for specialized knowledge. Antithyroid medication overuse needs to be avoided. Antithyroid medication blocking doses containing additional T_4 should never be used during pregnancy because the antithyroid medication crosses the placenta but the T_4 does not, which will inevitably result in a severely hypothyroid baby. Since propylthiouracil is more highly protein bound and ionized at pH 7:4, it may be somewhat less likely than carbimazole to have an effect on the infant. This lessens the amount that passes through the placenta and into milk. When pregnant or nursing, propylthiouracil should be used at the lowest possible effective doses.

8.2.5.4. Drug-Induced Thyroid Dysfunction

Thyroid hypofunction is known to be caused by other medications. Iodinated radiocontrast agents may result in a brief case of hyperthyroidism. Interleukins, amiodarone, and interferons can all result in hypo- or hyperthyroidism. Goiter and hypothyroidism are possible side effects of lithium and some of the new kinase inhibitors. The extent of thyroid dysfunction should be determined and the patient's need to continue taking the implicated medication should be assessed. The usual course of treatment, if medication therapy needs to be continued, is antithyroid or replacement thyroxine therapy combined with close monitoring of the thyroid axis. (Falkenstein et al, 2000; Schacke et al, 2002; Nelson, 2002; Nelson et al, 2002)

8.3. Calcium Metabolism

Calcium-sensitive receptors (CaSRs) in renal tubular cells and parathyroid hormone (PTH) sense plasma calcium, which is then kept within a limited physiological range by calcitonin, vitamin D, and PTH. The primary regulator of PTH secretion is the calcium concentration in plasma; a decrease in calcium concentration causes PTH release. PTH decreases the concentration of phosphate and increases plasma calcium. It affects the bones and kidneys. PTH induces phosphaturia and raises calcium reabsorption in the renal tubules, which together with the release of calcium from the bone raises the calcium concentration in plasma. PTH has three effects on bone: it stimulates osteoclast activity, forms new osteoclasts from progenitor cells, and temporarily reduces osteoblast activity. PTH is involved in the control of vitamin D metabolism as well. By promoting the synthesis of the active metabolite 1,25-dihydroxycholecalciferol, it increases the absorption of calcium in the gut indirectly.

Numerous significant metabolic disorders, including hyperparathyroidism, osteomalacia and rickets, Paget's disease, and osteoporosis, have an impact on the bones. Certain illnesses (e.g., osteomalacia) are linked to either normal or low levels of calcium in the plasma, some (e.g., hypercalcemia) and hyperparathyroidism) are linked, and some (e.g.osteoporosis) are linked to normal levels of calcium in plasma. The most prevalent of these conditions is post-menopausal osteoporosis, with iatrogenic glucocorticoids and excess thyroid hormone being major contributing factors. Those who are at risk should consume enough calcium and vitamin D through food (see below), and if at all feasible, have their contributing factors fixed. Due to an excess of thrombotic events, hormone replacement therapy (HRT) with estrogen is no longer the first line of defense against osteoporosis in women over 50, though it is at least momentarily effective if begun soon after menopause. An alternate is raloxifene. Postmenopausal osteoporosis can be effectively treated with bisphosphonates and teriparatide.

8.3.1. Vitamin D

The word "vitamin D" refers to a group of closely related substances that can both prevent and treat rickets. These consist of calcitriol (1,25-DHCC), α-calcidol (1-α-hydroxycholecalciferol), cholecalciferol (vitamin $D_{3)}$, and ergocalciferol (vitamin D_2). A summary of the vitamin D metabolic pathway can be found in Figure 8.1. In reaction to UV light, the skin produces vitamin D_3, which is then absorbed in the upper small intestine. Bile is required for its absorption because it is fat-soluble. Renal 1-α-hydroxylase is influenced by PTH and phosphate, which in turn affects the quantity of active 1,25-DHCC generated. In actuality, 1,25-DHCC is a hormone that the kidney produces. It increases calcium absorption in the intestines, releases calcium from bone, and (a minor side effect) increases calcium reabsorption in the kidney. A single large dose of vitamin D may be effective for several weeks because the body stores it.

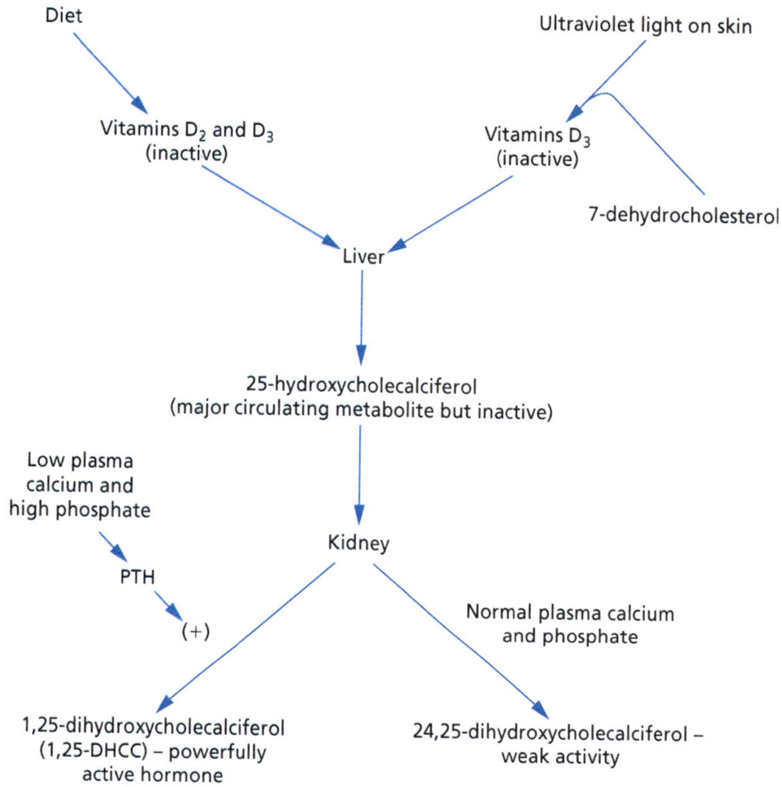

Figure 8.1. *Metabolic pathway of vitamin D. PTH, parathormone.*

Source: https://www.pharmaresearchlibrary.com/wp-content/uploads/2013/03/A-Textbook-of-Clinical-Pharmacology-and-Therapeutics-5th-edition.pdf.

- **Uses:** Poor diet and poverty are associated with dietary deficiency of vitamin D, which is further exacerbated by lack of sunlight. Elderly individuals living alone and Asian communities residing in the UK's northern regions are particularly vulnerable, as chapatis and other unleavened breads can hinder the absorption of vitamin D. Women who are expecting or nursing have greater needs. There are numerous vitamin D preparations with varying potencies and applications available.

1. Vitamin D is supplied in a physiological dose by calcium and ergocalciferol tablets, which are used to prevent osteomalacia and rickets. The small amount of calcium is not required, but there isn't a vitamin D preparation on hand.
2. Calciferol tablets are used to treat vitamin D-resistant rickets caused by intestinal malabsorption or chronic liver disease. They also provide a pharmacological dose of vitamin D.
3. α-Calcidol rapidly undergoes hydroxylation to 1,25- DHCC. It is used in:

- renal rickets, together with a phosphate-binding agent;
- hypoparathyroidism and (paradoxically) secondary hyperparathyroidism;

- vitamin D-resistant rickets;
- nutritional and malabsorptive rickets can be treated with small doses of α-calcidol instead of conventional vitamin D.

4. In addition, calcitriol (1,25-DHCC) is the recommended treatment for pseudohypoparathyroidism, an uncommon metabolic disorder in which low plasma calcium results from resistance to the biochemical action of PTH. It is also available for the treatment of vitamin D-resistant rickets.

- **Adverse Effects:** The primary issue is hypercalcemia, which can hasten renal dysfunction. It is crucial to take regular measurements of creatinine and plasma calcium (first every week).

8.3.2. Calcium

In addition to calciferol, calcium salts (lactate or gluconate) are used to treat hypocalcemic tetany, osteomalacia, and rickets. When it comes to potentially fatal cardiac dysrhythmias brought on by hyperkalemia, calcium chloride is a unique treatment. If a patient's daily intake of elemental calcium falls below 1 g, calcium and vitamin D supplements are used. Chewable or fizzy formulations are readily accessible and simple to consume.

8.3.3. Bisphosphonates

In terms of structure, bisphosphonates are similar to pyrophosphate, with the exception that carbon, not oxygen, connects the two phosphorus atoms. Such compounds are extremely stable due to their P-C-P backbone structure; no known enzyme can break them down.

- **Uses**

For the prevention and treatment of osteoporosis, alendronic acid or risedronate (taken orally) are the preferred bisphosphonates; etidronate is an alternate if these bisphosphonates are not tolerated. Bisphosphonates are also used to treat hypercalcemia caused by malignancy, Paget's disease of the bone, and skeletal complications from multiple myeloma and breast cancer that has metastasized to the bone. For postmenopausal and glucocorticoid-associated osteoporosis, they work well. Risedronate is prescribed for two months in patients with Paget's disease, and this can be repeated after a minimum of two months without treatment. Many patients achieve remission when taking etidronate at a low dosage for up to six months; in the event of a relapse, another course of treatment may be administered. Extended use beyond six months at a time does not maintain remission. Only when lower doses are ineffective or when quick disease control is required should high doses be used. During Paget's disease treatment, serum alkaline phosphatase, phosphate, and, if possible, urinary hydroxyproline are measured.

- **Mechanism of action**

By chemically adhering to the crystal surface of calcium hydroxyapatite, bisphosphonates alter its crystal growth, thereby impeding osteoclast turnover and remodeling of bone.

- **Adverse effects**

All bisphosphonates should be used with caution or in cases of renal impairment. Severe esophagitis and ulcers are possible. This can be reduced by taking risedronate or alendronic acid when standing or sitting, emptying the stomach 30 minutes before eating and taking these actions before breakfast. The whole range of gastrointestinal symptoms are among the other side effects. Patients with Paget's disease are more likely to fracture when taking etidronate.

- **Pharmacokinetics**

Only 10% of bisphosphonates are absorbed completely; absorption is further decreased by food and antacids. They spread to bone, where their effects persist for a long time, and quickly vanish from the blood. About half of the absorbed dose is eliminated unchanged in the urine in less than 24 hours, while the remaining portion is eliminated over several weeks.

8.3.4. Calcitonin

Thyroid parafollicular C-cells secrete this hormone, which is a polypeptide with 32 amino acids. The concentration of Ca_2 in the plasma primarily controls secretion.

- **Uses**

In addition to treating pain and some neurological side effects (such as deafness from severe Paget's disease due to VIII nerve compression), synthetic or recombinant salmon calcitonin (salcatonin) is also used to treat post-menopausal osteoporosis (in conjunction with calcium and vitamin D supplements, if the diet is inadequate). Calcitonin is administered as a nasal spray, by subcutaneous or intramuscular injection. Monitoring is done for plasma calcium, phosphate, alkaline phosphatase, and, if feasible, urine hydroxyproline excretion.

- **Mechanism of action**

The primary function of calcitonin is to inhibit bone resorption by attaching to a particular receptor on osteoclasts and preventing them from doing their job. It lessens the proximal tubules' ability to reabsorb phosphate and calcium in the kidney.

- **Adverse effects**

Adverse effects include the following: 1. pain at the injection site; 2. nausea and diarrhea; 3. flushing.

8.3.5. Strontium Ranelate

Strontium is a bone-seeking element that was used extensively in the 1950s to treat osteoporosis, but there were worries that it might lead to abnormal bone mineralization and inhibit the synthesis of calcitriol. These unfavorable outcomes might have been caused by an inadequate calcium diet and improper dosage. According to recent research, strontium ranelate helps women with post-menopausal osteoporosis by decreasing bone reabsorption, increasing bone formation, and lowering the risk of hip and vertebral fractures. When bisphosphonates are not tolerated or are contraindicated, it is taken orally at night by older women who have osteoporosis and a history of bone fractures. It has negative effects on the gastrointestinal tract.

8.3.6. Teriparatide

One PTH agonist is teriparatide. Experts in metabolic bone disease use this recombinant PTH fragment to treat postmenopausal osteoporosis. Use with caution if renal impairment or cardiac disease exists. It is contraindicated in patients with hyperparathyroidism, Paget's disease, or a history of radiation therapy to the skeleton. For up to 18 months, it is administered subcutaneously once a day, with serum calcium, phosphate, alkaline phosphatase, creatinine, and electrolytes being monitored.

8.3.7. Cinacalcet

A calcimimetic medication called cinacalcet improves signaling via the calcium sensing receptor (CaSR). It decreases PTH secretion and activates CaSR allostery. A slight drop in plasma calcium and phosphate is also present. It also lessens parathyroid hyperplasia and decreases PTH synthesis due to decreased PTH gene expression. It is taken orally in conjunction with serum calcium and PTH monitoring for the treatment of hypercalcemia brought on by parathyroid carcinoma and secondary hyperparathyroidism in dialysis patients with end-stage renal disease.

8.4. Adrenal Hormones

At the top of each kidney are the adrenal glands. They generate hormones that control metabolism, blood pressure, the immune system, and the stress response.

8.4.1. Glucocorticosteroids

Glucocorticosteroids are essential for the body's reaction to stress and have an impact on the metabolism of proteins and carbohydrates. Glucocorticosteroids facilitate amino acid transport to the liver, where it is converted to glucose (gluconeogenesis) and stored as glycogen by stimulating the mobilization of amino acids from skeletal muscle, bone, and skin. Glucocorticosteroids enhance catecholamines' ability to mobilize fat. The primary medical applications of glucocorticosteroids take advantage of their potent anti-inflammatory and immunosuppressive characteristics. They increase neutrophils in the blood while decreasing circulating eosinophils, basophils, and T lymphocytes. Strong steroids applied topically to the skin or mucous membranes can cause localized vasoconstriction, and large doses of steroids given systemically can cause generalized vasoconstriction, which can lead to hypertension.

8.4.1.1. Mechanism of Action

A phosphorylated heat shock protein complex is broken up by the cytoplasmic glucocorticosteroid receptor when it combines with glucocorticoids. After translocating to the nucleus, the receptor–glucocorticosteroid complex binds to DNA's glucocorticosteroid response elements (GREs) and functions as a transcription factor. As a result, more signal transduction proteins are transcriptionally active. Furthermore, the glucocorticosteroid receptor inhibits the transcription of numerous pro-inflammatory proteins by interacting with NFκB and AP-1. As a result, glucocorticosteroids have a significant but delayed anti-inflammatory effect.

8.4.1.2. Adverse Effects

We will talk about the group's common glucocorticosteroid adverse effects before moving on to the uses of the individual medications.

Chronic administration causes iatrogenic Cushing's syndrome. Features include:

- Cushingoid physical appearance;
- impaired resistance to infection;
- salt and water retention; hypokalemia;
- hypertension;
- hyperglycemia;
- osteoporosis;
- glucocorticosteroid therapy is weakly linked with peptic ulceration, and can mask the symptoms and signs of gastrointestinal perforation;
- mental changes: anxiety, elation, insomnia, depression and psychosis;
- posterior cataracts;
- proximal myopathy;
- growth retardation in children;
- aseptic necrosis of bone

After prolonged glucocorticosteroid administration, a rapid withdrawal may cause acute adrenal insufficiency. Withdrawing gradually is less dangerous. But even in patients who have been weaned off of long-term glucocorticosteroid treatment, stressful events (like trauma, surgery, or infection) can cause an acute adrenal crisis that requires high doses of sodium chloride, glucocorticosteroids, glucose, and water for a year or two after the event. If the daily dose of glucocorticosteroids is less than the amount normally secreted physiologically, then suppression of the adrenal cortex is unusual. Patients' ability to wean off of glucocorticosteroids at a given rate is contingent upon their underlying medical condition, therapy duration, and dosage. The patient should keep their steroid card on them for a minimum of a year after stopping long-term glucocorticosteroid therapy.

8.4.2. Hydrocortisone (Cortisol)

Although glucocorticoids are the main effect of hydrocortisone, it also exhibits strong mineralocorticoid activity. It has little to no effect on blood glucose regulation at physiological concentrations, but when used in pharmacological dosages, it can lead to hyperglycemia and even early onset of frank diabetes. This results from decreased insulin sensitivity paired with increased gluconeogenesis. In patients with adrenocortical insufficiency, hydrocortisone is administered as replacement therapy (typically in conjunction with fludrocortisone to replace mineralocorticoid).

For the short term, high-dose intravenous hydrocortisone is used to treat autoimmune inflammatory diseases (like acute inflammatory bowel disease) or acute severe asthma. Oral prednisolone is typically taken after the treatment. An insoluble suspension called hydrocortisone acetate can be injected into irritated bursae or joints to produce a targeted anti-inflammatory response. Because it is less potent than other steroids, hydrocortisone cream is especially useful for use on the face.

- **Pharmacokinetics**

Although hydrocortisone is quickly absorbed from the gastrointestinal tract, presystemic metabolism varies greatly amongst individuals, leading to significant variation in bioavailability. It is converted to tetrahydro metabolites in the liver (by CYP3A) and other tissues, where it is then coupled with glucuronide and eliminated in the urine. The biological $t_{1/2}$ is longer (six to eight hours) than the plasma $t_{1/2}$, which is roughly 90 minutes.

8.4.3. Prednisolone

Uses

Prednisolone, an analog of hydrocortisone, is marginally less active as a mineralocorticoid but about four times more potent than the natural hormone in terms of anti-inflammatory metabolic actions and involution of lymphoid tissue.

Its anti-inflammatory properties can lessen the inflammatory symptoms associated with connective tissue and vasculitic diseases, but it's frequently unclear if this improves the disease's underlying course. Thus, the course of treatment needs to be periodically reviewed, and if continued use is thought to be necessary, the dosage should be lowered to the lowest practical maintenance level. Less suppression of the pituitary–adrenal axis results from alternate-day dosing; however, not all diseases respond well to this kind of care (e.g. enormous cell arthritis). When alternative treatments for progressive rheumatoid arthritis have failed or as a stopgap until a disease-modifying medication, like methotrexate, has had time to take effect, prednisolone is taken into consideration. While intra-articular injections have potential benefits, there is a significant risk of joint damage if they are used frequently. For patients with severe articular symptoms from systemic lupus erythematosus, low doses of prednisolone may be helpful in the short term. For patients with steroid-responsive forms of glomerulonephritis or progressive central nervous system involvement, larger doses of prednisolone may be appropriate for a limited time.

Prednisolone may also be necessary in cases of severe asthma, certain interstitial lung diseases (fibrosing alveolitis, for example), some sarcoidosis patients, some types of acute and chronic active hepatitis, acute and chronic inflammatory bowel disease (which may require the use of suppositories or enemas), and minimal-change nephrotic syndrome. To prevent transplant rejection, prednisolone's immunosuppressive effect is further used, typically in conjunction with ciclosporin or azathioprine. Prednisolone is prescribed for benign hematological disorders such as idiopathic thrombocytopenic purpura and autoimmune hemolytic anemia. It is also a necessary part of chemotherapy regimens for lymphoma and Hodgkin's disease.

8.4.4. Dexamethasone

Dexamethasone is powerfully anti-inflammatory but is virtually devoid of mineralocorticoid activity. It is generally reserved for a few distinct indications, including:

- as a diagnostic agent in the investigation of suspected Cushing's syndrome (low- and high-dose dexamethasone suppression tests) as it does not cross-react with endogenous cortisol in conventional radioimmunoassays;
- in the symptomatic treatment of cerebral edema associated with brain tumors;
- to prevent respiratory distress syndrome in premature babies by administration to pregnant mothers;
- in combination with other anti-emetics to prevent cytotoxic chemotherapy-induced nausea and vomiting;
- when a corticosteroid is indicated, but fluid retention is problematic.

8.4.5. Mineralocorticoids

8.4.5.1. Aldosterone

The principal mineralocorticoid secreted by the adrenal cortex's zona glomerulosa is aldosterone. It is a mineralocorticoid that is approximately 1000 times more active than hydrocortisone, but it lacks glucocorticoid activity. The primary regulators of its release are angiotensin II, plasma potassium, and sodium. Pituitary failure permits the production of aldosterone despite the complete lack of cortisol secretion and ACTH.

Aldosterone promotes $Na+/K^+$ exchange in the distal nephron, which results in sodium retention and the excretion of potassium and hydrogen ions in the urine. A tumor or hyperplasia of the zona glomerulosa of the adrenal cortex are the causes of primary hyperaldosteronism, also known as Conn's syndrome. Nocturia, hypokalemia, hypomagnesemia, weakness, tetany, hypertension, and sodium retention are among the clinical manifestations. Aldosterone and other mineralocorticoids are in competition with spirolactone and eplerenone for the cytoplasmic mineralocorticosteroid receptor. They are used as diuretics that spare potassium and to treat primary or secondary hyperaldosteronism in patients with heart failure, hypertension, or both.

8.4.5.2. Fludrocortisone

Approximately 500 times more potent than hydrocortisone, fludrocortisone (9-α-fluorohydrocortisone) is a powerful synthetic mineralocorticoid. It functions similarly to aldosterone by binding to the mineralocorticoid steroid receptor. It has a substantial presystemic metabolism, but it can be taken orally, unlike aldosterone. In individuals with adrenocortical insufficiency, it serves as replacement therapy. Although it may result in the development of Conn's syndrome symptoms, it is occasionally used to treat patients with symptomatic postural hypotension.

8.4.6. Adrenal Medulla

The primary hormone that the adrenal medulla produces is adrenaline, also known as epiphany. It is utilized in critical circumstances like anaphylactic shock, cardiac arrest, and other life-threatening conditions requiring a combination of strong α- and β-agonist activity (e.g. beta-blocker overdose, shock). Through its vasoconstrictor action, it is used to extend the duration of local anesthetic effects. A prodrug form of adrenaline called dipivefrine is applied topically to treat open-angle chronic glaucoma. Surgery is used to treat phaeochromocytoma, tumors of the adrenal medulla that secrete adrenaline and other pharmacologically active catecholamines. For these patients, preoperative α- and β-blockade with phenoxybenzamine, a long-acting α-blocker, is crucial. (Falkenstein et al, 2000; Schacke et al, 2002; Nelson, 2002; Nelson et al, 2002)

8.5. Reproductive Endocrinology

The study of reproductive endocrinology focuses on the hormones and regulatory systems that govern sexual maturation, sexual function, and reproduction.

8.5.1. Female Reproductive Endocrinology

The cyclical processes of ovulation and menstruation, as well as appropriate sexual development during puberty, entail intricate interactions between endocrine and target organs. The anterior pituitary gland secretes gonadotrophins, luteinizing hormone (LH) and follicle-stimulating hormone (FSH), under the control of gonadotrophin releasing hormones (GnRH). LH and FSH encourage ovarian maturation and the release of progesterone and estrogen from the ovaries.

Cholesterol is the source of progesterone and estrogen. They produce both positive and negative feedback on the hypothalamic-pituitary-central nervous system (CNS), which inhibits and stimulates the secretion of gonadotrophin. They also stimulate the breast, uterus, and vagina.

Progesterone, androgens, oestradiol17β, and estrone are the primary hormones secreted by the ovary. Estrogens affect ovulation during the reproductive years and the development of secondary sexual characteristics, such as breast development and the distribution of fat in females.

8.5.1.1. Estrogens

- **Properties**

The properties of estrogens include the following:

- stimulation of endometrial growth;
- maintenance of blood vessels and skin;
- reduction of bone resorption and increase of bone formation;
- increase uterine growth;
- increase the hepatic production of binding proteins;
- increase circulating clotting factors II, VII, IX, X and plasminogen;
- increase high-density lipoprotein (HDL);
- increase biliary cholesterol;
- control salt and water retention

- **Uses**

Estrogens are used in:

- oral contraception;
- the treatment of symptoms of menopause;
- the prevention of osteoporosis. Fractures of the spine, wrist and hips are reduced by 50–70% and there is about a 5% increase in spinal bone

density in those women treated with estrogen within three years of the onset of menopause and for 5 to 10 years thereafter.

- the treatment of vaginal atrophy;
- the treatment of hypo-oestrogenism (as a result of hypogonadism, castration or primary ovarian failure);
- treatment of primary amenorrhea;
- treatment of dysmenorrhea;
- treatment of oligomenorrhoea;
- treatment of certain neoplastic diseases;
- treatment of hereditary hemorrhagic telangiectasia (Osler–Weber–Rendu syndrome);
- palliative treatment of prostate cancer.

For numerous indications listed above, ethylestradiol, a synthetic estrogen, serves as an alternative. The risk of thromboembolism has led to the discontinuation of the use of estrogens to suppress lactation. Instead, bromocriptine is employed.

- **Adverse effects**

Premenstrual symptoms, breast enlargement and tenderness, nausea and vomiting, abdominal cramps and bloating, and sodium and fluid retention are typical symptoms. Pharmacological doses may cause oedema, salt and water retention, hypertension, and an aggravation of heart failure. Gynecomastia and impotence in men are known to have dose-dependent effects. The risk of thromboembolism is elevated. Certain animals have been shown to develop cancer due to estrogens, and women who receive continuous treatment with exogenous estrogen without interference from progestogens have a higher risk of developing endometrial carcinoma.

- **Pharmacokinetics**

Estrogens are absorbed through the skin, mucous membranes, and mouth. Oestradiol-17β, the most powerful naturally occurring estrogen, is primarily oxidized to estrone and subsequently hydrated to produce estriol. The liver breaks down all three estrogens, which are then eliminated in the urine and bile as conjugates of glucuronide and sulphate. An indicator of ovarian function is the estimation of urinary estrogen excretion. Because of the sluggish hepatic metabolism, ethylestradiol has a prolonged half-life of roughly 25 hours.

8.5.1.2. Progestogens

A steroid hormone, progesterone affects the female menstrual cycle, pregnancy (helping with gestation), and embryogenesis. The precursor of 17-hydroxyprogesterone, which is transformed into androstenedione, which is then transformed into testosterone, estrone, and estradiol, is progesterone. The brain, the placenta, the corpus luteum, and the adrenal glands all produce progesterone.

Progesterones act on tissues that estrogens have primed, altering their effects. Progesterone and its analogs found in nature, as well as testosterone analogs like norethisterone and norgestrel, are the two main categories of progestogens. Progestogens vary in potency and adverse effects, but they all have antiestrogenic and anti-gonadotrophic qualities.

- **Uses of progesterone**

The uses of progesterone are:

- to control anovulatory bleeding;
- to prepare the uterine lining in infertility therapy and to support early pregnancy;
- for recurrent pregnancy loss due to inadequate progesterone production;
- in the treatment of intersex disorders, to promote breast development.

- **Uses of progestogens**

The uses of progestogens are:

- As part of the combined oral contraceptive and in the progestogen-only pill. Medroxyprogesterone acetate administered by depot injection is used when parenteral contraception is indicated.
- As an anti-androgen in androgen-sensitive tumors, such as prostate cancer, e.g. cyproterone acetate;
- As part of hormone replacement therapy in women with an intact uterus to counteract the effects of unopposed estrogen on the endometrium which can result in endometrial carcinoma;
- Endometriosis;
- In menstrual disorders, such as premenstrual tension, dysmenorrhea and menorrhagia;
- Progestogens that are frequently used include gestodene, levonorgestrel, norethisterone, desogestrel, and norgestimate. All of these substances are derived from norgestrel. The potencies of these vary significantly. Although studies have shown that oral contraceptives containing desogestrel and gestodene are associated with an approximately two-fold increase in the risk of venous thromboembolism compared to those containing other progestogens, they should be avoided in women with risk factors for thromboembolic disease. The newer progestogens, desogestrel, gestodene, and norgestimate, produce good cycle control and have a less marked adverse effect on plasma lipids. For women experiencing side effects from other progestogens, such as acne, headaches, depression, weight gain, breast symptoms, and breakthrough bleeding, desogestrel, drospirenone (a derivative of spironolactone with anti-androgenic and anti-mineralocorticoid properties), and gestodene should be taken into consideration. In a transdermal contraceptive patch, ethinylestradiol and the progestogen norelgestromin are combined.

- **Mechanism of action**

Progestogens stimulate the synthesis of new proteins by acting on intracellular cytoplasmic receptors. Their primary method of contraception involves making cervical mucus impenetrable to sperm. The extra anti-ovulatory effect of testosterone derivatives, which are partially metabolized estrogenic metabolites, may be explained. The endometrium undergoes a pseudodecidual alteration that deters zygote implantation even more.

- **Pharmacokinetics**

Progesterone works best when injected intramuscularly or sublingually, and it is metabolized by the presystemic hepatic system. Pregnenolone and pregnanediol are eliminated through the urine. It has a 25–50 hour elimination half-life and a prolonged absorption period. It is tightly bound to proteins. Oral absorption of norethisterone, a synthetic progestogen found in many oral contraceptives, is quick, and it has a half-life of seven to eight hours. It also has minimal presystemic hepatic metabolism.

8.5.1.3. The Combined Oral Contraceptive

This method has become the most popular form of contraception worldwide since the initial pilot trials in Puerto Rico demonstrated that steroid oral contraception was practical. In the UK, almost half of all women in their twenties use this type of contraception. Although it doesn't offer the same level of protection against STDs as condoms, it is the most consistently effective method of contraception and permits uninterrupted sexual relations. Ethinylestradiol is the most widely used estrogen. The combined oral contraceptive pill (COC) primarily suppresses ovulation by blocking the pituitary's release of gonadotrophin through negative feedback on the hypothalamus. By doing this, the mid-cycle rise in LH that starts ovulation is prevented.

Progestogens such as desogestrel, gestodene, and norgestimate are currently found in combination oral contraceptives. Compared to their predecessors, norethisterone, levonorgestrel, and ethynodiol, these "third-generation" progestogens are only weak anti-estrogens, exhibit less androgenic activity, and cause less disruption of lipoprotein metabolism. However, there is a chance of venous thrombo-embolism that is higher when using desogestrel and gestadene.

Endocrine effects of the combined oral contraceptive include:

1. Prevention of the normal premenstrual rise and mid-cycle peaks of LH and FSH and of the rise in progesterone during the luteal phase;
2. Increased hepatic synthesis of proteins, including thyroid-binding globulin, ceruloplasmin, transferrin, coagulation factors and renin substrate, while increased fibrinogen synthesis can raise the erythrocyte sedimentation rate;
3. Reduced carbohydrate tolerance;
4. Decreased albumin and haptoglobulin synthesis.

- **Adverse Effects of the COC**

The combined pill has an overall acceptability rate of about 80%, and mild side effects are frequently manageable with a modification in preparation. Users are more likely to develop venous thromboembolic disease; this risk is highest in women over 35, particularly if they smoke, are obese, or have been using oral contraceptives continuously for at least five years. It has become desirable to lower the estrogen dose as much as possible due to the increased risk of venous thromboembolism (VTE). Women who are more likely to develop thrombotic disease may benefit from taking progestogen-only pills.

The incidence of VTE in healthy, non-pregnant women not using oral contraceptives is approximately five cases per 100,000 women annually. The incidence for women taking the COC that contains a second-generation progestogen, like levonorgestrel, is 15 per 100,000 women per year of use. Studies involving COC preparations containing third-generation progestogens, such as gestodene and desogestrel, have reported incidences of approximately 25 per 100,000 women per year of use, suggesting a higher risk of VTE in these women. But since the overall risk is still very low and far lower than the risk of pregnancy, if women are aware of and accept the relative risks, the choice of a COC should be made collaboratively by the prescriber and the woman in question, taking into account the woman's specific medical history as well as any contraindications.

Increased blood pressure is a common side effect of the pill, and in roughly 5% of cases, it is clinically significant. Upon discontinuing medication, blood pressure typically returns to its pre-treatment level. There is no upper age limit for using the combined oral contraceptive in normotensive, nonsmoking women without other risk factors for vascular disease; however, it is advisable to use the lowest effective dose of estrogen, particularly in women 35 years of age or older. Rare but severe side effects associated with combined oral contraceptive use include mesenteric artery thrombosis and small bowel ischemia, as well as hepatic vein thrombosis and Budd-Chiari syndrome. These harmful effects on the cardiovascular system are linked to estrogen. Jaundice akin to cholestasis during pregnancy may manifest, typically during the initial several cycles. Detoxification from drugs is quick.

Oral contraceptives may affect migraine in the following ways:

1. Precipitation of attacks in the previously unaffected;
2. Exacerbation of previously existing migraine;
3. Alteration of the pattern of attacks – in particular, focal neurological features may appear;
4. Occasionally the incidence of attacks may decrease or they may even be abolished while the patient is on the pill.

An elevated risk of gallstones is one of the other significant side effects. A slight elevated risk of liver cancer exists. Both functional ovarian cysts and benign breast lesions are less common. The COC may cause the onset of diabetes mellitus. While amenorrhea following the cessation of combined oral contraceptive is not uncommon (occurs in approximately 5% of cases), it is rarely prolonged, and permanent sterility is extremely rare.

- **Risk–Benefit Profile**

There is a two-fold increase in ischemic stroke but no increased incidence of coronary artery disease due to COCs. According to data, there may be a slight increase in risk for breast cancer; however, 10 years after stopping the COC, this risk drops to zero. After five years of treatment, there is a slight increase in cervical cancer cases, and after 10 years, there is a twofold increase. For at least 10 years, there is a halving of the risk of endometrial and ovarian cancer.

- **Contraindications of the COC**

- Absolute contraindications: pregnancy, thrombo-embolism, multiple risk factors for arterial disease, ischemic heart disease, severe hypertension, migraine with focal neurological symptoms, severe liver disease, porphyria, otosclerosis, breast or genital tract carcinoma, undiagnosed vaginal bleeding and breast-feeding.
- Relative contraindications: uncomplicated migraine, cholelithiasis, hypertension, dyslipidemia, diabetes mellitus, varicose veins, severe depression, long-term immobilization, sickle-cell disease, inflammatory bowel disease.

- **Drug interactions with the COC**

Oral anticoagulant effectiveness is decreased and clotting factors are increased by estrogens. While pregnancy is highly undesirable in patients starting warfarin, this does not preclude their continued use; rather, it justifies more frequent monitoring of the international normalized ratio (INR).

Oral contraceptives may negatively impact antihypertensive therapy, at least in part due to elevated levels of circulating renin substrate.

Some examples of enzyme inducers that can reduce plasma levels of contraceptive estrogen include rifampicin, carbamazepine, phenytoin, nelfinavir, nevirapine, ritonavir, and St John's wort. This may lower the effectiveness of the combined contraceptive pill, leading to breakthrough bleeding and an increased risk of unwanted pregnancy.

Oral contraceptive steroids circulate through the liver, and conjugated steroids in the bile are converted to their parent steroids by gut bacteria and then reabsorbed. Antibiotics with broad spectrum (e.g. tetracycline and amoxicillin) can change the bacteria in the colon, increase the amount of estrogen excreted in the feces, and lower plasma concentrations, all of which can lead to the failure of contraceptives. It doesn't seem like progestogen-only pills cause this issue.

8.5.1.4. Post-Coital Contraception

One point five milligrams of levonorgestrel, also known as the "morning-after" pill, is administered as soon as possible—ideally, no later than 12 hours—following unprotected sexual activity. About 84% of anticipated pregnancies are avoided by doing this. The dose needs to be taken again if vomiting happens within three hours of consumption. Mifepristone, a progesterone antagonist, works very well with just one dose. The UK's use of post-coital contraception appears to be underutilized, based on abortion statistics.

8.5.1.5. Progestogen-Only Contraceptives

Progestogen-only contraception can be obtained through oral pills, depot injections given every 12 weeks, subcutaneous implants of a single flexible rod lasting up to three years in the lower arm, and intrauterine devices. Etonogestrel is released by a single flexible rod implant. The intrauterine device, or IUD, is approved for use as a contraceptive method, for treating primary menorrhagia, and to prevent endometrial hypoplasia while undergoing estrogen replacement therapy. It releases levonorgestrel directly into the uterine cavity. The effectiveness of this IUD is five years.

- **Uses**

Progestogen-only contraceptives, such as norgestrel or norethisterone, are linked to a high rate of menstrual disturbances, but they can be helpful if estrogen-containing pills are poorly tolerated or should not be used while nursing a baby or in women who have vascular disease risk factors, such as older smokers, diabetics, valvular heart disease patients, or migraineurs. Since only about 40% of women have their ovulation suppressed and the endometrium and cervical mucus are the main targets of contraception, the effectiveness of contraception is lower than it is with the combined pill. The pill should be taken at the same time every day, preferably three to four hours before the customary time of intercourse, as this effect peaks three to four hours after ingestion and diminishes over the following sixteen to twenty hours. Pregnancy rates are comparable to those utilizing barrier methods or intrauterine contraceptive devices (roughly 1–2 per 100 women annually, as opposed to 0–3 per 100 women annually for COCs). For certain patients, taking progestogen-only pills continuously throughout the menstrual cycle is convenient.

Oral progesterone preparations are not as effective as depot progesterone injections. With a failure rate of 0–25 per 100 women annually, a single intramuscular injection of medroxyprogesterone acetate offers contraception for 10 weeks. It is mostly used as a stopgap measure (for example, while waiting for a vasectomy to take effect), but in some cases, it is recommended for long-term use in women who are not candidates for other methods. The adverse effects bear close resemblance to those of oral progestogen-only formulations. Up to 40% of women experience amenorrhea and infertility after two years of treatment; consequently, pregnancy is unlikely for nine to twelve months following the last injection.

Treatment with depot progestogen injections should not be undertaken without full counseling of the patient.

- **Adverse effects**

The primary issues include sporadic breast tenderness, irregular menstrual bleeding (which can be heavy but usually subsides after a few cycles), and infrequently, nausea, headaches, disturbed appetite, weight fluctuations, and altered libido.

- **Contraindications**

These include liver adenoma, severe arterial disease, pregnancy, undetected vaginal bleeding, and porphyria.

8.5.1.5. Anti-Progestogens

The competitive antagonist is mifepristone. It is used as a medical substitute for surgical early pregnancy termination (currently effective up to 63 days gestation, though it can also be used in the second trimester). Unless the abortion is already complete, a single oral dose of mifepristone is followed by a vaginal pessary of gemeprost, a prostaglandin that ripens and softens the cervix. Since gemeprost can cause hypotension, blood pressure needs to be watched closely for six hours following the medication's administration. After eight to twelve days, the patient is checked on, and if a full abortion has not taken place, surgical termination is necessary. Ectopic pregnancy is one of the contraindications.

8.5.2. Male Reproductive Endocrinology

Testosterone is the main hormone secreted by the interstitial (Leydig) cells in the testis. In the bloodstream, testosterone is attached to a plasma globulin and circulates. Although it varies, the plasma concentration in adult males should be greater than 10 nmol/L. A 5-αreductase enzyme in target tissues changes testosterone into the more active androgen dihydrotestosterone. In the liver, testosterone and dihydrotestosterone are both inactivated.

Androgens have a wide range of activities, the most important of which include actions on:

- development of male secondary sex characteristics (including male distribution of body hair, breaking of the voice, enlargement of the penis, sebum secretion and male-pattern balding);
- protein anabolic effects influencing growth, maturation of bone and muscle development;
- spermatogenesis and seminal fluid formation.

Testicular function is controlled by the anterior pituitary.

- Follicle-stimulating hormone acts on the seminiferous tubules and promotes spermatogenesis.
- Luteinizing hormone stimulates testosterone production.

Gonadotrophin-releasing hormone is the mechanism by which the hypothalamus facilitates the pituitary's release of FSH and LH.

8.5.2.1. Androgens and Anabolic Steroids

- **Uses**

Treatment with androgens is inappropriate for many cases of impotence because they are psychogenic in nature. Replacement therapy improves secondary sex traits and may increase libido and erectile function in impotent patients with low circulating testosterone levels, but it does not increase fertility. Patients who want to become fertile but have hypogonadism due to hypothalamic or pituitary dysfunction can be treated with gonadotrophins or pulsatile gonadotrophin releasing hormone. The most dependable method of achieving replacement therapy is intramuscular injection of testosterone esters in oil, which come in a variety of preparations. Typically, they ought to be administered every two to three weeks to manage symptoms. As an alternative, oral medications such as mesterolone or testosterone undecanoate can be taken; their oil-based formulation promotes lymphatic absorption from the gastrointestinal tract.

Gonadotrophins or testosterone esters can be used to treat severe constitutional delays or delayed puberty brought on by primary or secondary gonadal deficiencies. Premature fusion of epiphyses can lead to short stature, so treatment is necessary and best overseen by specialized clinics.

Treatment with androgens is occasionally very beneficial in alleviating symptoms for patients with disseminated breast cancer.

Compared to other androgens, anabolic steroids (such as nandrolone, stanozolol, and danazol) have comparatively stronger anabolic and less virilizing effects. They have been extensively misused by bodybuilders and athletes, and their therapeutic effects have been largely disappointing. Although they have few accepted applications, they can be used to treat certain aplastic anemias, treat the vascular symptoms of Behçet's disease, and prevent recurrent episodes of hereditary angioneurotic edema.

- **Mechanism of action**

New protein synthesis is triggered by the interaction between intracellular receptors in responsive cells and testosterone and dihydrotestosterone.

- **Adverse effects**

Predictable outcomes include virilization in women and increased libido in men. Acne, facial hair growth, and deepening of the voice are common undesirable features in women that are caused by androgens. Menstrual irregularities and additional masculinizing effects may also emerge. Excessive masculinization in men can lead to priapism, frequent erections, and aggressive behavior. Epiphyses may fuse prematurely in children. Additional side effects include jaundice, especially cholestatic jaundice, for which methyltestosterone is no longer recommended as a result of this complication. Gonadotrophin secretion is inhibited, which results in azoospermia. An unidentified mechanism produces hypercalcemia, which can be severe, in patients receiving androgen therapy for malignant disease. Numerous gastrointestinal symptoms, such as anorexia, vomiting, flatus, diarrhea, and oily stools, are brought on by oral testosterone preparations in oil.

- **Pharmacokinetics**

Even though testosterone is easily absorbed when taken orally, the liver undergoes significant presystemic metabolism. It can also be taken under the tongue, though this is not very common. Although testosterone in oil is quickly metabolized, it is well absorbed when administered intramuscularly. Because of their longer-lasting effects, testosterone esters—which are far less polar—are administered via oily depot injections and released more gradually. The liver is where testosterone is rendered inactive. The primary metabolites, primarily eliminated in the urine, are androsterone and etiocholanolone. Six percent or so of the testosterone that is administered ends up in the feces after passing through the enterohepatic circulation.

8.5.2.2. Cyproterone

- **Uses**

To avoid the disease activity flare-up brought on by the initial spike in sex hormone release, men with inoperable prostatic carcinoma are treated with cyproterone acetate before starting gonadotrophin-releasing hormone analogs. Additionally, it has been used to lessen sexual drive in kids who hit puberty early and in cases of sexual deviation. It has been used to treat hyperandrogenic effects in women, such as acne, hirsutism, and male pattern baldness, which are frequently observed in polycystic ovarian disease. Cyproterone may have negative effects on HDL and LDL, so long-term use is discouraged. Before beginning treatment for relatively minor indications, one should carefully weigh the risk vs benefit.

- **Mechanism of action**

By competing with testosterone for its high affinity receptors, cyproterone inhibits the growth of the prostate, spermatogenesis, and the masculinization process. It also exhibits very little glucocorticoid effect and strong progestational activity.

- **Adverse effects**

Some side effects include spermatogenesis inhibition (which usually returns to normal six months after treatment cessation), fatigue and lassitude (which can be severe enough to make driving unsafe), and gynecomastia in about 20% of patients (occasionally with benign nodules and galactorrhea).

8.5.2.3. Dutasteride and Finasteride

- **Use**

Finasteride and dutasteride decrease prostate size and inhibit 5α-reductase, improving urinary flow rate and obstructive symptoms. These are helpful substitutes for alpha-blockers (e.g., doxazosin) in men with noticeably enlarged prostates in particular, as a treatment for benign prostatic hypertrophy. Measuring prostate-specific antigen is important because treatment shouldn't postpone prostate cancer diagnosis.

Impotence, reduced libido, problems with ejaculation, breast tenderness, and enlargement are among the side effects. Women who are or may become pregnant should not handle broken or crushed finasteride tablets or leaky dutasteride capsules.

A low strength of finasteride is licensed for treating male pattern baldness in men.

8.5.2.4. Drugs That Affect Male Sexual Performance

It is challenging to evaluate the impact of drugs on sexual function due to the intricate interaction between physiological and psychological factors that determine sexual desire and performance. A tiny but significant percentage of men who receive placebos in randomized, placebo-controlled, blinded studies stop taking part because they experience impotence, which they blame on the therapy. Sexual function can also be disrupted by drugs that alter the autonomic supply to the sex organs. In fact, in the Medical Research Council (MRC) trial of mild hypertension, bendroflumethiazide, a thiazide diuretic, caused significantly more impotence than propranolol, an β-adrenoceptor antagonist. Tricyclic antidepressants, butyrophenones, and phenothiazines are among the medications that can cause erectile dysfunction in addition to interfering with autonomic function. Nitric oxide is the neurotransmitter that the non-adrenergic, non-cholinergic nerves in the pelvis use to regulate erection. Certain cases of organic impotence, such as in diabetes mellitus, exhibit abnormal nitric oxide release from the endothelium in the corpus cavernosum.

Sildenafil, tadalafil, and vardenafil are phosphodiesterase type 5 inhibitors that are approved for the treatment of erectile dysfunction. They have completely changed how erectile dysfunction is treated. Patients with cardiovascular disease, those with anatomical deformities of the penis, such as Peyronie's disease, and those who are predisposed to prolonged erections, such as those with sickle-cell disease, should exercise caution. Patients on nitrates and those with a prior history of non-arteritic anterior ischemic optic neuropathy should not take them.

Dyspepsia, vomiting, headaches, flushing, myalgia, dizziness, elevated intraocular pressure, and nasal congestion are some of the side effects. Other treatments for erectile dysfunction include alprostadil (prostaglandin E1) applied urethrally or via intracavernosal injection. Side effects include hypotension and priapism. Only after treatable medical causes have been ruled out should erectile dysfunction treatment be started.

Idiopathic hyperprolactinemia is linked to a small number of cases of decreased libido and impotence in both males and females; in these cases, bromocriptine may help restore potency. Although androgens contribute to both male and female arousal, their use is not recommended outside of patients who have low levels of testosterone in their blood. (Falkenstein et al, 2000; Schacke et al, 2002; Nelson, 2002; Nelson et al, 2002)

8.6. Pituitary Hormones and Related Drugs

The pituitary gland, also known as the master gland, secretes many hormones that control different body processes.

8.6.1. Anterior Pituitary Hormones and Related Drugs

8.6.1.1. Growth Hormone: Physiology and Pathophysiology

The anterior pituitary's acidophil cells secrete growth hormone (GH), a 191-amino acid protein. The highest secretion happens while you sleep and happens in short bursts with a slower underlying diurnal variability. During growth, secretion is significantly higher than in older people. Hypoglycemia, fasting, stress, and agonists at dopamine, serotonin, and α- and β-adrenoceptors all stimulate secretion. Slow wave sleep is characterized by the stimulation of somatotropin release via the serotoninergic pathway. Eating, glucocorticosteroids, and estrogens all inhibit secretion. By secreting the GH-releasing hormone (GHRH), somatorelin, and the GH-release-inhibiting hormone, somatostatin, which is also produced in the D cells of the pancreatic islets of Langerhans, the hypothalamus regulates the pituitary's production of growth hormone (GH). Acromegaly in adults (gigantism in children) is caused by GH-secreting pituitary adenomas, while growth retardation and short stature are caused by GH deficiency in children.

8.6.1.2. Growth Hormone (Somatropin): Therapeutic Use

The synthetic, recombinant form of human growth hormone used for therapeutic purposes is called somatropin. It works in concert with insulin and encourages the synthesis of proteins. Somatomedin, a small peptide synthesized in the liver whose secretion is dependent on somatotropin, mediates its effect on skeletal growth. Children who have dwarfism as a result of isolated growth hormone deficiency or deficiency as a result of hypothalamic or pituitary disease are treated with somatropin. Diagnoses of this condition are frequently challenging and necessitate precise height measurements in combination with biochemical assessments of endogenous growth hormone during pharmacological (such as insulin, clonidine, glucagon, arginine, or L-dopa) or physiological (such as sleep, exercise) stimulation. Treatment with somatropin also causes children with Turner's syndrome to grow taller. To maximize linear growth, injections should begin well before puberty and continue until growth stops. Gonadotrophin or sex hormone replacement therapy is postponed until maximum growth has been attained. Additional indications include promoting growth in children with Prader-Willi syndrome, chronic renal failure, and small-for-gestational-age births. It is used to treat adults with severe hypogonadism that is accompanied by a pituitary hormone deficiency and lower quality of life. If, after nine months of treatment, the quality of life does not improve, it should be stopped in this situation. When an adult's growth is complete and they are under 25 years old, somatropin should be used to treat severe GH deficiency (such as after neurosurgery) until adult peak bone mass is reached.

8.6.1.3. Growth Hormone Excess

Treatment for over-GH secretion typically involves radiotherapy and neurosurgery, and it is typically linked to a functional adenoma of the acidophil cells of the adenohypophysis. When surgery is not successful in curing a patient, medical treatment should be used as a support measure while waiting for the effects of radiation therapy, which may take up to 10 years. Throughout such treatment, it is necessary to frequently evaluate the pituitary fossa's size and visual fields to look for signs of the tumor's continued growth. Acromegalics' GH levels are lowered by somatostatin, but it also inhibits many gut hormones and requires constant intravenous infusion. Long-acting somatostatin analogs that decrease somatotropin levels are octreotide and lanreotide. They are administered by sporadic injection. Pegvisomant is a GH receptor selective antagonist. It is a once-daily subcutaneous injection of a genetically altered GH analog. It is used to treat acromegaly when somatostatin analogs, radiation therapy, and surgery don't fully resolve the condition. It should only be used by doctors who have experience treating acromegaly, as it has many adverse effects, including neurological, metabolic, and gastrointestinal.

8.6.1.4. Octreotide

- **Uses**

Synthetic octapeptide analog of somatostatin, ocreotide prevents peptide release from pituitary and gastrointestinal tract tumors that secrete hormones. It is used to treat patients, such as those with carcinoid syndrome, insulinoma, VIPoma, or glucagonoma, whose symptoms are brought on by the release of pharmacologically active substances from gastro-enteropancreatic tumors. It lessens skin rash, diarrhea, and flushing symptoms but does not shrink the tumor. It works better than bromocriptinein to reduce somatotropin levels in acromegaly patients, but it needs to be given parenterally (usually subcutaneously three times a day) and is not usually a suitable substitute for surgery. Additionally, it works well for people who have adenohypophysis basophil tumors that secrete TSH and cause thyrotoxicosis, an extremely uncommon form of hyperthyroidism. In cases of portal hypertension, it lowers portal pressure and works well as an acute treatment for bleeding esophageal varices. Additionally, it is used to lessen diarrhea caused by ileostomy and diarrhea linked to cryptosporidiosis in patients with AIDS. When octreotide is taken in between meals, the likelihood of gastrointestinal side effects is reduced. Once a month, an intramuscular long-acting microsphere octreotide formulation in poly (alkyl cyanoacrylate) nano capsules is given.

- **Adverse effects**

These include:

- gastrointestinal upset, including anorexia, nausea, vomiting, abdominal pain, diarrhea and steatorrhea;

- impaired glucose tolerance, by reducing insulin secretion;
- increased incidence of gallstones and/or biliary sludge after only a few months of treatment, especially at higher doses. Ultrasound evaluation of the gall bladder is recommended before starting therapy and if biliary symptoms occur during therapy.

8.6.1.5. Gonadotrophins

Follicle-stimulating hormone (FSH) and luteinizing hormone (LH) are secreted by the human pituitary gland. FSH is a glycoprotein that increases spermatogenesis in males and regulates the development of the primary ovarian follicle in females. It also promotes the proliferation of granulosa cells and increases the production of estrogen. Another glycoprotein is LH. It triggers the initiation and maintenance of the female corpus luteum, promotes the production of thecal estrogen, and causes ovulation. LH plays a part in the maturation of spermatocytes and the development of secondary sex traits in males by stimulating Leydig cells to synthesize androgen.

Commercially available forms of human gonadotrophin (HMG), human chorionic gonadotrophin (HCG), synthetic leukotriene (LH), and recombinant FSH (follitropin alfa and beta) include HMG and HCG. When clomifene treatment fails, they are used to induce ovulation in anovulatory women with secondary ovarian failure. To prevent ovarian hyperstimulation and multiple pregnancies, treatment must be closely monitored with repeated pelvic ultrasound scans and overseen by specialists skilled in the use of gonadotrophins. Additionally useful in treating oligospermia brought on by secondary testicular failure are gonadotrophins. Naturally, they have no effect in cases of primary gonadal failure.

8.6.1.6. Gonadorelin Analogs

Gonadorelin (gonadotrophin-releasing hormone, GnRH) is the FSH/LH-releasing factor produced in the hypothalamus. It may be used in a single intravenous dose to assess anterior pituitary reserve. The hormone that releases LH and FSH is called gonadotrophin-releasing hormone, or GnRH. It is made in the hypothalamus. It can be administered intravenously as a single dose to evaluate anterior pituitary reserve. Prostate cancer, advanced breast cancer, endometriosis, and female infertility are among the conditions for which goserelin, buserelin, and leuprorelin—analogs of GnRH—are prescribed. Buserelin is administered intraperitoneally, while goserelin is typically injected subcutaneously or implanted into the anterior abdominal wall. Use in benign conditions should be restricted to no more than six months because low estrogen levels cause menopausal-like symptoms as well as decreased bone density. It is possible to prevent this for indications like endometriosis by combining a low-dose estrogen replacement therapy with a GnRH analog.

- **Mechanism of action**

GnRH analogs cause the pituitary stimulation of either the male or female gonads to be reduced, which effectively results in medical orchidectomy/ovariectomy (a condition of hypopituitary hypogonadism). Initially, GnRH analogs stimulate the release of FSH/LH, but they later downregulate this response (usually after two weeks) (Table 8.1).

Table 8.1. *GnRH Analogs*

Drug	Use and additional comments
Goserelin	Used to treat endometriosis, prostate cancer and advanced breast cancer
Leuprorelin	Used to treat endometriosis and prostate cancer
Buserelin	Used to treat endometriosis. Prostate cancer. Induction of ovulation prior to IVF

Source: https://www.pharmaresearchlibrary.com/wp-content/uploads/2013/03/A-Textbook-of-Clinical-Pharmacology-and-Therapeutics-5th-edition.pdf.

- **Adverse effects**

  Reduced trabecular bone density and local symptoms from buserelin-induced nasal mucosal irritation are also common menopausal symptoms.

- **Pharmacokinetics**

  Analogs of gonadorelin are administered parenterally and are peptides. Goserelin can be administered intravenously in pulses to resemble the natural release of gonadotropin. Depot preparations for inhibiting the release of FSH and LH are available. GnRH analogs are eliminated by the kidneys and liver through a combination of metabolism and excretion.

8.6.1.7. Adrenocorticotrophic Hormone

In the UK, adrenocorticotrophic hormone, also known as corticotropin, is no longer marketed for sale. Tetracosactide is a synthetic analog of ACTH that only has the first 24 amino acids. The remaining 15 amino acids of ACTH are species-specific and linked to antigenic activity, but this has full biological activity. Its $t_{1/2}$ (15 minutes) is marginally longer than ACTH's, but all other characteristics are the same. When assessing patients who may have Addison's disease (adrenal insufficiency), tetracosactide is used as a diagnostic test. After administering a single intravenous or intramuscular dose, venous blood is drawn to determine the plasma cortisol level. The possibility of anaphylaxis exists.

8.6.2. Posterior Pituitary Hormones

The related octapeptide hormones vasopressin (antidiuretic hormone, ADH) and oxytocin are produced in the paraventricular and supra-optic hypothalamic nuclei. Nerve fibers carry them to the pituitary gland's posterior lobe, where they are stored and then released (a process known as neurosecretion). Demeclocycline, an antagonist of ADH, has been administered to patients suffering from syndrome of inappropriate ADH secretion (SIADH)-related hyponatremia. More targeted ADH antagonists are being developed. (Falkenstein et al, 2000; Schacke et al, 2002; Nelson, 2002; Nelson et al, 2002)

A Closer Look

Thyroid Cancers and Their Treatment

Around 42 million South Asians are thought to be affected by thyroid disorders. While even a slight swelling may make certain thyroid diseases easy to diagnose, thyroid cancer may not be recognized in its early stages by many people. Thyroid conditions include autoimmune thyroiditis, goiter, hyperthyroidism, autoimmune thyroiditis, and thyroid cancer. Thyroid cancer is one of those that could be harmful if it is not identified and treated quickly.

Thyroid Cancer

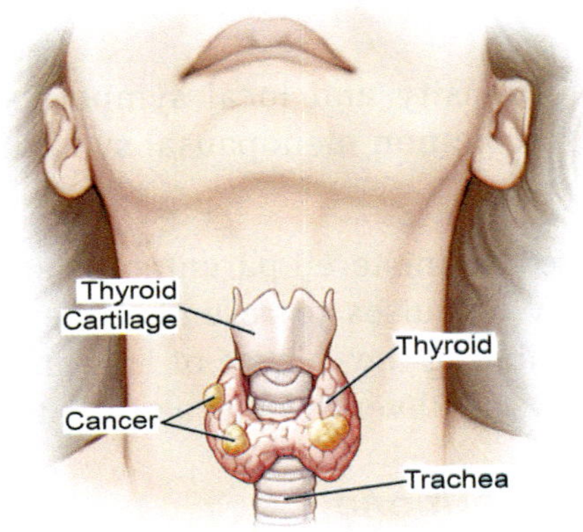

Source: https://my.clevelandclinic.org/health/diseases/12210-thyroid-cancer

Even though thyroid cancers make up over 90% of all endocrine cancers, they only make up 1% of all cancers in humans, with an annual incidence of about 1,40,000 cases worldwide. In women, thyroid cancer is more common.

Around 5% of women and 1% of men have thyroid nodules, which is a common condition. These nodules become clinically significant to rule out thyroid cancer. Of the various forms of thyroid cancer, papillary thyroid cancer is the most prevalent, making up 80% of cases and typically affecting fertile women. It spreads slowly and is the least dangerous type of thyroid cancer with the highest survival rate.

Ten to fifteen percent of cases of follicular thyroid cancer result in the cancer's recurrence and spread. Its victims are mostly elderly people, and it is more malignant in nature. Though it only affects 1% of thyroid cancer cases, anaplastic thyroid cancer is the most deadly type. This is an uncommon cancer that spreads quickly and is unresponsive to radioiodine therapy. Goiter and several years after the victim's initial radiation exposure are risk factors for this cancer.

Anti-cancer treatment regimens can lead to excellent long-term survival rates, which is why, in contrast to other cancers, the disease only causes a small number of deaths. The number of cases of thyroid cancer has increased globally, but research suggests that this may be more attributable to increased rates of detection than to an actual rise in the disease's incidence. Nevertheless, it makes sense to take the appropriate precautions and be aware of the signs and symptoms of thyroid cancer because the disorder may have a fatal outcome.

Summary

- The endocrine system helps to maintain internal homeostasis through the use of endogenous chemicals known as hormones.
- The use of drugs to help regulate and control endocrine function is an important area of pharmacology.
- Insulin is secreted by β-cells (also called B-cells) of the islets of Langerhans. It lowers blood glucose, but also modulates the metabolic disposition of fats and amino acids, as well as carbohydrate.
- Hypoglycemia is the most important and severe complication of insulin treatment. It is treated with an intravenous injection of glucose in unconscious patients, but sugar is given as a sweet drink in those with milder symptoms.
- Metformin is the only biguanide available in the UK. It is used in type 2 diabetic patients inadequately controlled by diet. Its anorectic effect aids weight reduction, so it is a first-choice drug for obese type 2 patients, provided there are no contraindications.
- Acarbose is used in type 2 diabetes mellitus in patients who are inadequately controlled on diet alone or diet and other oral hypoglycemic agents.
- The thyroid, or thyroid gland, is an endocrine gland in vertebrates. In humans, it is in the neck and consists of two connected lobes.
- Plasma calcium is sensed by a calcium-sensitive receptor (CaSR) in parathyroid and renal tubular cells and maintained within a narrow physiological range by parathyroid hormone (PTH), vitamin D and calcitonin.
- Glucocorticosteroids influence carbohydrate and protein metabolism and play a vital role in the stress response. Glucocorticosteroids stimulate the mobilization of amino acids from skeletal muscle, bone and skin, promoting their transport to the liver where they are converted into glucose (gluconeogenesis) and stored as glycogen.

References

1. Arlt, W., & Allolio, B. (2003). Adrenal insufficiency. *The Lancet, 361*(9372), 1881–1893. https://doi.org/10.1016/S0140-6736(03)13492-7.
2. Baird, D. T., & Glasier, A. F. (1999). Science, medicine, and the future: Contraception. *British Medical Journal, 319*(7215), 969–972. https://doi.org/10.1136/bmj.319.7215.969.
3. Birnbaumer, M. (2000). Vasopressin receptors. *Trends in Endocrinology and Metabolism, 11*(10), 406–410. https://doi.org/10.1016/S1043-2760(00)00311-7.
4. Cooper, M. S., & Stewart, P. M. (2003). Current concepts–Corticosteroid insufficiency in acutely ill patients. *New England Journal of Medicine, 348*(8), 727–734. https://doi.org/10.1056/NEJMra020529.
5. Drolet, G., & Rivest, S. (2001). Corticotropin-releasing hormone and its receptors: An evaluation at the transcription level in vivo. *Peptides, 22*(5), 761–767. https://doi.org/10.1016/S0196-9781(01)00393-4.

6. Falkenstein, E., Tillmann, H. C., Christ, M., Feuring, M., & Wehling, M. (2000). Multiple actions of steroid hormones–A focus on rapid, nongenomic effects. *Pharmacological Reviews, 52*(4), 513–556.

7. Feenstra, J., de Herder, W. W., ten Have, S. M., et al. (2005). Combined therapy with somatostatin analogues and weekly pegvisomant in active acromegaly. *The Lancet, 365*(9471), 1644–1646. https://doi.org/10.1016/S0140-6736(05)66574-0.

8. Freeman, M. E., Kanyicska, B., Lerant, A., & Nagy, G. (2000). Prolactin: Structure, function, and regulation of secretion. *Physiological Reviews, 80*(4), 1523–1631. https://doi.org/10.1152/physrev.2000.80.4.1523.

9. Ganguly, A. (1998). Current concepts–Primary aldosteronism. *New England Journal of Medicine, 339*(25), 1828–1834. https://doi.org/10.1056/NEJM199812173392507.

10. Goulding, N. J., & Flower, R. J. (2001). Glucocorticoids. In Parnham, M. J., & Bruinvels, J. (Series Eds.), *Milestones in Drug Therapy*. Berlin: Birkhäuser.

11. Hayashi, R., Wada, H., Ito, K., & Adcock, I. M. (2004). Effects of glucocorticoids on gene transcription. *European Journal of Pharmacology, 500*(1–3), 51–62. https://doi.org/10.1016/j.ejphar.2004.07.015.

12. Hays, R. M. (2006). Vasopressin antagonists–Progress and promise. *New England Journal of Medicine, 355*(21), 2146–2148. https://doi.org/10.1056/NEJMe068237.

13. Lamberts, S. W. J., Bruining, H. A., & de Jong, F. S. (1997). Corticosteroid therapy in severe illness. *New England Journal of Medicine, 337*(20), 1285–1292. https://doi.org/10.1056/NEJM199711133372007.

14. Lamberts, S. W. J., van der Lely, A. J., de Herder, W. W., & Hofland, L. J. (1996). Octreotide. *New England Journal of Medicine, 334*(4), 246–254. https://doi.org/10.1056/NEJM199601253340407.

15. Melmed, S. (2006). Medical progress: Acromegaly. *New England Journal of Medicine, 355*(24), 2558–2573. https://doi.org/10.1056/NEJMra062453.

16. Nelson, H. D. (2002). Assessing benefits and harms of hormone replacement therapy: Clinical applications. *Journal of the American Medical Association, 288*(7), 882–884. https://doi.org/10.1001/jama.288.7.882.

17. Nelson, H. D., Humphrey, L. L., Nygren, P., et al. (2002). Postmenopausal hormone replacement therapy: Scientific review. *Journal of the American Medical Association, 288*(7), 872–881. https://doi.org/10.1001/jama.288.7.872.

18. Okada, S., & Kopchick, J. J. (2001). Biological effects of growth hormone and its antagonist. *Trends in Molecular Medicine, 7*(3), 126–132. https://doi.org/10.1016/S1471-4914(01)01913-1.

19. Rhen, T., & Cidlowski, J. A. (2005). Anti-inflammatory action of glucocorticoids–New mechanisms for old drugs. *New England Journal of Medicine, 353*(16), 1711–1723. https://doi.org/10.1056/NEJMra050541.

20. Schacke, H., Docke, W. D., & Asadullah, K. (2002). Mechanisms involved in the side effects of glucocorticoids. *Pharmacology & Therapeutics, 96*(1), 23–43. https://doi.org/10.1016/S0163-7258(02)00297-8.

21. Tak, P. P., & Firestein, G. S. (2001). NF-kappaB: A key role in inflammatory diseases. *Journal of Clinical Investigation, 107*(1), 7–11. https://doi.org/10.1172/JCI11830.

22. Thibonnier, M., Coles, P., Thibonnier, A., et al. (2001). The basic and clinical pharmacology of nonpeptide vasopressin receptor antagonists. *Annual Review of Pharmacology and Toxicology, 41*(1), 175–202. https://doi.org/10.1146/annurev.pharmtox.41.1.175.

23. Trainer, P. J., Drake, W. M., Katznelson, L., et al. (2000). Treatment of acromegaly with the growth hormone-receptor antagonist pegvisomant. *New England Journal of Medicine, 342*(16), 1171–1177. https://doi.org/10.1056/NEJM200004203421603.

24. US Preventive Services Task Force. (2005). Hormone therapy for the prevention of chronic conditions in postmenopausal women: Recommendations from the US Preventive Services Task Force. *Annals of Internal Medicine, 142*(10), 855–860. https://doi.org/10.7326/0003-4819-142-10-200505170-00010.

25. Vance, M. L., & Mauras, N. (1999). Growth hormone therapy in adults and children. *New England Journal of Medicine, 341*(16), 1206–1216. https://doi.org/10.1056/NEJM199910143411606.

26. Wathen, C. N., Feig, D. S., Feightner, J. W., & The Canadian Task Force on Preventive Health Care. (2004). Hormone replacement therapy for the primary prevention of chronic diseases: Recommendation statement from the Canadian task force on preventive health care. *Canadian Medical Association Journal, 170*(10), 1535–1537. https://doi.org/10.1503/cmaj.1031604.

27. Wenzel, V., Krismer, A. C., Arntz, H. R., et al. (2004). A comparison of vasopressin and epinephrine for out-of-hospital cardiopulmonary resuscitation. *New England Journal of Medicine, 350*(2), 105–113. https://doi.org/10.1056/NEJMoa025493.

28. White, P. C. (1994). Mechanisms of disease–Disorders of aldosterone biosynthesis and action. *New England Journal of Medicine, 331*(4), 250–258. https://doi.org/10.1056/NEJM199407283310407.

Chapter

9

PHARMACOLOGICAL MANAGEMENT OF URINARY INCONTINENCE: CURRENT AND EMERGING TREATMENTS

Contents

Introduction

Urinary incontinence (UI) is the term used to describe any involuntary urine leakage, according to the International Continence Society (ICS). An estimated 20 million women and 6 million men in the US are thought to have experienced urine incontinence at some point in their lives. Urge urinary incontinence (UUI), mixed urinary incontinence (MUI), and stress urinary incontinence (SUI) are the three categories of urinary incontinence. UUI is the complaint of involuntary leakage that is preceded or accompanied by urgency, whereas SUI is the complaint of involuntary leakage that occurs during effort or exertion, such as when sneezing or coughing. MUI is the complaint of involuntary leakage related to exertion, effort, coughing, or sneezing in addition to urgency.

Over half of all women 60 years of age or older suffer from stress urinary incontinence (SUI), the most prevalent type of incontinence in women. In men, where it frequently occurs as a side effect after prostate surgery like a radical prostatectomy or transurethral resection of the prostate (TURP), suicidal ideation is less common. The current state of pharmaceutical therapy for SUI is inadequate, and new, effective medications are desperately needed to address this condition.

If there is no known infection or other evident pathology, overactive bladder syndrome (OAB) is characterized by urinary urgency, with or without urgency urinary incontinence, and typically increased frequency during the day and at night. Because of the aging population, associated comorbidities, and higher risk of hospitalization, OAB is primarily a chronic condition that primarily affects the elderly population and is associated with a very high socioeconomic burden. Many pathophysiological mechanisms have been proposed, including urothelial dysfunction, overactivity of the afferent arm of the micturition reflex, primary dysfunction of higher central nervous system (CNS) inhibitory centers, and primary detrusor dysfunction (shown as detrusor overactivity during urodynamic studies). When behavioral therapy fails or only provides partial symptom relief, pharmaceutical therapy becomes critical to the management of OAB patients. The global market for OAB treatment has grown due to the availability of several pharmacological principles; estimates indicate that the market will reach USD 4.19 billion by 2022 from USD 3.63 billion in 2017. For many years, antimuscarinic agents were the cornerstone of pharmacological treatment; however, in the modern era, beta-3-agonists are acknowledged as a reliable and secure substitute. Injections of botulinum toxin A detrusors are a useful but more intrusive treatment option for patients who are not responding well to oral medications. Preclinical research has been conducted on a wide range of investigational compounds, some of which have progressed to the clinical stage with varying degrees of success.

Orientation and Directional Terms

Term	Definition	Illustration
Urinary incontinence (UI)	Urinary incontinence (UI) is the involuntary loss of bladder control, or the unintentional leakage of urine. It can range from a minor issue to something that significantly impacts your quality of life.	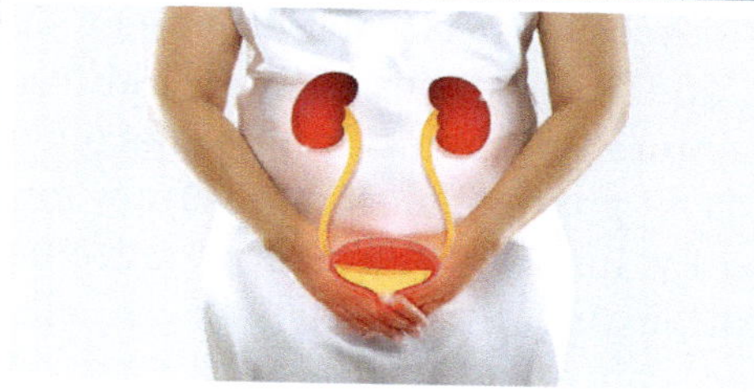
Blood–brain barrier (BBB)	The blood–brain barrier (BBB) is a highly selective semipermeable border of endothelial cells that regulates the transfer of solutes and chemicals between the circulatory system and the central nervous system, thus protecting the brain from harmful or unwanted substances in the blood.	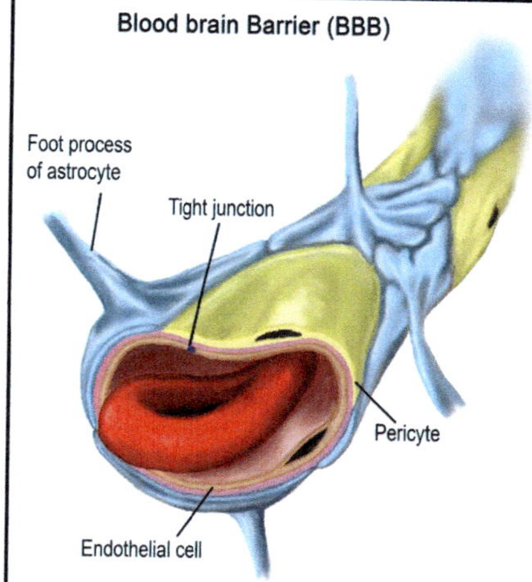
Ovarian cancer	Ovarian cancer is a cancerous tumor that develops in the ovaries, the female reproductive glands that produce eggs and hormones. It can originate in the ovaries or nearby structures, such as the fallopian tubes or the lining of the abdomen	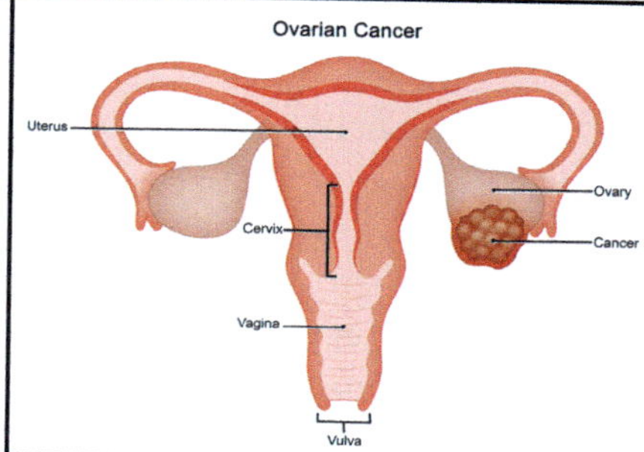
Bladder outlet obstruction (BOO)	Bladder outlet obstruction (BOO) is a blockage at the base of the bladder. It reduces or stops the flow of urine into the urethra. The urethra is the tube that carries urine out of the body.	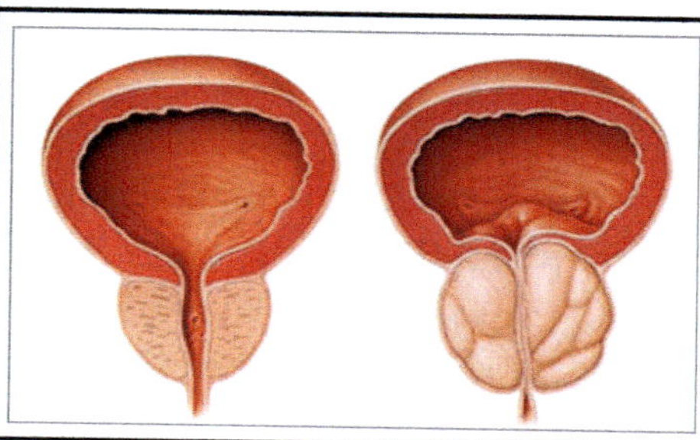

9.1. Antimuscarinics

The primary mechanism of human voiding contractions is mediated by muscarinic receptor stimulation caused by acetylcholine (ACh), which is released from cholinergic nerves. Muscarinic receptor subtypes (M^1–M^5) have been divided into five groups. The human bladder contains both the M_2 and M_3 subtypes. Although M^2 receptors are more common, some research has shown that M_3 receptors with specific pharmacological properties are also involved in bladder contraction. Nowadays, pharmacological therapy for overactive bladder (OAB) and/or urgency incontinence frequently involves the use of antimuscarinics (AMs). An overview of the most widely used medications is provided in Table 9.1, all of which have shown their efficacy and safety in carefully planned, controlled trials.

Table 9.1. *Characteristics of Antimuscarinic Drugs for Urgency Urinary Incontinence*

Medication	Selectivity	Ability to Cross BBB
Darifenacin	M_3	Low
Fesoterodine	Nonselective	Low
Imidafenacin	Predominantly M3	Low
Oxybutynin	Nonselective	High
Propiverine	Nonselective	Moderate
Solifenacin	Predominantly M3	Moderate
Tolterodine	Nonselective	Moderate
Trospium	Nonselective	Low

Abbreviation: BBB: blood–brain barrier.

Source: https://www.ncbi.nlm.nih.gov/pmc/articles/PMC8630428/.

9.1.1. Adverse Effects

While anticholinergic agents have proven effective in patients with OAB, they are associated with several bothersome adverse effects (AEs), including dry mouth, constipation, somnolence, drowsiness, and blurred vision, which impact on both compliance and persistence with long-term treatments, dry mouth being the most common.

While the effectiveness of all antimuscarinic medications is similar, immediate-release (IR) oral oxybutynin was linked to a higher number of side effects. In comparison to the immediate release (IR) formulations of both drugs (68% and 28.8%, respectively), a meta-analysis of adverse event reports (AEs) revealed statistically significant lower rates of dry mouth for extended-release (ER) formulations of oxybutynin (40%) and tolterodine (18%). Compared to the 40.0% meta-analyzed rates for oral oxybutynin ER and the 68.0% rates for oral oxybutynin IR, transdermal oxybutynin (patch and gel) demonstrated lower rates of dry mouth. Given that other results were comparable and that the primary cause of discontinuing AM use is dry mouth, ER and transdermal formulations might be a suitable place to start for treatment. However, skin reactions were the most frequent cause of treatment discontinuation among transdermal oxybutynin users.

A growing concern is neurological adverse events (AEs), especially in older patients due to increased permeability of the blood-brain barrier (BBB) with aging. More cumulative anticholinergic use has been linked to an increased risk of dementia and Alzheimer's disease, according to recent research. As stated by Dmochowski et al. When compared to non-use, the average estimated risk of dementia increases by 46% when anticholinergic agents are used for at least three months. There is also inconsistent data regarding the effects of individual AMs on cognition. Short-term studies in older adults have shown little to no cognitive impairment associated with fesoterodine, solifenacin, or trospium. In contrast, oral oxybutynin has been linked in the short term to cognitive impairment in the elderly and, when combined with tolterodine, to a higher risk of incident dementia. Yonguc et al. demonstrated that fesoterodine 4 mg significantly reduced OAB symptoms in idiopathic Parkinson's disease patients with OAB without statistically significant impairment of cognitive functions when compared with placebo in a randomized, double-blind, placebo-controlled trial.

9.1.2. Latest Developments

In an effort to improve side-effect profiles and achieve a higher M_3 affinity, new antimuscarinic compounds were created.

Since 2007, imidafenacin (Uritos; Kyorin Pharmaceutical Co., Japan) has been used as a novel antimuscarinic agent to treat ovarian cancer (OAB) in Japan. Its lower affinity for the M_2 subtype and higher affinity for the M_1 and M_3 receptor subtypes have made it more tolerable as a therapy. The effectiveness and safety of imidafenacin for the treatment of OAB in Japanese patients were shown in a placebo-controlled clinical trial. Pushkar et al. conducted a randomized, open-label, tolterodine-controlled trial that showed imidafenacin's effectiveness and safety in patients who were Caucasian. Twelve weeks into the treatment, the mean number of incontinence episodes changed; in the imidafenacin group, it was −2.1 ± 2.2, and in the tolterodine group, it was −1.9 ± 1.8 (p=0.001); in the case of the daytime incontinence episodes, it changed to −1.7 ± 1.7 and −1.5 ± 1.4 (p=0.01). Gastrointestinal problems were the most common medication-associated adverse events (AEs), with no discernible variations between the groups. Imidafenacin and other AMs were found to have similar efficacy in a recent systematic review and meta-analysis of all published RCTs comparing it to other ADs. However, imidafenacin caused fewer nocturia episodes and demonstrated lower rates of dry mouth, constipation, and withdrawals, making it the preferred medication for patients who require long-term use.

Tarafenacin is a novel quinuclidinol derivative. It has the best selectivity between the human M_3 and M_2 subtypes of all reference antagonists tested. Additionally, it shows a very favorable selectivity index between the two tissues, with the submandibular gland and bladder showing less significant inhibition of M_3 activation. In a Phase II study that was double-blind, randomized, and placebo-controlled, Song et al. showed that tarafenacin 0.4 mg significantly reduced OAB symptoms compared to placebo. It's interesting to note that tarafenacin had a somewhat higher rate of dry mouth (64.2%) than other anticholinergics that have been reported (29.6%), but a relatively lower rate of constipation (2.1%) than other agents (7.7%). (Lightner et al, 2019; Peyronnet et al, 2019)

9.2. Beta-3-Agonists

The most prevalent subtype of β-ARs in the human bladder is beta-3 adrenergic receptor (β_3-AR), which mediates noradrenaline-induced detrusor relaxation. The initial goal of developing β_3-AR agonists was to treat diabetes mellitus. The first oral medication substitute for AMs for the treatment of OAB, mirabegron, was approved for commercialization in 2012 after a comprehensive international clinical development program. While mirabegron 50 mg was considerably better tolerated than antimuscarinic treatments, it demonstrated comparable overall efficacy in multiple studies. In patients with OAB who were dissatisfied with previous antimuscarinic treatment, mirabegron significantly improved the rates of treatment satisfaction and symptoms, according to the results of a recent multicenter prospective study (the FAVOR study). At 12 weeks, the response rate for treatment satisfaction was 69.3% (275/397).

9.2.1. Adverse Effects

In clinical trials lasting up to a year, the most frequent adverse events (AEs) linked to mirabegron were hypertension (7.3%), nasopharyngitis (3.4%), and urinary tract infections (3–0%). Due to the exclusion of patients with poorly controlled hypertension, arrhythmia, or cardiac heart failure from prior studies, data on patients with severe uncontrolled high blood pressure (systolic ≥180 mm Hg and/or diastolic ≥110 mm Hg) is currently missing from the product label of mirabegron. However, no evidence of an increased cardiovascular risk was found when comparing mirabegron to a placebo in an analysis of pooled safety data from over 13,000 patients across 13 studies.

Regarding constipation and urine retention, the rate of dry mouth associated with mirabegron 50 mg was comparable to that of placebo and considerably lower than that of nearly all other active treatments. Whether used as the first- or second-line drug, treatment persistence with mirabegron was noticeably longer than that with AMs.

The PILLAR trial assessed the safety and tolerability of mirabegron in patients with OAB-wet who were 65 years of age or older. Treatment-emergent adverse events (TEAEs), most of which were mild or moderate in severity, were reported in 39.4% of patients who received a placebo and 44.2% and 49.8% of patients who received 25 mg or 50 mg of mirabegron, respectively. These results are consistent with the safety profile of mirabegron. In patients treated with mirabegron, urinary tract infection, headache, and diarrhea were the most frequent TEAEs. When comparing patients under 75 years old to those over 75 years old, the incidence of TEAEs was marginally higher in the former group. The Montreal Cognitive Assessment test (MoCA), which was used in the same trial, demonstrated that mirabegron treatment has no effect on drug-related cognitive side effects. Specifically, there was no statistically significant difference in the adjusted mean MoCA total score between the placebo group (−0.1 [0.1]) and the mirabegron group (−0.2 [0.1]) between the baseline and end of treatment.

9.2.2. Latest Developments

Urovant Sciences GmbH's Vibegron (MK-4618) is a potent, novel, and selective β_3-AR agonist that is derived from MK-0634, an β_3-AR agonist developed in the early 2000s for the treatment of obesity. Although the compound's efficacy in treating obesity was not realized, it was instead investigated for treating OAB, for which human proof-of-concept was shown. Yoshida et al.

showed that vibegron 50 mg (V50) and 100 mg (V100) once daily for 12 weeks produced superior efficacy over placebo in the treatment of Japanese patients with OAB in a double-blind, placebo-controlled Phase 3 RCT. With regard to vibegron groups ($p<0.001$), the estimated differences in mean micturitions/d, urgency incontinence episodes/day, and incontinence episodes/day were −0.86, −0.27, and −0.30, respectively, and −0.81, −0.39, and −0.43, respectively, for v100 ($p<0.001$). Constipation and dry mouth were vibegron's most frequent drug-related adverse events (TEAEs); however, the incidence of dry mouth was comparable to that of placebo. Vibegron considerably increased the voided volume/micturition and significantly decreased the number of UUI episodes/day in patients with OAB, according to a post hoc analysis of the same RCT. The response rate was higher than 50%. The V50, V100, and placebo groups had reductions in the number of UUI episodes at week 12 of −1.35, −1.47, and −1.08 in all patients, and −2.95, −3.28, and −2.10 in the severe UUI subgroup.

A recent Phase III randomized, double-blind, placebo and active-controlled study found that once daily 75 mg vibegron (V75) provided statistically significant reductions in micturition, urgency episodes, and urgency incontinence, and increased the volume per micturition. At 12 weeks, urgency incontinence episodes decreased by an adjusted mean of 2.0 episodes per day for V75 vs 1.4 for placebo ($p<0.0001$) and 1.8 for tolterodine. An international Phase IIb dose finding RCT in the Caucasian population also concluded that once-daily V50 and V100 improved OAB symptoms. After a 12-week period, the V75 group had a 52.4% reduction in UUI episodes per day (75% or more fewer than the baseline) compared to the placebo group's 36.8% ($p<0.0001$). Tolterodine accounted for 47.6% of the proportion. Vibegron demonstrated a good safety record, with a 1% incidence of hypertension comparable to that of a placebo.

Regarding the safety profile, vibegron did not exhibit any induction or inhibitory effects on CYP enzymes, suggesting no risk of drug–drug interactions. On the other hand, mirabegron is known to inhibit CYP2D6, a cytochrome P450 (CYP450) enzyme, so drug–drug interaction should be taken into consideration.

The Japanese PMDA approved Vibegron for the treatment of OAB in September 2018, and the US FDA approved it in December 2020.

Kennely et al. conducted an indirect treatment comparison of vibegron and mirabegron in the absence of head-to-head trials. When compared to mirabegron, visbegron was linked to a significantly higher improvement from baseline in volume voided at 12 and 52 weeks ($p<0.05$, each) and total incontinence episodes at 4 and 52 weeks ($p<0.05$, each). The frequency of adverse events was largely similar.

Solabegron, previously known as GW427343, is a highly selective β_3-AR agonist designed for treating OAB and irritable bowel syndrome. Ohlstein et al conducted a randomized, double-blind study to assess the effectiveness and safety of solabegron 50 mg and 125 mg taken twice a day compared to a placebo in women with OAB. The results showed that Solabegron 125 mg had a significant impact on reducing incontinence episodes over 24 hours, micturitions over 24 hours, and increasing urine volume voided compared to placebo. Solabegron was well-tolerated with no significant differences in adverse events compared to placebo. Additionally, there were no significant differences in blood pressure or heart rate changes during the 24-hour ambulatory measurement.

Maruyama et al. examined the effects of ritabegron, a novel β_3-AR agonist, on salivary secretion and bladder function in rats, comparing it to tolterodine. Cystometrography was used to assess the effects of drugs on bladder functions following a 6-week partial bladder outlet obstruction (BOO). Ritobegron did not alter micturition pressure, residual volume, or salivary secretion induced by carbachol; instead, it reduced the frequency and amplitude of non-voiding contractions (NVC). Tolterodine decreased the amplitude of NVC, but it also significantly inhibited salivary secretion induced by carbachol and markedly increased residual volume. (Lightner et al, 2019; Peyronnet et al, 2019)

9.3. Phosphodiesterase-5 Inhibitors

Inhibitors of phosphodiesterase 5 (PDE5i) have long been used to treat erectile dysfunction. Through the inhibition of cGMP degradation, a crucial mediator of smooth muscle tone, PDE-5i prolongs the physiological effects of nitric oxide (NO)/cyclic guanosine monophosphate (cGMP) signaling in tissues. Tadalafil in particular, which is a 5-PDEi, has demonstrated potential therapeutic utility in treating OAB and male LUTS in many studies. Research on animals revealed that a drop in detrusor cGMP and urinary NO levels may inhibit detrusor relaxation, resulting in an overactive bladder.

Daily tadalafil intake may reduce bladder overactivity by increasing nitric oxide synthase (eNOS) activity in the bladder mucosa, restoring urinary NO availability, and raising the detrusor cGMP level, according to recent results by Lee et al. in rats with metabolic syndrome.

Dell'Atti demonstrated that tadalafil 5 mg/d, in contrast to fesoterodine 8 mg/d, significantly improved urgency incontinence episodes (1.7 ± 1.3 to 0.5 ± 1.3 vs 1.7 ± 1.3 to 1.0 ± 1.4; $p<0.001$) in a prospective randomized controlled trial (RCT) involving men over 65 with OAB. Additionally, the tadalafil group experienced a greater improvement in erectile function and QoL scores.

Likewise, Chen et al.'s double-blind, placebo-controlled randomized clinical trial (RCT) in females with overactive bladder (OAB) showed that tadalafil 5 mg/d significantly reduced the frequency, urgency, and incontinence episodes when compared to placebo. Tadalafil 5 mg/d was well tolerated, and no significant side effects were seen—perhaps as a result of the medication's low dosages.

9.3.1. Latest Developments

In a multicenter, double-blind, placebo-controlled RCT, Giuliano et al. examined the modified release (MR) formulation of a novel PDE5i called gistandenafil (UK-369003, by Pfizer) as a potential treatment for men with a clinical diagnosis of OAB. Regretfully, no clinically significant treatment variations were observed for any of the UK-369003 MR doses in terms of nocturia, urgency episode frequency, mean voided volume, or frequency of voiding. (Lightner et al, 2019; Peyronnet et al, 2019)

9.4. Combination Therapy

Combining various medications is becoming more common in clinical practice and is believed to have a role in the treatment of refractory OAB/UI, much like it is in the management of other medical conditions (like refractory hypertension, benign prostatic hyperplasia, and cancer treatments). The benefit of combination therapy is its ability to act concurrently on several pharmacological pathways, producing additive and/or synergistic effects.

Combining an anticholinergic drug with mirabegron is the combination therapy that has received the most research. The BESIDE, SYNERGY, and SYMPHONY trials were the three largest randomized controlled trials (RCTs) on the topic. They all showed that, when compared to solifenacin or mirabegron monotherapy, combination therapy of the two improves urine frequency, urgency, and urgency incontinence in a statistically significant way. Specifically, mirabegron add-on therapy to solifenacin was assessed by Drake et al. (BESIDE) in patients with incontinent overactive bladders who did not respond well to the first four weeks of solifenacin monotherapy. They discovered that when mirabegron 50 mg was added to solifenacin 5 mg, OAB symptoms were significantly better than when solifenacin 5 or 10 mg was used alone. Compared to solifenacin 5 mg (37.9%) and 10 mg (40.2%), considerably more patients experienced dryness when using the combination. Gibson et al. discovered in a predetermined analysis of the BESIDE trial that older (>65 yr) and elderly (>75 yr) patients treated with a combination of solifenacin and mirabegron maintain efficacy and safety in the general population.

Yamanishi et al. assessed the effectiveness of tadalafil and mirabegron combined versus tadalafil monotherapy in the CONTACT study for the management of men's persistent overactive bladder symptoms. Combination therapy significantly reduced the overall OAB symptoms score ($p<0.001$) from monotherapy by 1.78 (95% CI 1.05–2.50) points.

Alternative approaches include antimuscarinic cycling (where patients alternate multiple anticholinergic molecules one after the other) or combining two antimuscarinics in patients who are not responding to first-line antimuscarinic monotherapy. In 129 patients who were resistant to monotherapy, Wang et al. assessed the safety and effectiveness of combining two distinct antimuscarinic medications by flexibly adding on oxybutynin ER (5–15 mg once a day). Only 31 (24.0%) patients continued the combined medication for up to 12 months, whereas 25 (19.4%) patients reported successful therapeutic effect at three months. In 28 patients (21.7%), the combined medication was stopped due to adverse events. Urinary urgency and urgency incontinence are reduced when trospium and solifenacin are combined, as shown by Kosilov et al. when compared to placebo. In particular, continuous therapy with standard doses of trospium and solifenacin resulted in low adherence and high rates of treatment withdrawal (⍰66%) despite satisfactory clinical and urodynamic results. In contrast, one-year cyclic therapy with a combination of trospium and solifenacin provided a high compliance level (76–84%). Chancellor et al. evaluated that UI symptom burden did not change as patients tried more anticholinergic therapies based on a one-time cross-sectional survey of 620 patients with wet-OAB. This suggests that cycling on additional anticholinergics may not be beneficial for patients who remain incontinent after attempting an anticholinergic. (Lightner et al, 2019; Peyronnet et al, 2019)

9.5. Botulinum Toxin

There are seven subtypes of botulinum toxin (BoNT), of which subtype A (BoNT-A) is clinically the most relevant. Four different commercial forms of BoNT-A are available: onabotulinumtoxin A, abobotulinumtoxin A, incobotulinumtoxin A and prabotulinumtoxin A. The majority of preclinical and clinical studies have focused on onabotulinumtoxinA (Botox®, Allergan, Inc., Irvine, CA). OnabotulinumtoxinA (onaBoNT-A) intradetrusor injections are currently the only FDA-approved botulinum toxin treatment for patients with OAB and/or UUI, who have failed first-line pharmacological treatment. The mechanism of action of BoNT in the nerve terminals has been well-established: BoNT protease activity degrades the SNARE complex protein SNAP-25, thus preventing neurosecretory vesicles from docking/fusing and releasing ACh and other neurotransmitters from the axon endings, with a long-lasting neuronal blockade leading to decreased muscle contractility and chemical denervation at the injection site

Two Phase III trials demonstrated the effectiveness and safety of onaBoNT-A for treating OAB and urgency incontinence. This led to the approval of a starting dose of 100 U (10 mL) for patients with idiopathic OAB. OnaBoNT-A was found to provide greater reductions in UI compared to AMs in both patients with idiopathic OAB and those with neurogenic OAB.

During a 3.5-year study, patients who received up to 6 treatment administrations found that the treatment was safe and effective for the long term. The median duration of the treatment's effect was 7.6 months. The most frequent adverse event was a urinary tract infection, occurring in 17% of patients after the first treatment. Catheterization after the first treatment was 4.0%, and subsequent treatments had rates ranging from 0.6% to 1.7%. Discontinuations due to lack of efficacy or treatment-related adverse events were 5.7% and 0.5%, respectively. In the treatment of antimuscarinic-experienced patients with OAB, a recent network meta-analysis compared the safety and effectiveness of mirabegron and onaBoNT-A. It discovered that onaBoNT-A was linked to better outcomes, such as fewer episodes of incontinence. On the other hand, mirabegron was linked to a lower incidence of UTIs than onaBoNT-A.

The FDA has not approved the use of botulinumtoxin A to treat OAB and UUI due to a lack of large multicenter randomized controlled trials to support this use. Nonetheless, abobotulinumtoxin A (aboBoNT-A) intradetrusor injections have been suggested as a potential treatment option in many series. In 211 patients with neurogenic detrusor overactivity, Peyronnet al. compared the effects of the first intradetrusor injections of aboBoNT-A 750U and onaBoNT-A 200 and 300U. While there were similar success rates in the aboBoNT-A 750U and onaBoNT-A 300U groups (65.4% vs 65%; p=0.91) but with a trend towards longer intervals between the first and second injection in the onaBoNT-A 300U group (12.4 vs 9.3 months; p=0.09), patients treated with aboBoNT-A 750U had higher success rates compared to those who received onaBoNT-A 200U. When intradetrusor injections of onaBoNT-A failed, Bottet et al. observed in a multicenter study involving 57 patients that switching to aboBoNT-A may be helpful in the treatment of neurogenic detrusor overactivity. 52.63% of patients had a significant decrease in the number of UI episodes per day (p<0.001), a mean increase in maximum cystomanometric capacity of 41.2 mL (p=0.02) was observed, and at week 6, following aboBoNT-A injections, the proportion of patients with no uninhibited detrusor contractions increased significantly (from 15.79% to 43.9%; p=0.0002).

9.5.1. Latest Developments

Since the discovery that the depth and volume of an injection can affect the potency of intradetrusor onaBoNT-A injections, there has been a surge in interest in the hunt for novel drug delivery strategies (Figure 9.1).

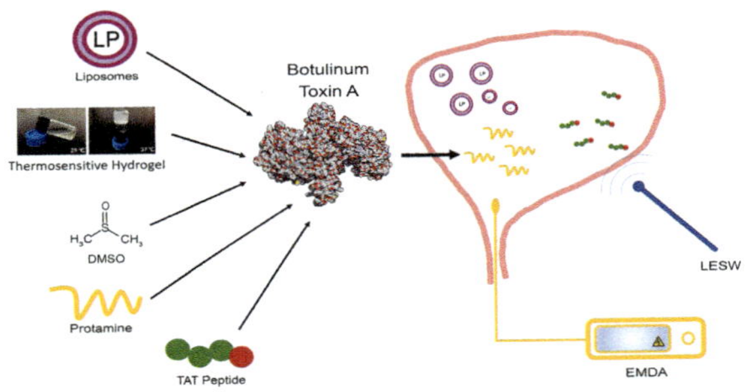

Figure 9.1. *Different approaches for intravesical delivery of botulinum toxin.*

Abbreviations: DMSO: dimethyl sulfoxide; EMDA: electromotive drug administration; and LESW: low energy shock waves.

Source: https://www.ncbi.nlm.nih.gov/pmc/articles/PMC8630428/.

Many studies have been conducted on liposomes (lipid vesicles) as a drug delivery mechanism for anticancer medications, and the FDA has recently approved several of these products. According to *in vitro* research, urine proteases did not cause onaBoNT-A complexed with liposomes to undergo proteolytic degradation. To evaluate the safety and effectiveness of onaBoNT-A complexed with liposomes in men and women with OAB, a multi-center placebo-controlled trial was carried out following compelling results of tests in animal models. When lipo-botulinum toxin was administered four weeks after treatment, there was no urinary retention, a comparable risk of UTI, and a statistically significant decrease in micturition events per three days (−4.64 vs. −0.19 for placebo, p=0.02). There was also a statistically significant decrease in urgency severity scores when compared to placebo (p=0.01).

Drugs can stay in the bladder longer thanks to the development of intravesical thermosensitive hydrogels. Because of thermosensitive hydrogels' special rheological characteristic, the instillation can be liquid at room temperature (25°C) and semi-solid at body temperature. Thermosensitive hydrogel enhanced the intravesical delivery of onaBoNT-A in patients with painful bladder syndrome, according to a clinical study of TC-3 Gel/BTX-A combination. Unlike saline instillation, which typically takes two hours, the hydrogel in the bladder allowed for a gradual release of 200U of onaBoNT-A for up to six or eight hours. According to preliminary results, there was a brief, mild adverse event (AE) period of a few weeks, along with a transient and common side effect (constipation).

Dimethyl sulfoxide (DMSO) is an organic solvent that has been used to increase the permeability of the urothelium in animal bladders to facilitate the delivery of several anticancer drugs. In the work of Petrou et al., onaBoNT-A mixed with DMSO was administered to 25 women who had idiopathic OAB and were resistant to antimuscarinics (22 patients received OnaBoNT-A 300U mixed with 50 mL of 50% DMSO, while three patients received two-thirds of that dose). The median number of UUI episodes rose back to 4 at 3 months after declining from 4 at baseline to 2 at 1 month (p=0.004). There was also a noticeable drop in symptom scores from baseline, and there were no major adverse events reported.

Protamine is a polycationic peptide rich in arginine that is used as a complexing agent for long-acting insulin and as an antidote to heparin overdoses. Several studies have reported that protamine instillation at concentrations of 10–30 mg/mL denudes the urothelium. Protamine internalizes into cells through heparin sulfate mediated endocytosis. Rats with spinal cord injuries had better absorption of onaBoNT-A into their bladders thanks to this action on the urothelium. Protein transduction allows cationic peptides like protamine to pass through membranes. Protein transduction domains (PTDs) are small segments (10–16 residues long) of these proteins.

PTDs help fused materials move across cellular membranes by facilitating protein transduction across membranes. PTDs can enter any type of cell without the help of receptors or transporters by covalently attaching to onaBoNT-A. Human immunodeficiency virus (HIV) TAT peptide is a PTD that has been successfully used to facilitate the uptake of conjugated peptide nucleic acids into rat bladders. Thus, it is easy to imagine onaBoNT-A being delivered intravesically into the bladder after conjugation with TAT peptide.

A gel application developed by Revance Therapeutics (Newark, CA, USA) successfully delivered onaBoNT-A conjugated to PTDs transdermally and reduced skin wrinkles in 45 patients by 44.5%. The physical method of electromotive drug administration (EMDA) increases the permeability of the bladder to drug molecules injected through electromotive forces (EMF). To create a potential difference that could drive the diffusion of instilled drugs, EMF involves placing electrodes on the abdomen and inside the bladder. This BoNT-A delivery method (BoNTA/EMDA) was assessed for treating refractory neurogenic detrusor overactivity in 15 children who received 10 IU/kg of electromotive BoNT-A. A pulsed current generator delivered 10 mA for 15 minutes while the children were attached to a specially made indwelling catheter and two dispersive pads. At post-treatment urodynamics, mean maximal detrusor pressure and end-fill pressure significantly decreased (75 ± 16 cmH2O vs 39 ± 10 cmH2O and 22 ± 7 cmH2O vs 13 ± 2 cm H2O), but maximal bladder capacity increased significantly (121 ± 39 mL vs 262 ± 41 mL; $p<0.001$). In 12 patients, the urinary incontinence improved in 80% of cases. Also, 10 (83.3%) of the 12 kids had their fecal incontinence resolved. Six children had burning sensations and erythema on their skin. In an animal study, Kajbafzadeh et al. discovered that BoNTA can be found via a trans-axonal retrograde transfer mechanism in bladder and bowel structures, as well as the upper and lower spinal cord, after intravesical BoNTA/EMDA. This new mechanism of action explains why children's bowel and bladder functions have improved at the same time.

Low energy shock wave (LESW) is another route of administration based on increasing cell permeability. Kodama et al. claim that LESW can increase the permeability of the plasma membrane by generating shear forces due to liquid movement in relation to cells. Huang et al. examined the viability of employing LESW for intravesical BoNT-A delivery and assessed its effectiveness for acetic acid-induced bladder hyperactivity in rats. Without sacrificing their ability to void, rats given BoNT-A plus LESW exhibited a markedly decreased response (48 point 6% decreased intercontraction interval) to acetic acid instillation.

9.6. Duloxetine

Duloxetine blocks norepinephrine (NE) and serotonin (5-HT) from being taken up synaptically again. The concentration of 5-HT and NE in the synaptic cleft of the sacral spinal cord increases the stimulation of 5-HT and NE receptors on the pudendal motor neurons. This, in turn, increases the urethral striated sphincter's contraction strength and resting tone. In a recent study using a rat model, Wrobel et al. discovered that while solifenacin and mirabegron primarily act via peripheral pathways, duloxetine acts via central pathways to reverse the symptoms of overactive bladder coexisting with depression. When surgery is not an option, duloxetine has been studied as a temporary improvement for adult patients' SUI. With doses of 80 mg/d, a 10% cure rate may be attained; however, data regarding improvements in quality of life are inconsistent. Long-term treatment was associated with a high rate of patient withdrawal due to ineffectiveness and a high frequency of adverse events, such as nausea and vomiting (40% or more of patients). 60 female patients with idiopathic OAB participated in a single-blinded interventional randomized clinical trial conducted by Mirzaet al. to assess the safety and effectiveness of duloxetine 20 mg/daily versus solifenacin 10 mg/daily. The mean ICIQ-OAB questionnaire score one month after treatment commenced revealed no statistically significant difference (p-value=0.148) between duloxetine and solifenacin (duloxetine vs. solifenacin: 8.76 vs. 9.66 from 13.90 vs. 14.86 before treatment). The solifenacin group experienced higher rates of AEs (dry mouth, blurred vision, anorexia, sleep disturbance, and anxiety); only the frequency of blurred vision was statistically significant (p-value=0.042) (Mariappan et al, 2007).

9.7. New Agents

An overview of the most appealing new medications for the pharmacological treatment of urine incontinence can be found in Table 9.2.

Table 9.2. *Overview of the Most Attractive New Agents for Pharmacological Treatment of Urinary Incontinence*

Agent	Molecular Pathway	Drug Component	Localization	Effect on Bladder Activity	Experimental Phase	Notes
DA-8010	Cholinergic system	M3 receptor antagonist	Bladder smooth-muscle and urothelial cells	Inhibitory	Human Phase II	Highly selective for the urinary bladder over salivary glands, intestine and heart
URO-902	Big potassium (BK) channels	Plasmid DNA vector expressing BK channel α subunit	Bladder smooth-muscle cells	Inhibitory	Human Phase I	No significant AEs; significant reduction in urgency and UUI episodes
SN003	CRF peptides and receptors	Reversible antagonist of CRF1	CNS (pontine micturition center)	Inhibitory	Animal	Improved cystometric parameters in a rat model of DO
KPR-5714	TRPM8 channels	TRPM8 antagonist	PNS (bladder afferent nerves)	Inhibitory	Animal	Combination of KPR-5714 and β3-AR agonist or AM additively reduced bladder contractions and voiding frequency
O-1602	Cannabinoid receptor	GPR55 and GPR18agonist	Bladder	Inhibitory	Animal	Alleviates DO without impairing voiding function, in rats
Retigabine	Voltage-gated potassium channels (Kvs)	Kv7 Channel Activator	Bladder smooth-muscle cells	Inhibitory	Animal	Inhibited the frequency of RBCs and mechanosensitive primary bladder afferent activities, in rats
Eliapixant	P2 purinergic receptor family	P2X3 receptor antagonist	Bladder and PNS (bladder sensory nerves)	Inhibitory	Human Phase I	Antagonized bladder overactivity in rats. Research on humans is ongoing

Abbreviations: AEs, adverse effects; UUI, urgency urinary incontinence; DO, detrusor overactivity; CRF, corticotropin-releasing factor; CNS, central nervous system; PNS, peripheral nervous system; β3-AR, beta3-adrenergic receptor; AM, antimuscarinic; TRPM, transient receptor potential cation channel subfamily M (melastatin); GPR, G protein-coupled receptor.

Source: https://www.ncbi.nlm.nih.gov/pmc/articles/PMC8630428/.

DA-8010 (by the Dong-A ST Pharmaceutical Company, Yongin, Korea) is a novel, highly potent M3 antagonist, which appeared more highly selective for the urinary bladder over the salivary glands, large intestine and heart in preclinical studies compared with other antimuscarinic agents. In the work of Choi et al, oral administration of DA-8010 improved findings in an OAB rat model induced by partial BOO. In a recent randomized, double-blind, human Phase II study, a total of 306 patients (69.93% female) were randomized to 12 weeks of treatment in 1 of 4 groups: two experimental groups (DA8010 2.5 mg or 5 mg), an active reference group (solifenacin 5 mg), or a placebo group. The mean values (standard deviation) of the changes (Δ) in 24 hr frequency at 12 weeks were −1.01 (2.44) for placebo, −1.22 (2.05) for DA8010 2.5 mg, and −1.67 (2.25) for DA8010 5 mg, with a significant difference between DA8010 5 mg and placebo ($p=0.0413$). In the solifenacin 5 mg group, Δ 24 hr frequency at 12 weeks was −1.56 (2.17), showing no significant difference from either DA8010 2.5 mg ($p=0.4098$) or DA8010 5 mg ($p=0.8540$). AEs were observed in 3.95% of placebo, 6.67% of DA8010 2.5 mg, 18.42% of DA8010 5 mg, and 17.33% of solifenacin 5 mg groups.

A naked plasmid DNA vector, URO-902 (hMaxi-K), double-stranded and nonviral, expresses the α subunit of the human big potassium (BK) channel. The BK channel controls the function of the bladder detrusor muscle and is highly expressed on smooth muscle cells in the bladder. The excitability of smooth muscle cells is decreased by BK channel activation. Two Phase I double-blind, placebo-controlled trials (NCT00495053 and NCT01870037) assessed the safety and possible effectiveness of URO-902 administered by intravesical instillation (ION-02) and direct injection into the bladder wall (ION-03), respectively, in healthy women with OAB and urodynamically demonstrated DO. Among the safety results, neither trial had any dose-limiting toxicities or noteworthy adverse events (AEs), and no participant withdrew because of an AE. When it came to efficacy, ION-02 (N=21) showed a downward trend in mean urgency incontinence episodes and involuntary detrusor contractions at 24 weeks; ION-03 (N=13) showed a significant reduction in urgency episodes and number of voids compared to placebo 1 week after injection.

Reversible antagonist SN003 blocks the G-protein coupled corticotropin-releasing factor (CRF) receptor CRF1. The CRF family of peptides and receptors, which is highly expressed in the parts of the central nervous system that regulate voiding (Barrington's nucleus), coordinates the endocrine, autonomic, and behavioral responses of mammals to stress. In a DO model, it was discovered that inhibiting CRF1 improved cystometric parameters. SN003 showed promise as a treatment for wet OAB in a recent study by Wrobel et al., as it reduced changes in nearly all cystometric parameters in rats with induced DO.

A brand-new, highly specific transient receptor potential melastatin 8 (TRPM8) antagonist is KPR-5714. Primary afferent neurons express TRPM8 channels primarily in response to cold temperature and/or chemical agents. According to earlier research, mechanosensitive C fibers in the bladder may be a pathogenic source of afferent hyperactivity, which is related to the TRPM8 channels. In rats with OAB, Aizawa et al. studied the effects of TRPM8 antagonist in combination with β3-adrenoceptor agonist or anticholinergic agent. They found that when KPR-5714 and mirabegron or tolterodine tartrate were administered together, bladder contractions and frequency of voiding were significantly reduced compared to when monotherapy was used.

O-1602 is a novel cannabinoid receptor agonist that modulates bladder afferent information peripherally. It specifically binds to the GPR55 and GPR18 cannabinoid receptors, which are expressed in the bladder. Oral medications that alter cannabinoid receptor activity have been suggested as an alternate treatment for OAB patients in many clinical trials. According to Wrobel et al., O-1602 affects the storage phase of rats with DO without affecting the voiding phase. It alleviates or reverses the changes in cystometric and biochemical parameter characteristic of DO/OAB. O-1602 does not affect the cystometric parameters in normal rats.

It has been proposed that Kv7 voltage-gated potassium channels regulate nociception and mechano-afferent transduction in the bladder. The effects of retigabine, a Kv7 channel activator, on single-unit afferent activities of the primary bladder mechanosensitive afferent nerve fibers in rats as well as rhythmic bladder contractions (RBCs) were studied by Aizawa et al. The frequency of RBCs and mechanosensitive primary bladder afferent activities were shown to be inhibited by retigabine, indicating that Kv7 channel activation may be a promising treatment for bladder hypersensitive disorders like OAB.

Eliapixant is a purinergic P2X3 receptor antagonist that is being studied in the OVADER trial (NCT04545580), a double-blind, randomized, placebo-controlled, proof-of-concept trial that aims to evaluate the safety and effectiveness of the drug in patients with OAB and UUI. P2X3 ionotropic receptors (P2X3R) are members of the P2 purinergic receptor family and play a significant role in nociception and sensory hypersensitization. They are expressed in sensory neurons and are activated by extracellular ATP. P2X3Rs are also expressed in the lamina propria, urothelium, and detrusor smooth muscle of the urinary bladder. In conscious rats, it has been shown that ATP dose-dependently induced bladder hyperactivity, an effect that TNP-ATP counteracted. P2X3R antagonists are therefore acknowledged as possible medications to treat overactive bladder. (Lightner et al, 2019; Peyronnet et al, 2019)

A Closer Look

Estrogen

The class of sex hormone known as estrogen (British English: estrogen; spelling variations may apply) is in charge of the maturation and control of the female reproductive system as well as secondary sexual characters. Estrone (E1), estradiol (E2), and estriol (E3) are the three main endogenous estrogens with estrogenic hormonal activity. The strongest and most common estrane is estradiol. Estetrol (E4) is an additional estrogen that is only generated during pregnancy.

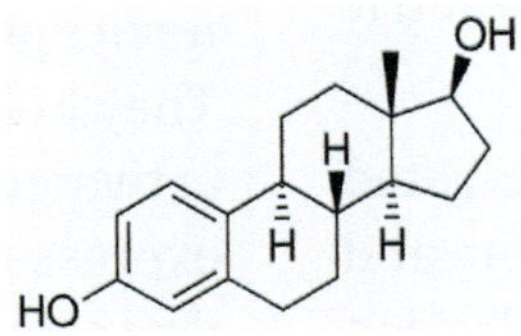

Source: https://upload.wikimedia.org/wikipedia/commons/thumb/0/00/Estradiol.svg/1024px-Estradiol.svg.png

In certain insects and all vertebrates, estrogens are synthesized. In both men and women, the quantitative levels of estrogens in the blood are lower than those of androgens. Even though men have much lower estrogen levels than women do, estrogens still play vital physiological roles in men.

Estrogens easily permeate through cell membranes, just like all other steroid hormones. Once within the cell, they attach to and activate estrogen receptors (ERs), which subsequently change how many genes are expressed. Furthermore, rapid-signaling membrane estrogen receptors (mERs), like GPER (GPR30), are bound and activated by estrogens.

Apart from their inherent hormone function, estrogens are also used as pharmaceuticals in the treatment of menopause, hormonal birth control, and feminizing hormone therapy for transgender, intersex, and nonbinary individuals.

Xenoestrogens are natural and synthetic estrogens that have been discovered in the environment. Among the many different types of endocrine-disrupting chemicals (EDCs) are estrogens, which can affect human and animal health and reproductive function.

Summary

- Acetylcholine (ACh) released from cholinergic nerves stimulates muscarinic receptors and mediates the main part of voiding contractions in humans.
- While anticholinergic agents have proven effective in patients with OAB, they are associated with several bothersome adverse effects (AEs), including dry mouth, constipation, somnolence, drowsiness, and blurred vision, which impact both compliance and persistence with long-term treatments, dry mouth being the most common.
- Novel antimuscarinic molecules were developed with the intention of attaining better M3 affinity and improving side-effect profiles.
- Beta-3 adrenergic receptor (β3-AR) represents the most common subtype of β-ARs in the human bladder where it mediates noradrenaline-induced detrusor relaxation.
- Phosphodiesterase 5 inhibitors (PDE5i) have traditionally been used in the treatment of erectile dysfunction. PDE-5i prolong the physiological effects of nitric oxide (NO)/cyclic guanosine monophosphate (cGMP) signaling in tissues through the inhibition of cGMP degradation, an important mediator of smooth muscle tone.
- Liposomes (lipid vesicles) have been widely studied as a drug delivery tool for anticancer drugs, and several such products are now FDA approved.
- Intravesical thermosensitive hydrogels have been developed to increase the residence time of drugs within the bladder.

References

1. Abrams, P., Andersson, K. E., Buccafusco, J. J., et al. (2006). Muscarinic receptors: Their distribution and function in body systems, and the implications for treating overactive bladder. *British Journal of Pharmacology, 148*(5), 565–578. https://doi.org/10.1038/sj.bjp.0706780.
2. Abrams, P., Cardozo, L., Fall, M., et al. (2002). The standardization of terminology of lower urinary tract function: Report from the standardization sub-committee of the international continence society. *Neurourology and Urodynamics, 21*(2), 167–178. https://doi.org/10.1002/nau.10052.
3. Abrams, P., Kelleher, C., Staskin, D., et al. (2015). Combination treatment with mirabegron and solifenacin in patients with overactive bladder: Efficacy and safety results from a randomized, double-blind, dose-ranging, phase 2 study (Symphony). *European Urology, 67*(3), 577–588. https://doi.org/10.1016/j.eururo.2014.02.012.
4. Aizawa, N., Fujimori, Y., Nakanishi, O., et al. (2021). Efficacy of the combination of KPR-5714, a novel transient receptor potential melastatin 8 (TRPM8) antagonist, and β3-adrenoceptor agonist or anticholinergic agent on bladder dysfunction in rats with bladder overactivity. *European Journal of Pharmacology, 899*, 173995. https://doi.org/10.1016/j.ejphar.2021.173995.
5. Aizawa, N., Wakamatsu, D., Kida, J., et al. (2017). Inhibitory effects of retigabine, a Kv7 channel activator, on mechanosensitive primary bladder afferent activities and nociceptive behaviors in rats. *Neurourology and Urodynamics, 36*(2), 280–285. https://doi.org/10.1002/nau.22920.

6. Anderson, R. U., Mobley, D., Blank, B., Saltzstein, D., Susset, J., & Brown, J. S. (1999). Once daily controlled versus immediate release oxybutynin chloride for urge urinary incontinence. OROS Oxybutynin Study Group. *Journal of Urology, 161*(6), 1809–1812. https://doi.org/10.1016/S0022-5347(05)68810-6.
7. Andersson, K. E. (2004). Antimuscarinics for treatment of overactive bladder. *Lancet Neurology, 3*(1), 46–53. https://doi.org/10.1016/S1474-4422(03)00622-7.
8. Asai, T., Tsuzuku, T., Takahashi, S., et al. (2014). Cell-penetrating peptide-conjugated lipid nanoparticles for siRNA delivery. *Biochemical and Biophysical Research Communications, 444*(4), 599–604. https://doi.org/10.1016/j.bbrc.2014.01.107.
9. Bientinesi, R., & Sacco, E. (2018). Managing urinary incontinence in women–A review of new and emerging pharmacotherapy. *Expert Opinion on Pharmacotherapy, 19*(18), 1989–1997. https://doi.org/10.1080/14656566.2018.1532502.
10. Bientinesi, R., Mancuso, C., Martire, M., et al. (2017). KV7 channels in the human detrusor: Channel modulator effects and gene and protein expression. *Naunyn-Schmiedeberg's Archives of Pharmacology, 390*(2), 127–137. https://doi.org/10.1007/s00210-016-1312-9.
11. Bottet, F., Peyronnet, B., Boissier, R., et al. (2018). Switch to abobotulinum toxin A may be useful in the treatment of neurogenic detrusor overactivity when intradetrusor injections of onabotulinum toxin A failed. *Neurourology and Urodynamics, 37*(1), 291–297. https://doi.org/10.1002/nau.23291.
12. Bump, R. C., Voss, S., Beardsworth, A., Manning, M., Zhao, Y. D., & Chen, W. (2008). Long-term efficacy of duloxetine in women with stress urinary incontinence. *BJU International, 102*(2), 214–218. https://doi.org/10.1111/j.1464-410X.2008.07577.x.
13. Buser, N., Ivic, S., Kessler, T. M., Kessels, A. G., & Bachmann, L. M. (2012). Efficacy and adverse events of antimuscarinics for treating overactive bladder: Network meta-analyses. *European Urology, 62*(6), 1040–1060. https://doi.org/10.1016/j.eururo.2012.08.060.
14. Cannon, T., & Chancellor, M. (2003). Pharmacotherapy for stress urinary incontinence. *Reviews in Urology, 5*, 135–141.
15. Cartwright, R., & Cardozo, L. (2007). Transdermal oxybutynin: Sticking to the facts. *European Urology, 51*(4), 907–914. https://doi.org/10.1016/j.eururo.2006.11.033.
16. Caulfield, M. P., & Birdsall, N. J. (1998). International union of pharmacology. XVII. Classification of muscarinic acetylcholine receptors. *Pharmacological Reviews, 50*(2), 279–290.
17. Cetinel, S., Ercan, F., Sirvanci, S., et al. (2003). The ameliorating effect of melatonin on protamine sulfate induced bladder injury and its relationship to interstitial cystitis. *Journal of Urology, 169*(4), 1564–1568. https://doi.org/10.1097/01.ju.0000049649.80549.17.
18. Chancellor, M. B., Yehoshua, A., Waweru, C., et al. (2016). Limitations of anticholinergic cycling in patients with overactive bladder (OAB) with urinary incontinence (UI): Results from the CONsequences of Treatment Refractory Overactive bLadder (CONTROL) study. *International Urology and Nephrology, 48*(7), 1029–1036. https://doi.org/10.1007/s11255-016-1277-0.
19. Chapple, C. R., Cardozo, L., Nitti, V. W., Siddiqui, E., & Michel, M. C. (2014). Mirabegron in overactive bladder: A review of efficacy, safety, and tolerability. *Neurourology and Urodynamics, 33*(1), 17–30. https://doi.org/10.1002/nau.22505.

20. Chapple, C. R., Khullar, V., Gabriel, Z., Muston, D., Bitoun, C. E., & Weinstein, D. (2008). The effects of antimuscarinic treatments in overactive bladder: An update of a systematic review and meta-analysis. *European Urology, 54*(3), 543–562. https://doi.org/10.1016/j.eururo.2008.06.047.

21. Chapple, C., Sievert, K. D., MacDiarmid, S., et al. (2013). OnabotulinumtoxinA 100 U significantly improves all idiopathic overactive bladder symptoms and quality of life in patients with overactive bladder and urinary incontinence: A randomized, double-blind, placebo-controlled trial. *European Urology, 64*(2), 249. https://doi.org/10.1016/j.eururo.2013.04.001.

22. Chen, D., Song, D., Wientjes, M. G., & Au, J. L. (2003). Effect of dimethyl sulfoxide on bladder tissue penetration of intravesical paclitaxel. *Clinical Cancer Research, 9*(1), 363–369.

23. Chen, H., Wang, F., Yu, Z., et al. (2017). Efficacy of daily low-dose tadalafil for treating overactive bladder: Results of a randomized, double-blind, placebo-controlled trial. *Urology, 100*, 59–64. https://doi.org/10.1016/j.urology.2016.11.008.

24. Choi, J. B., Jeon, S. H., Kwon, E. B., et al. (2020). The effects of oral administration of the novel muscarinic receptor antagonist DA-8010 on overactive bladder in rat with bladder outlet obstruction. *BMC Urology, 20*(1), 41. https://doi.org/10.1186/s12894-020-00611-8.

25. Chuang, Y. C., Huang, T. L., Tyagi, P., & Huang, C. C. (2016). Urodynamic and immunohistochemical evaluation of intravesical botulinum toxin A delivery using low energy shock waves. *Journal of Urology, 196*(2), 599–608. https://doi.org/10.1016/j.juro.2015.12.078.

26. Chuang, Y. C., Kaufmann, J. H., Chancellor, D. D., Chancellor, M. B., & Kuo, H. C. (2014). Bladder instillation of liposome encapsulated onabotulinumtoxinA improves overactive bladder symptoms: A prospective, multicenter, double-blind, randomized trial. *Journal of Urology, 192*(6), 1743–1749. https://doi.org/10.1016/j.juro.2014.07.008.

27. Chuang, Y. C., Tyagi, P., Huang, C. C., et al. (2009). Urodynamic and immunohistochemical evaluation of intravesical botulinum toxin A delivery using liposomes. *Journal of Urology, 182*(2), 786–792. https://doi.org/10.1016/j.juro.2009.03.083.

28. Coelho, A., Cruz, F., Cruz, C. D., & Avelino, A. (2012). Spread of onabotulinumtoxinA after bladder injection. Experimental study using the distribution of cleaved SNAP-25 as the marker of the toxin action. *European Urology, 61*(6), 1178. https://doi.org/10.1016/j.eururo.2012.01.046.

29. Dell'Atti, L. (2015). Efficacy of tadalafil once daily versus fesoterodine in the treatment of overactive bladder in older patients. *European Review for Medical and Pharmacological Sciences, 19*(9), 1559–1563.

30. Dmochowski, R. R., Thai, S., Iglay, K., et al. (2021). Increased risk of incident dementia following use of anticholinergic agents: A systematic literature review and meta-analysis. *Neurourology and Urodynamics, 40*(1), 28–37. https://doi.org/10.1002/nau.24536.

31. Drake, M. J., Chapple, C., Esen, A. A., et al. (2016). Efficacy and safety of mirabegron add-on therapy to solifenacin in incontinent overactive bladder patients with an inadequate response to initial 4-week solifenacin monotherapy: A randomized double-blind multicentre phase 3B study (BESIDE). *European Urology, 70*(1), 136–145. https://doi.org/10.1016/j.eururo.2016.02.030.

32. Ebbesen, M. H., Hunskaar, S., Rortveit, G., et al. (2013). Prevalence, incidence and remission of urinary incontinence in women: Longitudinal data from the Norwegian HUNT study (EPINCONT). *BMC Urology, 13*(1), 27. https://doi.org/10.1186/1471-2490-13-27.

33. Edmondson, S. D., Zhu, C., Kar, N. F., et al. (2016). Discovery of vibegron: A potent and selective β3 adrenergic receptor agonist for the treatment of overactive bladder. *Journal of Medicinal Chemistry, 59*(2), 609–623. https://doi.org/10.1021/acs.jmedchem.5b01372.

34. Fantl, A. J. (1996). *Urinary Incontinence in Adults: Acute and Chronic Management/Urinary Incontinence in Adults. Guideline Panel Update*. Rockville, MD: U.S. Department of Health and Human Services; Agency for Health Care Policy and Research; Clinical Practice Guideline Number 2: AHCPR publication no. 96-0682.

35. Ferreira, R. S., D'Ancona, C. A. L., Oelke, M., & Carneiro, M. R. (2018). Intradetrusor onabotulinumtoxinA injections are significantly more efficacious than oral oxybutynin for treatment of neurogenic detrusor overactivity: Results of a randomized, controlled, 24-week trial. *Einstein, 16*(3), eAO4207. https://doi.org/10.1590/S1679-45082018AO4207.

36. Ford, A. P., & Undem, B. J. (2013). The therapeutic promise of ATP antagonism at P2X3 receptors in respiratory and urological disorders. *Frontiers in Cellular Neuroscience, 7*, 267. https://doi.org/10.3389/fncel.2013.00267.

37. Freeman, R. M., Adekanmi, O., Waterfield, M. R., Waterfield, A. E., Wright, D., & Zajicek, J. (2006). The effect of cannabis on urge incontinence in patients with multiple sclerosis: A multicenter, randomized placebo-controlled trial (CAMS-LUTS). *International Urogynecology Journal, 17*(6), 636–641. https://doi.org/10.1007/s00192-006-0086-x.

38. Gibson, W., MacDiarmid, S., Huang, M., et al. (2017). Treating overactive bladder in older patients with a combination of mirabegron and solifenacin: A prespecified analysis from the BESIDE study. *European Urology Focus, 3*(6), 629–638. https://doi.org/10.1016/j.euf.2017.08.008.

39. Giuliano, F. A., Lamb, J., Crossland, A., Haughie, S., Ellis, P., & Tamimi, N. A. (2010). A placebo-controlled exploratory study investigating the efficacy and safety of the phosphodiesterase type 5 inhibitor UK-369,003 for the treatment of men with storage lower urinary tract symptoms associated with a clinical diagnosis of overactive bladder. *BJU International, 106*(5), 666–673. https://doi.org/10.1111/j.1464-410X.2010.09205.x.

40. Glogau, R., Blitzer, A., Brandt, F., Kane, M., Monheit, G. D., & Waugh, J. M. (2012). Results of a randomized, double-blind, placebo-controlled study to evaluate the efficacy and safety of a botulinum toxin type A topical gel for the treatment of moderate-to-severe lateral canthal lines. *Journal of Drugs in Dermatology, 11*(1), 38–45.

41. Goepel, M., Gronewald, A., Krege, S., & Michel, M. C. (1998). Muscarinic receptor subtypes in porcine detrusor: Comparison with humans and regulation by bladder augmentation. *Urological Research, 26*(2), 149–154. https://doi.org/10.1007/s002400050038.

42. Griebling, T. L., Campbell, N. L., Mangel, J., et al. (2020). Effect of mirabegron on cognitive function in elderly patients with overactive bladder: MoCA results from a Phase 4 randomized, placebo-controlled study (PILLAR). *BMC Geriatrics, 20*(1), 109. https://doi.org/10.1186/s12877-020-1474-7.

43. Herbison, P., & McKenzie, J. E. (2018). Which anticholinergic is best for people with overactive bladders? A network meta-analysis. *Neurourology and Urodynamics, 38*(2), 1–10.

44. Herschorn, S., Chapple, C. R., Abrams, P., et al. (2017). Efficacy and safety of combinations of mirabegron and solifenacin compared with monotherapy and placebo in patients with overactive bladder (SYNERGY study). *BJU International, 120*(4), 562–575. https://doi.org/10.1111/bju.13882.

45. Herschorn, S., Kohan, A., Aliotta, P., et al. (2017). The efficacy and safety of onabotulinumtoxinA or solifenacin compared with placebo in solifenacin naïve patients with refractory overactive bladder: Results from a multicenter, randomized, double-blind Phase 3b trial. *Journal of Urology, 198*(1), 167–175. https://doi.org/10.1016/j.juro.2017.01.069.

46. Herschorn, S., Staskin, D., Schermer, C. R., Kristy, R. M., & Wagg, A. (2020). Safety and tolerability results from the PILLAR study: A Phase IV, double-blind, randomized, placebo-controlled study of mirabegron in patients ≥ 65 years with overactive bladder-wet. *Drugs & Aging, 37*(9), 665–676. https://doi.org/10.1007/s40266-020-00783-w.

47. Homma, Y., Yamaguchi, T., & Yamaguchi, O. (2008). A randomized, double-blind, placebo-controlled Phase II dose-finding study of the novel anti-muscarinic agent imidafenacin in Japanese patients with overactive bladder. *International Journal of Urology, 15*(9), 809–815. https://doi.org/10.1111/j.1442-2042.2008.02104.x.

48. Kajbafzadeh, A. M., Ahmadi, H., Montaser-Kouhsari, L., Sabetkish, S., Ladi-Seyedian, S., & Sotoudeh, M. (2021). Intravesical electromotive administration of botulinum toxin type A in improving the bladder and bowel functions: Evidence for novel mechanism of action. *Journal of Spinal Cord Medicine, 44*(1), 89–95. https://doi.org/10.1080/10790268.2019.1603490.

49. Kajbafzadeh, A. M., Ahmadi, H., Montaser-Kouhsari, L., Sharifi-Rad, L., Nejat, F., & Bazargan-Hejazi, S. (2011). Intravesical electromotive botulinum toxin type A administration–part II: Clinical application. *Urology, 77*(2), 439–445. https://doi.org/10.1016/j.urology.2010.06.003.

50. Kavia, R., De Ridder, D., Constantinescu, C., Stott, C., Fowler, C. J., & Constantinescu, C. S. (2010). Randomized controlled trial of Sativex to treat detrusor overactivity in multiple sclerosis. *Multiple Sclerosis Journal, 16*(11), 1349–1359. https://doi.org/10.1177/1352458510378020.

51. Kelleher, C., Hakimi, Z., Zur, R., et al. (2018). Efficacy and tolerability of mirabegron compared with antimuscarinic monotherapy or combination therapies for overactive bladder: A systematic review and network meta-analysis. *European Urology, 74*(3), 324–333. https://doi.org/10.1016/j.eururo.2018.03.020.

52. Kennelly, M. J., Rhodes, T., Girman, C. J., Thomas, E., Shortino, D., & Mudd, P. N. Jr. (2021). Efficacy of vibegron and mirabegron for overactive bladder: A systematic literature review and indirect treatment comparison. *Advances in Therapy, 38(11), 5452–5464*. https://doi.org/10.1007/s12325-021-01902-8.

53. Khera, M., Somogyi, G. T., Salas, N. A., Kiss, S., Boone, T. B., & Smith, C. P. (2005). In vivo effects of botulinum toxin A on visceral sensory function in chronic spinal cord-injured rats. *Urology, 66*(1), 208–212. https://doi.org/10.1016/j.urology.2005.01.055.

54. Ko, K. J., Choo, M. S., Chang, Y. S., Kim, J. C., & Lee, K. S. (2020). A multicenter prospective study for overactive bladder patient treatment satisfaction with mirabegron after being unsatisfied with antimuscarinic therapy (FAVOR study). *Neurourology and Urodynamics, 39*(8), 2417–2424. https://doi.org/10.1002/nau.24505.

55. Kodama, T., Tomita, Y., Koshiyama, K., & Blomley, M. J. (2006). Transfection effect of microbubbles on cells in superposed ultrasound waves and behavior of cavitation bubble. *Ultrasound in Medicine & Biology, 32*(6), 905–914. https://doi.org/10.1016/j.ultrasmedbio.2006.03.004.

56. Kosilov, K. V., Loparev, S. A., Ivanovskaya, M. A., & Kosilova, L. V. (2014). Randomized controlled trial of cyclic and continuous therapy with trospium and solifenacin combination for severe

overactive bladder in elderly patients with regard to patient compliance. *Therapeutic Advances in Urology, 6*(6), 215–223. https://doi.org/10.1177/1756287214544896.

57. Lee, M. J., Moon, J. H., Lee, H. K., Cho, C. H., Choi, S. H., & Im, W. B. (2019). Pharmacological characterization of DA-8010, a novel muscarinic receptor antagonist selective for urinary bladder over salivary gland. *European Journal of Pharmacology, 843*, 240–250. https://doi.org/10.1016/j.ejphar.2018.11.037.
58. Lee, W. C., Chiang, P. H., Tain, Y. L., et al. (2012). Sensory dysfunction of bladder mucosa and bladder oversensitivity in a rat model of metabolic syndrome. *PLoS One, 7*(9), e45578. https://doi.org/10.1371/journal.pone.0045578.
59. Lee, W. C., Leu, S., Wu, K. L. H., Tain, Y. L., Chuang, Y. C., & Chan, J. Y. H. (2021). Tadalafil ameliorates bladder overactivity by restoring insulin-activated detrusor relaxation via the bladder mucosal IRS/PI3K/AKT/eNOS pathway in fructose-fed rats. *Scientific Reports, 11*(1), 8202. https://doi.org/10.1038/s41598-021-87505-3.
60. Li, M., Wang, Y., Banerjee, R., et al. (2019). Molecular mechanisms of human P2X3 receptor channel activation and modulation by divalent cation bound ATP. *eLife, 8*, e47060. https://doi.org/10.7554/eLife.47060.
61. Lightner, D. J., Gomelsky, A., Souter, L., & Vasavada, S. P. (2019). Diagnosis and treatment of overactive bladder (non-neurogenic) in adults: AUA/SUFU guideline amendment 2019. *Journal of Urology, 202*(3), 558–563. https://doi.org/10.1097/JU.0000000000000309.
62. Lozano-Ortega, G., Walker, D., Rogula, B., et al. (2019). The relative efficacy and safety of mirabegron and onabotulinumtoxinA in patients with overactive bladder who have previously been managed with an antimuscarinic: A network meta-analysis. *Urology, 127*, 1–8. https://doi.org/10.1016/j.urology.2019.02.005.
63. Malde, S., Apostilidis, A., Selai, C., et al. (2020). Botulinum toxin A for refractory OAB and idiopathic urinary retention: Can phenotyping improve outcome for patients: ICI-RS 2019? *Neurourology and Urodynamics, 39*(Suppl 3), S104–S112. https://doi.org/10.1002/nau.24207.
64. Mangera, A., Andersson, K. E., Apostolidis, A., et al. (2011). Contemporary management of lower urinary tract disease with botulinum toxin A: A systematic review of Botox (onabotulinumtoxinA) and Dysport (abobotulinumtoxinA). *European Urology, 60*(4), 784–795. https://doi.org/10.1016/j.eururo.2011.07.001.
65. Mariappan, P., Alhasso, A., Ballantyne, Z., Grant, A., & N'Dow, J. (2007). Duloxetine, a serotonin and noradrenaline reuptake inhibitor (SNRI) for the treatment of stress urinary incontinence: A systematic review. *European Urology, 51*, 67–74.
66. Maruyama, I., Yonekubo, S., Tatemichi, S., et al. (2012). Effects of ritobegron (KUC-7483), a novel β3-adrenoceptor agonist, on both rat bladder function following partial bladder outlet obstruction and on rat salivary secretion: A comparison with the effects of tolterodine. *Journal of Smooth Muscle Research, 48*(5–6), 115–124. https://doi.org/10.1540/jsmr.48.115.
67. Mirzaei, M., Daneshpajooh, A., Anvari, S. O., Dozchizadeh, S., & Teimorian, M. (2021). Evaluation of the clinical efficacy and complications of duloxetine in comparison to solifenacin in the treatment of overactive bladder disease in women: A randomized clinical trial [published online ahead of print, 2021 Aug 3]. *Urology Journal*. https://doi.org/10.22037/uj.v18i.6274.
68. Mitcheson, H. D., Samanta, S., Muldowney, K., et al. (2019). Vibegron (RVT-901/MK-4618/KRP-

114V) administered once daily as monotherapy or concomitantly with tolterodine in patients with an overactive bladder: A multicenter, Phase IIb, randomized, double-blind, controlled trial. *European Urology, 75*(2), 274–282. https://doi.org/10.1016/j.eururo.2018.10.006.

69. Mukerji, G., Yiangou, Y., Corcoran, S. L., et al. (2006). Cool and menthol receptor TRPM8 in human urinary bladder disorders and clinical correlations. *BMC Urology, 6*(1), 6. https://doi.org/10.1186/1471-2490-6-6.

70. Mushrush, D. J., Koteiche, H. A., Sammons, M. A., Link, A. J., McHaourab, H. S., & Lacy, D. B. (2011). Studies of the mechanistic details of the pH-dependent association of botulinum neurotoxin with membranes. *Journal of Biological Chemistry, 286*(30), 27011–27018. https://doi.org/10.1074/jbc.M111.256982.

71. Nagai, J., Komeda, T., Katagiri, Y., Yumoto, R., & Takano, M. (2013). Characterization of protamine uptake by opossum kidney epithelial cells. *Biological and Pharmaceutical Bulletin, 36*(12), 1942–1949. https://doi.org/10.1248/bpb.b13-00553.

72. Nambiar, A. K., Bosch, R., Cruz, F., et al. (2018). EAU guidelines on assessment and nonsurgical management of urinary incontinence. *European Urology, 73*(4), 596–609. https://doi.org/10.1016/j.eururo.2017.12.031.

73. National Library of Medicine (U.S.). (2020). A randomized, placebo-controlled, double-blind, parallel-group, multi-center, proof-of-concept study to assess the efficacy and safety of BAY 1817080 in patients with overactive bladder (OAB) over a 12-week treatment period. Identifier NCT04545580; (September 2020–February 2022). Available from: https://clinicaltrials.gov/ct2/show/NCT04545580 (accessed on 30 July 2024).

74. Nitti, V. W., Dmochowski, R., Herschorn, S., et al. (2013). OnabotulinumtoxinA for the treatment of patients with overactive bladder and urinary incontinence: Results of a Phase 3, randomized, placebo-controlled trial. *Journal of Urology, 189*(6), 2186. https://doi.org/10.1016/j.juro.2012.12.022.

75. Nitti, V. W., Ginsberg, D., Sievert, K. D., et al. (2016). Durable efficacy and safety of long-term onabotulinumtoxinA treatment in patients with overactive bladder syndrome: Final results of a 3.5-year study. *Journal of Urology, 196*(3), 791–800. https://doi.org/10.1016/j.juro.2016.03.146.

76. Ohlstein, E. H., von Keitz, A., & Michel, M. C. (2012). A multicenter, double-blind, randomized, placebo-controlled trial of the β3-adrenoceptor agonist solabegron for overactive bladder. *European Urology, 62*(5), 834–840. https://doi.org/10.1016/j.eururo.2012.05.053.

77. Ouslander, J. G., & Wood, A. J. J. (2004). Management of overactive bladder. *New England Journal of Medicine, 350*(8), 786–799. https://doi.org/10.1056/NEJMra032662.

78. Pakulski, C., Drobnik, L., & Millo, B. (2000). Age and sex as factors modifying the function of the blood-cerebrospinal fluid barrier. *Medical Science Monitor, 6*, 314–318.

79. Petrou, S. P., Parker, A. S., Crook, J. E., Rogers, A., Metz-Kudashick, D., & Thiel, D. D. (2009). Botulinum A toxin/dimethyl sulfoxide bladder instillations for women with refractory idiopathic detrusor overactivity: A phase 1/2 study. *Mayo Clinic Proceedings, 84*(8), 702–706. https://doi.org/10.1016/S0025-6196(11)60520-X.

80. Peyronnet, B., Castel-Lacanal, E., Roumiguie, M., et al. (2017). Intradetrusor injections of onabotulinum toxin A (Botox®) 300 U or 200 U versus abobotulinum toxin A (Dysport®) 750

U in the management of neurogenic detrusor overactivity: A case-control study. *Neurourology and Urodynamics, 36*(3), 734–739. https://doi.org/10.1002/nau.23009.

81. Peyronnet, B., Mironska, E., Chapple, C., et al. (2019). A comprehensive review of overactive bladder pathophysiology: On the way to tailored treatment. *European Urology, 75*(6), 988–1000. https://doi.org/10.1016/j.eururo.2019.02.038.

82. Pushkar, D. Y., Kasyan, G. R., Kolontarev, K. B., Sharvadze, G. G., & Mukhametshina, E. I. (2019). Randomized, open-label, tolterodine-controlled, comparative study of the novel antimuscarinic agent imidafenacin in patients with overactive bladder. *Neurourology and Urodynamics, 38*(5), 1313–1321. https://doi.org/10.1002/nau.23980.

83. Rappaport, Y. H., Zisman, A., Jeshurun-Gutshtat, M., et al. (2018). Safety and feasibility of intravesical instillation of botulinum toxin-A in hydrogel-based slow-release delivery system in patients with interstitial cystitis-bladder pain syndrome: A pilot study. *Urology, 114*, 60–65. https://doi.org/10.1016/j.urology.2017.12.028.

84. Richardson, K., Fox, C., Maidment, I., et al. (2018). Anticholinergic drugs and risk of dementia: Case–control study. *BMJ, 361*, k1315. https://doi.org/10.1136/bmj.k1315.

85. Risacher, S. L., McDonald, B. C., Tallman, E. F., et al. (2016). Association between anticholinergic medication use and cognition, brain metabolism, and brain atrophy in cognitively normal older adults. *JAMA Neurology, 73*(6), 721–732. https://doi.org/10.1001/jamaneurol.2016.0580.

86. Rosa, G. M., Ferrero, S., Nitti, V. W., Wagg, A., Saleem, T., & Chapple, C. R. (2016). Cardiovascular safety of β3-adrenoceptor agonists for the treatment of patients with overactive bladder syndrome. *European Urology, 69*(2), 311–323. https://doi.org/10.1016/j.eururo.2015.09.007.

87. Rovner, E., Chai, T. C., Jacobs, S., et al. (2020). Evaluating the safety and potential activity of URO-902 (hMaxi-K) gene transfer by intravesical instillation or direct injection into the bladder wall in female participants with idiopathic (non-neurogenic) overactive bladder syndrome and detrusor overactivity from two double-blind, imbalanced, placebo-controlled randomized phase 1 trials. *Neurourology and Urodynamics, 39*(2), 744–753. https://doi.org/10.1002/nau.24272.

88. Sacco, E. (2012). Physiopathology of overactive bladder syndrome. *Urologic, 79*(1), 24–35. https://doi.org/10.5301/RU.2012.8972.

89. Sacco, E., & Bientinesi, R. (2012). Mirabegron: A review of recent data and its prospects in the management of overactive bladder. *Therapeutic Advances in Urology, 4*(6), 315–324. https://doi.org/10.1177/1756287212457114.

90. Sacco, E., Bientinesi, R., & Tienforti, D., et al. (2014). Discovery history and clinical development of mirabegron for the treatment of overactive bladder and urinary incontinence. *Expert Opinion on Drug Discovery, 9*(4), 433–448. https://doi.org/10.1517/17460441.2014.892923.

91. Sacco, E., Pinto, F., & Bassi, P. (2008). Emerging pharmacological targets in overactive bladder therapy: Experimental and clinical evidences. *International Urogynecology Journal and Pelvic Floor Dysfunction, 19*(4), 583–598. https://doi.org/10.1007/s00192-007-0529-z.

92. Sacco, E., Prayer-Galetti, T., Pinto, F., et al. (2006). Urinary incontinence after radical prostatectomy: Incidence by definition, risk factors and temporal trend in a large series with a long-term follow-up. *BJU International, 97*(6), 1234–1241. https://doi.org/10.1111/j.1464-410X.2006.06185.x.

93. Sacco, E., Tienforti, D., D'Addessi, A., et al. (2010). Social, economic, and health utility considerations in the treatment of overactive bladder. *Open Access Journal of Urology, 2*, 11–24. https://doi.org/10.2147/OAJU.S4166.

94. Salcedo, C., Davalillo, S., Cabellos, J., et al. (2009). In vivo and in vitro pharmacological characterization of SVT-40776, a novel M3 muscarinic receptor antagonist, for the treatment of overactive bladder. *British Journal of Pharmacology, 156*(5), 807–817. https://doi.org/10.1111/j.1476-5381.2008.00082.x.

95. Soda, T., Tashiro, Y., Koike, S., Ikeuchi, R., & Okada, T. (2020). Overactive bladder medication: Persistence, drug switching, and reinitiation. *Neurourology and Urodynamics, 39*(8), 2527–2534. https://doi.org/10.1002/nau.24527.

96. Son, H., Kim, J., Kim, H., et al. (2021). Efficacy and safety of DA8010, a novel M3 antagonist, in patients with overactive bladder: Randomized, double-blind, Phase 2 study. *Journal of Urology, 206*(Supplement 3), e19. https://doi.org/10.1097/ju.0000000000001963.18.

97. Song, M., Kim, J. H., Lee, K. S., et al. (2015). The efficacy and tolerability of tarafenacin, a new muscarinic acetylcholine receptor M3 antagonist in patients with overactive bladder; Randomized, double-blind, placebo-controlled phase 2 study. *International Journal of Clinical Practice, 69*(2), 242–250. https://doi.org/10.1111/ijcp.12540.

98. Staskin, D., Frankel, J., Varano, S., Shortino, D., Jankowich, R., & Mudd, P. N. Jr. (2020). International Phase III, randomized, double-blind, placebo and active controlled study to evaluate the safety and efficacy of vibegron in patients with symptoms of overactive bladder: EMPOWUR. *Journal of Urology, 204*(2), 316–324. https://doi.org/10.1097/JU.0000000000000807.

99. Staskin, D., Kay, G., Tannenbaum, C., et al. (2010). Trospium chloride has no effect on memory testing and is assay undetectable in the central nervous system of older patients with overactive bladder. *International Journal of Clinical Practice, 64*(9), 1294–1300. https://doi.org/10.1111/j.1742-1241.2010.02433.x.

100. Tyagi, P., Banerjee, R., Basu, S., Yoshimura, N., Chancellor, M., & Huang, L. (2006). Intravesical antisense therapy for cystitis using TAT-peptide nucleic acid conjugates. *Molecular Pharmaceutics, 3*(4), 398. https://doi.org/10.1021/mp050093x.

101. Tyagi, P., Li, Z., Chancellor, M., De Groat, W. C., Yoshimura, N., & Huang, L. (2004). Sustained intravesical drug delivery using thermosensitive hydrogel. *Pharmaceutical Research, 21*(5), 832. https://doi.org/10.1023/B:PHAM.0000026436.62869.9c.

102. Tzoumas, N., Farrah, T. E., Dhaun, N., & Webb, D. J. (2020). Established and emerging therapeutic uses of PDE type 5 inhibitors in cardiovascular disease. *British Journal of Pharmacology, 177*(24), 5467–5488. https://doi.org/10.1111/bph.14920.

103. Wagg, A., Arumi, D., Herschorn, S., et al. (2017). A pooled analysis of the efficacy of fesoterodine for the treatment of overactive bladder, and the relationship between safety, co-morbidity and polypharmacy in patients aged 65 years or older. *Age and Ageing, 46*, 620–626.

104. Wagg, A., Dale, M., Tretter, R., Stow, B., & Compion, G. (2013). Randomized, multicenter, placebo-controlled, double-blind crossover study investigating the effect of solifenacin and oxybutynin in elderly people with mild cognitive impairment: The SENIOR study. *European Urology, 64*(1), 74–81. https://doi.org/10.1016/j.eururo.2013.01.002.

105. Wang, C. C., Jiang, Y. H., & Kuo, H. C. (2017). Efficacy and adherence of flexibly adding on a second antimuscarinic agent for patients with refractory overactive bladder. *Low Urinary Tract Symptoms, 9*(1), 27–32. https://doi.org/10.1111/luts.12103.

106. Warren, K., Burden, H., & Abrams, P. (2016). Mirabegron in overactive bladder patients: Efficacy review and update on drug safety. *Therapeutic Advances in Drug Safety, 7*(5), 204–216. https://doi.org/10.1177/2042098616659412.

107. White, W. B., Siddiqui, E., Tat, T., Franks, B., & Schermer, C. R. (2018). Cardiovascular safety of mirabegron: Analysis of an integrated clinical trial database of patients with overactive bladder syndrome. *Journal of the American Society of Hypertension, 12*(11), 768–778.e1. https://doi.org/10.1016/j.jash.2018.08.001.

108. Wróbel, A., Doboszewska, U., Rechberger, E., Wlaź, P., & Rechberger, T. (2017). SN003, a CRF1 receptor antagonist, attenuates depressive-like behavior and detrusor overactivity symptoms induced by 13-cis-retinoic acid in rats. *European Journal of Pharmacology, 812*, 216–224. https://doi.org/10.1016/j.ejphar.2017.07.010.

109. Wróbel, A., Serefko, A., Poleszak, E., & Rechberger, T. (2016). Fourteen-day administration of corticosterone may induce detrusor overactivity symptoms. *International Urogynecology Journal, 27*(11), 1713–1721. https://doi.org/10.1007/s00192-016-3027-3.

110. Wróbel, A., Serefko, A., Woźniak, A., et al. (2020). Duloxetine reverses the symptoms of overactive bladder co-existing with depression via the central pathways. *Pharmacology Biochemistry and Behavior, 189*, 172842. https://doi.org/10.1016/j.pbb.2019.172842.

111. Wróbel, A., Szopa, A., Serefko, A., & Poleszak, E. (2020). A novel alternative in the treatment of detrusor overactivity? In vivo activity of O-1602, the newly synthesized agonist of GPR55 and GPR18 cannabinoid receptors. *Molecules, 25*(6), 1384. https://doi.org/10.3390/molecules25061384.

112. Wu, J. P., Peng, L., Zeng, X., et al. (2020). Is imidafenacin an alternative to current antimuscarinic drugs for patients with overactive bladder syndrome? *International Urogynecology Journal, 32*(5). https://doi.org/10.1007/s00192-020-04329-x.

113. Yamanishi, T., Kaga, K., Fuse, M., Shibata, C., Kamai, T., & Uchiyama, T. (2015). The role of muscarinic receptor subtypes on carbachol-induced contraction of normal human detrusor and overactive detrusor associated with benign prostatic hyperplasia. *Journal of Pharmacological Sciences, 128*(2), 65–70. https://doi.org/10.1016/j.jphs.2015.05.005.

114. Yamanishi, T., Kaga, K., Sakata, K., et al. (2020). A randomized controlled study of the efficacy of tadalafil monotherapy versus combination of tadalafil and mirabegron for the treatment of persistent overactive bladder symptoms in men presenting with lower urinary tract symptoms (CONTACT Study). *Neurourology and Urodynamics, 39*(2), 804–812. https://doi.org/10.1002/nau.24285.

115. Yonguc, T., Sefik, E., Inci, I., et al. (2020). Randomized, controlled trial of fesoterodine fumarate for overactive bladder in Parkinson's disease. *World Journal of Urology, 38*(8), 2013–2019. https://doi.org/10.1007/s00345-019-02981-7.

116. Yoshida, M., Takeda, M., Gotoh, M., et al. (2020). Efficacy of vibegron, a novel β3-adrenoreceptor agonist, on severe urgency urinary incontinence related to overactive bladder: Post hoc analysis of a randomized, placebo-controlled, double-blind, comparative Phase 3 study. *BJU International, 125*(5), 709–717. https://doi.org/10.1111/bju.15020.

Chapter 10

LOWER URINARY TRACT DISORDERS DUE TO ADVERSE DRUG REACTIONS

Contents

Introduction

Being safe and effective is pharmacotherapy's main objective. Demonstrating an acceptable risk-benefit ratio for the medications that are currently on the pharmaceutical market is necessary to achieve this goal. This does not, however, imply that drug use is impervious to adverse effects, which can appear in a variety of organs and systems, including the kidneys and urinary tract. Consequently, drug-induced disturbances may be the cause of lower urinary tract disorders.

The term "side effect of the drug," also known as "adverse drug reaction" is defined in different ways. The World Health Organization (WHO) defines an adverse drug reaction (ADR) as "a response to a medicine which is noxious and unintended, and which occurs at doses normally used in man."

Another commonly accepted definition of an ADR is that of Ivor Ralph Edwards: "an appreciably harmful or unpleasant reaction, caused by an intervention related to the use of a medicinal product, which predicts hazard from future administration and warrants prevention or specific treatment, or the alteration of the dosage regimen, or the withdrawal of the product." A similar characterization of an ADR was given by Schatz and Weber: "an unwanted, undesirable effect of a medication that occurs during usual clinical use." Thus, researchers define the concept of an adverse drug reaction differently, and various definitions highlight different aspects of this phenomenon. However, the common denominator of all definitions of an ADR is the direct causal relationship between the use of the medicine and the disorder present. The causes and nature of adverse drug events are often complex and multifactorial.

Because ADRs are thought to be a cause of unplanned hospital admissions that may continue after hospital discharge, their prevalence is a serious clinical issue. Despite numerous preventative measures, it is estimated that 5–10% of patients experience an ADR at admission, during admission, or after discharge. Patients who are older, have a higher baseline pathophysiological burden, and are receiving polypharmacotherapy are more likely to experience adverse reactions. Approximately 11.0% of older adults experience ADRs. The percentage of ADRs that result in an urgent hospital stay is 3.3%. To sum up, adverse drug reactions (ADRs) are thought to be the most prevalent iatrogenic illness, complicating between 5% and 15% of therapeutic drug courses.

Agents used to treat cardiovascular disorders (beta-adrenergic blocking agents, diuretics, and angiotensin-converting enzyme inhibitors); antiplatelets; warfarin and other anticoagulants; antipsychotic agents; non-opioid and opioid analgesics; cytotoxics; immunosuppressants; antidiabetics; and antibiotics are among the drug classes thought to be most frequently linked to adverse drug reactions (ADRs).

Gastrointestinal disturbances (including loss of appetite, nausea, abdominal pain, bloating sensation, constipation, and diarrhea) are common types of adverse drug reactions (ADRs) because many medications are administered via the per os route and pass through the digestive tract. Adverse drug reactions are also common in a variety of dermatological disorders. Adverse drug reactions, however, have the potential to appear in any system or organ. Drug-induced disruptions of the urinary system are among the 21 anatomical and physiological areas that the CIOMS report identifies for ADR reporting purposes.

Around 11 of the drug-related disturbances of the urinary system (SOC1300) identified in this report were found to primarily affect the kidneys and urinary tract: renal tubular disorder, kidney vasculitis, glomerular vasomotor disorder, acute or chronic glomerulonephritis, acute or chronic nephritis interstitial, nephropathy analgesic, nephropathy toxic, nephrotic syndrome, acute kidney failure, kidney tubular disorder, and urinary retention (UR).

Certain disturbances like acute tubular necrosis and glomerulonephritis can have severe effects on the kidneys, while others may affect the kidneys as part of a larger systemic disorder like vasculitis. Drugs can lead to kidney dysfunction through various mechanisms such as pre-kidney effects, obstructive uropathy, allergic or immunological damage, and direct nephrotoxicity. These mechanisms can cause issues like water or electrolyte loss, tubular blockage, inflammation, and acute kidney damage.

Many lower urinary tract disorders besides UR are not included in the list of drug-induced urinary tract disorders mentioned above, but the report does note that drugs can also have negative effects on the bladder or urothelium, such as hemorrhagic cystitis or urinary tract carcinoma.

Using the search terms "adverse drug reactions" and "lower urinary tract" or "urological," the PubMed database searches, conducted in June 2023 and restricted to English-language records from the previous 10 years, produced 170 and 576 results, respectively. Simultaneously, a far greater number of publications were discovered when searching the PubMed database for records on adverse drug reactions in the gastroenterology or dermatology fields. (Dobrek et al, 2023)

Orientation and Directional Terms

Term	Definition	Illustration
Adverse drug reaction (ADR)	An adverse drug reaction (ADR) can be defined as 'an appreciably harmful or unpleasant reaction resulting from an intervention related to the use of a medicinal product; adverse effects usually predict hazard from future administration and warrant prevention, or specific treatment, or alteration of the dosage regimen, or withdrawal of the product'.	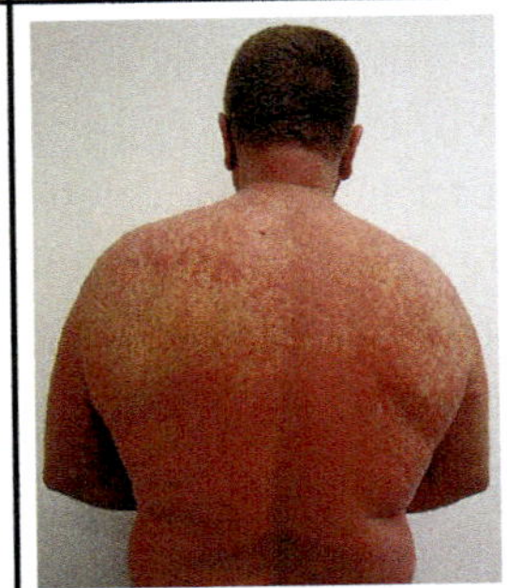
Human urinary system	The human urinary system, also known as the urinary tract or renal system, consists of the kidneys, ureters, bladder, and the urethra. The purpose of the urinary system is to eliminate waste from the body, regulate blood volume and blood pressure, control levels of electrolytes and metabolites, and regulate blood pH.	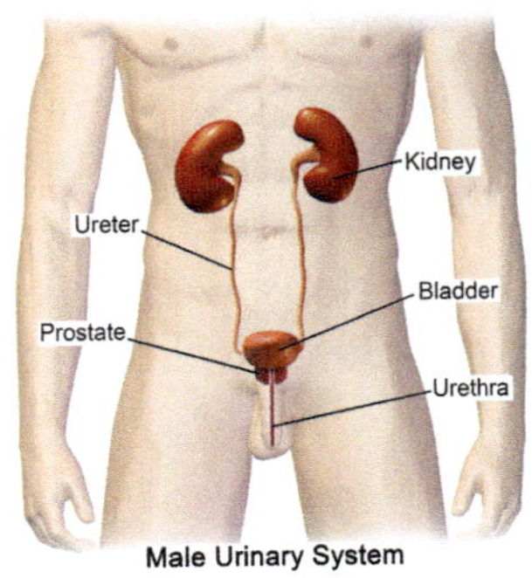
Periaqueductal gray (PAG),	The periaqueductal gray (PAG), also known as the central gray, is a brain region that plays a critical role in autonomic function, motivated behavior and behavioural responses to threatening stimuli. PAG is also the primary control center for descending pain modulation. It has enkephalin-producing cells that suppress pain.	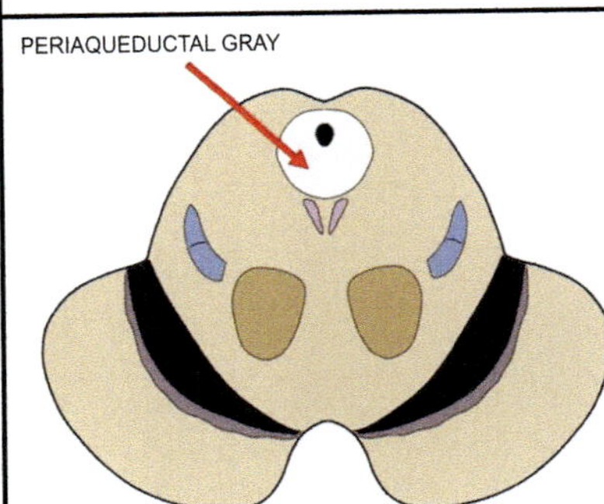
Benzodiazepines	Benzodiazepines are a class of medications that slow down activity in your brain and nervous system. They're most often used for treating anxiety and related mental health conditions, as well as brain-related conditions like seizures. These medications are tightly regulated and are only available with a prescription.	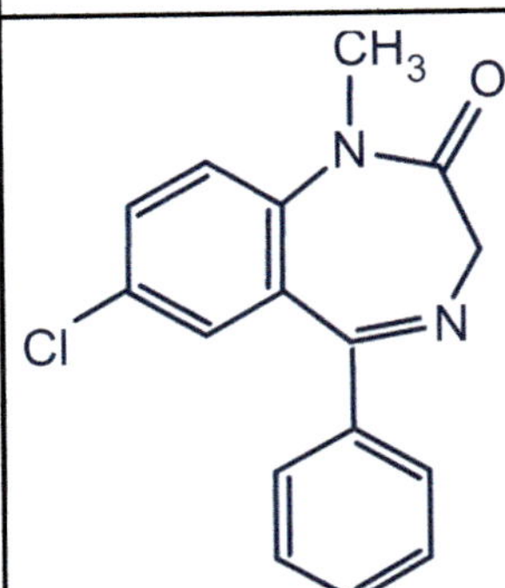

10.1. Urinary Retention or Urinary Incontinence

Urine excretion of drugs and their metabolites, along with metabolic wastes, is the primary role of the kidneys and urinary tract. This is a vital bodily function. Complex peripheral neural pathways that are regulated by cell groups in the brain, brainstem, and spinal cord govern the voiding process. The stages of micturition, which include bladder emptying and urinary outlet (which is made up of the bladder neck, urethra, and urethral sphincters), and the storage of urine inside the bladder ("filling") are complementary. The distention of the bladder that permits bladder filling is the basis for the storage reflex that preserves continence. In adults, the bladder can typically hold 300–400 mL. Additionally, the voluntary contraction of the external urethral sphincter and the sympathetic contraction of the inner urethral sphincter define the filling phase.

Afferent activity is triggered during bladder filling by the smooth muscle and urothelium's distention. The pelvic (parasympathetic nervous system) and hypogastric (sympathetic nervous system) carry the afferents from stretch and volume receptors found at myelinated Aδ sensory fibers, while the pudendal (somatic nervous system) and hypogastric nerves transmit impulses from the urethra and neck of the bladder. Furthermore, in certain ailments like hyperactive bladder or UTIs, unmyelinated C-sensory fibers are involved in afferent activity. These fibers have a high mechanical threshold in a physiological state, but they react to numerous neurotransmitters and other inflammatory mediators. These neuromodulators cause symptoms like urgency, frequent urination, and urinary incontinence (UI) by lowering the threshold for bladder contraction. The periaqueductal gray (PAG) matter and pontine micturition center (PMC; Barrington's nucleus) are located in the medial dorsal pons, either adjacent to or encompassing the lateral dorsal tegmental nucleus and locus coeruleus. The afferent signals are transmitted to the spinal cord and subsequently travel via the spinothalamic tract. The PAG's function in bladder function regulation includes connections with higher brain regions involved in decision-making and the start of urination, in addition to downstream connections.

Via the PAG matter, the higher brain centers responsible for micturition interact with the PMC to either trigger or inhibit the voiding reflex. When the bladder distends, the afferent signal from the bladder's stretch receptors reaches the pons, which then alerts the brain. The sensation of a full bladder or the urge to urinate is the outcome of this afferent signal. The higher brain makes the decision about when to trigger the voiding reflex (prefrontal cortex and anterior cingulate). The PAG matter is primarily used by the higher brain to transmit reciprocal inhibitory signals, which suppress PMC. It eliminates the urge to urinate and permits postponing urination until a time and location that are acceptable in society. The micturition reflex is activated when the suppression of PMC vanishes, marking the proper moment and location to start voiding. In addition to somatic fibers, the efferent pathways also involve parasympathetic and sympathetic fibers. The hypogastric nerve contains sympathetic fibers that connect to the base of the bladder and the urethra. These fibers originate from the T_{11}-L_2 spinal segments. Noradrenaline, which is released from the postganglionic sympathetic terminals, acts on the alpha-1 adrenergic receptors in the proximal urethra, which causes it to contract, and on the beta-3 adrenergic receptors in the bladder, which helps to relax the detrusor muscle during the bladder's filling phase. The S_2–S_4 spinal segments are the source of the parasympathetic preganglionic fibers, which pass through the pelvic nerves and attach to the bladder wall. Acetylcholine is released from parasympathetic terminals during bladder emptying, causing an increase in parasympathetic efferent drive. The result is the activation of M_1–M_3 muscarinic receptors. The M_3 muscarinic receptor is the most common one, and when it is activated, the bladder contracts. M_2 receptor activation inhibits detrusor relaxation by reducing sympathetic activity, whereas M_1 receptors seem to promote additional acetylcholine release. The detrusor response to M_3 receptor activation is improved as a result. Additionally, the external urethral sphincter's striated muscles are linked to the somatic motor nerves from the S_2–S_4 motor neurones via nicotinic receptors, which strengthens the sphincter's contraction. This process occurs in the pudendal nerves. The striated muscle that makes up the external sphincter is comparable to skeletal muscle that is controlled voluntarily. Figure 10.1 illustrates how the micturition reflex is organized.

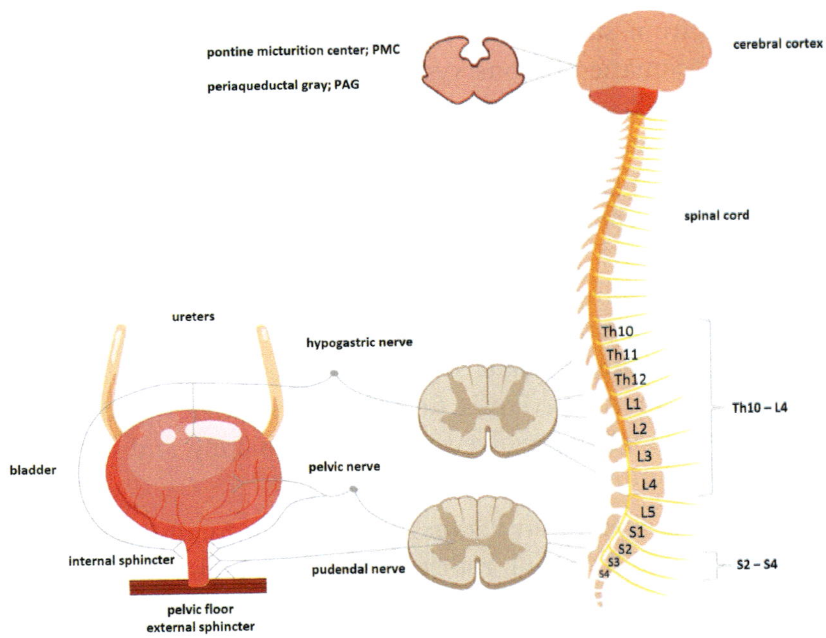

Figure 10.1. *The neurological control of the lower urinary tract.*

Source: Dobrek L. Lower Urinary Tract Disorders as Adverse Drug Reactions-A Literature Review. Pharmaceuticals (Basel). 2023 Jul 20;16(7):1031. doi: 10.3390/ph16071031. PMID: 37513941; PMCID: PMC10383968.

Therefore, it follows that the proper coordination of the bladder's contraction and relaxation—that is, the bladder outlet and bladder contraction—coordinated by the central nervous system is necessary for the expulsion of urine. Incontinence and uremia are both classified as "lower urinary tract symptoms," or LUTS, which includes voiding, storage, and post-voiding symptoms. The phrases "failure to store" and "failure to empty" have been replaced with LUTS.

Urinary retention (UR) is caused by an inefficient bladder emptying mechanism. It is a clinical condition that can be either chronic or acute. The incapacity to urinate and a sudden onset linked to suprapubic pain are characteristics of acute urinary retention. On the other hand, since the body may still leak small amounts of urine, chronic UR is not linked to pain. Paradoxically, after passing the critical urine volume and intravesical pressure, patients with chronic UR may exhibit UI symptoms. Men are more likely than women to have UR, and the condition is becoming more common as people age. Many disturbances can cause urinary reflux (UR), but the most common one is a bladder outflow obstruction (this can be caused by tumors, blood clots, calculi, benign prostatic hyperplasia, calculi, prostate carcinoma, or stones, strictures, diverticulum, posterior urethral valves, surgery, at the bladder level). Acute pain, neurogenic factors (also known as "neurogenic bladder") in the context of focal lesions (such as stroke, tumors, traumatic spinal cord injuries), disseminated lesions (such as Parkinson's disease, brain trauma, multiple sclerosis), peripheral neuropathies (such as diabetes mellitus), and idiopathic myogenic factors that interrupt ion storage and exchange, excitation-contraction coupling, calcium storage, and energy generation are some of the other etiological factors of UR. In clinical practice, post-operative complications and recumbency are two other common causes of UR. It should be noted at this point that several terms, including detrusor areflexia, hypotonic bladder, detrusor failure, and chronic retention, have been proposed to describe a dysfunctional bladder. The phrase "underactive bladder; UAB," which is characterized by detrusor underactivity (DU) and comparable to overactive bladder (OAB) and detrusor overactivity, has also been introduced to describe chronic UR. The International Continence Society defines DU as a contraction of reduced strength and/or duration that results in prolonged bladder emptying within a normal time span, whereas UAB is defined as a complex symptom suggesting DU, characterized by prolonged urination time with or without a sensation of incomplete bladder emptying, typically with hesitancy, reduced sensation on filling, and a slow stream.

Given the above-described intricate mechanism of voiding, classes of drugs that can obstruct this process and cause UR or UI can be identified. Opioid drugs (by affecting opioid receptors); non-opioid analgesics (by affecting tachykinin receptors); benzodiazepines (by affecting GABA receptors); and serotonin reuptake inhibitors (by potentiating serotonin-dependent increased sympathetic activity that increases bladder compliance) all disrupt the mutual afferent and efferent signalling between the bladder and urethra and the central nervous system, which contributes to urine retention. Conversely, medications known as anticholinergics that block muscarinic receptors affect the bladder's cholinergic-mediated contractility. Similarly, calcium channel blockers directly affect smooth muscle by inhibiting calcium channels, which in turn impairs bladder contractility. Alpha-1 adrenergic receptor stimulation can also cause drug-induced urine retention by contracting the internal urethral sphincter and impairing urine outflow. Figure 10.2 provides a schematic representation of the aforementioned mechanisms that may contribute to drug-induced urinary retention.

Considering the autonomic regulation of urination, it can be inferred that medications that impact the reciprocal transmission of signals between the central nervous system and the lower urinary tract, such as those that block the parasympathetic system (muscarinic M_3 receptor antagonists) or activate the sympathetic nervous system (alpha-1 receptor agonists), may impede the micturition process and consequently lead to drug-induced UR. It should be noted that the majority of the medications listed above are also used to treat bladder overactivity, which is the opposite condition of UR. Table 10.1 lists the medications that have a higher chance of causing UR along with the specific mechanisms that lead to this disorder.

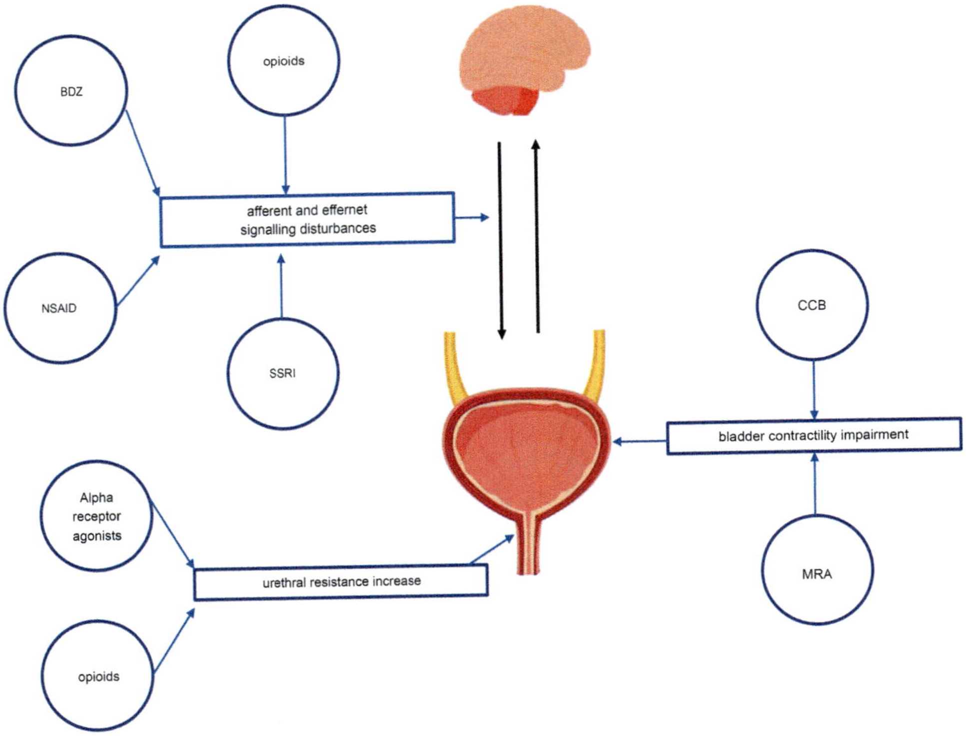

Figure 10.2. *The main mechanisms contributing to potential drug-induced urinary retention (BDZ–benzodiazepines; NSAID–non-steroidal anti-inflammatory drugs; SSRI–selective serotonin reuptake inhibitors; CCB–calcium channel blockers, MRA–muscarinic receptor antagonists (anticholinergics).*

Source: Dobrek L. Lower Urinary Tract Disorders as Adverse Drug Reactions-A Literature Review. Pharmaceuticals (Basel). 2023 Jul 20;16(7):1031. doi: 10.3390/ph16071031. PMID: 37513941; PMCID: PMC10383968.

Table 10.1. *Drugs Associated With an Increased Risk of Urinary Retention*

Drug Class		**Examples**	**Postulated Mechanism Contributing to Urinary Retention**
Drugs with anticholinergic effects–muscarinic receptor antagonists (MRA)	Tricyclic antidepressants	Amitriptyline, Imipramine, Clomipramine, Nortriptyline	Drugs with antimuscarinic effect can cause or exacerbate urinary retention due to the failure of cholinergic-mediated bladder contraction (especially in patients with a pre-existing bladder outlet obstruction, e.g., benign prostate hyperplasia).
	Classic antipsychotics	Thioridazine, Chlorpromazine, Chlorprothixene, Risperidone, Clozapine	

	H1-antihistamines (1st generation)	Chlorpheniramine, Triprolidine Cyproheptadine, Clemastine, Dimenhydrinate, Diphenhydramine, Doxylamine	
	Antispasmodics	Dicyclomine, Propantheline, Oxybutynin	
	Antiparkinsonian agents	Benzatropine, Orphenadrine, Procyclidine	
	Antiarrhythmic drugs class I	Disopyramide, Flecainide	
	Antimuscarinic bronchodilators	Ipratropium, Tiotropium, Glycopyrronium	
	Anticholinergic drugs used to treat overactive bladder	Oxybutynin, Fesoterodine, Solifenacin, Trospium, Tolterodine	
Premedication drugs (cholinolytics)		Atropine, Hyoscine	
Anesthetics		Bupivacaine, Propofol, Ketamine, General anesthetics of duration greater than 60 min	Inhibitory effects on the contraction of the bladder (inhibition of micturition reflex).
Opioids		Morphine, Pethidine, Pentazocine, Fentanyl	Urinary retention occurs due to the mu-receptor-mediated blockade of the sensory input from the bladder and the volume-evoked micturition reflex that results in decreasing the usual sensation of bladder fullness and bladder overdistention, and partially the anticholinergic effect of opioids. In addition, opioids can increase bladder sphincter tone due to excessive sympathetic stimulation, resulting in a bladder outlet restraint.

Non-steroidal anti-inflammatory drugs		Diclofenac, Ketoprofen	Impairment of the direct prostaglandin-induced bladder contractility and by the impairment of tachykinins stimulating neurokinin receptors on afferent nerves and detrusor smooth muscle.
Benzodiazepines		Diazepam, Clonazepam	Probably caused by detrusor muscle relaxation
Selective serotonin reuptake inhibitors (SSRI)		Fluoxetine, Sertraline, Citalopram	Serotonin is an important neurotransmitter that facilitates storage by increasing sympathetic activity and inhibiting parasympathetic control over voiding; thus, SSRI may cause an increase in the post-voiding residual volume (the volume of urine left in the bladder at the end of micturition).
Calcium channel blockers (CCB)		NDHP blockers: Diltiazem and Verapamil DHP blockers: Amlodipine and Nifedipine (the highly vascular selective DHP Felodipine and Lercanidipine seem to have less effect on micturition	Reduce bladder smooth muscle contractility via the inhibition of the calcium influx.
Alpha-1-agonists		Methoxamine, Phenylephrine, Ethylephrine	Binding to the alpha-1A/D adrenergic receptors of the internal urethral sphincter resulting in a higher tone of the internal sphincter.
Non-selective alpha-agonists		Pseudoephedrine (e.g., found in many over-the-counter cold remedies)	

Source: Dobrek L. Lower Urinary Tract Disorders as Adverse Drug Reactions-A Literature Review. Pharmaceuticals (Basel). 2023 Jul 20;16(7):1031. doi: 10.3390/ph16071031. PMID: 37513941; PMCID: PMC10383968.

UI is the opposite disorder of UR. Urine loss that is not voluntary is one of the symptoms of this condition. Although UI is typically diagnosed in patients over 40 and worsens with age, it can also be diagnosed in children and may go away with growth. UI is thought to primarily affect women. According to the estimates, the prevalence of UI is roughly 19% in women under 45 and reaches approximately 29% in women who are 80 years of age or older. Despite the fact that UI primarily affects women, a sizable portion of men also experience UI. It has been reported that the incidence rate of UI rises with age, affecting 12–17% of males. In addition to age, other risk factors include diabetes, smoking, obesity, parity, and hysterectomy. It is possible to distinguish between acute, frequently transitory UI and chronic UI. Transient UI appears out of the blue, lasts for less than six months, and goes away when the underlying illness gets better. There are four primary types of incontinence that can be identified based on the pathomechanism: stress, urge, mixed, and overflow forms. Stress urinary incontinence (UI) is primarily seen in females and is caused by weaker bladder sphincteric mechanisms that are not strong enough to completely stop urine leaks. This type of UI is seen when someone sneezes, coughs, or exhibits other symptoms that are linked to elevated abdominal pressure. Urine leaks uncontrollably when the increased abdominal pressure surpasses the intravesical pressure and there is insufficient bladder outlet and sphincter resistance. Both genders are affected by urge UI, which is characterized by an overwhelming urge to urinate that is impossible to put off because of involuntary detrusor contractions that occur when the bladder fills. A hybrid user interface (UI) combines the two mechanisms mentioned above. The main symptom of overflow urinary integument (UI) in men is overfilling of the bladder that cannot be emptied. Additionally, there is a primary idiopathic OAB, which is a functional lower urinary tract disease. This clinical entity is characterized by nocturia, increased daily frequency of voiding episodes, urinary urgency with or without UI, and nocturia. Some pathomechanisms have been proposed to explain the development of OAB in the absence of a clear and obvious pathology. These include primary, myogenic detrusor overactivity, which has been observed in urodynamic recordings; dysfunction of the afferent arm of the micturition reflex, which lowers the threshold of afferent fiber excitation); and dysfunction at the level of the higher central nervous system (CNS), which is responsible for the perception of the bladder filling phase.

UI may be the only symptom of an underlying illness that affects the nervous system and the autonomic regulation of urination, such as neuropathies, Parkinson's disease, Alzheimer's disease, multiple sclerosis, stroke, or myelomeningoceles. Furthermore, benign prostatic hyperplasia, prostate cancer, and associated surgery or radiation therapy are some of the specific causes of male UI.

The collective term for these forms of UI is incontinence after prostate treatment (IPT). It is important to consider that UI may also result from the administration of certain medications when making a differential diagnosis. The basic mechanism of drug-induced UI involves increasing intravesical pressure or lowering bladder outlet resistance to impair the bladder storage phase. The intrabladder filling pressure during filling is still less than the urethral and sphincter's resistance under physiological conditions. Therefore, the time between micturitions depends critically on the functioning of the bladder's compliance and sphincter mechanisms; any malfunction affecting these systems may cause the involuntary loss of urine. Many medications have been directly linked to disruptions of the storage phase, which are caused by a general sphincter tone weakening that contributes to stress UI, e.g. adrenergic alpha receptor antagonists or antipsychotics (through intricate interactions with the muscarinic, serotonin, GABA, and central and peripheral adrenergic receptors).

Additionally, some medications cause complex CNS actions or direct stimulation of muscarinic receptors in the bladder, resulting in uninhibited bladder contraction activity (urge UI). Additionally, UI may be indirectly conditioned through decreased bladder emptying, which results in overdistention of the bladder (overflow UI). Therefore, medications that have been identified as potential causes of UR may also subsequently cause UI. The primary mechanisms causing urine incontinence (UI) are illustrated in Figure 10.3, along with a list of the primary drug classes for each type of UI (Dobrek et al, 2023).

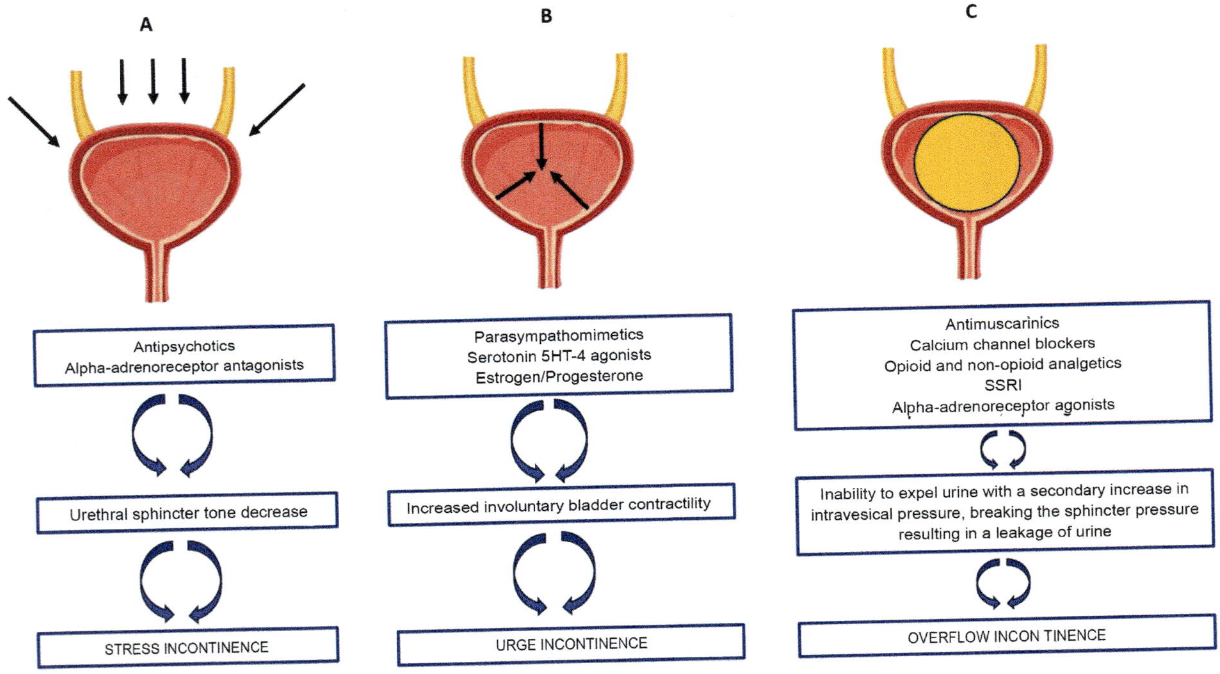

Figure 10.3. *The main types of urinary incontinence based on the prevailing pathomechanism, along with listing the most important classes of drugs contributing to the development of urinary incontinence (SSRI–selective serotonin reuptake inhibitors). The arrows in panel (**A**) show the increase in intra-abdominal pressure; the arrows in the panel (**B**) show the spontaneous increase in bladder contractile activity; panel (**C**) shows the bladder overfilling with urine.*

Source: Dobrek L. Lower Urinary Tract Disorders as Adverse Drug Reactions-A Literature Review. Pharmaceuticals (Basel). 2023 Jul 20;16(7):1031. doi: 10.3390/ph16071031. PMID: 37513941; PMCID: PMC10383968.

Several drug classes have the potential to cause UI, based on the pathophysiological principles previously discussed. Only a few classes of drugs have strong evidence of drug-induced UI, and there is still little and unclear information regarding the connection between the administration of many drugs and UI. Furthermore, it should be mentioned that the medications mentioned in the previous paragraph that cause UR may also result in overflow incontinence. It's also important to remember that diuretics can cause excessive urine production, which can result in UI. Table 10.2 contains a list of medications that are more likely to result in UI.

Table 10.2. *Drugs Associated With an Increased Risk of Urinary Incontinence*

Drug Class	Examples	Postulated Mechanism Contributing to Urinary Incontinence
Antipsychotics	Chlorpromazine, Thioridazine, Chlorprothixene, Trifluoperazine, Fluphenazine, Haloperidol	Stress urinary incontinence: These drugs decrease urethral sphincter tone (e.g., via the inhibition of alpha-adrenoreceptors or as a result of a complex action on the central and peripheral serotonin or muscarinic or GABA receptors); thus, situations related to increased intra-abdominal pressure may result in a breakdown of the sphincter pressure and the possibility of urine leakage.
Alpha-adrenoreceptor antagonists	Prazosin, Doxazosin, Terazosin, Phenoxybenzamine, Phentolamine	
Benzodiazepines and non-benzodiazepine sedatives	Diazepam, Zopiclone, Zolpidem	
Other drugs	Reserpine, Misoprostol, Urapidil	
Parasympathomimetic (direct and indirect)	Acetylcholine esterase inhibitors	Urge urinary incontinence: These drugs may increase involuntary detrusor contractility during the storage phase of the bladder, resulting from the stimulation of muscarinic receptors or as a result of a complex action on other central and peripheral receptors (e.g., serotonin ones) or estrogen/progesterone receptors located in the urethra, vesical triangle, sacrouterine ligament, levator ani muscles and pubocervical fascia.
Antidepressants	Amitriptyline, Nortriptyline, Desimipramine	
Serotonin 5-HT4 receptor agonists	Cisapride, Tegaserod, Prucalopride	
Hormone replacement therapy	Estrogen/Progesterone preparations	
Drugs listed in Table 10.1 (e.g., antimuscarinics, antihistamines, antiparkinsonian agents, beta-adrenergic agonists, calcium channels blockers, opioids, sedatives)		Overflow urinary incontinence: These drugs contribute to an inability to expel urine and consequently, a secondary increase in intravesical pressure, breaking the sphincter pressure and causing a leakage of urine. Angiotensin receptor blockade also decreases both detrusor contractility and urethral sphincter tone, leading to increased stress urinary incontinence, which may be worsened by a cough related to the use of these drugs.
Angiotensin-converting enzyme inhibitors/ Angiotensin receptor antagonists	Benazepril, Captopril, Enalapril, Perindopril, Quinapril	

Miscellaneous	Alcohol, Caffeine, Diuretics	These compounds contribute to excessive urine production by inhibiting the reabsorption of electrolytes and water from primary urine or by enhancing glomerular filtration. Thus, they cause the bladder to fill faster and increase the frequency of urination.

Source: Dobrek L. Lower Urinary Tract Disorders as Adverse Drug Reactions-A Literature Review. Pharmaceuticals (Basel). 2023 Jul 20;16(7):1031. doi: 10.3390/ph16071031. PMID: 37513941; PMCID: PMC10383968.

10.2. Urinary Tract Infections

An infection of the lower urinary tract (urethra and bladder) is known as an uncomplicated urinary tract infection (UTI). It occurs in patients who do not have structural abnormalities or comorbidities, such as diabetes, immunocompromised states, pregnancy, kidney transplants, urinary catheter use, or other conditions that could make the infection more complicated to treat. It is also referred to as lower UTI or cystitis, and its typical symptoms include dysuria, suprapubic discomfort, urgency, and frequency of urination. Enteric coliforms, which normally reside in the periurethral vaginal introitus, are the usual cause of UTIs. The majority of UTIs are caused by *Escherichia coli*, which is followed in etiology by Klebsiella and additional organisms (Proteus, Enterobacter, and Enterococcus). A simple UTI affects the bladder and begins with bacterial invasion of the mucosal wall through the use of adhesins on the surface of the bacteria that enable them to adhere to the urothelial mucosal surface. Moreover, a short urethra facilitates the uropathogen's entry into the urinary tract, which explains why UTIs are noticeably more common in women.

According to estimates, between 40 and 60% of women will experience a UTI episode at some point in their lives. This implies that women experience UTIs four times more frequently than men do. Further complications from a UTI can include developing urinary calculi, urinary infection (UI), chronic prostatitis, and problems with the upper urinary tract (pyelonephritis, kidney abscess, kidney failure). The pathophysiology of infectious UTI is covered in some papers in this field and is outside the purview of this chapter. Nonetheless, the patient's medication regimen may also contribute to the development of a UTI.

Thus, urological manifestations of adverse drug reactions may include urinary tract infections. Because they prevent glucose from the urine from being reabsorbed, gliflozins (inhibitors of kidney sodium-glucose co-transporters, SGLT2) are among the drug classes with the most research on their impact on the onset of UTIs. This leads to glycosuria, which is the root cause of ascending urinary and genital tract infections that are urogenic. Other medications, though, also increase the risk of developing UTIs.

The other primary mechanisms underlying a drug-induced UTI are immunodeficiency in the lower urinary tract (caused by systemically or topically acting immunosuppressive and cytotoxic drugs); impairment of the neurogenic control of the bladder; and impairment of micturition and bladder emptying (caused by the cholinolytic activity or the increase in bladder outlet resistance evoked by the aforementioned drugs). (Dobrek et al, 2023). Figure 10.4 provides a summary of them.

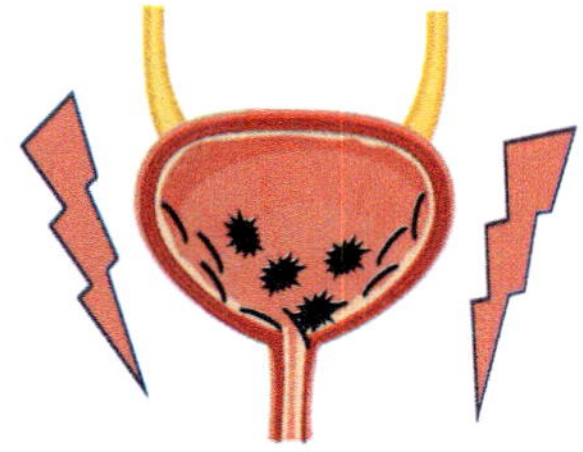

Figure 10.4. *The main drug-related mechanisms contributing to urinary tract infection development. "Lightning bolts" indicate the development of inflammation; uropathogens colonizing the bladder are marked in black.*

Source: Dobrek L. Lower Urinary Tract Disorders as Adverse Drug Reactions-A Literature Review. Pharmaceuticals (Basel). 2023 Jul 20;16(7):1031. doi: 10.3390/ph16071031. PMID: 37513941; PMCID: PMC10383968.

Additionally, the intensification and promotion of the bacterial colonization of urine (due to medications that intensify glycosuria) as well as urine stagnation and retention secondary to urinary stone formation in the urinary tract are complementary mechanisms that contribute to urinary tract infections. Table 10.3 lists the medications that may result in UTIs.

Table 10.3. *Drugs Associated with an Increased Risk of Urinary Tract Infection Development*

Drug Class	Examples	Postulated Mechanism Contributing to Urinary Tract Infections
Gliflozins–inhibitors of kidney sodium-glucose transport proteins 2 (SGLT2)	Canagliflozin, Dapagliflozin, Empagliflozin	Gliflozins cause glycosuria, with subsequent bacterial colonization of the urinary tract and genital area.
Immunosuppressive agents	Glucocorticoids, Azathioprine, Cyclosporin A, Sirolimus–rapamycin, Mycophenolate mofetil	These drugs cause the impairment of local and systemic immune mechanisms, thereby facilitating bacterial colonization.
Drugs with anticholinergic effects listed in Table 10.1 (e.g., antimuscarinics, antihistamines, antiparkinsonian agents, beta-adrenergic agonists, calcium channels blockers, opioids, sedatives)		These drugs affect the micturition by inhibiting the contractile activity of the bladder, dependent on the activation of muscarinic receptors, resulting in urinary retention in the bladder, which facilitates the bacterial colonization of the bladder and the reduced evacuation of bacteria along with the urine stream.

Benzodiazepines, Calcium channel antagonists, Opioids, and Non-steroidal anti-inflammatory drugs (NSAIDs) are listed in Table 10.2.		These drugs may impair micturition through detrusor muscle relaxation and contribute to voiding reflex disturbances, either on a spinal or supraspinal level, resulting in reducing and delaying the emptying of the bladder, which provides better conditions for bacterial colonization.
Miscellaneous	Antibacterial agents (Sulphonamides, Ciprofloxacin, Ampicillin), Antacids, Calcium, Vitamin D and/or C, Laxatives, Loop diuretics (Furosemide), Anhydrase inhibitors (Acetazolamide), Xanthine oxidase inhibitors (Allopurinol)	These drugs or their metabolites may precipitate in the urinary tract and/or these drugs change the pH of the urine, contributing to the crystallization of endogenous lithogenic substances in the urinary tract, thereby enabling the formation of urinary stones.

Source: Dobrek L. Lower Urinary Tract Disorders as Adverse Drug Reactions-A Literature Review. Pharmaceuticals (Basel). 2023 Jul 20;16(7):1031. doi: 10.3390/ph16071031. PMID: 37513941; PMCID: PMC10383968.

Furthermore, cystitis can manifest as severe hemorrhagic bladder damage and be non-infectious. Therefore, medications that result in the development of hemorrhagic cystitis (HC), a complication of chemical cystitis (CC), should receive particular attention. A variety of chemical agents can cause CC, including immunologic or chemotherapeutic medications like ifosfamide or cyclophosphamide (oxazophosphorine compounds), mitomycin C, ketamine, tiaprofenic acid, danazol, or agents applied intravenously (e.g., diluted gentian violet is used to assess bladder injury after herniorrhaphy, BCG as prophylactic immunotherapy for intermediate or high-risk non-muscle-invasive bladder cancer, or transurethral resection of bladder tumors). Other forms of cystitis also present with symptoms similar to those of CC/HC, including suprapubic pain, dysuria, frequency, urgency, and microscopic or macroscopic hematuria. The hepatic byproduct acrolein, which is produced when oxazaphosphorines are metabolized, is linked to the pathophysiology of HC caused by cyclophosphamide and ifosfamide. The kidneys filter acrolein, which then builds up in the bladder where it causes a complex reaction with pyroptotic effects in the urothelium, exposing the blood vessels and muscularis mucosa and causing ulceration. Additionally, acrolein can damage DNA structure and break down proteins, which produces a metabolite that triggers apoptosis. Oxazaphosphorine-induced hyperproduction of highly reactive oxygen and nitrogen-free radicals as well as the aggravation of oxidative stress constitute a significant part of the pathophysiology of HC. A thorough explanation of the pathophysiology causing HC caused by oxazaphosphine is available in some of the reviews related to this topic. Ketamine is a dissociative anesthetic and psychotomimetic drug that is an antagonist of the N-Methyl-D-aspartate receptor. Significant ketamine-induced cystitis (KIC), which presents with LUTS and includes frequent urination, urgency, and excruciating bladder pain, can result from long-term ketamine abuse. A contracted bladder, thickening of the bladder wall, mucosal bleeding in the bladder, and ureteral stricture with hydronephrosis occur as the disease worsens. Ulcerative cystitis with readily bleeding mucosa is a common finding. Manypathomechanisms, including the direct toxic effect of ketamine, the activation of inflammatory cells, the disruption of the bladder-urothelial barrier, the dysregulation of neurotransmission, the overexpression of carcinogenic genes, cell apoptosis, and oxidative stress, are hypothesized to contribute to the pathophysiology of KIC. (Dobrek et al, 2023)

10.3. Urolithiasis

Research shows that the overall prevalence of urolithiasis, also known as nephrolithiasis or kidney stone disease, varies between 1 and 5% in Asia, 5–8% in Europe, 13% in the USA, and even 20% in Middle Eastern countries. Urolithiasis is a relatively common clinical entity. One can differentiate between infectious and non-infectious stones based on their general etiology: those resulting from genetic defects and those brought on by unfavorable drug reactions. Urinary stone formation generally arises from three main disturbances: (1) an excess of certain compounds in the urine that exceeds their solubility in the urine; (2) promoters present concurrently with a lack of inhibitors of precipitation; and (3) abnormalities of the urothelium that allow an attachment and subsequent growth of rising crystals. Urolithiasis has a complicated pathophysiology that is split into the nucleation phase and the crystal growth that follows. The microcrystals carry out the overgrowth in the second step, which is achieved by the aggregation of preformed crystals or secondary nucleation of the crystal on the matrix.

The association and fixation of the crystals in the renal tubule cell lining constitute the last stage. The size, location, and potential presence of a urinary tract infection are the primary determinants of urolithiasis symptomatology. Stones less than 5 mm have the potential to flow through the urinary tract without any problems. The symptoms of kidney stones appear as the stone passes through the urinary tract. The movement of a stone through the urinary tract can cause excruciating cramping pain known as kidney stone pain, which is made worse by ureteral spasm and potential blockage.

In addition to nausea, vomiting, and macro-or at least micro-hematuria, the pain is typically unrelated to one's posture and is frequently accompanied by symptoms of bladder overactivity, such as urgency and frequency of urination. Additional reviews contain a more thorough explanation of the pathophysiology and symptomatology of urolithiasis, which is outside the purview of this chapter.

One can differentiate between infectious and non-infectious stones, those brought on by genetic flaws, and those brought on by unfavorable drug reactions based on general etiology. However, the chemical composition described above can be used to classify five main types of stones: calcium, urate or uric acid, magnesium ammonium phosphate, struvite or urate, cystine, and rare stones (including drug-induced ones).

Two primary types of drug-induced urinary stones can be distinguished based on the main pathomechanism (Figure 10.5).

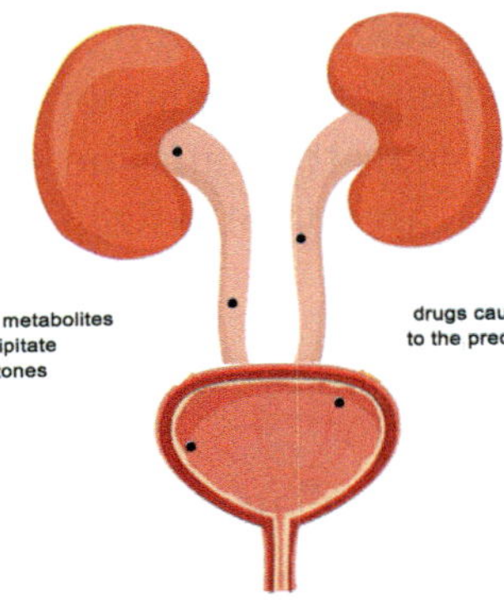

Figure 10.5. *The main mechanisms responsible for the formation of drug-induced urinary stones. The dots represent urinary stones in the lower urinary tract.*

Source: Dobrek L. Lower Urinary Tract Disorders as Adverse Drug Reactions-A Literature Review. Pharmaceuticals (Basel). 2023 Jul 20;16(7):1031. doi: 10.3390/ph16071031. PMID: 37513941; PMCID: PMC10383968.

The first category consists of stones that are primarily made of the drug and/or the metabolites that are released into the urine. These are poorly soluble substances that are primarily eliminated by the kidneys. According to the overall pathophysiology of urolithiasis, these medications may therefore be characterized in supersaturated urine by surpassing the solubility equilibrium. The second category of drug-induced urinary stones is referred to as "metabolic stones" because the use of these medications causes metabolic disruptions that can lead to the crystallization of endogenous lithogenic substances. Numerous medications have the potential to cause the development of urinary stones by altering the pH of urine (to the point where many endogenous substances become less soluble), interfering with the balance and function of crystallization promoters/inhibitors, or alternating the glomerular filtration and tubular secretion/reabsorption of the endogenous substances. Table 10.4 lists the medications that can cause kidney stones to form as a result of drug use. (Dobrek et al, 2023)

Table 10.4. *Drugs Associated with an Increased Risk of Kidney Stone Development*

Drug Class	**Examples**	**Postulated Mechanism Contributing to Kidney Stone Development**
Drug-containing stones		
Sulfonamides	Sulfadiazine, Sulfaguanidine, Sulfamethoxazole, Sulfasalazine	These drugs and their metabolites are poorly soluble in urine; in the case of long-term treatment, they may precipitate in urine.
Aminopenicillins Cephalosporins	Ampicillin, Amoxicillin, Ceftriaxone	

Quinolones	Pipemidic acid, Ciprofloxacin, Norfloxacin	
Other antibacterial drugs	Nitrofurantoin	
Protease inhibitors	Indinavir, Nelfinavir, Atazanavir	
Antacids aluminum hydroxide	Magnesium trisilicate, Aluminum hydroxide	
Miscellaneous	Triamterene, Allopurinol, Ephedrine, Acyclovir, Methotrexate	
Drug-induced "metabolic stones"		
Calcium-containing supplements	Many preparations are commercially available, also as dietary supplements	These drugs enhance intestinal calcium absorption, leading to hypercalcemia and the hypercalciuric state.
Vitamin D-containing supplements		
Loop diuretics	Furosemide	
Anhydrase inhibitors	Acetazolamide, Zonisamide, Topiramate	These drugs inhibit bicarbonate reabsorption and hydrogen ion excretion in proximal tubules, leading to systemic metabolic acidosis, an increase in urinary pH and a decrease in urinary citrates.
Laxative drugs (when abused)	Hyperosmotic or stimulant agents	These drugs, when abused, cause increased gastrointestinal fluid and potassium loss and low urinary output. The potassium depletion contributes to intracellular acidosis, compensated by ammonia genesis enhancement in kidney proximal tubules and increased citrate reabsorption, potentiated by increased expression of the H^+/K^+ activity in the distal tubules.
Corticosteroids	Cortisol	These drugs promote the release of calcium from the bones and lead to the hypercalciuria and hyperphosphaturia state.
Ascorbic acid (vitamin C)	Many preparations are commercially available, also as dietary supplements	The excess of vitamin C is metabolized to form oxalates and it increases the urinary oxalates excretion. Moreover, high doses of vitamin C cause acidification of the urine.

Xanthine oxidase inhibitors	Allopurinol	The drug inhibits the biotransformation of hypoxanthine into xanthine and the final synthesis of uric acid, leading to the formation of xanthine-containing purine stones.
Uricosuric drugs	Benzbromarone, Probenecid	These drugs reduce hyperuricemia by enhancing urinary uric acid excretion, leading to the formation of uric acid-containing purine stones.

Source: Dobrek L. Lower Urinary Tract Disorders as Adverse Drug Reactions-A Literature Review. Pharmaceuticals (Basel). 2023 Jul 20;16(7):1031. doi: 10.3390/ph16071031. PMID: 37513941; PMCID: PMC10383968.

10.4. Erectile Dysfunction

Men can develop erectile dysfunction (ED) for a variety of reasons, including psychological and pathophysiological (diabetes, hypertension, and hyperlipidemia). Drugs are one of the iatrogenic causes of ED, though. Numerous drug-dependent processes have been suggested as possible contributors to the emergence of ED. Among these are an antiandrogenic effect, the development of hyperprolactinemia, a reduction in androgen levels, autonomic innervation disorders, or poor peripheral circulation (Figure 10.6).

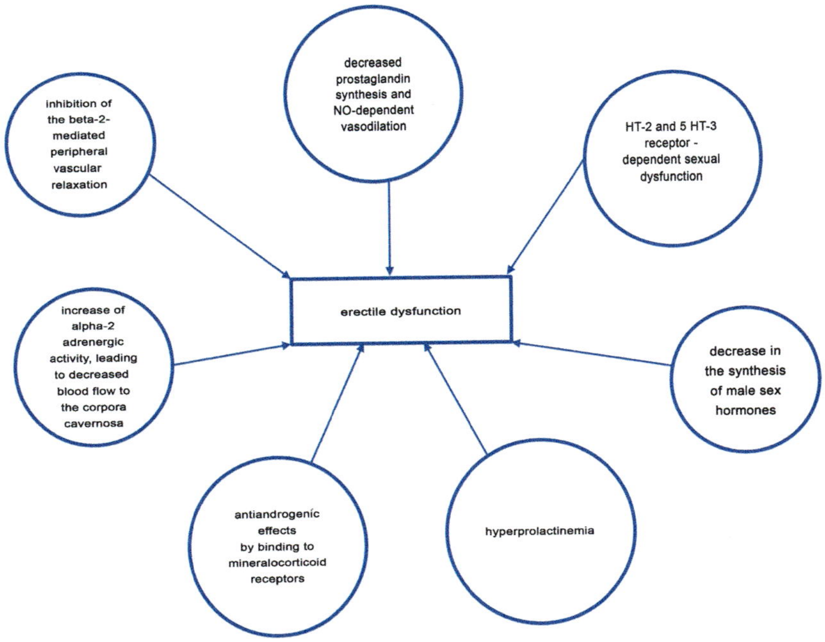
inhibition of the beta-2-mediated peripheral vascular relaxation
decreased prostaglandin synthesis and NO-dependent vasodilation
HT-2 and 5 HT-3 receptor - dependent sexual dysfunction
erectile dysfunction
increase of alpha-2 adrenergic activity, leading to decreased blood flow to the corpora cavernosa
decrease in the synthesis of male sex hormones
antiandrogenic effects by binding to mineralocorticoid receptors
hyperprolactinemia

Figure 10.6. *The main drug-related mechanisms contributing to erectile dysfunction.*

Source: Dobrek L. Lower Urinary Tract Disorders as Adverse Drug Reactions-A Literature Review. Pharmaceuticals (Basel). 2023 Jul 20;16(7):1031. doi: 10.3390/ph16071031. PMID: 37513941; PMCID: PMC10383968.

Various medications can impact sexual functioning, leading to significant consequences for patients' overall quality of life. In men, sexual dysfunction can also hinder the effectiveness of treatment by reducing adherence to medication regimens. This issue is particularly critical when dealing with drugs that need to be administered precisely to achieve the desired pharmacological effects, such as anti-HIV medications, anticonvulsants, and immunosuppressants. Additionally, the true incidence of erectile dysfunction (ED) as an adverse drug reaction is often underestimated due to the embarrassing nature of the condition. ED frequently leads to the premature discontinuation of antidepressant treatment, which ideally should continue for at least 6 months. Studies suggest that approximately 42% of men stop taking antidepressants once they experience sexual side effects. ED is commonly seen in patients with benign prostatic hyperplasia and lower urinary tract symptoms, with over 70% of these patients experiencing sexual dysfunction. Treatment with 5-alpha-reductase inhibitors may worsen this issue. Cardiovascular drugs, antidepressants, certain antipsychotics, antiepileptics, non-steroidal anti-inflammatory drugs, muscle relaxants, and H2-receptor antagonists are among the drug classes known to have the most significant impact on ED. (Dobrek et al, 2023) (Table 10.5)

Table 10.5. *Drugs That May Cause Erectile Dysfunction*

Drug Class	Examples	Postulated Mechanism Contributing to Erectile Dysfunction
Beta-adrenergic antagonists	Non-selective (Propranolol, Sotalol, Oxyprenolol)	Beta-blockers suppress the sympathetic outflow and inhibit the beta-2-mediated peripheral relaxation, indirectly predisposing patients to the stimulation of alpha-adrenergic receptors that promote vasoconstriction. Non-selective beta-antagonists have a higher potential to cause ED resulting from the vasoconstriction within the corpora cavernosa.
	Beta1-selective agents (Metoprolol, Atenolol)	
Thiazide diuretics	Chlorthalidone Hydrochlorothiazide	Thiazides can cause sexual dysfunction through direct effects on vascular smooth muscles or by interfering with catecholamine responsiveness. Moreover, the thiazide-induced sodium loss and lower blood pressure may contribute to increased alpha-2 adrenergic activity, leading to decreased blood flow to the corpora cavernosa.
Potassium-sparing diuretics (aldosterone inhibitors)	Spironolactone, Eplerenone	These agents exhibit strong antiandrogenic effects by binding to mineralocorticoid receptors, causing gynecomastia, mastodynia and ED.
Statins	Simvastatin	The statin-induced decrease in cholesterol synthesis may negatively impact the male steroidal hormone level (androgens–testosterone). Moreover, statins inhibit not only HMG-CoA but also 17-ketosteroid-oxidoreductase that catalyzes the synthesis of androstenedione and testosterone. Thus, a decrease in serum testosterone level is observed in males with hypercholesterolemia treated with statins.

Tricyclic antidepressants	Imipramine, Clomipramine	The increased availability of serotonin due to the inhibition of its reuptake evoked by SSRI/SNRI leads to the increased binding of this neurotransmitter to the 5-HT2 and 5-HT3 receptors which disturbs sexual functions. Moreover, the complex, multi-receptor effect of tricyclic antidepressants also contributes to peripheral circulatory disturbances. In general, antidepressants with lower affinity to dopamine and noradrenaline receptors have a lower influence on ED.
Selective serotonin or noradrenalin reuptake inhibitors (SSRI/SNRI)	Sertraline, Citalopram, Paroxetine, Escitalopram, Duloxetine, Venlafaxine	
First generation antipsychotics	Haloperidol, Clozapine, Thioridazine	First-generation antipsychotics block central D2 receptors, decreasing the inhibition of prolactin production in the anterior pituitary gland, resulting in secondary disturbances in testosterone synthesis. Moreover, antipsychotics may also impair peripheral vasodilatation via cholinergic antagonism
Antiepileptics	Phenytoin, Phenobarbital, Carbamazepine	Both antiepileptic drugs and seizures interfere with the hypothalamic-pituitary-gonadal axis and alter sex steroid hormone production. Moreover, some antiepileptics induce hepatic enzymes resulting in increases of sex hormone binding globulin, which leads to lower free testosterone levels.
Non-steroidal anti-inflammatory drugs	Naproxen, Diclofenac, Ibuprofen	Cyclooxygenase inhibition decreases the production of prostanoids (prostaglandins and thromboxanes) with a subsequent decrease of vasodilatory, and the erectile effect of nitric oxide (NO).
Muscle relaxants	Baclofen	The inhibition of afferent stimulation from the penis, somatic motor efferents mediating perineal muscle contraction and visceral motor efferents controlling the penile vasculature.
H2 receptor antagonists	Cimetidine, Ranitidine, Famotidine	H2 receptors are strongly associated with the relaxation of the corpus cavernosum; thus, H2 receptor antagonism results in decreased relaxation, increased contraction and a decreased potential for erection. Moreover, cimetidine exhibits anti-androgen, which affects and causes hyperprolactinemia
5-alpha reductase inhibitors	Finasteride, Dutasteride	These drugs inhibit type II 5-alpha reductase–the enzyme that catalyzes the conversion of testosterone into more biologically potent dihydrotestosterone (DHT), with the subsequent decrease in nitric oxide synthase activity

Cancer drugs	Cisplatin, Vincristine, Vinblastine	Chemotherapy is known to cause ED by causing neural and vasculature damage. Moreover, long-acting gonadotrophin-releasing hormone agonists used for prostate and breast cancer cause hypogonadism, leading to a reduction in sexual desire and ED.
Miscellaneous	Antiandrogens (cyproterone), Digoxin, Steroids, Immunosuppressants (Sirolimus, Everolimus), Protease inhibitors in HIV	Various, complex mechanisms: the blocking of the androgen receptors, the lowering of serum testosterone and the impairment of gonadal functions.

Source: *Dobrek L. Lower Urinary Tract Disorders as Adverse Drug Reactions-A Literature Review. Pharmaceuticals (Basel). 2023 Jul 20;16(7):1031. doi: 10.3390/ph16071031. PMID: 37513941; PMCID: PMC10383968.*

10.5. Retroperitoneal Fibrosis

A rare disorder known as retroperitoneal fibrosis (RPF) is characterized by persistent inflammation and fibrosis in the retroperitoneum, which leads to the development of a midline plaque, typically at the aortic bifurcation. RPF resembles a smooth, flat, dense mass with a tan color that surrounds the retroperitoneal structures, which are typically centered at the fourth and fifth lumbar vertebrae. The ureters are frequently impacted by the extensive fibrotic process, which can result in ureteric obstruction. RPF is seen in patients between the ages of 40 and 60, with a male predominance (approximately 2:1 or 3:1 male-to-female ratio). It is estimated that the disease affects one in 200,000 to 500,000 people annually. RPF can cause back pain, stomach pain, hydrocoele, edema, or anuria as a clinical symptom. Although the exact cause of RPF is unknown, an idiopathic mechanism of development is primarily thought to be responsible in 70% of cases. Assuming the best, an idiopathic RPF is considered a sign of a systemic autoimmune disease. This condition can also develop from primary aortitis, which causes a periaortic fibro-inflammatory response. Ceroid, a complex polymer of oxidized lipids and protein found in atherosclerotic plaques with cellular infiltration including IgG4-positive plasma cells and lymphocytes, is the factor suspected of initiating and maintaining the immune response and fibrosis. Approximately thirty percent of RPF cases have a known cause. Secondary causes of retroperitoneal fibrosis have also been identified, including malignancy (carcinoid, Hodgkin and non-Hodgkin lymphoma, sarcomas); infections (tuberculosis, histoplasmosis, actinomycosis); radiation therapy for testicular seminoma, colon and pancreatic cancer; and surgery. Apart from cancer, autoimmune conditions, or radiation therapy, chronic use of specific medications is another potential cause of iatrogenic RPF. Drug-induced RPF's precise pathogenesis has not been adequately explained, but it may involve a drug-haptenic role or, conversely, be connected to the release of fibrotic markers (transforming growth factor-1; TGF-1, basic fibroblast growth factor; bFGF, platelet-derived growth factor; PDGF) and phlogogenic mediators (histamine, kinins, prostaglandins). Last but not least, the overproduction of extracellular matrix (ECM) components such as collagen, fibronectin, tenascin, and glycosaminoglycans is brought about by the TGF/Smads cascade-mediated enhancement of myofibroblast proliferation. According to observational studies, the risk of developing RPF is most commonly associated with the use of ergot derivatives such as methysergide, which is only prescribed to prevent severe headaches, and other ergot derivatives like cabergoline, pergolide, lisuride, and bromocriptine that are used to treat Parkinson's disease. The remaining medications that are thought to be connected to RPF are mentioned in Table 10.6.

Table 10.6. *Drugs with Suggested Association with Retroperitoneal Fibrosis*

Drug Class	Examples	Postulated Mechanism Contributing to Retroperitoneal Fibrosis
Non-opioid and opioid analgesics	Aspirin, Paracetamol, Codeine	Drugs may initiate an immune response in the retroperitoneum followed by a progression to a chronic inflammatory process in the form of the proliferation of fibroblasts and the deposition of collagen, fibronectin, tenascin and glycosaminoglycans. The process of fibrosis involves the adjacent organs, including the ureters, causing their compression and possible symptoms of obstructive uropathy.
Antihypertensives	Hydralazine, Methyldopa, Reserpine, Hydrochlorothiazide	
Beta-adrenergic antagonists	Non-selective (Propranolol, Sotalol, Oxyprenolol)	
	Beta1-selective agents (Metoprolol, Atenolol)	
Cytostatics	Carboplatin, Methotrexate	
Biological drugs	Etanercept (TNF-alpha receptor blocker), Infliximab (anti-TNF-alpha monoclonal antibody)	
Miscellaneous	Egrot derivatives, Haloperidol, Ampicillin, Glibenclamide,	

Source: Dobrek L. Lower Urinary Tract Disorders as Adverse Drug Reactions-A Literature Review. Pharmaceuticals (Basel). 2023 Jul 20;16(7):1031. doi: 10.3390/ph16071031. PMID: 37513941; PMCID: PMC10383968.

10.6. Clinical Examples of Drug-Induced Urological Disorders

After receiving treatment with centrally acting drugs, adverse drug reactions affecting the lower urinary tract are most frequently observed in clinical practice, according to a review of clinical reports on the subject. Trinchieri et al.'s meta-analysis in the context of a systematic review. analysis of urological conditions brought on by antidepressant and antipsychotic medication shows that antidepressant medication use is linked to a higher risk of micturition disorders (disturbances in both storage and emptying). Serotonin and norepinephrine reuptake inhibitors (SNRIs) and tricyclic antidepressants were associated with an increased risk of voiding dysfunction. The effect was not as strong in the case of SSRIs. Numerous urinary disorders, such as incontinence and urinary retention, were reported in the analysis of antipsychotics. These disorders were primarily associated with atypical antipsychotics like clonazine or conventional antipsychotics like phenothiazines and thioxanthenes (chlorprothixene). Drawings similar to these can be made from Winkler et al.'s analysis. on urological conditions evaluated in patients receiving psychotropic medications in hospitals. UR (129 cases, 0.028 %) was the most common drug-induced LUTS among 462,661 in patients treated with psychotropic drugs in 99 psychiatric hospitals between 1993 and 2016, followed by incontinence (23 cases, 0.005 %). A thorough investigation revealed that trimipramine, amitriptyline, clomipramine, and paroxetine were the antidepressants that carried the greatest risk of UR development. Patients receiving venlafaxine, duloxetine, mirtazapine, doxepin, escitalopram, sertraline, citalopram, and trazodone have been reported to have these disorders to a lesser extent. When it came to antipsychotics, patients receiving promethazine, haloperidol, pipamperone, olanzapine, perazine, levomepromazine, flupentixol, and chlorprothixene had a higher incidence of UR.

The literature review on sertraline also included case reports of patients who experienced both UR and U when using the drug. Elderly patients are more susceptible to urological disorders, especially if they are receiving antidepressant therapy and have multiple medical conditions. An amitriptyline dose of 10 mg per day was found to cause urine retention in an 86-year-old patient with benign prostatic hyperplasia; the patient's symptoms were less severe when the medication was stopped. Another case of acute urine retention was in a patient receiving TCAs for postpartum depression and also taking an antimuscarinic spasmolytic medication for dysmenorrhea.

A case of a 62-year-old patient with a medical history noteworthy for bipolar I disorder, nephrogenic diabetes insipidus, and metastatic colorectal cancer was also discovered through the literature review. The patient's chief complaint was non-radiating suprapubic abdominal pain. After developing nephrogenic insipidus, the patient's lithium treatment was changed to lamotrigine, and then to olanzapine three weeks before the start of the UR episode. After conducting a differential diagnosis, it was determined that the patient's UR was caused by olanzapine's antimuscarinic effect in conjunction with reduced micturition. Another patient, 51 years old, developed chronic urine retention (UR) after receiving 22 points5 mg of olanzapine for four years. The patient also experienced worsening psychotic symptoms, blurred vision, and difficulty urinating.

In actual clinical practice, the use of a class of medications known as opioids is also linked to an increased risk of UR. In an upcoming research project, Panicker et al. revealed that UR episodes were seen in 13 out of 61 patients receiving treatment with opioids (morphine, tramadol, or oxycodone) because of the range of pain syndromes (mostly back pain brought on by a mechanical derangement of the spine, musculoskeletal pain, or abdominopelvic pain). Buprenorphine and urinary retention are also related, especially when used in conjunction with intrathecal or epidural delivery. A 49-year-old patient with a history of alcoholism, bipolar disorder, opiate dependence, and borderline personality disorder was shown to have the acute UR caused by buprenorphine. Buprenorphine (8–12 mg daily) was used to treat his opioid dependency. The patients arrived at the emergency department (ED) on the third day following the start of treatment, complaining of suprapubic discomfort and an inability to urinate. An ED examination resulted in the drainage of 800 mL of urine.

The next class of centrally acting drugs whose use is linked to disturbances in voiding is benzodiazepines. In a planned investigation, Landi et al. showed that 475 people who were taking benzodiazepines at the time (21% of patients aged 60–74 years and 38% of patients aged > 75 years) had UI. The effect was primarily linked to agents with a long half-life elimination, and the estimated global risk of UI during benzodiazepine treatment was close to 45%. However, the use of benzodiazepines can also cause UR to develop. A 67-year-old male patient was described as having alprazolam-induced UR. The patient had a prostatectomy for BPH and was also prescribed 1 mg of alprazolam per day for sleeplessness. After the second dosage, the patient started experiencing difficulty voiding, and an organic pathology could not account for the urine retention that was already present in the table.

In actual clinical practice, drug-induced UI was also examined by Hall et al. among the 5503 men and women in Boston who are between the ages of 30 and 79. According to their estimates, 4 points6% of men and 9 points0% of women experienced UI overall. The mean age of both men and women with UI was significantly higher than that of those without. The incidence was highest among women who used angiotensin II receptor blockers (ARBs) (22.9%) and specific antihistamines (28.4%). The incidence was highest in men among those who used ARBs (22%) and loop diuretics (19 points 1%).

Among cardiovascular medications, calcium channel blockers are the group most commonly associated with causing voiding disorders. These drugs impact voiding by weakening the detrusor muscle's ability to contract effectively. A study by Elhebir et al. examined 278 medical inpatients, including 85 users of calcium channel blockers, with an average age of 72.1. After adjusting for various factors, it was found that patients taking amlodipine/nifedipine and diltiazem/verapamil were more likely to experience lower urinary tract symptoms (LUTS) compared to non-users, while those on felodipine/lercanidipine were less likely to have LUTS. Additionally, 22.4% of patients on calcium channel blockers were also being treated for LUTS, compared to 9.3% of those not taking these medications. This study reinforced the link between using calcium channel blockers and developing LUTS. A systematic review by Salman et al., analyzing five relevant studies, found that three of them showed a significant connection between calcium channel blocker use and LUTS development. The remaining study suggested that using calcium channel blockers alone was associated with a higher occurrence of nocturia and voiding symptoms, particularly in young females.

The class of medications known to be most commonly reported in clinical reports when it comes to predisposing to UTIs is sodium-glucose co-transporter 2 (SGLT2) inhibitors (gliflozins). In a study conducted by Uitrakul et al. According to a study done in actual clinical settings with patients diagnosed with type 2 diabetes, the overall incidence rate of UTI was 33.49% higher in the group treated with SGLT2 inhibitors than in the control group. 11 points72% in the patient population not receiving gliflozin therapy. There was no significant difference in the incidence rates of UTI between the dapagliflozin and empagliflozin treatment groups (34.00% and 34.03%, respectively). A review conducted by Figueiredo et al. based on a review of 23 clinical trials, also revealed a higher rate of UTIs in gliflozin-using patients, whether they were receiving SGLT2i monotherapy or combination therapy. Furthermore, the review noted that, regardless of dosage, the use of dapagliflozin, canagliflozin, and tofogliflozin was primarily linked to increased risk. Additionally, dapafliflozin was examined in a Khan et al. cross-sectional study involving 400 diabetes patients receiving dapagliflozin as an add-on medication for type 2 diabetes, either at a dose of 5 mg or 10 mg. Five percent of diabetic patients receiving dapagliflozin (5 mg or 10 mg) had a UTI worldwide. UTIs were more common in patients over 50 (85.7%) than in any other age group, and women were more affected than men (76.2%).

Tasian et al. conducted a thorough investigation of anti-infective chemotherapy drugs. indicated a higher chance of kidney stones for particular drug classes. 13 million adult and pediatric patients seen by general practitioners between 1994 and 2015 had their medical records examined. Approximately 26,000 kidney stone patients and nearly 260,000 control subjects had histories of antibiotic exposure. The study found that five classes of drugs—sulpha drugs, cephalosporins, fluoroquinolones, broad-spectrum penicillins, and nitrofurantoin—were linked to a diagnosis of kidney stone disease in clinical practice. The use of these agents is linked to an increased risk of nephrolithiasis, with the highest odds for exposure occurring recently and at a younger age, according to the authors' additional conclusion.

Patients who use medications that cause autonomic imbalance predominate in case studies pertaining to drug-induced ED. Therefore, medications that affect the adrenergic and cholinergic systems, such as nonselective beta-blockers, alpha-blockers, anticholinergic medications, and other medications, as well as other antihypertensive medications, are frequently implicated in ED. Clinical reports also suggest that centrally acting medications contribute to the development of drug-induced ED.

Hydralazine, ampicillin, hydrochlorothiazide, and pergolide given to Parkinson's disease patients have all been linked to drug-related entities of retroperitoneal fibrosis. RPF has previously been documented as a side effect of methysergide therapy for migraines and headaches. The new drug class used in melanoma-anti-programmed cell death 1 (anti-PD-1) antibodies, which are used in personalized therapy for lung cancer, has also been shown to increase the risk of developing RPF.

Numerous medication uses may be linked to the emergence of iatrogenic kidney and urinary tract disorders. When a patient receives pharmacotherapy, it may result in UR or UI, UTIs, urolithiasis, ED, or RPF, among other LUTS. Clinical reports most frequently list centrally acting medications, antihypertensive agents, certain antibacterial chemotherapy drugs, gliflozins, and medications that affect the autonomic nervous system as among the medications that may predispose to urological disorders. (Dobrek et al, 2023)

A Closer Look At Erectile Dysfunction Causes, Solutions

Men's erections are a complex issue, involving both psychological and physiological factors. Erectile dysfunction, or ED, is a prevalent sexual dysfunction that sex therapists often come across. Men experiencing ED may have trouble achieving or sustaining an erection. According to the Johns Hopkins Bloomberg School of Public Health, approximately 18 million men over the age of 20 in the United States are affected by ED.

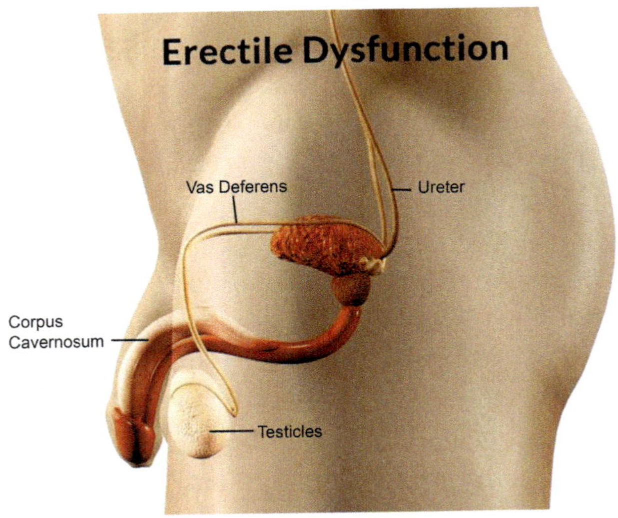

Source: https://siiut.com/erectile-dysfunction-treatment/

Physiological problems may be the cause of erectile dysfunction. It is frequently linked to advanced age, diabetes, heart disease, and inactivity. Nearly 90% of men with ED had at least one cardiovascular disease risk factor, according to a Johns Hopkins Bloomberg School of Public Health study (diabetes, hypertension, poor cholesterol, smoker). Other physiological problems, such as endocrine abnormalities and drug side effects, are also closely linked to ED.

A medical professional can assist in determining which lifestyle modifications, such as dieting, exercise, stress reduction, or quitting smoking, will be beneficial if erectile dysfunction is linked to physiological issues. A medical professional may also recommend drugs like Cialis, Levitra, or Viagra to treat ED. These medications function by boosting blood flow to the penis during intercourse. About 35% of men with ED are not responsive to this kind of medication, according to the National Institutes of Health. In those situations, additional therapies might be suggested, like penile injection therapy, which involves injecting a medication into the penis to enhance blood flow. According to research by the NIH, up to 80% of men with ED who tried this therapy reported improvement in erection. Usually, 10 to 20 minutes after the injection, an erection happens. There is a 12-month maximum for the number of injections.

An interesting alternative for treating erectile dysfunction in men is a vacuum constriction device, also known as a penis pump. Blood rushes into a man's penis when air is removed from a plastic tube that is attached to a pump, creating a vacuum. After the penis is filled with blood, the blood cannot exit using a plastic ring placed at the base. Men's satisfaction with vacuum devices varies according to research, with results ranging from 35 to 84%.

ED can also be brought on by psychological factors, which can be divided into two primary groups: situational psychological blocks and generalized psychological blocks. These psychological factors include stress, anxiety, and depression. Generalized problems concern the individual in their entirety. For example, a man who is getting older may have less sexual desire as a result of a drop in testosterone. If his issue was situational, his ED might be related to issues at work or a lack of interest in his partner.

Summary

- The primary goal of pharmacotherapy is to be effective and safe. Attaining this goal is related to demonstrating an acceptable risk–benefit ratio of the drugs that are currently on the pharmaceutical market.
- The most important function of the kidneys and urinary tract is the excretion of urine containing metabolic wastes and drugs with their metabolites, which is one of the vital functions of the human body.
- The opposite disorder of UR is UI. It is a condition characterized by the involuntary loss of urine. UI can be diagnosed in childhood and may resolve itself with growth; however, it usually occurs in patients over 40 years of age and increases with aging.
- An uncomplicated urinary tract infection (UTI) is an infection of the lower urinary tract (urethra and bladder), developing in patients without structural abnormality and comorbidities, such as diabetes, immunocompromised state, pregnancy, kidney transplants, the presence of a urinary catheter or other factors predisposing them to a complicated course of the infection.
- Urolithiasis (nephrolithiasis; kidney stone disease) is a relatively common clinical entity and research indicates that the general prevalence of the disease varies between 1 and 5% in Asia, 5–9% in Europe, 13% in the USA to even 20% in Middle Eastern countries.
- There are many causes of erectile dysfunction (ED) development in men, including pathophysiological (hypertension, hyperlipidemia, diabetes) and psychological factors.

References

1. Abrams, P. (1994). New words for old: Lower urinary tract symptoms for "prostatism". *BMJ, 308*, 929–930. https://doi.org/10.1136/bmj.308.6934.929.
2. Alberti, C. (2012). Revisiting the retroperitoneal fibroses: Are there any significant news about their aetiopathogenesis and diagnostic approaches? *European Review for Medical and Pharmacological Sciences, 16*, 1078–1094.
3. Alberti, C. (2015). Drug-induced retroperitoneal fibrosis: Short aetiopathogenetic note, from the past times of ergot-derivatives large use to currently applied bio-pharmacology. *Giornale Italiano di Chirurgia, 36*, 187–191. https://doi.org/10.11138/gchir/2015.36.4.187.
4. Alelign, T., & Petros, B. (2018). Kidney stone disease: An update on current concepts. *Advances in Urology, 2018*, 3068365. https://doi.org/10.1155/2018/3068365.
5. Amarenco, G., Sheikh Ismael, S., Chesnel, C., Charlanes, A., & Le Breton, F. (2017). Diagnosis and clinical evaluation of neurogenic bladder. *European Journal of Physical and Rehabilitation Medicine, 53*, 975–980. https://doi.org/10.23736/S1973-9087.17.04992-9.
6. Aykut, D. S., & Uysal, R. A. E. (2018). Acute urinary retention after alprazolam use: A case report. *Psychiatry and Clinical Psychopharmacology, 28*, 220–221. https://doi.org/10.1080/24750573.2017.1400936.
7. Baydal, K., Anton, C., & Ferner, R. (2017). Adverse drug reactions and urological disease. *Trends in Urology and Men's Health, 8*, 21–25. https://doi.org/10.1002/tre.581.

8. Beckel, J. M., & Holstege, G. (2011). Neurophysiology of the lower urinary tract. *Handbook of Experimental Pharmacology, 202*, 149–169.

9. Begum, S., Madani, M., & Hassan, M. (2019). Nephrolithiasis: An update on current concepts. *IAJPS, 6*, 14073–14087.

10. Bilici, A., Karadag, B., Doventas, A., Erdincler, D. S., Cetinkaya, S., Ogut, G., Tezcan, V., & Beger, T. (2004). Retroperitoneal fibrosis caused by pergolide in a patient with Parkinson's disease. *Netherlands Journal of Medicine, 62*, 389–392.

11. Bishop, K., Momah, T., & Ricks, J. (2020). Nephrolithiasis. *Primary Care, 47*, 661–671. https://doi.org/10.1016/j.pop.2020.08.005.

12. Brasselet, D., Chouchana, L., Vial, T., Damin-Pernik, M., & Lebrun-Vignes, B. (2020). Drug-induced retroperitoneal fibrosis: A case/non-case study in the French PharmacoVigilance Database. *Expert Opinion on Drug Safety, 19*, 903–914. https://doi.org/10.1080/14740338.2020.1766022.

13. Chapple, C. R., Wein, A. J., Abrams, P., Dmochowski, R. R., Giuliano, F., Kaplan, S. A., McVary, K. T., & Roehrborn, C. G. (2008). Lower urinary tract symptoms revisited: A broader clinical perspective. *European Urology, 54*, 563–569. https://doi.org/10.1016/j.eururo.2008.03.109.

14. Chen, C. L., Wu, S. T., Cha, T. L., Sun, G. H., & Meng, E. (2022). Molecular pathophysiology and potential therapeutic strategies of ketamine-related cystitis. *Biology (Basel), 11*, 502. https://doi.org/10.3390/biology11040502.

15. Cichon, G. J., & Qadri, S. F. (2023). Risperidone-induced sexual dysfunction: Case report. *Cureus, 15*, e35357. https://doi.org/10.7759/cureus.35357.

16. Coleman, J. J., & Pontefract, S. K. (2016). Adverse drug reactions. *Clinical Medicine (London), 16*, 481–485. https://doi.org/10.7861/clinmedicine.16-5-481.

17. Conaglen, H. M., & Conaglen, J. V. (2013). Drug-induced sexual dysfunction in men and women. *Australian Prescriber, 36*, 42–46. https://doi.org/10.18773/austprescr.2013.021.

18. Das, A. K., Kucherov, V., Glick, L., & Chung, P. (2020). Male urinary incontinence after prostate disease treatment. *Canadian Journal of Urology, 27*, 36–43.

19. Daudon, M., & Jungers, P. (2004). Drug-induced renal calculi: Epidemiology, prevention, and management. *Drugs, 64*, 245–275. https://doi.org/10.2165/00003495-200464030-00003.

20. Daudon, M., Frochot, V., Bazin, D., & Jungers, P. (2018). Drug-induced kidney stones and crystalline nephropathy: Pathophysiology, prevention, and treatment. *Drugs, 78*, 163–201. https://doi.org/10.1007/s40265-017-0853-7.

21. Denisenko, A. A., Clark, C. B., D'Amico, M., & Murphy, A. M. (2021). Evaluation and management of female urinary incontinence. *Canadian Journal of Urology, 28*, 27–32.

22. Dobrek, Ł. (2020). Kidney stone disease with special regard to drug-induced kidney stones—A contemporary synopsis. *Wiadomości Lekarskie, 73*, 2031–2039. https://doi.org/10.36740/WLek202009226.

23. Dobrek, Ł. (2021). Drug-related urinary tract infections. *Wiadomości Lekarskie, 74*, 1728–1736. https://doi.org/10.36740/WLek202107130.

24. Dobrek, Ł. (2023). A synopsis of current theories on drug-induced nephrotoxicity. *Life, 13*, 325. https://doi.org/10.3390/life13020325.

25. Dobrek, L. (2023). Lower urinary tract disorders as adverse drug reactions: A literature review. *Pharmaceuticals (Basel), 16*(7), 1031. https://doi.org/10.3390/ph16071031.

26. Dobrek, Ł., & Thor, P. J. (2012). Bladder urotoxicity pathophysiology induced by the oxazaphosphorine alkylating agents and its chemoprevention. *Postępy Higieny i Medycyny Doświadczalnej (Online), 66*, 592–602. https://doi.org/10.5604/17322693.1009703.

27. Dobrek, Ł., Juszczak, K., Wyczółkowski, M., & Thor, P. J. (2011). Overactive bladder—Current definition and basic pathophysiology concepts. *Advances in Clinical and Experimental Medicine, 20*, 119–129.

28. Drake, M. J., Nixon, P. M., & Crew, J. P. (1998). Drug-induced bladder and urinary disorders: Incidence, prevention, and management. *Drug Safety, 19*, 45–55. https://doi.org/10.2165/00002018-199819010-00004.

29. Edwards, I. R., & Aronson, J. K. (2000). Adverse drug reactions: Definitions, diagnosis, and management. *Lancet, 356*, 1255–1259. https://doi.org/10.1016/S0140-6736(00)02799-9.

30. Edwards, R. T., McCormick-Deaton, C., & Hosanagar, A. (2014). Acute urinary retention secondary to buprenorphine administration. *American Journal of Emergency Medicine, 32*, 109.e1–109.e2. https://doi.org/10.1016/j.ajem.2013.08.022.

31. Elhebir, E. S., Hughes, J. D., & Hilmi, S. C. (2013). Calcium antagonists use and its association with lower urinary tract symptoms: A cross-sectional study. *PLoS ONE, 8*, e66708. https://doi.org/10.1371/journal.pone.0066708.

32. Fecik, S. E. (1998). Drug-induced sexual dysfunction. *Medical Update Psychiatry, 3*, 176–181. https://doi.org/10.1016/S1082-7579(98)00024-7.

33. Figueiredo, I. R., Rose, S. C. P., Freire, N. B., Patrocínio, M. S., Pierdoná, N., & Bittencourt, R. J. (2019). Use of sodium-glucose cotransporter-2 inhibitors and urinary tract infections in type 2 diabetes patients: A systematic review. *Revista da Associação Médica Brasileira, 65*, 246–252. https://doi.org/10.1590/1806-9282.65.2.246.

34. Flores-Mireles, A. L., Walker, J. N., Caparon, M., & Hultgren, S. J. (2015). Urinary tract infections: Epidemiology, mechanisms of infection, and treatment options. *Nature Reviews Microbiology, 13*, 269–284. https://doi.org/10.1038/nrmicro3432.

35. Fujiu, K., Utsumi, Y., Omi, F., Suzuki, M., & Suzuki, H. (2022). Two cases of retroperitoneal fibrosis during anti-programmed cell death 1 antibody treatment. *Japanese Journal of Lung Cancer, 62*, 1044–1047. https://doi.org/10.2482/haigan.62.1044.

36. Gandi, C., & Sacco, E. (2021). Pharmacological management of urinary incontinence: Current and emerging treatments. *Clinical Pharmacology, 13*, 209–223. https://doi.org/10.2147/CPAA.S289323.

37. Gani, J., & Hennessey, D. (2017). The underactive bladder: Diagnosis and surgical treatment options. *Translational Andrology and Urology, 6*(Suppl. S2), S186–S195. https://doi.org/10.21037/tau.2017.04.07.

38. Gordijn, R., Teichert, M., Nicolai, M. P. J., Elzevier, H. W., & Guchelaar, H. J. (2019). Adverse drug reactions on sexual functioning: A systematic overview. *Drug Discovery Today, 24*, 890–897. https://doi.org/10.1016/j.drudis.2019.01.012.

39. Graham, J. R., Suby, H. I., LeCompte, P. R., & Sadowsky, N. L. (1966). Fibrotic disorders

associated with methysergide therapy for headache. *New England Journal of Medicine, 274*, 359–368. https://doi.org/10.1056/NEJM196602172740701.

40. Halbgewachs, C., & Domes, T. (2015). Postobstructive diuresis. *Canadian Family Physician, 61*, 137–142.

41. Hall, S. A., Yang, M., Gates, M. A., Steers, W. D., Tennstedt, S. L., & McKinlay, J. B. (2012). Associations of commonly used medications with urinary incontinence in a community-based sample. *Journal of Urology, 188*, 183–189. https://doi.org/10.1016/j.juro.2012.02.2575.

42. Howard, R. (2008). Amitriptyline in BPH: Increased risk of post-void residual and urinary retention. *Prescriber, 19*, 42–45.

43. Hu, J. S., & Pierre, E. F. (2019). Urinary incontinence in women: Evaluation and management. *American Family Physician, 100*, 339–348.

44. Jayaraman, U. C., & Gurusamy, A. (2018). Review on uro-lithiasis pathophysiology and aesculapian discussion. *IOSR Journal of Pharmacy, 8*, 30–42.

45. Jhang, J. F., Hsu, Y. H., & Kuo, H. C. (2015). Possible pathophysiology of ketamine-related cystitis and associated treatment strategies. *International Journal of Urology, 22*, 816–825. https://doi.org/10.1111/iju.12841.

46. Jiang, S., Burke, H., Hernandez, M., & Ruth, L. (2022). Sertraline-induced urinary retention reversed by mirtazapine in an adolescent. *Primary Care Companion for CNS Disorders, 24*, 22cr03254. https://doi.org/10.4088/PCC.22cr03254.

47. Kamei, J., & Fujimura, T. (2023). Urinary tract infection in patients with lower urinary tract dysfunction. *Journal of Infection and Chemotherapy, 29*, 744–748. https://doi.org/10.1016/j.jiac.2023.04.019.

48. Khalil, H., & Huang, C. (2020). Adverse drug reactions in primary care: A scoping review. *BMC Health Services Research, 20*, 5. https://doi.org/10.1186/s12913-019-4651-7.

49. Khan, S., Hashmi, M. S., Rana, M. A., Zafar, G. M., Asif, S., Farooq, M. T., & Zahoor, S. (2022). Frequency of urinary tract infections in type 2 diabetic patients taking dapagliflozin. *Cureus, 14*, e21720. https://doi.org/10.7759/cureus.21720.

50. Kumar, R., Singh, S., Arora, S., & Bhati, S. (2018). Adverse drug reactions: A comprehensive review. *Journal of Drug Delivery and Therapy, 8*, 103–107. https://doi.org/10.22270/jddt.v8i1.1658.

51. Landi, F., Cesari, M., Russo, A., Onder, G., Sgadari, A., Bernabei, R., & Silvernet-HC Study Group. (2002). Benzodiazepines and the risk of urinary incontinence in frail older persons living in the community. *Clinical Pharmacology & Therapeutics, 72*, 729–734. https://doi.org/10.1067/mcp.2002.129318.

52. Maehara, M., & Sugiyama, M. (2021). A community pharmacist's intervention in antipsychotic drug-induced sexual dysfunction in a patient with schizophrenia. *Clinical Case Reports, 9*, 2074–2076. https://doi.org/10.1002/ccr3.3946.

53. Mancuso, G., Midiri, A., Gerace, E., Marra, M., Zummo, S., & Biondo, C. (2023). Urinary tract infections: The current scenario and future prospects. *Pathogens, 12*, 623. https://doi.org/10.3390/pathogens12040623.

54. Matlaga, B. R., Shah, O. D., & Assimos, D. G. (2003). Drug-induced urinary calculi. *Reviews in Urology, 5*, 227–231.

55. Matz, E. L., & Hsieh, M. H. (2017). Review of advances in uroprotective agents for cyclophosphamide- and ifosfamide-induced hemorrhagic cystitis. *Urology, 100*, 16–19. https://doi.org/10.1016/j.urology.2016.07.030.
56. Mirzakhani, H., Rahim, M., & Mathew, J., Jr. (2020). Expanding our understanding of atypical antipsychotics: Acute urinary retention secondary to olanzapine. *Case Reports in Psychiatry, 2020*, 6157548. https://doi.org/10.1155/2020/6157548.
57. Olawale, O. O., Kezeli, T., Nikoleishvili, E., & Sulashvili, N. (2018). Adverse drug reaction. *Caucasian Journal of Health Sciences and Public Health, 2*(Suppl. S3), 1–4.
58. Osborne, C. A., Lulich, J. P., Swanson, L. L., & Albasan, H. (2008). Drug-induced urolithiasis. *Veterinary Clinics of North America: Small Animal Practice, 39*, 55–63. https://doi.org/10.1016/j.cvsm.2008.09.004.
59. Osman, N., Mangera, A., Hillary, C., Inman, R., & Chapple, C. (2016). The underactive bladder: Detection and diagnosis. *F1000Research, 5*, 102. https://doi.org/10.12688/f1000research.7344.1.
60. Ozdemir, P. G., Aydin, A., Gulec, M., & Cim, E. F. A. (2023). Switching to fluoxetine in a case of sertraline-induced urinary incontinence: A case report. *Düşünen Adam: The Journal of Psychiatry and Neurological Sciences, 26*, 117–118. https://doi.org/10.5350/DAJPN2013260116.
61. Panesar, K. (2014). Drug-induced urinary incontinence. *US Pharmacist, 39*, 24–29.
62. Panicker, J. N., Game, X., Khan, S., Kessler, T. M., Gonzales, G., Elneil, S., & Fowler, C. J. (2012). The possible role of opiates in women with chronic urinary retention: Observations from a prospective clinical study. *Journal of Urology, 188*, 480–484. https://doi.org/10.1016/j.juro.2012.04.011.
63. Payne, H., Adamson, A., Bahl, A., Borwell, J., Dodds, D., Heath, C., Huddart, R., McMenemin, R., Patel, P., Peters, J. L., et al. (2013). Chemical- and radiation-induced haemorrhagic cystitis: Current treatments and challenges. *BJU International, 112*, 885–897. https://doi.org/10.1111/bju.12291.
64. Pease, E., Singh, B., Ziegelmann, M., & Betcher, H. (2021). Dose-dependent urinary incontinence with sertraline use in obsessive-compulsive disorder. *Psychopharmacology Bulletin, 51*, 117–121.
65. Petca, R. C., Popescu, R. I., Toma, C., Dumitrascu, M. C., Petca, A., Sandru, F., & Chibelean, C. B. (2021). Chemical hemorrhagic cystitis: Diagnostic and therapeutic pitfalls (Review). *Experimental and Therapeutic Medicine, 21*, 624. https://doi.org/10.3892/etm.2021.10056.
66. Purohith, A. N., Ramesh, P., Vaidya, B. P., Shenoy, S., & Sharma, P. S. V. N. (2023). Olanzapine-associated chronic urinary retention and ciliochoroidal effusion: Rare adverse effects of a commonly prescribed antipsychotic. *Indian Journal of Psychological Medicine, 45*, 96–97. https://doi.org/10.1177/02537176221111581.
67. Ramello, A., Vitale, C., & Marangella, M. (2000). Epidemiology of nephrolithiasis. *Journal of Nephrology, 13*(Suppl. S3), S45–S50.
68. Razdan, S., Greer, A. B., Patel, A., Alameddine, M., Jue, J. S., & Ramasamy, R. (2018). Effect of prescription medications on erectile dysfunction. *Postgraduate Medical Journal, 94*, 171–178. https://doi.org/10.1136/postgradmedj-2017-135233.

69. Riedl, M. A., & Casillas, A. M. (2003). Adverse drug reactions: Types and treatment options. *American Family Physician, 68*, 1781–1791.

70. Runowska, M., Majewski, D., & Puszczewicz, M. (2016). Retroperitoneal fibrosis—The state-of-the-art. *Reumatologia, 54*, 256–263. https://doi.org/10.5114/reum.2016.63667.

71. Salman, M., Khan, A. H., Syed Sulaiman, S. A., Khan, J. H., Hussain, K., & Shehzadi, N. (2017). Effect of calcium channel blockers on lower urinary tract symptoms: A systematic review. *Biomedical Research International, 2017*, 4269875. https://doi.org/10.1155/2017/4269875.

72. Samajdar, S. S., Mukherjee, S., Saha, D., Jumani, D., & Tripathi, S. K. (2021). Drug-induced erectile dysfunction: Two interesting cases. *Journal of Pharmacology & Pharmacotherapy, 12*, 177–179.

73. Sherif, I. (2020). Uroprotective mechanisms of natural products against cyclophosphamide-induced urinary bladder toxicity: A comprehensive review. *Acta Scientiarum Polonorum. Technologia Alimentaria, 19*, 333–346. https://doi.org/10.17306/J.AFS.0832.

74. Sighinolfi, M. C., Eissa, A., Bevilacqua, L., Zoeir, A., Ciarlariello, S., Morini, E., Puliatti, S., Durante, V., Ceccarelli, P. L., Micali, S., et al. (2019). Drug-induced urolithiasis in pediatric patients. *Paediatric Drugs, 21*, 323–344. https://doi.org/10.1007/s40272-019-00355-5.

75. Stamatiou, K., Alevizos, A., Petrakos, G., Lentzas, I., Mariolis, A., & Panagopoulos, P. (2007). Tricyclic antidepressant-induced acute urine retention in a young woman with postpartum depression: Case report. *Clinical and Experimental Obstetrics & Gynecology, 34*, 60.

76. Tanaka, T., & Masumori, N. (2020). Current approach to diagnosis and management of retroperitoneal fibrosis. *International Journal of Urology, 27*, 387–394. https://doi.org/10.1111/iju.14218.

77. Tasian, G. E., Jemielita, T., Goldfarb, D. S., Copelovitch, L., Gerber, J. S., Wu, Q., & Denburg, M. R. (2018). Oral antibiotic exposure and kidney stone disease. *Journal of the American Society of Nephrology, 29*, 1731–1740. https://doi.org/10.1681/ASN.2017111213.

78. Trinchieri, M., Perletti, G., Magri, V., Stamatiou, K., Montanari, E., & Trinchieri, A. (2021). Urinary side effects of psychotropic drugs: A systematic review and meta-analysis. *Neurourology and Urodynamics, 40*, 1333–1348. https://doi.org/10.1002/nau.24695.

79. Tsakiris, P., Oelke, M., & Michel, M. C. (2008). Drug-induced urinary incontinence. *Drugs & Aging, 25*, 541–549. https://doi.org/10.2165/00002512-200825070-00001.

80. Uitrakul, S., Aksonnam, K., Srivichai, P., Wicheannarat, S., & Incomenoy, S. (2022). The incidence and risk factors of urinary tract infection in patients with type 2 diabetes mellitus using SGLT2 inhibitors: A real-world observational study. *Medicines, 9*, 59. https://doi.org/10.3390/medicines9120059.

81. Verhamme, K. M., Sturkenboom, M. C., Stricker, B. H., & Bosch, R. (2008). Drug-induced urinary retention: Incidence, management and prevention. *Drug Safety, 31*, 373–388. https://doi.org/10.2165/00002018-200831050-00002.

82. Viljoen, A., Chaudhry, R., & Bycroft, J. (2019). Renal stones. *Annals of Clinical Biochemistry, 56*, 15–27. https://doi.org/10.1177/0004563218781672.

83. Wagenlehner, F. M. E., Bjerklund Johansen, T. E., Cai, T., Koves, B., Kranz, J., Pilatz, A., & Tandogdu, Z. (2020). Epidemiology, definition, and treatment of complicated urinary tract infections. *Nature Reviews Urology, 17*, 586–600. https://doi.org/10.1038/s41585-020-0362-4.

84. Waters, V. V. (1989). Hydralazine, hydrochlorothiazide and ampicillin associated with retroperitoneal fibrosis: Case report. *Journal of Urology, 141*, 936–937. https://doi.org/10.1016/S0022-5347(17)41059-7.

85. Winkler, D., Grohmann, R., Friedrich, M. E., Toto, S., Bleich, S., Seifert, J., Konstantinidis, A., Shariat, S. F., Kasper, S., & Pjrek, E. (2021). Urological adverse drug reactions of psychotropic medication in psychiatric inpatients—A drug surveillance report from German-speaking countries. *Journal of Psychiatric Research, 144*, 412–420. https://doi.org/10.1016/j.jpsychires.2021.10.026.

86. Woo, S. D., Yoon, J., Doo, G. E., Park, Y., Lee, Y., Lee, S. H., Lee, Y. H., & Ye, Y. M. (2020). Common causes and characteristics of adverse drug reactions in older adults: A retrospective study. *BMC Pharmacology and Toxicology, 21*, 87. https://doi.org/10.1186/s40360-020-00464-9.

87. Zare, A., Jahanshahi, A., Rahnama'I, M. S., Schipper, S., & van Koeveringe, G. A. (2019). The role of the periaqueductal gray matter in lower urinary tract function. *Molecular Neurobiology, 56*, 920–934. https://doi.org/10.1007/s12035-018-1131-8.

88. Zhou, J., Scott, C., Miab, Z. R., & Lehmann, C. (2023). Current approaches for the treatment of ketamine-induced cystitis. *Neurourology and Urodynamics, 42*, 680–689. https://doi.org/10.1002/nau.25148.

89. Živković, D., Franić, D., & Kojović, V. (2022). Urinary incontinence—From childhood onwards. *Acta Clinica Croatica, 61*, 115–123. https://doi.org/10.20471/acc.2022.61.01.14.

INDEX

B

C

F

G

H

R

Printed and bound by CPI Group (UK) Ltd, Croydon, CR0 4YY
18/09/2026
14965065-0002